MOSBY'S
HANDBOOK OF
PATIENT TEACHING

Visit our website at **www.mosby.com**

MOSBY'S
HANDBOOK OF
PATIENT TEACHING

MARY M. CANOBBIO, RN, MN, FAAN
Cardiovascular Clinical Specialist
Lecturer, UCLA School of Nursing
Los Angeles, California

SECOND EDITION

 Mosby

A Harcourt Health Sciences Company

St. Louis   London   Philadelphia   Sydney   Toronto

M Mosby

OCT 1 9 2000

A Harcourt Health Sciences Company

Editor-in-Chief: Sally Schrefer
Executive Editor: Barbara Nelson Cullen
Senior Developmental Editor: Sandra Clark Brown
Project Manager: Patricia Tannian
Production Editor: Richard Hund
Book Design Manager: Gail Morey Hudson
Cover Designer: Teresa Breckwoldt

Mosby, Inc.
A Harcourt Health Sciences Company
11830 Westline Industrial Drive
St. Louis, Missouri 63146

Printed in the United States of America

International Standard Book Number 0-323-01103-9

00 01 02 03 04 GW/FF/KPT 9 8 7 6 5 4 3 2 1

Contributors

Theresa S. Ayer, MS, RN, CNAA
Ayer Associates
Annandale, Virginia

Patricia Ann Carter, PhD, RN, CNS
Assistant Professor
School of Nursing
University of Texas-Austin
Austin, Texas

Angela Garrido, BSN, OCN
Oncology Nurse Educator
Oncology Education Services
Simi Valley, California

Margaret Karwecki, RN, MSN, C-ACNP, CCRN
Acute Care Nurse Practitioner
Cardiovascular Institute
Los Angeles, California

Betty Y.F. Lee, RN, MN, CCRN
Clinical Nurse Specialist
Cardiothoracic Surgery
UCLA Medical Center
Los Angeles, California

Mei-Sheng Lu, RN, MSN, ACNP
Acute Care Nurse Practitioner
Vencor Hospital
Researcher, Department of Neurology
UCLA Medical Center
Los Angeles, California

Margaret A. Marinow, RN, BSN
Commander
United States Navy, Retired

Reviewers

Cindy L. Boyer, MA, MSN, RN, SCCRN
Manager of the Sara Cole Hirsh Institute
For Best Nursing Practices Based on Evidence
Frances Payne Bolton School of Nursing
Case Western Reserve University
Cleveland, Ohio

Bonnie Faherty, PhD, FNP, CS
Associate Professor
Department of Health Sciences
California State University, Northridge
Northridge, California

Ruth M. Kleinpell, PhD, RN, CCRN
Associate Professor
College of Nursing
Rush University
Chicago, Illinois

Teri A. Murray, PhD, RN
Barnes College of Nursing
University of Missouri, St. Louis
St. Louis, Missouri

Kathy Russell, RNC, MSN
Nursing Professor
Front Range Community College
Westminster, Colorado

To

our patients and **their families**

who have the right to know . . .

and

To my husband **John G. Colias** and **family**

for putting up with all the rush deadlines,

lost weekends, and postponed vacations

Preface

For health care, the final decades of the 20th century ended much like it began. In the early 1900s, nurses were sent to care for the sick at home. For the sick, visiting nurses brought care and relief from the burden of illness. The focus of health care was then on prevention in the spread of disease. Today nurses and other health care providers are once again providing care and relief from the burden of illness to the patient and the family in the home setting. Today the shift of health care to the home and community is largely the result of economic forces that have resulted in earlier discharges and increased community and home-based health care. Consequently, ensuring that patient education occurs places a greater responsibility onto health care providers.

Assessing and meeting informational needs of patients and their families are integral parts of health care practice. Over the past years, the focus of patient education has been largely on the pathophysiology and treatment of disease. Today, however, patients are being asked to assume greater responsibility for all aspects of their care, including caring for their incisions and catheters and practicing disease prevention and health promotion. Therefore the intent of *Mosby's Handbook of Patient Teaching* is to help health care providers ensure that their patients are well informed about every aspect of home care management.

As **hospital** lengths of stay decrease and same-day surgeries increase, it becomes essential to maintain safe and consistent standards of practice that lead to positive patient outcomes within any health care delivery system. Regulatory agencies such as the Joint Commission on Accreditation of Healthcare Organizations (JCAHO) have long recognized the importance of patient and family education. A number of JCAHO standards statements* for patient education have been incorporated into this text and are summarized here:

    1. Provide the patient and family/significant other with

Joint Commission on Accreditation of Healthcare Organizations: *The Joint Commission's 1996 accreditation manual for hospitals: the new care of the patient standards,* Washington, DC, 1996, American Hospital Association.

information that will enhance their knowledge and skills necessary to promote recovery and improve function.

2. Encourage patient participation in decision making, and include the family in the teaching process.

3. Use an educational program that begins with an assessment and addresses the identified learning needs, abilities, and preferences.

4. Consider cultural, religious, physical and cognitive limitations, language, and financial barriers in education assessment.

5. Educate patients about the safe and effective use of their medications according to their needs.

6. Educate patients about the safe and effective use of equipment and supplies and means of obtaining them.

7. Counsel patients as to foods and diets appropriate to illness, as well as possible food-drug interactions.

8. Provide patients leaving a facility with information on obtaining follow-up care and accessing community resources.

Based on the preceding standards, this text provides guidelines for information the caregiver should cover with the patient and his or her family or primary caregiver. The guidelines are written as broad statements that will remind the health care provider of what to include in the individualized educational discharge plan. For example, because occupation varies from patient to patient, a reminder statement is made to "urge the patient to ask questions about occupational as well as recreational activities." In this way, patients are assured of receiving important information about allowances or limitations related to their clinical problems.

Community-based health care has historically focused on health promotion and disease prevention, but along with public and private **ambulatory settings** that deal with chronic illness, the acuity level has risen, placing an additional burden on the provider to ensure greater understanding by their clients about disease management in the home setting. Furthermore, technologic advances have made it possible to perform most diagnostic and many surgical procedures on an outpatient basis. This book can be useful in developing teaching protocols for ambulatory settings.

Patient teaching has always been an integral component of health care delivery, but the timing (when to teach) and the content (what to teach) have always been problematic. Today patient education begins with the initial contact between patient and provider, be it in the hospital, office or clinic, or home. What to teach is more of a challenge given the brevity of time allowed per visit. *Mosby's Handbook of Patient Teaching* attempts to provide the provider with some guidelines. As in the ambulatory care setting, **home health providers** may use this text to develop patient education standards and protocols for their staff and for the client.

It is not the intent of this book to teach readers about diseases, disorders, or procedures. This knowledge is assumed. The purpose is simply to remind the health care provider of what is essential to discuss with the patient.

The second edition of *Mosby's Handbook of Patient Teaching* is divided into two parts. The first part focuses on diseases, disorders, and surgical procedures. Home care procedures that require direct patient/caregiver participation have been moved to the second part, and a number of new procedures have been added including glucose monitoring, percutaneous indwelling catheters, and how to care for the dying in the home. Each disease or procedure begins with a **Definition. Signs/Symptoms** of the disease or disorder are those a patient would be taught to expect or observe for. Similarly, the **Complications** are those directly associated with the disease (that is, complications for which the patient should be alert). **Diagnostic Tests** are listed with a brief explanation of their purpose. A reminder to provide detailed information about each of the ordered tests is given at the beginning of each list. A general listing of **Medical Management** specific to the disease, disorder, or procedure follows.

The **Home Care** section includes key points to teach, review, and discuss with the patient in home care management. Using principles of adult education, the text's consistent, structured format serves to remind the health care provider to include the patient's family or caregiver in the teaching and to provide supportive materials such as written information and telephone numbers for follow-up questions. When demonstrating care is important in preparing the patient, the text reminds the reader to do so.

To assist health care workers in preparing the patient for discharge, the home care section addresses the elements to include in every discharge plan: description of the disorder or procedure, causes or risk factors, symptoms to report, diet counseling, medications, activities, and any specific instructions related to the disease or procedure. Finally, readers are reminded to provide home care referral, including community resources. A list of organizational resources for patient information is provided in the Appendixes.

I gratefully acknowledge and thank Kimberly Shimabukuro, student volunteer at the University of California, Los Angeles, for helping with manuscript preparation.

Mary M. Canobbio

Contents

Teaching Guidelines

Although patient education has long been a cornerstone of health care practice, the shortening of stays has increased the need for a discharge teaching plan that includes home care. Today's patients are assuming responsibility for aspects of care previously handled in the hospital. Therefore health care providers must broaden their assessment of patients' educational needs to include not only the disease or disorder, but also the environment to which patients will be returning and the available resources.

In developing an individual teaching plan, the care provider must incorporate basic principles of adult learning into the assessment of the patient. Some of the issues to be considered in developing an educational discharge plan for home care follow.

EDUCATIONAL ASSESSMENT

Patient education begins with an assessment of what the patient *needs to know* to achieve recovery and return to function. Because of anxiety and discomfort, patients retain little of the instruction in the hospital. Therefore nurses should limit the information to specific content, skills, and behaviors necessary to learn before discharge. What the patient *wants* to know and what can be learned in the limited time available should be factored into the assessment of necessary information to cover.

An assessment plan considers all factors that will influence the teaching and learning process. Age, sex, education, cultural, language skills, and religious practices, occupation, and previous life experiences influence the patient's ability and readiness to learn. The nurse must attempt to assess the patient's lifestyle, preferences, and attitudes toward health and illness. Barriers to learning, such as physical limitations, finances, and type of health care coverage, must also be evaluated, particularly when prescribing home care equipment and supplies and making referrals.

ENVIRONMENTAL ASSESSMENT

In preparing the patient for home care, the nurse must assess the physical and community environment to which the patient will be discharged. If the patient is discharged to home, the nurse must make certain that the home environment is safe and suitable for the patient to carry out the instructions given. For example, can the patient maneuver safely, or does he live in a second-story apartment with no elevator to reach the ground floor? If instructed to weigh daily, does the patient own a scale? The external environment includes both hospital-based and community resources available and affordable to the patient. The health care provider must become familiar with community resources, such as self-help programs, home health agencies, and professional organizations to which the patient can be referred. Appendix F provides a partial list of resources available to patients.

LEVEL OF INFORMATION

The information given to the patient should be appropriate for the patient's age, literacy level, education, and language skills. Patient materials should be geared between sixth- and eighth-grade reading levels. Use of medical terminology or jargon should be avoided. For example, the terms "myocardial infarction" and "MI" should not be used in place of "heart attack" unless they have already been defined for the patient.

USE OF PATIENT EDUCATION MATERIALS

With shorter lengths of stay and limited time for teaching, print and audiovisual materials are important adjuncts for any discharge teaching plan. They are, however, just adjuncts and should not replace individualized instruction.

Printed material can vary from comprehensive booklets to single-topic tearsheets. Printed materials are useful for reinforcing information provided to patients while in the hospital and also serve as a ready resource. Because of the low retention and recall levels of hospitalized patients, printed material is an important reminder of key points after patients return home.

The end of the 20th century brought attention to the broad access the public can have to health information via the Internet. As health educators, we cannot lose sight of this potentially valuable source of information, but we must be alert to what information our clients are obtaining so that we can identify and correct any misinformation. Incorporating sites that have been reviewed and recommended as part of an educational protocol provides yet another source of patient information. The benefit of using websites is that the patient is self-directed and learning takes place in a self-paced, nonstressful environment such as the home. A series of websites for professional organizations that offer patient education materials is included in the appendixes.

FAMILY PARTICIPATION

As hospital stays shorten, discharged patients may not feel prepared for or physically capable of performing self-care activities. Consequently, family members are the vital links in the transition from hospital to home care. Families must be included in all discussions and demonstrations.

For purposes of this book the term "family" is used in the broadest sense to include any person who plays an important role in the patient's life. The "family member" may not be an individual who is legally related to the patient but simply the one who will assume primary responsibility for the care of the patient at home. Therefore it is important to apply the previously discussed principles of learning to this family member, who now also becomes a client.

TEACHING OF SKILLS

To maximize patient self-care skills, the health care provider must permit sufficient time and opportunity for the patient to practice the skills. Practice should be integrated into all encounters with the patient, not saved up until the patient is ready for discharge. Every effort must be made to ensure that learning takes place in incremental steps and that patients are not overwhelmed with too much information at one time.

TIMING OF PATIENT EDUCATION

Providing ample time for patient teaching has always been a problem, but with shorter hospital stays, health care providers must develop a variety of strategies to ensure that patient educational needs are met. For example, in a **hospital setting,** the education plan must begin with the admission and be incorporated into the daily management plan that provides frequent patient encounters. Classroom activities may have to be scheduled more frequently during the week to provide additional opportunities for the patient and family to participate. Early involvement and teaching of the family or caretaker are essential, particularly if the patient's clinical condition precludes them from learning.

Providing postdischarge telephone numbers and resources to call for clarification or further information is an essential component of discharge planning.

In the **ambulatory setting,** utilization of waiting room time may be an opportunity to provide patient education. For example, materials may be developed to prepare the patient to ask questions regarding disease, medications, or diet. If space is available, a room can be provided that has educational and audiovisual materials for patients and families to use before or after their appointment. Organizing community-based patient education classes or activities at different times during the week is one means of reaching a large number of patients. In recent years, specific clinics, such as for anticoagulation therapy, hypertension, or chemotherapy, have been organized for follow-up to ensure patient safety and compliance. Staffed by advanced practice nurses, these clinics provide a good opportunity to implement teaching protocols in an unhurried but timely manner. They also are often covered by health care plans.

REFERENCES

DeMuth JS: Patient teaching in ambulatory setting, *Nurse Clin North Am* 24:645-654, 1989.

Johnson EA, Jackson JE: Teaching the home care client, *Nurs Clin North Am* 24:687-693, 1989.

Joint Commission on Accreditation of Healthcare Organizations: *The Joint Commission's 1996 accreditation manual for hospitals: the new care of the patient,* Washington, DC, 1996, American Hospital Association.

Knowles MS: The modern practice of adult education. In *Pedagogy to andragogy,* ed 2, Chicago, 1980, Follett.

Redman B: *The process of patient education,* ed 7, St Louis, 1993, Mosby.

Ruzicki DA: Realistically meeting the educational needs of hospitalized acute and short-stay patients, *Nurs Clin North Am* 24:629-637, 1989.

Winthrop E: *Mosby's patient teaching tips,* St Louis, 1994, Mosby.

MOSBY'S
HANDBOOK OF
PATIENT TEACHING

Diseases, Disorders, and Treatments

Abdominal Aneurysm

—Abdominal aneurysm: an outpouching sac that forms at a weak point in the aortic wall. Most abdominal aneurysms are found below the bifurcation (take-off) of the renal arteries. Aneurysms can grow, but they are asymptomatic until they begin to press on adjacent organs or tears develop within the blood vessel (dissection).

CAUSES/CONTRIBUTING FACTORS/RISK FACTORS

- Hereditary lack of elastin
- Vessel wall trauma
- Congenital defect
- Loss of vessel wall elasticity
- Atherosclerosis
- Elderly men with hypertension, coronary artery disease, or peripheral vascular disease

SIGNS/SYMPTOMS

- Asymptomatic
- Painless, pulsating sensation or throbbing abdominal mass
- Chronic pain in middle or lower back or flank area
- With expansion or dissection: sudden onset of severe abdominal or back pain

COMPLICATIONS

- Dissection
- Rupture
- Exsanguination
- Insufficient blood supply to the kidneys, bowels, and/or lower extremities
- Thromboemboli (blood clots in the lower extremities)
- Heart attack (high incidence in older men)
- Compression of adjacent structures (i.e., ureter, duodenum, vena cava, or vertebral column)

DIAGNOSTIC TESTS

- Describe each procedure, its purpose, and the normal feelings or sensations that are likely, as well as any preprocedural or postprocedural care.
- Abdominal ultrasonography: to determine the size and shape of the aneurysm
- Chest x-ray: to detect calcification and gauge the size of the aneurysm
- Computed tomography/magnetic resonance imaging: to locate an arterial tear and to determine the size of the aneurysm
- Aortography: to determine the condition of the vessel above and below the aneurysm

TREATMENT
Medical

- Indications
  —Aneurysm <6 cm. The goal of medical treatment is to prevent enlargement of the aneurysm and to monitor its growth.
- Drugs
  —Antihypertensives: to lower and/or control blood pressure (BP)
  —Beta blockers: to reduce the force of the heart's pumping action and to decrease the pulsating feeling of the aneurysm
  —Analgesics: to relieve pain
  —Antilipid medications: for elevated cholesterol

Surgical

- Indications
  —Aneurysm >4 to 6 cm; emergence of symptoms (abdominal tenderness or pain); emergency procedure for dissection and rupture
- Procedure
  —Resection and grafting with autogenous graft (see Abdominal Surgery, p. 6)

⌂ HOME CARE

- Give both patient and caregiver *verbal* and *written* instructions. Provide them with the name and telephone number of a physician or nurse to call if questions arise.
- *General information*
  —Describe and explain dissection and rupture.

- *Warning signs*
  —Stress the importance of seeking emergency care if the following occur:
    Sudden onset of severe pain (ripping or tearing) in the abdomen, back, or groin
    Pallor, sweating, and/or sudden loss of consciousness
- *Special instructions*
  —Stress the importance of adopting a lifestyle that prevents acceleration of the aneurysm's growth.
    Controlling weight to ease the work of the circulatory system
    Limiting fat to prevent progression of atherosclerosis
    Reducing or eliminating salt to control BP
    Stopping smoking
  —Teach the patient how to care for the incision (review the signs of infection, thrombus, or embolism); instruct him or her to report any problems to a physician or nurse.
- *Medications*
  —Explain the purpose, dosage, and schedule of the prescribed medications, as well as side effects to report to a physician or nurse.
  —Emphasize that the patient should not stop taking the medications without first checking with a physician or nurse.
- *Activity*
  —Advise the patient to alternate mild to moderate exercise with periods of rest; the patient should avoid vigorous exercise and heavy lifting.
  —Encourage the patient to discuss allowances or limitations related to occupation and to favorite recreational sports or activities.
- *Diet*
  —Encourage the patient to follow a low-fat, low-cholesterol, and low-salt diet.

FOLLOW-UP CARE

- Stress the importance of regular follow-up visits. Make sure the patient has the necessary names and telephone numbers.
  —Medical patients: ultrasound scans to monitor the size of the aneurysm
  —Surgical patients: monitoring to ensure the patency of the graft and/or to detect a new aneurysm early

Abdominal Surgery

—Abdominal surgery: surgical incision into the abdomen. Abdominal surgery is performed for a number of reasons, such as to treat gastrointestinal disorders, to remove parts of an organ or a whole organ (gastrectomy), to transplant organs, or to monitor the progression of disease.

PREPROCEDURAL TEACHING

- Using illustrations, review the physician's explanation of the procedure.
- Explain the need for written consent for surgery, anesthesia, and blood transfusions.
- Explain that the patient usually is admitted to the hospital the day of surgery, rather than before, unless extensive bowel preparation is needed.

Review of Preprocedural Care

- The patient must not eat or drink anything after midnight the night before surgery.
- The patient may need to be shaved from the nipple line to the thigh (including the perineal area) to prevent infection of the surgical wound.
- A small cleansing enema, done at home, may be required the night before surgery.
- Before coming to the hospital, the patient may be instructed to shower with a bactericidal soap (e.g., Hibiclens).

Review of Postprocedural Care

- Stress the importance of turning, coughing, and deep breathing.
- Discuss the purpose of the incentive spirometer, and demonstrate how to use it.
- Explain the importance of getting out of bed the first day after surgery.
- Explain the reason for wearing thigh-high elastic stockings and for alternating them with pressure stockings while in bed.
- Explain the importance of moving the arms and legs while in bed.
- Explain that pain is expected after surgery, but that analgesics are available to control it. Discuss the types of pain control:

—Patient-controlled analgesia (PCA): the patient self-administers pain medication by pushing a button on a device regulated by a computerized time and dose schedule

—Intramuscular injection: pain medication is injected as prescribed

• Explain that hydration is maintained by the IV line until the patient is allowed to eat and drink.

• Explain that a variety of tubes and suction systems may be used after surgery to drain excess blood and fluid around the incision. These may include: nasogastric (NG) tube, until bowel sounds return; urethral catheter; Penrose drain; Jackson-Pratt self-suction bulb drainage system; Hemovac self-suction drain.

COMPLICATIONS

• Wound infection
• Wound dehiscence
• Deep vein thrombosis
• Paralytic ileus
• Fluid-electrolyte imbalance
• Bowel obstruction
• Urinary tract infection
• Pulmonary complications
• Hemorrhage
• Acute renal failure

HOME CARE

• Give both patient and caregiver *verbal* and *written* instructions. Provide them with the name and telephone number of a physician or nurse to call if questions arise.

• *Wound/incision care*

—Teach the patient how to change the dressings and how to care for the tubes and drains.

—Help the patient obtain the necessary supplies, and make sure he or she knows what supplies to get and where to get them after discharge from the hospital.

• *Warning signs*

—Review the signs and symptoms the patient should report to a physician or nurse.

Wound infection: redness, tenderness, warmth, and swelling around the incision site; increased drainage; fever

Changes in bowel habits: diarrhea, constipation, flatulence

- *Medications*
  —Explain the purpose, dosage, schedule, and route of administration of the prescribed medications, as well as side effects to report to a physician or nurse.
- *Special instructions*
  —Review pain management techniques.
  —Instruct the patient to splint the abdomen when coughing or sneezing.
  —Reassure the patient that as activity level increases, the pain and soreness will diminish.
- *Activity*
  —Explain the need for frequent rest periods and the avoidance of prolonged sitting or lying in bed.
  —Stress the need for the patient to increase activity gradually as tolerated.
  —Instruct the patient to avoid heavy lifting (>10 pounds) and strenuous work or sports for 4 to 6 weeks or longer, as the physician advises.
- *Diet*
  —Explain that diet may be dictated by the underlying condition or diagnosis. If no diet is prescribed, instruct the patient to maintain a diet low in residue and high in protein and calories.
  —Instruct the patient on administration of enteral or parenteral therapy if ordered (p. 734).

FOLLOW-UP CARE AND REFERRALS

- Stress the importance of regular follow-up visits. Make sure the patient has the necessary names and telephone numbers.

Acquired Immune Deficiency Syndrome

—**Acquired immune deficiency syndrome (AIDS): a progressive, incurable disease caused by the human immunodeficiency virus (HIV). AIDS destroys the CD4+ T cells, impairing the immune system and predisposing the individual to a number of opportunistic infections and cancers. HIV is transmitted through intimate sexual contact, use of contami-**

nated needles, and exposure to HIV-tainted blood, body fluids that contain blood, and blood products. It also can be transmitted from mother to newborn.

CDC CLASSIFICATION OF HIV INFECTION

- Stage I: acute infection; a mononucleosis-like syndrome develops at the time of exposure; HIV-antibody seroconversion occurs about 3 months later
- Stage II: no symptoms are present, but the individual tests positive for HIV antibody
- Stage III: persistent, generalized lymphadenopathy appears; decrease in CD4+ T cells
- Stage IV: HIV-related diseases develop
  —Constitutional symptoms (persistent fever, weight loss, diarrhea)
  —Neurologic disease
  —Secondary infectious diseases
  —Secondary cancers
  —Associated conditions

RISK FACTORS

- Homosexual/bisexual men
- Heterosexuals engaging in high-risk behavior (e.g., IV drug use; sharing of needles and syringes; unprotected sex with multiple partners)
- Neonates born to infected women
- Infants, children, and adults who receive HIV-contaminated blood or blood products (e.g., those with hemophilia)

SIGNS/SYMPTOMS

- Prolonged period of silent infection, often lasting >10 years
- Viral syndrome resembling mononucleosis or influenza within a few days or weeks of infection
- Persistent, generalized swelling of the lymph nodes
- Skin disorders (e.g., seborrhea)
- Opportunistic infections
  —Bacterial *(Mycobacterium avium)*
  —Fungal (candidiasis, cryptococcosis, histoplasmosis)
  —Protozoal (cryptosporidiosis, pneumocystosis, toxoplasmosis)
  —Viral (cytomegalovirus, herpes simplex)

- Malignancies
  —Kaposi's sarcoma
  —Non-Hodgkin's lymphoma
  —Primary central nervous system (CNS) lymphoma
  —Cervical cancer
  —Anal carcinoma
  —Malignant melanoma
  —Hepatocellular carcinoma
  Metastasis to central nervous system, skin, mucous membranes, respiratory and gastrointestinal tracts. End-stage disease: unexplained weight loss, persistent fever, diarrhea, or night sweats

DIAGNOSTIC TESTS

- Describe each procedure, its purpose, and the normal feelings or sensations that are likely, as well as any preprocedural or postprocedural care.
- To confirm HIV infection
  —Enzyme-linked immunosorbent assay (ELISA)
  —Western blot
  —Polymerase chain reaction
- To measure severity of immunosuppression
  —T-cell count: <400,000 or depressed
  —White blood cells: depressed
  —Lymphocytes: depressed
- To evaluate symptoms of opportunistic infection or malignancy

TREATMENT
Medical

- Drugs
  —Antiretrovirals: to slow progression of the disease or inactivate HIV
      Azidothymidine
      Zidovudine (Retrovir)
  —Antiinfectives: as prophylaxis against opportunistic infections; also, to treat such infections as they arise
The treatment of AIDS is directed by the type of infection or malignancy that develops. It may include the following:
- Kaposi's sarcoma: chemotherapy, surgical excision, electrodesiccation, radiation therapy
- Non-Hodgkin's lymphoma: chemotherapy (mBACOD: metho-

trexate, bleomycin, doxorubicin, cyclophosphamide, vincristine, dexamethasone, folic acid); hematopoietic growth factors
• Primary CNS lymphoma: radiation therapy, corticosteroids
• Cervical cancer: radical hysterectomy, pelvic lymphadenectomy; chemotherapy, radiation therapy for advanced or
systemic disease
• Anal carcinoma: fulguration or cryotherapy; chemotherapy;
possibly radiation therapy

HOME CARE

• Give both patient and caregiver *verbal* and *written* instructions.
Provide them with the name and telephone number of a
physician or nurse to call if questions arise.
• *General information for HIV-positive patients*
—Explain how HIV is transmitted and the disease process.
• *Warning signs*
—Review the signs and symptoms of infection (flulike
symptoms, stiff neck) and cancers that should be reported to
a physician or nurse.
• *Special instructions*
—Stress the importance of preventing further exposure to or
transmission of the virus by avoiding exchange of body fluids
(e.g., vaginal or anal intercourse, oral sex) without using a
latex condom, sharing of IV needles or sex toys, blood
contact of any kind.
—Discuss the importance of avoiding large crowds, as well as
individuals who may be infectious or who have been
vaccinated recently.
—Teach the patient and caregiver the precautions they should
take at home to prevent transmission of HIV.
   Wash hands meticulously before and after patient care.
   Use disposable gloves whenever contact with the patient's
   blood or body fluids is likely.
   Separate any bedding or clothing soiled by secretions or
   excretion, and wash it in a 10% bleach solution (¼ cup
   of bleach for each gallon of water).
   Wash dishes and eating utensils in hot, soapy water (no
   special handling is required).
   Dispose of dry waste (e.g., tissues, napkins) contaminated
   by blood or body fluids in a separate container, and bag
   securely.

> Put all needles used to administer drugs in a sturdy, closed container before disposing of them.

—See the specific malignancy for further care guidelines.

PSYCHOSOCIAL CARE

- Encourage verbalization regarding fears and concerns about disease and prognosis; encourage questions and expressions of anger and grief.
- Provide information to patient, partner/caretaker regarding counseling and support groups.
- Encourage and permit self-care as tolerated.

FOLLOW-UP CARE

- Stress the importance of regular visits for medical care and laboratory tests. Make sure the patient has the necessary names and telephone numbers.
- Discuss the importance of informing health care providers about the HIV diagnosis.
- Explain the importance of refraining from donating blood or semen.

REFERRALS

- Provide and assist with referrals as needed for home health care, supplies, equipment, social service, and financial help.
- Assist patient and partner to obtain referrals for community support (self-help support groups, hospice care).

Adrenal Insufficiency
(Addison's Disease, Secondary Adrenocortical Insufficiency)

—Adrenal insufficiency: a chronic disorder of the adrenal glands. Hypofunctioning of the adrenal cortex leads to a deficiency of adrenocortical hormones (glucocorticoid, aldosterone) and androgens. These hormones regulate fluid blance, glucose formation, and secondary sex characteristics, particularly in women. *Addison's disease* is a primary adrenocortical insufficiency; *secondary adrenocortical insufficiency* is a consequence of other conditions.

CAUSES

- Addison's disease: damage to the adrenal glands, which may result from an autoimmune factor, trauma, infection, or surgery
- Secondary adrenocortical insufficiency: reduced secretion of the pituitary adrenocorticotropic hormone (ACTH) caused by a pituitary tumor, head trauma, or optic gliomas

SIGNS/SYMPTOMS

- *Early*
  —Fatigue
  —Muscle weakness that worsens through the day
  —Orthostatic hypotension
  —Hyperpigmentation (bronze skin color)
  —Loss of or decrease in body hair
  —Vitiligo
- *Midcourse*
  —Anorexia
  —Nausea, vomiting
  —Diarrhea
  —Salt craving
  —Abdominal pain
  —Headache
  —Dizziness, fainting
  —Intolerance to cold
- *Late*
  —Weight loss
  —Dehydration
  —Postural hypotension
  —Confusion, restlessness
  —Emotional lability
- Women: amenorrhea, infertility, reduced libido

COMPLICATIONS

- Addisonian (adrenal) crisis: a rapid drop in cortisol and aldosterone levels, which can result in shock, coma, and death. It can be precipitated by any stressor (e.g., emotion, infection, minor surgery, or trauma). *This is a medical emergency.*

DIAGNOSTIC TESTS

- Describe each procedure, its purpose, and the normal feelings or sensations that are likely, as well as any preprocedural or postprocedural care.
  - —Cortisol, ACTH levels; ACTH stimulation test: to confirm adrenocortical insufficiency and identify type
  - —Blood chemistry, electrolytes (potassium, glucose, sodium, chloride, bicarbonate, blood urea nitrogen)
  - —Urinalysis: 24-hour urinalysis to detect sodium and/or free cortisol
  - —Complete blood count with differential: in crisis to detect neutropenia, lymphocytosis, and elevated eosinophils
  - —Computed tomography/magnetic resonance imaging: to determine decrease in adrenal or pituitary size

TREATMENT
Medical

- Diet
  - —Diet high in calories, carbohydrates, protein, and vitamins
- Drugs
  - —Corticosteroid replacement (e.g., cortisone, hydrocortisone)
  - —Antibiotics for infection
  - —Adrenal crisis
    - IV hydrocortisone
    - IV fluid replacement (with severe dehydration)
    - Vasopressors to maintain blood pressure
    - Cardiac monitoring

HOME CARE

- Give both patient and caregiver *verbal* and *written* instructions. Provide them with the name and telephone number of a physician or nurse to call if questions arise.
- *General information*
  - —Explain the underlying disorder, its cause, and contributing factors.
  - —Discuss the effect stress can have on hormone levels.
  - —Instruct the patient to notify the physician or a nurse during periods of heightened emotional stress, before elective surgery, or after a traumatic event so that drug dosages can be adjusted.

—Explain the increased risk for infection. Instruct the patient to avoid individuals who have communicable illnesses (e.g., cold or flu).

—Stress the importance of proper handwashing.

• *Warning signs of addisonian crisis*
  —Review the signs and symptoms of addisonian crisis (i.e., profound weakness, fatigue, dizziness, nausea, vomiting, abdominal pain, and cool, clammy skin).

  —Emphasize the importance of seeking immediate medical care if the above signs appear.

  —Make sure the patient and caregiver know the quickest way to an emergency department from home and from work.

  —Help the patient organize or obtain an emergency kit containing alcohol sponges and syringes with 100 mg of hydrocortisone.

  —Advise the patient to carry the emergency kit when traveling and to check the supplies regularly for expiration dates.

  —Teach the patient and caregiver how to prepare and administer a hydrocortisone (IM) injection in the event of adrenal crisis.

• *Special instructions*
  —Women: instruct the patient to report any changes in her menstrual pattern, such as amenorrhea.

  —Discuss other methods of dealing with stressful events (e.g., relaxation techniques, guided imagery, diversional activities).

• *Medications*
  —Explain the purpose, dosage, schedule, and route of administration of the prescribed medications, as well as side effects to report to a physician or nurse.

  —Emphasize that hormone replacement is a lifelong commitment.

• *Activity*
  —Instruct the patient to avoid strenuous exercise in hot, humid weather.

  —Advise the patient to increase intake of fluid and salt if he or she is sweating heavily.

  —Caution the patient to change position gradually to minimize postural drainage.

• *Diet*
  —Caution the patient not to skip meals during periods of activity.

—Urge the patient not to use salt-restricted foods or salt substitutes.

—Advise an anorexic patient to eat small, frequent meals to enhance the nutritional condition.

PSYCHOSOCIAL CARE

• Encourage the patient to verbalize concerns and fears about disease progression.

• Assist the patient to adjust to lifestyle changes by encouraging participation in planning home care.

FOLLOW-UP CARE AND REFERRALS

• Stress the importance of regular follow-up visits. Make sure the patient has the necessary names and telephone numbers.

• Assist the patient and caregiver to identify community emergency numbers.

• Advise the patient to inform all physicians, dentists, and health care providers about the disease *before* a treatment or procedure.

• Help the patient obtain a MedicAlert bracelet and identification card listing the diagnosis and medications and emergency treatment.

• Provide referrals for home care and medical social work services as indicated.

Adrenalectomy

—**Adrenalectomy: surgical removal of one or both adrenal glands.**

INDICATIONS

• Adrenal hyperfunction (Cushing's syndrome) and hyperaldosteronism

• Benign adrenal adenomas or malignant ACTH-producing tumors

• Secondary treatment of prostate and breast cancers dependent on adrenal hormone secretion

A

PREPROCEDURAL TEACHING

- Review the physician's explanation of the procedure and the reason for surgery, the skin preparation process, and the location of the incision; encourage the patient to ask questions and to discuss any fears or anxieties.
- If both glands are to be removed, explain that the patient will need lifelong cortisone treatment; if only one gland is to be removed, the patient will take cortisone for 6 months to 2 years.
- Explain that the patient may be admitted to the hospital the day of surgery rather than before.
- Explain the need for written consent for surgery and anesthesia.

Review of Preprocedural Care

- The patient should not eat or drink anything after midnight the night before surgery.
- The patient will be carefully monitored after surgery to prevent complications (e.g., adrenal crisis, infection, hypertension) that may result from removal of one or both adrenals. (Refer to the primary disease for specific medications to be given, such as antihypertensives and glucose.)

Review of Postprocedural Care

- Stress the importance of turning, coughing, and deep breathing.
- Show the patient how to splint his or her side to reduce pain when coughing.
- Discuss the purpose of the incentive spirometer, and demonstrate how to use it.

COMPLICATIONS

- Adrenal crisis (see p. 13)
- Hemorrhage
- Infection
- Hypoglycemia
- Electrolyte imbalance
- Hypotension

 HOME CARE

- Give both patient and caregiver *verbal* and *written* instructions. Provide them with the name and telephone number of a physician or nurse to call if questions arise.

- *Wound/incision care*
  —Teach the patient how to care for the incision.
  —Instruct the patient not to wear tight or restrictive clothing (e.g., belts, suspenders) over the incision because this may irritate the wound.
- *Warning signs*
  —Review the signs and symptoms that should be reported to a physician or nurse.
    Wound infection: redness, swelling, and increasing tenderness around the incision; increased drainage; fever
- *Special instructions*
  —Emphasize the importance of seeking immediate medical care if a crisis is suspected. Review the signs and symptoms of crisis: profound weakness, fatigue, dizziness, nausea, vomiting, abdominal pain, and cool, clammy skin. Make sure the patient and caregiver know the quickest way to an emergency department from home and from work.
  —Advise the patient to carry the emergency kit when traveling and to check the supplies regularly for expiration dates.
  —Help the patient organize or obtain an emergency kit containing alcohol sponges and syringes with 100 mg of hydrocortisone.
  —Teach the patient and caregiver how to prepare and administer a hydrocortisone injection in the event of crisis.
- *Medications*
  —Explain the purpose, dosage, schedule, and route of administration of prescribed medications, as well as side effects to report to a physician or nurse.
  —If the patient has had a unilateral adrenalectomy, explain that steroid replacement will be necessary until the remaining adrenal gland begins to function adequately. Steroid replacement will continue for a period ranging from 6 months to up to 2 years.
  —Patients who have a bilateral adrenalectomy require lifelong steroid replacement therapy; review the long-term management of adrenal insufficiency.
  —Emphasize that hormone replacement is a lifelong commitment, and that discontinuing the drug suddenly can precipitate adrenal crisis.
  —Stress the importance of not discontinuing the steroid medication suddenly.

- *Activity*
  - —Instruct the patient to allow for frequent rest periods, gradually increasing the activity level as tolerated.
  - —Tell the patient to avoid heavy lifting (>10 pounds) and strenuous work, exercise, and sports for 4 to 6 weeks or longer as the physician advises.
  - —Encourage the patient to discuss allowances and limitations regarding occupation and favorite recreational sports and activities.
- *Diet*
  - —Tell the patient to follow the diet prescribed by the primary physician for the underlying disorder.

FOLLOW-UP CARE AND REFERRALS

- Stress the importance of regular follow-up visits. Make sure the patient has the necessary names and telephone numbers.
- Help the patient obtain a MedicAlert bracelet and identification card listing the surgery, medications, and emergency treatment.
- See Home Care under Adrenal Insufficiency (p. 12) for additional guidelines.

Aldosteronism, Primary

(Hyperaldosteronism, Conn's Syndrome)

—Primary aldosteronism: overproduction of aldosterone by the adrenal glands, resulting in an excess of mineralocorticoids and, consequently, increases in sodium reabsorption and total body sodium. The most common cause is adrenal adenoma (60% of cases), but the disorder also may be caused by adrenal hyperplasia or adrenal carcinoma. It is three times more likely to occur in women aged 30 to 50 years.

SIGNS/SYMPTOMS

- Hypertension
- Postural hypotension
- Polydipsia, polyuria (especially nocturnal)

- Muscle weakness, fatigue
- Tetany
- Paresthesia

COMPLICATIONS

- Transient paralysis
- Heart failure
- Renal failure

DIAGNOSTIC TESTS

- Describe each procedure, its purpose, and the normal feelings or sensations that are likely, as well as any preprocedural or postprocedural care.
  —Serum studies
    Electrolytes: sodium, potassium
    Aldosterone, plasma renin activity cortisol
  —Urine studies: 24-hour urinary aldosterone levels
  —Computed tomography: scans of the adrenal glands
  —Venous catheterization of the adrenal glands

TREATMENT
Medical

- Therapy
  —Low-sodium, high-potassium diet
- Drugs
  —Spironolactone (Aldactone): to control blood pressure

Surgical

- Adrenalectomy: unilateral for adenoma, bilateral for hyperplasia

HOME CARE

- Give both patient and caregiver *verbal* and *written* instructions. Provide them with the name and telephone number of a physician or nurse to call if questions arise.
- *General information*
  —Review the physician's explanation of the disease and its underlying causes. Explain adrenalectomy (see p. 16) if the procedure has been scheduled.

A

- *Warning signs*
  —Review the signs and symptoms that should be reported to a physician or nurse.

  Hyperaldosteronism: headache, fatigue, muscle weakness
  Hypokalemia: weakness, paresthesia, tetany, palpitation
- *Medications*
  —Explain the purpose, dosage, schedule, and route of administration of the prescribed medications, as well as side effects to report to a physician or nurse.
  —Emphasize that the patient should not stop taking the medications without first checking with a physician or nurse.
- *Activity*
  —Encourage the patient to discuss allowances and limitations regarding occupation and favorite recreational sports and activities.
  —Emphasize the importance of alternating exercise with rest periods.
- *Diet*
  —Stress the importance of following a low-sodium, high-potassium diet; the patient should avoid foods high in salt (most processed foods, luncheon meats, bacon, ham, and fast foods).
  —Encourage the patient to eat foods high in potassium (bananas, citrus fruit, tomatoes, dates).
  —Instruct the patient to read food labels for sodium content; suggest the use of herbs, spices, and sodium-free salt substitutes for flavoring.

FOLLOW-UP CARE AND REFERRALS

- Stress the importance of regular follow-up visits. Make sure the patient has the necessary names and telephone numbers.
- Help the patient obtain a MedicAlert bracelet and identification card listing the diagnosis and medications and emergency treatment.

Allergy

—Allergy: a hypersensitivity reaction to intrinsic antigens, most of which are environmental. It is estimated that 1 out of 6 Americans has a severe allergy and that more than 20 million have allergic reactions to airborne or inhaled allergens such as cigarette smoke, house dust, and pollen. Common allergies are divided into two types of reactions: immediate (or antibody-mediated) reactions, which occur within minutes of exposure as the result of release of a substance (e.g., histamine, bradykinin, or immunoglobulin) into the circulation (type I reactions); and delayed (or cell-mediated) reactions, which develop over 24 to 48 hours and are caused by antigens (type IV reactions).

COMMON ALLERGIES/REACTIONS

- Allergic conjunctivitis: hyperemia (reddening, warmth) of the conjunctivae, caused by allergens such as pollen, grass, topical medications, air pollutants, occupational irritants, and smoke
- Allergic dermatitis: an acute inflammation of the skin that occurs upon exposure to an allergen to which the individual is hypersensitive (e.g., poison ivy, nickel compounds)
- Allergic rhinitis: inflammation of the nasal passages, producing watery nasal discharge and itching of the nose and eyes, which is associated with airborne allergens such as house dust, animal dander, or an antigen (commonly pollen)

SIGNS/SYMPTOMS

- Mild
    - —Conjunctivitis
    - —Urticaria (hives)
    - —Nasal congestion and drainage
    - —Bronchial congestion
    - —Erythema (redness), edema, scaling
    - —Vomiting
- Severe
    - —Anaphylaxis

DIAGNOSTIC TESTS

- Describe each procedure, its purpose, and the normal feelings or sensations that are likely, as well as any preprocedural or postprocedural care.
  —Allergy skin tests: to identify offending allergens
    Intradermal test
    Scratch test
    Patch text
  —Blood tests: Complete blood count, eosinophil count, smear; serum IgE levels
  —Radioallergosorbent test (RAST) to identify specific IgE antibodies
  For allergic rhinitis
  —Sinus x-ray: to rule out other disorders (e.g., nasal polyps), infection, and structural defects
  —Computed tomography: scan of the sinuses to rule out other disorders and structural defects

TREATMENT
Medical

- Therapy
  —Immunotherapy (hyposensitization): for inhalant antigens (e.g., tree, grass, and weed pollens)
  —Desensitization: to modify the hyperactivity of allergen
  —Environmental control: to eliminate or modify offending allergens in the environment
- Drugs
  —Antihistamines: via inhaler, nebulizer, or oral or nasal administration
  —Sympathomimetic agents: oral or topical decongestants
  —Corticosteroids: systemic, topical, or ocular
  —Antiinfective agents
  —Analgesics

HOME CARE

- Give both patient and caregiver *verbal* and *written* instructions. Provide them with the name and telephone number of a physician or nurse to call if questions arise.
- *General information*
  —Discuss the chronic nature of allergies; help the patient identify allergens that are a problem, and discuss ways to

prevent symptoms through the use of medication and/or environmental control.

* *Specific instructions*
  —Explain environmental control as a means of preventing and treating symptoms.
  —Teach the patient how to assess home, work, and social environments for offending allergens; urge the patient to eliminate or avoid them if possible.
  —Explain that allergens may be seasonal (i.e., pollen counts are high in spring or after heavy rains) or may be more prominent in certain areas (e.g., open fields, woods, rural areas).
  —Review measures to eliminate or control common allergens:
      Trees, grass, weeds, and pollens: keep windows closed during the pollen season and use air conditioning.
      Mold spores: remove the source (e.g., plants, dirt); apply mold-retardant solutions in damp areas such as the bathroom; use high-efficiency particulate-arresting (HEPA) air filters or electrostatic air cleaners.
      House dust, animal dander, mites: prevent household items from becoming "dust catchers": wash bedding frequently; encase mattresses in plastic; remove rugs and drapes, or vacuum them frequently; use damp dusting, and wear a face mask while dusting; use air filters; remove or avoid pets and other animals.
  —Stress the importance of avoiding foods containing allergens (e.g., nuts). Ask how foods were prepared when eating away from home.
  —Instruct the patient to monitor response to treatments (medications, environmental control, immunotherapy, desensitization), to record any problems, new symptoms, or side effects, and to report them to the physician or a nurse.
  —If anaphylaxis is possible, help patient to organize or obtain an emergency kit containing alcohol sponges and syringes with epinephrine, diphenhydramine, or corticosteroids as directed by physician.
* *Medications*
  —Explain the purpose, dosage, schedule, and route of administration of the prescribed medications, as well as side effects to report to a physician or nurse.
  —If an oral inhaler or nebulized drugs are prescribed, teach the patient how to use them (see Aerosol Therapy, p. 645).

—Stress the importance of not overusing or abusing prescribed or over-the-counter medications, since these drugs may have a cumulative effect.
- Activity
  —For allergic rhinitis, or conjunctivitis, instruct the patient to avoid or curtail strenuous work or exercise on days when the pollen count is high, especially if the allergens trigger an attack. If prescribed, medication may be taken before exercise or activity to prevent an attack.

FOLLOW-UP CARE AND REFERRALS

- Stress the importance of any prescribed follow-up care, including allergy testing and laboratory tests. Make sure the patient has the necessary names and telephone numbers.
- Help the patient obtain a MedicAlert bracelet and identification card listing allergies, medications, and emergency treatment.
- Advise patient to carry the emergency kit when traveling and to check the supplies regularly for expiration dates.

Alzheimer's Disease

—Alzheimer's disease: progressive deterioration of the intellect, memory, and personality, leading to severe dementia. The specific cause is unknown, but the disorder is believed to arise from a deficiency in the brain's neurotransmitter. Immunologic, genetic, and environmental factors have been implicated. The onset of the disease is insidious, affecting people in their forties; the lifetime risk of developing Alzheimer's disease is between 12% and 17%.

SIGNS/SYMPTOMS

- Intellectual loss
  —Memory loss (initially the patient cannot remember recent events but can recall early life events)
  —Loss of sense of time
  —Poor decision-making ability
  —Loss of train of thought during conversations
  —Requires repetitive directions

—Inability to perform arithmetic calculations
—Shortened attention span
—Inability to recognize family and friends
- Personality or affective loss
  —Personality changes
  —Apathy, loss of initiative
  —Anxiety, fear, belligerence, stubbornness
  —Suspicion, progressing to paranoia
  —Loss of sense of humor
  —Insensitivity to others
  —Inattentiveness
  —Conversation changes (slow speech, loss of words, use of clichés)
  —Easily fatigued
  —Reactive depression
  —Crying spells
  —Lethargy
  —Neglect of self-care
  —Nocturnal wandering
- Advanced stage
  —Apathy, muteness
  —Inability to recall recent or remote events
  —Disorientation/confusion
  —Inability to perform activities of daily living (ADLs)
  —Incontinence

COMPLICATIONS

- Physical and/or psychologic dependence
- Injury
- Bladder and bowel incontinence
- Dehydration/malnutrition
- Infection
- Aspiration pneumonia

DIAGNOSTIC TESTS

- Describe each procedure, its purpose, and the normal feelings or sensations that are likely, as well as any preprocedural or postprocedural care.
  —Computed tomography: to detect progressive brain atrophy and ventricular enlargement and to rule out other neurologic problems

—Magnetic resonance imaging: used in early stage to detect any biochemical and anatomic changes
—Electroencephalography: to detect slowed brain wave activity
—Brain biopsy: to identify neurofibril tangles and neuritic plaques
—Psychometric, behavioral rating scales (Mini-Mental State, Mental Status Questionnaire, Hamilton Depression Scale): to establish baseline and monitor changes or progression of mental and behavioral disorders

TREATMENT
Medical

- No specific treatment is available; the prescribed treatment is directed toward controlling the symptoms and providing physiologic and psychologic support for the patient and family to enhance their ability to cope with the progressively deteriorating effects of the disease.
- Drugs
    —For treatment of cognitive symptoms:
    > Donepezil (Aricept)
    > Tacrine HCl (Cognex)
    —For treatment of behavioral symptoms such as agitation, aggression, paranoia, delusions, depression:
    > *Antipsychotics (neuroleptics)*
    > ○ Haloperidol (Haldol)
    > ○ Olanzapine (Zyprexa)
    > ○ Quetiapine (Seroquel)
    > ○ Risperidone (Risperdal)
    > *Antianxiety drugs*
    > ○ Alprazolam (Xanax)
    > ○ Buspirone (Buspar)
    > ○ Diazepam (Valium)
    > ○ Lorazepam (Ativan)
    > *Antidepressants*
    > ○ Amitriptyline (Elavil or Endep)
    > ○ Bupropion (Wellbutrin)
    > ○ Desipramine (Norpramin or Pertofrane)
    > ○ Fluoxetine (Prozac)
    > ○ Fluvoxamine (Luvox)
    > ○ Nefazodone (Serzone)
    > ○ Nortriptyline (Pamelor or Aventyl)

○ Paroxetine (Paxil)
○ Sertraline (Zoloft)
○ Trazodone (Desyrel)

HOME CARE

- Give both patient and caregiver *verbal* and *written* instructions. Provide them with the name and telephone number of a physician or nurse to call if questions arise.
- *General information*
  —Discuss the disease and explain its progressive nature. To direct home care, help the caregiver identify the patient's functional stage (see box on p. 29).
  —Explain that behavioral symptoms often result from treatable problems such as physical discomfort, medication side effects, pain, or infection.
  —Assist caregiver to begin to identify signs or symptoms.
- *Special instructions*
  —Teach the caregiver how to help the patient with reality orientation and stimulation.
    Introduce all caregivers by name each time, and have them wear name tags (encourage consistent use of caregivers).
    Writing down instructions and directions may be helpful.
    Put a clock with a large face and a calendar where the patient can see them; remind the patient of the time for a scheduled activity.
    Be consistent and use repetition.
    Give single-step, simple instructions.
    Frequently remind the patient of the day and the hour and where he or she is.
    Place familiar personal objects within reach.
  —Encourage the caregiver to structure and plan the day's activities so the patient will know what to expect, which will assist in focusing the patient's attention on tasks such as bathing, dressing, and cleaning.
  —Provide scheduled time for leisure activities such as painting and walking.
  —Encourage the patient's participation in organizing activities.
  —Teach the caregiver how to deal with an agitated patient by modifying the environment.
    Speak in quiet tones.

STAGES OF FUNCTIONAL LOSS

Stage I: Early confusion
- Forgetful, loses things
- Expresses awareness of loss (depression not uncommon)

Stage II: Late confusion
- Increased difficulty with money management, work, driving, housekeeping, and shopping
- Social withdrawal from clubs, routine activities with friends
- Depression, increased fatigue
- Denies symptoms but may state, "I feel like I'm losing my mind"
- May require placement in an adult care center or, if living alone, may need to move into a residential care center

Stage III: Ambulatory dementia
- Increased loss of activities of daily living
- Worsening of symptoms as day progresses
- Withdrawal from family and friends
- Appears unaware of losses
- Increased stress threshold behavior (nocturnal wakefulness; wandering, pacing; agitation, belligerence)
- Speech and writing difficult to understand

Stage IV: Late-stage dementia
- No longer ambulates; cannot remember to eat, swallow, or chew
- Little purposeful activity
- No recognition of caregivers or family
- Muteness or possibly spontaneous screaming
- Incontinent; may be totally dependent for physical hygiene
- Becoming increasingly vegetative

Maintain a quiet, calm environment and avoid rushing; reduce the amount and complexity of stimuli if the patient shows signs of frustration and agitation.

Be alert for factors that may precipitate agitation such as loud and erratic noise, so as to eliminate or modify them.

—Discuss the potential for injury as the patient's condition progressively deteriorates. Encourage the caregiver to establish home safety precautions.

Provide supervision to protect the patient from being injured, humiliated, or lost.

Keep the patient's surroundings free of clutter and hazardous equipment.

Keep the area free of sharp objects and flammable items (e.g., lighter fluid).

Remove or dismantle door locks.

Have the patient use an electric razor, not a straight or safety razor.

Do not allow the patient to participate in potentially dangerous activities, such as smoking or cooking.

Put labels with the patient's name and telephone number in his or her clothing.

Provide assistance with daily routines (e.g., hygiene, diet, toileting). Medical supply stores carry special equipment for showers, bars for the toilet, and other devices.

Consider installing alarm systems or signal devices to alert the family when the patient wanders out the door.

—Discuss the patient's need for regular physical hygiene (i.e., bathing, shampooing, skin and oral care). Discuss the possibility of employing an attendant to help with daily care as dependency progresses.

—Provide direction in use of aids for dressing such as Velcro closures, elastic waists, or zippers.

—Explain that the patient needs to establish regular bowel and bladder habits.

—Discuss ways to prevent constipation.

Determine the patient's normal patterns.

Remind the patient to go to the bathroom at scheduled times.

Provide stool softeners and laxatives per prescription.

Encourage the patient to drink fluids and eat high-fiber foods.

A

Be alert for signs of impaction: no formed stool for 3 days, semiliquid stools, and restlessness (discuss the treatment for impaction: laxatives, suppositories, and enemas).
—Discuss ways to prevent urinary incontinence.
  Assess the patient's routine voiding patterns.
  Remind the patient to go to the bathroom q2h.
  Do not give the patient fluids before bedtime.
  Use disposable diapers and pads as indicated.
* *Medications*
  —Explain the purpose, dosage, schedule, and route of administration of the prescribed medication, as well as side effects to report to a physician or nurse.
  —Explain that certain drugs such as donepezil require regular laboratory monitoring.
* *Diet*
  —Alzheimer's patients need a properly balanced, high-fiber, high-calorie diet.
  —Present one course at a time (e.g., salad first, then entree); help the patient cut food as needed.
  —Use the following measures to prevent aspiration.
    Evaluate the patient's alertness.
    Monitor the patient's chewing and swallowing ability.
    Remind the patient to eat slowly, take small bites, and swallow each bite before taking another.

PSYCHOSOCIAL CARE

* Encourage verbalization regarding fears and concerns about disease and prognosis.
* Provide reality orientation as indicated.
* Encourage questions and expressions of anger and grief by patient and family.
* Provide information to patient and family/caretaker regarding counseling and support groups.
* Assist and encourage participation in self-care as long as possible; focus on strengths and intact roles.
* Provide family with referrals for counseling and support as they begin to develop a long-term plan of care.

FOLLOW-UP CARE

* Stress the importance of regular follow-up visits. Make sure the patient has the necessary names and telephone numbers.

REFERRALS

- Provide the names and telephone numbers of referral services, such as support groups for caregivers; social services for financial concerns and potential placement; home care services for possible in-home assistance and/or residential care centers.
- Refer to the Alzheimer's Association, 919 N. Michigan, Suite 1000, Chicago, IL 60611-1676.

Amputation

—**Amputation: surgical removal of a body part (fingers, toes, upper extremity, or lower extremity). Most amputations are performed on the legs. The surgical goal in amputation is to remove the least amount of tissue, leaving enough for a flap with which to create a stump that will allow fitting of a prosthesis.**

INDICATIONS

- Most common
  - —Severe trauma
  - —Crush injuries
  - —Severe sepsis (e.g., gas gangrene)
  - —Gangrene due to loss of arterial or venous circulation
- Less common
  - —Severe or recurrent osteomyelitis
  - —Musculoskeletal tumors
  - —Intractable pain from limb paralysis

TYPES OF AMPUTATION

- Forequarter: removal of the entire arm, forearm, and hand; the extremity is disarticulated at the shoulder joint
- Arm: amputation above the elbow or along the forearm
- Hemipelvectomy: removal of the entire thigh, leg, and foot (also called hindquarter amputation)
- Thigh: above-knee amputation (AKA)
- Lower leg: below-knee amputation (BKA)

- Foot: amputation of the toes and part of the foot at the metatarsal joints
- Finger or toe: amputation of part or all of one or more fingers or toes
- Disarticulation: amputation through a joint
- Closed amputation: creation of a weight-bearing stump, in which a flap composed of skin and soft tissues serves as padding over the bone end (also called definitive end-bearing amputation)
- Open (guillotine) amputation: creation of open stump surfaces as tissues are cut perpendicularly across with little initial incisional closure due to infection; the incision is closed later in another operation

PREPROCEDURAL TEACHING

- Review the surgeon's explanation of the procedure and the reasons for it.
- Explain the need for written consent to surgery and anesthesia.

Review of Preprocedural Care

- Explain that the patient may be admitted to the hospital the day of surgery, rather than before.
- Explain that the patient must have nothing to eat or drink after midnight of the night before surgery.
  —Explain that the patient's skin will be cleansed with a bactericidal soap or antiseptic solution to remove bacteria.
  —Explain that a complete blood count and urinalysis will be done to check for infection and bleeding.
- If lower extremity amputation is involved, instruct the patient in proper crutch walking when possible.
- Encourage the patient to ask questions and discuss any fears, concerns, and grief over losing a limb.
- For psychologic support, try to arrange for a preoperative visit from a person who has adjusted well to a similar amputation.

Review of Postprocedural Care

- Explain the care of the stump area and dressing.
  —The extremity will be elevated for 24 hours, then kept flat and extended (a longer period of elevation may be required, depending on the amount of swelling).

—The stump will be checked often to note color, drainage, swelling, bleeding, and wound and to check the pulses proximal to the incision.

—The drainage around the incision may be scant or moderate; tubes and drains are used to drain fluid.

• Discuss the phenomenon of phantom pain, painful or irritating sensations that feel as if they arise from the amputated part. Explain that medications are available to control pain.

• Review the type of prosthesis prescribed by the surgeon.

—Delayed fitting: a dressing and an elastic bandage are applied to the stump after surgery, and a prosthesis is fitted in 2 to 3 months, once the swelling has diminished.

Teach the patient and caregiver the proper method of wrapping the stump to help shape it for the prosthesis. Tell them that an orthotic technician will measure the stump to ensure a proper fit for the prosthesis.

Immediate postsurgical fitting and immediate postoperative prosthesis: these are prescribed to allow immediate or early ambulation and weight bearing. A cast is applied to the stump, and the prosthesis is attached to the cast.

• Explain that the patient will be kept on bed rest with the stump elevated for the length of time prescribed by the surgeon (24 to 48 hours). If the patient has had a lower extremity amputation, he or she then will be gotten up on crutches.

• Explain and demonstrate the adduction and extension exercises to be done on the amputated extremity to prevent contracture.

• For lower extremity amputations:

—Stress the importance of range-of-motion exercises for the unaffected extremities.

—Stress the importance of turning to the prone position for 1 hour three times daily to prevent flexion contractures of the knee and hip.

—Teach the patient exercises to increase strength of muscle extensors to avoid flexion contractures.

• For lower extremity amputations without a prosthesis:

—Explain that the patient should avoid long periods of sitting in a chair; teach the patient how to use ambulation aids (e.g., crutches or a walker).

—Encourage the patient to wear a good walking shoe and to keep the stump in a normal position (i.e., relaxed and in a downward position).

- For lower extremity amputations with a prosthesis:
  - —Teach the patient how to use ambulation aids (e.g., crutches or a walker).
  - —Explain that the periods of ambulation will be increased with the prescribed amount of weight bearing.
- Stress the importance of conditioning exercises (trunk flexion, sit-ups, hopping in place, hopping with the walker).
- Review medications, and discuss alternate methods to control phantom pain, such as distraction; behavior modification; relaxation; biofeedback; hypnosis; whirlpool; ultrasound; acupressure; cutaneous stimulation with oil of wintergreen, heat, and massage; and transcutaneous electrical nerve stimulation.
- Instruct the patient to report prolonged or chronic phantom pain for possible exploration and resection of a neuroma at the site of resection of the stump.

SIDE EFFECTS/COMPLICATIONS
- Hemorrhage, dehiscence
- Wound infection
- Phantom pain
- Contracture
- Abduction deformity

HOME CARE
- Give both patient and caregiver *verbal* and *written* instructions; use visual aids to assist in explanations. Provide the patient and caregiver with the name and telephone number of a physician or nurse to call if other questions arise.
- *Warning signs*
  - —Review the signs of infection to report to a physician or nurse: fever; chills; redness and swelling around the incision; drainage; or a foul odor from the incision or dressing.
  - —Emphasize that prolonged phantom limb pain is unusual and should be reported to the physician or surgeon.
- *Special instructions*
  - —Ensure that the patient receives complete instructions in the care of the prosthesis by the prosthetist-orthotist.
  - —Delayed fitting technique: teach the patient how to apply the elastic sleeve or wrap the stump for molding and shaping, and allow time for the patient to return the demonstration. Emphasize that the stump should not be wrapped too tightly, since this will impair circulation.

—Teach and demonstrate stump care.

Discuss the importance of daily hygiene to prevent infection and skin breakdown: wash the stump daily with soap and water and dry it well before applying the dressing, sleeve, or prosthesis. Caution against the use of emollients, which can create skin maceration beneath the prosthesis.

Stress the importance of inspecting and cleaning the stump daily; explain use of a handheld mirror to check for signs of infection, pressure sores, skin irritation, or drainage. Advise the patient to report to the physician or surgeon any sign of skin irritation: blisters (blebs), abrasions, or red or tender areas.

Explain that when molding is complete, the patient will be fitted with a residual limb sock to allow air to circulate around the stump.

- *Medications*
—Explain the purpose, dosage, schedule, and route of administration of prescribed drugs (antibiotics, analgesics, sedatives) and side effects to report to the physician or nurse.
- *Activity*
—Stress the importance of participating in the prescribed rehabilitation program: physical therapy, daily conditioning, and stump-strengthening exercises.
—Explain the need to exercise unaffected joints.
—Assess the need for assistive devices for bathing, toileting, dressing, and eating.

PSYCHOSOCIAL CARE

- Assess response of amputation on body image on patient or family/caregiver.
- Encourage expression of feelings regarding amputation: grief, anger, loss.
- Encourage patient/caregiver to participate in dressing changes and care of stump.
- Encourage and permit self-care as tolerated.
- Discuss phantom limb pain sensations; explain causes and pain-relieving techniques.
- Encourage and provide referrals for counseling as indicated.

FOLLOW-UP CARE

- Discuss the importance of making and keeping follow-up appointments: physical therapy, occupational therapy. Make sure the patient has the necessary names and telephone numbers.

REFERRALS

- Provide referrals for home-health care, rehabilitation, and medical social services as indicated.
- Assist patient/caregiver to obtain necessary home supplies and equipment.
- Provide names and phone numbers of community-based support programs.
- Refer to home health care for assistance with ADLs as needed.
- Evaluate and provide referral for medical social work services as indicated.

Amyloidosis

—Amyloidosis: a rare and incurable chronic disease characterized by accumulation of a proteinaceous material (amyloid) in the soft tissues. Amyloid can infiltrate one or more body organs, compromising organ function. Amyloidosis can occur as a primary disease, which may be familial, or as a secondary disorder stemming from a long-term, chronic inflammatory, infectious, or neoplastic disease. The cause of amyloidosis is unknown, but immunobiologic factors are believed to be involved.

SIGNS/SYMPTOMS

The signs and symptoms of amyloidosis reflect organ system involvement and its complications.

- Neuropathy: decreased temperature, pain sensation; inability to sweat
- Gastrointestinal (GI) system: difficulty talking, swallowing, and eating due to macroglossia (swollen tongue); abdominal pain, constipation, diarrhea, GI bleeding

- Respiratory system: dyspnea, cough, wheezing, nasal lesions, vocal cord lesions
- Skin: waxy, indurated papules and purpura, thickening of the skin, alopecia
- Joints: early morning stiffness, fatigue

COMPLICATIONS

- Cardiac system
  —Restrictive cardiomyopathy
  —Myocardial infarction
  —Congestive heart failure
- Renal system
  —Nephrotic syndrome
  —Renal failure
- Gastrointestinal system
  —Malabsorption syndrome
  —Hemorrhage
  —Protein-losing enteropathy
  —Perforation, ischemic necrosis
  —Hepatomegaly
- Skeletal system
  —Rheumatoid arthritis and osteomyelitis
- Respiratory system
  —Lung abscess, bronchiectasis, pneumonia
- Neurologic system
  —Peripheral, sensorimotor neuropathy

DIAGNOSTIC TESTS

- Describe each procedure, its purpose, and the normal feelings or sensations that are likely, as well as any preprocedural or postprocedural care.
  —Serum and urine electrophoresis
  —Tissue biopsy (sites may include gingiva, skin, abdominal fat pad, and rectal mucosa)

TREATMENT
Primary

- Treatment aimed at controlling symptoms

Secondary

- Treat underlying disease

Medical

- Therapy
  —Plasmapheresis: to stop dissemination of amyloid chains
- Drugs
  —Antineoplastics: to reduce the concentration of amyloid
  —Colchicine, dimethyl sulfoxide (DMSO)
  —Corticosteroids: to treat underlying inflammatory disorder
  —Antibiotics

 HOME CARE

- Give both patient and caregiver *verbal* and *written* instructions. Provide them with the name and telephone number of a physician or nurse to call if questions arise.
- *General information*
  —Review the physician's explanation of the disorder, its causes, and associated involvement of other body organs.
- *Warning signs*
  —Review the signs and symptoms of disease progression that should be reported to the physician or a nurse: chest pain, dyspnea, shortness of breath, peripheral edema, bleeding, abdominal pain, and diarrhea.
- *Special instructions*
  —Teach the patient how to care for skin lesions if present; stress the importance of reporting to the physician any signs of skin infection, such as reddened, warm, painful, draining lesions.
  —Discuss the need for safety measures at home if the patient has peripheral or sensory impairment:
    Test the temperature of the bathwater before getting into the tub.
    Do not use heating pads.
    Avoid wearing tight, constricting clothing (e.g., socks, stockings).
- *Medications*
  —Explain the purpose, dosage, schedule, and route of administration of the prescribed medication, as well as side effects to report to a physician or nurse.
  —If steroids are prescribed, emphasize that the patient should not abruptly stop taking the drugs without first checking with the physician.

- *Activity*
  —Encourage the patient to discuss allowances and limitations regarding occupation and favorite recreational sports and activities.
  —Stress the importance of rest if fatigue or weakness occurs.
  —Encourage the patient to continue with ADLs, but limitations may be required during periods of illness (colds, flu).
- *Diet*
  —Tell the patient to follow a regular diet or one ordered for the associated disease.
  —If the tongue is affected, instruct the patient to take small bites, to chew thoroughly, and to swallow each bite completely before taking another.
  —If the patient suffers from malnutrition, encourage the addition of high-calorie food supplements to the diet.

FOLLOW-UP CARE

- Stress the importance of regular follow-up visits. Make sure the patient has the necessary names and telephone numbers.
- Help the patient obtain a MedicAlert bracelet and identification card listing the diagnosis and medications.

Amyotrophic Lateral Sclerosis
("Lou Gehrig's Disease")

—Amyotrophic lateral sclerosis (ALS): a progressive lower motor neuron disorder that results in muscle wasting and weakness. The weakness begins in the upper extremities (upper arms and shoulders) and progressively involves the muscles of the neck and throat. The trunk and legs usually are not affected until late in the disease.

SIGNS/SYMPTOMS

- Irregular muscle fasciculations with weakness
- Cramping
- Incoordination of movement of the hands and fingers

- Muscle weakness, wasting, and atrophy of the hands, arms, and shoulders
- Spastic gait
- Progressive weakness, flaccidity, and atrophy of the legs
- Slurred speech (dysarthria)
- Difficulty swallowing (dysphagia)
- Excessive drooling
- Dyspnea
- Hyperreflexia and muscle spasticity

COMPLICATIONS

- Neuromuscular deficit (mild to severe)
- Respiratory infection
- Aspiration
- Atelectasis
- Respiratory failure
- Injury

DIAGNOSTIC TESTS

- Describe each procedure, its purpose, and the normal feelings or sensations that are likely, as well as any preprocedural or postprocedural care. Explain that the following diagnostic procedures help confirm the diagnosis.
  —Computed tomography scan
  —Muscle biopsy
  —Electromyelography
  —Nerve conduction studies
  —Laboratory tests
      Creatinine phosphokinase (CPK): elevated
      Cerebrospinal fluid analysis: elevated protein

TREATMENT
Medical

- Therapy
  —Physical therapy
  —Occupational, speech therapy
  —Oxygen/ventilatory support
  —Swallowing therapy
- Drugs
  —Riluzole (Rilutek): slows the progression of disease
  —Muscle cramping: quinidine, baclofen

—Antidepressants
—Excessive salivation: amitriptyline, benadryl, glycopyrrolate (Rokinul)
—Muscle relaxants

Surgical

- Transtympanic neuroectomy
- Cricopharyngeal myotomy: to alleviate dysphagia
- Cervical esophagostomy
- Tracheostomy

HOME CARE

- Give both patient and caregiver *verbal* and *written* instructions. Provide them with the name and telephone number of a physician or nurse to call if questions arise. Use visual aids to assist in instruction.
- *General information*
  —Review the physician's explanation of the disorder, as well as the symptoms and the progression of the disease.
  —Discuss the importance of skin care to prevent skin breakdown (back rubs, frequent changes of position, use of air mattress, sheepskin, and footboard).
  —Explain the need to maintain good oral and eye hygiene. Explain the need for oral suctioning as the disease progresses, and demonstrate the procedure.
- *Warning signs*
  —Review the signs and symptoms of disease progression that should be reported to the physician or a nurse: excessive salivation, weakening voice, difficulty swallowing.
  —Explain to the patient and caregiver that cognitive processes are not affected. Emphasize the importance of expressing feelings about the progressive muscular wasting and weakness.
- *Special instructions*
  —Explain to the patient and caregiver the respiratory support equipment to be kept in the home (oxygen therapy, suction setup), and show household members how to use it. Ask the physician for a prescription, and help the patient and caregiver obtain equipment from a medical supply store or pharmacy.

A

—A noninvasive ventilatory assistive device (Bi DAP) may be recommended when vital capacity decreases below 70%.

—Provide guides to facilitate breathing:

Instruct the patient not to lie down after eating.

Avoid eating large meals that can increase abdominal pressure and interfere with expansion of the diaphragm.

Sleep with the head elevated 15 to 30 degrees.

—Demonstrate how to use an electrolarynx to facilitate vocalization.

—Discuss the need to develop alternative methods of communication (using the eyes, blinking) when the voice no longer functions.

- *Medications*

    —Explain the purpose, dosage, schedule, and route of administration of the prescribed medication, as well as side effects to report to a physician or nurse.

- *Activity*

    —Teach the patient to balance passive or active range-of-motion activities with rest periods and to avoid strenuous exercise or activity; encourage participation in family activities.

    —Review the purpose of braces, splints, and cervical collars to support the hands, ankles, and neck, and demonstrate how to use them properly.

    —Review strengthening exercises to maintain function.

    —Demonstrate to the caregiver procedures for positioning and transfer and techniques for turning.

- *Diet*

    —Advise a high-calorie, high-protein soft diet as tolerated.

    —Instruct the patient to weigh himself or herself weekly at the same time wearing the same clothing and report progressive loss.

    —Teach the patient and caregiver how to assess swallowing ability and manage as the disease progresses.

    Place pureed foods on the posterior aspect of the tongue.

    If solid foods are still possible, cut food into small pieces, chew thoroughly, and swallow each bite completely before taking another, to avoid aspiration.

    —Clean the corners of the patient's mouth after eating and prn.

    —Have the patient use a bib.

—If nasogastric (NG) or gastrostomy feedings must be considered, demonstrate the procedure for NG tube feeding, as well as care of the equipment.

—Explain the need to provide for and anticipate elimination; explain that the patient can prevent constipation by adding fiber to diet, drinking fluids, and using suppositories or stool softeners daily.

PSYCHOSOCIAL CARE

• Encourage verbalization about fears and concerns about disease progression and body image changes.

• Encourage consultation with a mental health counselor for the patient, family, and children soon after diagnosis.

• Encourage the patient to participate in home care planning.

FOLLOW-UP CARE

• Stress the importance of regular medical and laboratory follow-up visits. Explain that the patient should have vital capacity tested regularly. Make sure the patient has the necessary names and telephone numbers.

• Encourage and help the patient to obtain a MedicAlert bracelet and identification card listing diagnosis and medications.

REFERRALS

• Provide the patient and caregiver with the names and telephone numbers of referral services, such as home health care, physical and occupational therapy centers, social services, and a skilled nursing facility as indicated.

• Refer the patient and caregiver to the Amyotrophic Lateral Sclerosis Association and to a local ALS support group.

Anaphylaxis

—Anaphylaxis: a rapid, systemic, antigen-antibody hypersensitivity reaction that affects a number of organs throughout the body. It often is an immediate, life-threatening event that occurs with seconds to minutes of exposure to a causative allergen. The most common causes are insect venom (bees, wasps, hornets, yellow jackets), drugs (e.g., penicillin, iodine, and sulfonamides), blood products, and foods (e.g., shellfish and eggs).

SIGNS/SYMPTOMS

- Early (within seconds of exposure)
  —Sweating
  —Weakness
  —Feeling of impending doom or fright
  —Shortness of breath
  —Pruritus, urticaria
  —Angioedema of the eyes, lips, and tongue
- Late (within minutes of exposure)
  —Respiratory
     Bronchospasm
     Dyspnea
     Wheezing
     Laryngeal edema
     Cyanosis
     Hypoxia
     Respiratory arrest
  —Cardiovascular
     Lightheadedness (due to hypotension)
     Rapid, weak pulse
     Arrhythmias
  —Neurologic
     Confusion
     Seizures
     Coma

COMPLICATIONS

- Shock
- Respiratory failure
- Cardiac arrest
- Death

DIAGNOSTIC TESTS

- No specific tests are used to diagnose anaphylaxis; the patient's history, signs, and symptoms direct the diagnosis and treatment (skin and scratch tests may be done to identify allergens in patients considered at risk for an anaphylactic reaction).

TREATMENT
Medical

Anaphylaxis is *always* an emergency; treatment involves immediate, aggressive management of symptoms.

- Therapy
  —Intubation: to establish an airway
  —Admission to an intensive care unit for monitoring and management
- Drugs
  —Epinephrine: to counter the effects of the allergen
  —Vasopressors: to maintain blood pressure
  —Diphenhydramine (Benadryl): to treat angioedema and urticaria
  —Aminophylline: for bronchospasm

Surgical

- Tracheostomy: for severe airway obstruction

HOME CARE

- Give both the patient and the caregiver *verbal* and *written* instructions. Provide them with the name and telephone number of a physician or nurse to call if questions arise.
- *General information*
  —Review the physician's explanation of the disorder, making sure the patient understands what caused the anaphylactic episode.
  —Stress the importance of avoiding known allergens in the future.
    If food was the allergen: help the patient list other foods that also may cause a reaction (e.g., if shrimp caused the reaction, the patient should avoid all shellfish, such as oysters, lobster, and mussels).
    If insect venom was the allergen: instruct the patient to avoid outdoor areas that may have a high concentration of insects during a particular season or to have the area sprayed.
- *Warning signs*
  —See Signs/Symptoms for early and late manifestations.

- *Special instructions*
  —Discuss the need to always carry an auto-injector (such as EpiPen or Anaki) that delivers a subcutaneous dose of epinephrine. If one is ordered, teach the patient and family members, including older children, how to administer the medication. Instruct the patient to check the kit regularly for expiration dates.

FOLLOW-UP CARE

- Discuss the need for any follow-up appointments, including future allergy testing when indicated. Make sure the patient has the necessary names and telephone numbers.
- Emphasize that the patient should inform health care providers about the allergy before any procedures are done.
- Explain the importance of obtaining a MedicAlert bracelet and identification card listing the specific allergen.
- Advise the patient to identify the emergency department nearest home and work.

Anorectal Abscess, Fistula, and Fissure

—**Anorectal abscess:** a localized infection caused by inflammation of soft tissue of the anal canal, rectum, or perianal skin. Initially appearing as a collection of pus, an anorectal abscess may progress to a fistula in the soft tissues and perianal skin.

—**Anorectal fistula:** an abnormal opening between the perianal area and rectum.

—**Anal fissure:** a small tear in the lining of the anus.

CAUSES/CONTRIBUTING FACTORS/RISK FACTORS

- Abrasion, trauma, or tearing of the lining of the anal canal, rectum, or perianal skin, with subsequent infection with *Escherichia coli,* staphylococci, or streptococci
- Infection of submucosal hematomas, sclerosed hemorrhoids, or anal fissures

- Obstruction of glands in the anal area
- Cryptitis
- Infection of apocrine glands
- Folliculitis in the perianal area
- Ulcerative colitis
- Crohn's disease

SIGNS/SYMPTOMS

- Rectal pain (usually described as throbbing or dull and aching, depending on the abscess's location)
- Erythematous lump or swelling in the anal area
- Aggravation of pain with sitting, walking, or defecation
- Discharge or bleeding
- Anal pruritus
- Fever, chills, nausea, vomiting, malaise
- If fistula present: pink or red, elevated ulcer that produces a discharge on perianal skin

COMPLICATIONS

- Perineal cellulitis
- Formation of scar tissue
- Anal stricture
- Peritonitis

DIAGNOSTIC TESTS

- Describe each procedure, its purpose, and the normal feelings or sensations that are likely, as well as any preprocedural and postprocedural care.
    —Digital rectal examination
    —Proctoscopy: to visualize lesions
    —Additional procedures that may be performed to rule out other conditions
        Sigmoidoscopy
        Barium enema
        Colonoscopy

TREATMENT
Medical

- Therapy
    —Diet high in fiber and fluids
    —Sitz baths

A

- Drugs
  —Stool softeners
  —Antibiotics
  —Analgesics

Surgical

- For anorectal abscess: surgical incision and drainage
- For fistulas: fistulotomy (removal of the fistula and granulated tissue) or fistulectomy (removal of the fistulous tract and drainage)

 HOME CARE

- Give both the patient and the caregiver *verbal* and *written* instructions. Provide them with the name and telephone number of a physician or nurse to call if questions arise.
- *General information*
  —Explain how an anorectal abscess, fistula, and tears develop, and discuss the causes and contributing factors, diagnostic tests, care, and treatment.
- *Warning signs*
  —Review the signs and symptoms that should be reported to a physician or nurse.
    Infection (fever, purulent drainage from the incision, redness, swelling, tenderness)
  —Instruct the patient to note the time of the first bowel movement after surgery and to notify the physician or nurse if no bowel movement occurs or if constipation develops.
- *Special instructions*
  —Help the patient obtain the appropriate supplies (dressings, perineal pads, mesh panties) to aid complete healing of the infected area after surgery.
  —Demonstrate proper wound care and dressing changes (procedure, frequency, packing, irrigation). Show the patient how to use a mirror to inspect the area and to change the dressing.
  —Instruct the patient to check the dressing after bowel or bladder elimination and to replace it if it becomes soiled. Advise the patient to dispose of soiled dressings in a plastic bag and to wash hands thoroughly.
  —Advise the patient to shave the perianal area weekly to keep hair out of the affected area (a caregiver may need to help the patient with this).

—Encourage defecation to prevent fecal impaction.

—Advise the patient to sit on thick foam pillows or pads and to avoid air or rubber donuts because they spread the buttocks apart.

—Teach the patient to avoid straining during a bowel movement, since this may increase discomfort and put pressure on the affected area.

—Stress the importance of perianal cleanliness at all times; explain that proper hygiene helps prevent infection.

—Provide warm sitz baths to cleanse the perianal region and to relieve the patient's discomfort; show the patient how to prepare one.

—Explain that anorectal infections tend to recur and that anorectal sexual activities need to be modified to control recurrences or complications.

- *Medications*

—Explain the purpose, dosage, schedule, and route of administration of the prescribed drugs, as well as side effects to report to the physician or a nurse.

—Teach the patient that stool-softening laxatives, along with a high-fiber diet, will help prevent constipation.

- *Diet*

—Help the patient plan a diet high in fiber and fluids, which helps produce regular bowel movements.

FOLLOW-UP CARE

- Stress the importance of regular follow-up visits and make sure the patient has the necessary names and telephone numbers.
- Explain that follow-up visits are important because perianal fistulas can take 4 to 5 weeks to heal; deeper wounds may take 12 to 16 weeks.

Aortic Aneurysm

—Aortic aneurysm: an abnormal widening of the aorta, either at the beginning of the vessel (ascending) or after it curves toward the abdomen (descending). In a dissecting aneurysm,

A

blood makes its way between the layers of the blood vessel, causing them to separate. An aneurysm can involve the full circumference of the vessel or only a weak patch on one side of the arterial wall. Blood pools in the pouch, causing blood clots.

—The patient may be asymptomatic or may have symptoms that result from pressure on adjacent structures or from intimal tears or rupture.

CAUSES/CONTRIBUTING FACTORS/RISK FACTORS
- Atherosclerosis (ascending aorta)
- Infection (aortic arch and descending aorta)
- Coarctation of the aorta
- Trauma (descending aorta)
- Syphilis (ascending aorta)
- Hypertension (in dissecting aneurysm)
- Marfan's syndrome
- Men aged 50 to 70 years
- African-Americans

SIGNS/SYMPTOMS
- Wheezing
- Hoarseness
- Numbness (paresthesia)
- Neuralgia
- Sudden onset of pain in anterior chest, extending to the neck, shoulder, lower back, or abdomen
- Syncope
- Pallor
- Sweating
- Shortness of breath
- Increased pulse rate
- Duskiness
- Leg weakness (involvement of the aortic valve, ascending aneurysm)

COMPLICATIONS
- Dissection, rupture
- Bleeding
- Embolization

DIAGNOSTIC TESTS

- Explain that the following diagnostic procedures confirm the diagnosis. Explain each procedure as it is ordered. Describe each procedure, its purpose, and the normal feelings or sensations that are likely, as well as any preprocedural or postprocedural care.
  —Aortography: to show location of the aneurysm, its form, and whether the walls of the artery are separating (dissecting aneurysm)
  —Electrocardiogram: to differentiate pain of thoracic aneurysm from that of a myocardial infarction
  —Echocardiogram: to help identify dissecting aneurysm (separation of the arterial walls)
  —Computed tomography: to locate and confirm the location of the aneurysm or to determine the size of an intimal tear and monitor progression
  —Magnetic resonance imaging: to confirm the diagnosis
  —Transesophageal echocardiogram: to locate the aneurysm from the back of the aorta
  —Hemoglobin: to detect loss of blood

TREATMENT
Medical

- Drugs
  —Antihypertensive drugs such as beta blockers: to keep blood pressure under control and alleviate undue pressure on the vessels, including the site of repair

Surgical

- Resection of the aneurysm and restoration of normal blood flow by using Dacron or Teflon graft replacement. If the aortic valve is involved or is insufficient, replacement is necessary (see Valve Repair/Replacement, p. 635).

 HOME CARE

- Give both patient and caregiver *verbal* and *written* instructions. Provide them with the name and telephone number of a physician or nurse to call if questions arise.
- *General information*
  —Review the indications and causes of the patient's aneurysm. Discuss any factors that will help to prevent future

A

aneurysms, such as controlling blood pressure and slowing the atherosclerotic process.

- *Specific instructions*
  —Review symptoms of tears or rupture: sudden onset of severe pain, pallor, diaphoresis, loss of consciousness.
  —Stress the importance of seeking emergency care should signs occur.
  —Teach hypertensive patients how to monitor blood pressure and keep a record. Provide blood pressure parameters. Include information on where to obtain necessary equipment and supplies as indicated.
  —After surgery:
    Instruct the patient in care of the incisional wound, reviewing signs of wound infection and thrombus formation within the graft.
- *Medications*
  —Explain the purpose, dosage, schedule, and route of administration of the prescribed medications, as well as side effects and drug-drug interactions to report to a physician or nurse.
- *Activity*
  —Advise the patient to alternate exercise with rest and avoid vigorous exercise or heavy lifting.
  —Encourage the patient to discuss allowances or limitations with respect to occupation, sports, and activities.
  —Caution the patient to avoid sudden outbursts of activity associated with stress.
  —Emphasize that the patient should not shovel snow, change a tire, or push a car.
- *Diet*
  —Advise the patient to follow a low-salt, low-fat, and low-cholesterol diet.
  —Instruct the patient to limit alcohol consumption because of alcohol's effect on blood pressure.

FOLLOW-UP CARE AND REFERRALS

- Make sure that the patient has scheduled a follow-up visit. Check that the patient has the necessary names and telephone numbers of health care providers and emergency services in the area.

- Discuss the importance of not delaying surgery if recommended.
- Stress the importance of not smoking because nicotine has negative effects on the blood vessels and blood pressure.

Aortic Insufficiency
(Incompetence, Regurgitation)

—**Aortic insufficiency: incompetence or insufficiency of the aortic valve, which permits blood to flow (leak) back into the left ventricle. This causes decreased flow of blood outward into the tissues and increased volume in the left ventricle, adding to the work of the heart and resulting in a hypertrophic left ventricle. The cusps are unable to close because of the presence of lesions, perforations, or tears or the development of eroded or scarred tissue because of infection or fibrosis.**

CAUSES/CONTRIBUTING FACTORS

- Rheumatic fever
- Syphilis
- Hypertension
- Endocarditis
- Idiopathic
- Associated with Marfan's syndrome
- Dissection of aortic aneurysm
- Ankylosing spondylitis
- Congenital bicuspid aortic valve
- Chest trauma

SIGNS/SYMPTOMS

- Palpitations
- Awareness of the heartbeat, especially when lying down
- Tachycardia
- Dyspnea
- Orthopnea
- Paroxysmal nocturnal dyspnea

- Fatigue
- Exertional angina

COMPLICATIONS

- Heart rhythm abnormalities
- Congestive heart failure
- Ventricular hypertrophy
- Endocarditis
- Pulmonary edema
- Sudden death

DIAGNOSTIC TESTS

- Describe each procedure, its purpose, and the normal feelings or sensations that are likely, as well as any preprocedural or postprocedural care.
  - —Electrocardiogram: to detect evidence of left ventricular hypertrophy
  - —Chest x-ray: to detect aortic valve calcification, left ventricle enlargement, and dilation of the ascending aorta
  - —Echocardiogram: to detect rhythm abnormalities, the presence of left ventricle enlargement, and ischemic changes
  - —Radionuclide studies: to determine ejection fraction
  - —Cardiac catheterization: to determine severity of valve incompetence, assess ventricular function, and look for involvement of other valves

TREATMENT
Medical

- Drugs
  - —Inotropic drugs (e.g., digitalis)
  - —Vasodilators
  - —Diuretics
  - —Calcium channel blockers
  - —Antiarrhythmic agents

Surgical

- Aortic valve replacement

HOME CARE

- Give both patient and caregiver *verbal* and *written* instructions. Provide them with the name and telephone number of a physician or nurse to call if questions arise.

- *General information*
  —Use heart models or diagrams to assist in instruction. Show the patient the location of the affected valve.
  —Discuss the disease process and causes, explaining that appearance of signs and symptoms may reflect disease progression.
  —Explain the risk of endocarditis, discussing causes and means of prevention including alerting the dentist and other medical personnel (urologist, gynecologist) of valve disease. Explain the importance of good oral hygiene and regular dental care. Stress the importance of antibiotic prophylaxis before dental care or any invasive procedures (i.e., dilation and curettage, cystoscopy) for prevention.
  —Describe the need for valve replacement, if recommended (see p. 635).
- *Warning signs*
  —Review the signs and symptoms that should be reported to a physician or nurse.
  > Exertional dyspnea
  > Orthopnea
  > Paroxysmal nocturnal dyspnea
  > Fatigue
  > Palpitations
- *Specific instructions*
  —Provide female patients with instructions regarding pregnancy and appropriate forms of contraception (e.g., avoid estrogen-based oral contraceptives and intrauterine devices). Emphasize the importance of planning all pregnancies.
- *Medications*
  —Explain the purpose, dosage, schedule, and route of administration of the prescribed medications, as well as side effects to report to a physician or nurse.
- *Activity*
  —Stress the importance of avoiding strenuous activities. Encourage the patient to discuss allowances and limitations with respect to occupation and recreational sports activities. Explain the need for moderate activity. Encourage frequent rest periods and avoid fatigue. Discuss measures that minimize fatigue (e.g., shower with a chair rather than take a tub bath).

A

- *Diet*
  —Discuss the need to restrict salt intake. Explain that further sodium restrictions may be necessary in the presence of heart failure.

FOLLOW-UP CARE AND REFERRALS

- Stress the importance of any prescribed follow-up care, including allergy testing and laboratory tests. Make sure the patient has the necessary names and telephone numbers.
- Stress the importance of not smoking or using tobacco products. Provide information and referrals to smoking cessation programs as necessary.

Aortic Valve Stenosis

—Aortic valve stenosis: narrowing of the three-leaflet aortic valve from the normal 2.6 to 3.5 cm opening to as little as 0.4 cm. The narrowing is due to the accumulation of plaque (calcification). This narrowing or obstruction restricts the flow of blood across the valve into the aorta, depriving the heart and other organs of circulation and increasing the workload of the heart.

CAUSES/CONTRIBUTING FACTORS/RISK FACTORS

- Congenital bicuspid valve
- Rheumatic fever
- Male sex
- Degenerative calcific changes (persons older than 60 years of age)

SIGNS/SYMPTOMS

- Symptoms appear late in the course of the illness
- Angina
- Syncope (faintness) with exertion
- Orthopnea, dyspnea, shortness of breath
- Fatigue
- Cool extremities
- Palpitations
- Dizziness

COMPLICATIONS

- Arrhythmias
  —Atrial fibrillation
  —Conduction defects
- Heart failure
- Sudden cardiac death
- Infective endocarditis
- Embolization

DIAGNOSTIC TESTS

- Describe each procedure, its purpose, and the normal feelings or sensations that are likely, as well as any preprocedural and postprocedural care.
  —Electrocardiogram: to detect rhythm abnormalities and identify left ventricular hypertrophy
  —Echocardiography: to determine severity of the obstruction and assess ventricular function
  —Cardiac catheterization and coronary angiography: to assess degree of obstruction across the valve, ventricular function, coronary blood flow
  —Chest x-ray: to detect valvular calcification, heart enlargement, and lung congestion

TREATMENT
Medical

- Therapy
  —Catheter balloon aortic valvuloplasty
- Drugs
  —Digitalis
  —Diuretics
  —Antiarrhythmic agents

Surgical

- Aortic valve replacement
- Percutaneous aortic valvuloplasty

 HOME CARE

- Give both the patient and the caregiver verbal and written instruction. Provide them with the name and telephone number of a physician or nurse to call if questions arise.

- *General information*
  - —Use heart models or diagrams to assist in instruction. Show the patient the location of the affected valve and explain its role in the arterial circulation.
  - —If balloon angioplasty or surgery is recommended, help the patient understand why and explain what is involved in these procedures (see Valve Repair/Replacement, p. 635).
  - —Discuss the disease process, contributing factors, the cause of obstruction, and the signs and symptoms of disease progression.
  - —Explain the risk of endocarditis and discuss its causes and means of preventing it, including alerting the dentist and any other medical personnel (urologist, gynecologist) that the patient has valve disease, maintaining good oral hygiene, and receiving regular dental care. Explain the importance of antibiotic prophylaxis before dental care and other invasive procedures (dilation and curettage, cystoscopy).
- *Warning signs*
  - —Review the signs and symptoms that should be reported to a physician or nurse.
    Faintness
    Palpitations
    Shortness of breath
    Dyspnea on exertion
    Signs of systemic emboli: muscle weakness, paresthesias, confusion
- *Special instructions*
  - —Provide female patients with instruction regarding contraception and risk of pregnancy (e.g., avoid estrogen-based oral contraception or intrauterine devices). Stress the importance of pregnancy planning.
- *Medications*
  - —Explain the purpose, dosage, schedule, and route of administration of any prescribed drugs, as well as side effects to report to the physician or nurse.
- *Activity*
  - —Emphasize the importance of avoiding strenuous activity, such as vacuuming, pushing a car, changing a tire, or engaging in competitive sports.
  - —Encourage the patient to discuss limitations with respect to occupation and recreational activities.

—Explain the need for moderate activity, such as walking for conditioning.

—Encourage the patient to rest frequently and avoid fatigue.

• *Diet*

—Discuss the need to restrict salt intake to <2000 mg per day.

—Explain that further sodium restrictions may be necessary in the presence of heart failure.

FOLLOW-UP CARE AND REFERRALS

• Stress the importance of regular follow-up visits. Make sure the patient has the necessary names and telephone numbers.

• Advise the patient with severe asymptomatic aortic stenosis that he or she may require electrocardiogram (EKG), echocardiogram, and clinical examination every 6 to 12 months.

• Emphasize the importance of not smoking or using tobacco products. Provide information about and referrals to smoking cessation programs as necessary.

Aplastic Anemia
(Hypoplastic)

—Aplastic anemia: results from inability of the bone marrow to produce erythrocytes (RBCs). Usually the onset of aplastic anemia is insidious, but when it develops suddenly, it has a poor prognosis. Hypoplastic anemia most often involves the depression of production of all three bone marrow elements: erythrocytes, platelets, and granulocytes (pancytopenia).

CAUSES

• Antineoplastic or antimicrobial agents
• Infectious processes
• Pregnancy
• Hepatitis
• Radiation

SIGNS/SYMPTOMS

- Fatigue
- Shortness of breath
- Headache
- Weakness
- Pallor
- Dysphagia
- Numbness and tingling in extremities
- Easy bruising and bleeding
- Dizziness
- Fever
- Infection
- Oral ulcerations

COMPLICATIONS

- Bleeding or infection

DIAGNOSTIC TESTS

- Describe each procedure, its purpose, and the normal feelings or sensations that are likely, as well as any preprocedural and postprocedural care.
  - —Complete blood count with differential
  - —Platelet count
  - —Bleeding time
  - —Bone marrow aspiration
  - —Reticulocyte count
  - —Peripheral blood smear
  - —Cultures (if infection is suspected)

TREATMENT
Medical

- Therapy
  - —Oxygen if anemia is severe
  - —Transfusions
    - RBCs, packed red cells
    - Platelets
    - Granulocytes
- Drugs
  - —Steroids (see Steroid Therapy, p. 590)
  - —Colony-stimulating factors
  - —Antibiotics
  - —Androgens

Surgical

- Bone marrow transplantation

🏠 HOME CARE

- Give both the patient and the caregiver *verbal* and *written* instructions. Provide them with the name and telephone number of a physician or nurse to call if questions arise.
- *General information*
  —Explain aplastic anemia, its causes, and contributing factors to the patient.
- *Warning signs*
  —Review the signs and symptoms that should be reported to a physician or nurse.

  > Infections: systemic: fever, malaise, fatigue; urinary tract: cloudy, malodorous urine; burning; frequency; urgency; upper respiratory: malodorous, purulent, colored, copious secretions; productive cough

  > Bleeding/hemorrhage: melena, hematuria, epistaxis, ecchymosis, bleeding of gums

  > Anemia: fatigue, weakness, paresthesias

- *Special instructions*
  —Teach the patient how to self-monitor laboratory values. Identify the patient's baseline levels to monitor further decreases or changes.
  —Stress the importance of avoiding exposure to individuals known to have acute infections.
  —Teach the patient to avoid trauma, abrasions, and breakdown of the skin, which could lead to infection.
  —Discuss methods of preventing hemorrhage, such as using an electric razor and soft-bristled toothbrush and avoiding activities that might traumatize the tissues.
- *Medications*
  —Explain the purpose, dosage, schedule, and route of administration of any prescribed drugs, as well as side effects to report to the physician or nurse.
  —See Steroid Therapy (p. 590).
  —Explain that antibiotics must be taken for the entire period prescribed to prevent superinfection.
  —Advise the patient to avoid the use of aspirin, aspirin products, nonsteroidal antiinflammatory drugs (NSAIDs), and ibuprofen products in the presence of a bleeding disorder.

- *Activity*
  —Encourage the patient to discuss limitations with respect to occupation, recreational sports, and activities.
  —Advise the patient to limit activities when fatigued and during episodes of infection.
  —Discourage smoking and excessive alcohol consumption.
- *Diet*
  —Discuss the need to maintain a well-balanced diet to enhance resistance to infection.
  —Discuss the need to increase dietary fiber (e.g., fresh fruit and vegetables) to prevent constipation and straining at stool.

FOLLOW-UP CARE

- Stress the importance of regular follow-up visits. Make sure the patient has the necessary names and telephone numbers.

Appendicitis/Appendectomy

—Appendicitis: obstruction of the appendix, a small, finger-like pouch attached to the cecum of the colon, causing inflammation, distention, decreased blood supply, necrosis, and sometimes perforation. If untreated, appendicitis causes generalized peritonitis or localized abscess.

—Appendectomy: surgical removal of the appendix.

RISK FACTORS

- Incidence highest in adolescent and young adult males
- Familial tendencies

SIGNS/SYMPTOMS

- Early stage
  —Vague abdominal pain in periumbilical area
  —Nausea and vomiting
  —Fever
  —Sensitivity over appendix area (right lower abdomen)

- Intermediate or acute stage
  - —Pain over right lower abdomen aggravated by walking or coughing
  - —Feeling of constipation, urge to defecate
  - —Loss of appetite
  - —Malaise
  - —Sometimes diarrhea
  - —Decreased bowel sounds
  - —Rapid pulse
  - —Fever
  - —Rigidity of abdomen when palpated

COMPLICATIONS

- Perforated appendix
  - —Sudden relief of pain with perforation, then development of peritonitis
- Peritonitis
  - —Increased, generalized pain over abdomen
  - —Recurrence of vomiting
  - —Side-lying position with knees flexed
  - —Rapid pulse, shallow respirations, low blood pressure
  - —Chills, fever
  - —Pallor or flushing
  - —Irritability, restlessness, anxiety
  - —Progressive abdominal distention and rigidity
  - —Failure to pass flatus or stool
  - —Decreased or absent bowel sounds
  - —Loss of appetite
- Dehydration
- Sepsis
- Abdominal abscess
- Electrolyte imbalance

DIAGNOSTIC TESTS

- Describe each procedure, its purpose, and the normal feelings or sensations that are likely, as well as any preprocedural and postprocedural care.
  - —Blood studies: increase in white blood cells (WBCs) seen on differential
  - —X-ray of abdomen

—Intravenous pyelography: to eliminate kidney stones or pyelitis from the diagnosis (see Urolithiasis, p. 630)
—Urinalysis: to rule out genitourinary conditions mimicking appendicitis
—Abdominal ultrasound: to rule out Crohn's disease, diverticulitis, or gastroenteritis
—Abdominal computed tomography: may reveal an appendiceal abscess or acute appendicitis

TREATMENT
Medical *(until taken to surgery)*

* Therapy
  —Nothing by mouth (NPO)
  —Hydration, intravenous
  —Comfort measures
  —Nasogastric tube if excessive distention and vomiting
  —Bed rest
* Drugs
  —Antibiotics

Surgical

* Surgery is performed within 24 to 48 hours of onset of symptoms or when patient is stabilized.
* See Abdominal Surgery (p. 6) for preoperative and postoperative care.
* Appendectomy procedures
  —Laparoscopic approach (used if appendix has not ruptured)
     Incision is made below umbilius with three or four abdominal punctures to permit insertion of laparoscope for viewing and removal of appendix.
     Procedure requires general anesthesia and overnight stay.
  —Abdominal surgical approach
     Right lower quadrant abdominal incision is performed under general anesthesia and requires 2-day hospital stay.
     If appendix is ruptured, drain remains in place and patient stays in hospital 5 days or more.

HOME CARE

* Give both the patient and the caregiver *verbal* and *written* instructions. Provide them with the name and telephone number of a physician or nurse to call if questions arise.

- *Warning signs*
  - —Review the postoperative signs and symptoms that should be reported to a physician or nurse.
  - —Inspect the incisional site
    Redness
    Swelling
    Tenderness
    Skin warm to touch
    Purulent drainage
- *Special instructions*
  - —Review any restrictions: avoid enemas until approved by physician; avoid tub baths, showers permitted.
  - —Advise patient on how and where to obtain wound care supplies.
  - —Teach patient how to take care of wound and dressing changes. If appendix is ruptured, irrigation with sterile saline and sterile dressings may be required.
  - —Teach the patient and caregiver to care for drains if the patient is discharged with them.
- *Medications*
  - —Explain the purpose, dosage, schedule, and route of administration of any prescribed drugs, as well as side effects to report to the physician or nurse.
- *Activity*
  - —Instruct the patient to avoid lifting anything over 10 pounds for the first 6 weeks (less time for laparoscopy), to rest when fatigued, and to increase activities as tolerated.
  - —Normal activities can usually be resumed within 4 weeks. Ask the patient to check with the physician or nurse before driving, returning to work, or engaging in recreational sports.

FOLLOW-UP CARE

- Stress the importance of regular follow-up visits. Make sure the patient has the necessary names and telephone numbers.

Arterial Insufficiency

—Arterial insufficiency: impaired arterial blood flow. Arterial insufficiency can occur in any part of the arterial system but generally affects the lower extremities (legs and feet). There are two forms: acute and chronic. *Acute arterial insufficiency* is a sudden decrease in arterial blood supply to an area, resulting in thrombus (clot), embolism, and trauma. *Chronic arterial insufficiency* is most commonly caused by arteriosclerosis (calcification of the arteries resulting from progressive narrowing, thickening, and loss of vessel elasticity) or atherosclerosis (gradual accumulation of plaque resulting from hardening of the arteries that occurs with age).

CONTRIBUTING FACTORS
- Atherosclerotic plaque
- Thrombus (blood clots)
- Aneurysms
- Trauma or fracture
- Embolism

RISK FACTORS
- Familial tendency
- Diabetes
- Elevated cholesterol levels
- Diet high in animal fats
- Hypertension
- Sedentary lifestyle
- Tobacco use
- Age older than 50 years
- Male sex
- Myocardial infarction
- Atrial fibrillation

SIGNS/SYMPTOMS
- Acute ("six P's")
  —Paresthesias
  —Pain: sudden severe
  —Paralysis, numbness

—Pallor: pale yellow skin color
—Pulselessness (absence of pulse)
—Poikilothermy

- Chronic
  —Intermittent claudication: severe cramps or burning sensation in calf (leg) muscle, buttock, or thigh that occurs with exercise and is relieved by rest; symptoms are constant and reproducible
  —Sores and cuts that are slow to heal
  —Discoloration and decreased sensation of the affected extremities
  —Thickened nails
  —Shiny skin
  —Decreased temperature
  —Absence of pulse

COMPLICATIONS

- Leg ulcers
- Gangrene
- Thrombosis
- Limb amputation
- Neurologic deficit

DIAGNOSTIC TESTS

- Describe each procedure, its purpose, and the normal feelings or sensations that are likely, as well as any preprocedural and postprocedural care.
  —Doppler ultrasound: identifies abnormal blood flow patterns proximal to occlusion
  —Plethysmography: records decrease in blood flow distal to occlusion
  —Echocardiography: determines whether an embolus from the heart is the source of obstruction
  —Arteriography: determines the location, type, and degree of obstruction; can be used to evaluate degree of collateral circulation
  —Duplex imaging: using ultrasound to assess arteries for plaque formation; measures flow and pressure
  —Digital subtraction angiography: visualizes arteries radiologically to determine presence and extent of occlusion

—Exercise testing: to determine the level of exercise that precipitates the symptoms of lack of blood flow

—Oscillometry: using a blood pressure cuff connected to a manometer to find occlusive sites, as evidenced by decreased pressure readings

—Ankle-brachial index: to assess blood flow to lower extremity and to measure ratio of ankle to brachial systolic blood pressure

TREATMENT
Chronic Obstruction
Medical

- Therapy
  —Risk-reduction program: control of blood pressure, elimination of smoking, weight reduction, lowering of cholesterol and lipids
  —Program of daily walking
- Drugs
  —Antiplatelet therapy (dipyridamole and aspirin): to prevent arterial occlusion
  —Pentoxifylline (Trental): to improve blood flow through capillaries; used to increase the distance patients with claudication can walk
  —Aspirin: to relieve pain and prevent thromboembolism
  —Calcium channel blockers: to reduce vasospasm
  —Thrombolytic agents (urokinase, streptokinase, alteplase): to dissolve clots and relieve obstruction caused by thrombus
  —Vitamins E and C: to defend against vascular injury

Surgical

- Amputation: surgical removal of limb if gangrene, uncontrollable infection, or intractable pain develops
- Atherectomy: shaving and removal of plaque from an artery by special catheters

Acute Obstruction
Medical

- Therapy
  —Percutaneous transluminal angioplasty: compression of the obstruction using balloon inflation catheter

—Laser angioplasty: use of a hot-tip laser to vaporize (dissolve) the obstruction
—Stents: insertion of a mesh wire that will stretch and mold to the arterial wall to prevent occlusion
- Drugs
  —Heparin
  —Intra-arterial infusion of fibrinolytic agents (for thrombus)

Surgical

- Embolectomy: to remove clot from affected artery
- Thromboembolectomy: surgical opening of the artery to remove the athetotic plaque or thrombus
- Patch grafting: removal of the affected arterial segment with an autologous vein (e.g., saphenous vein) or with a Dacron graft
- Bypass graft: use of an autologous vein (e.g., saphenous vein) or a Dacron graft to bypass the affected arterial segment
- Lumbar sympathectomy

HOME CARE

- Give both patient and caregiver *verbal* and *written* instructions. Provide them with the name and telephone number of a physician or nurse to call if questions arise.
- *General information*
  —Discuss the arteriosclerotic and atherosclerotic process and its roles in producing arterial occlusive disease. Review causes and contributing factors. Show the patient the location of the suspected obstruction and describe collateral circulation. Explain intermittent claudication and how it develops.
  —Teach the patient how to inspect the affected limb for color, warmth, and presence of pulses.
- *Warning signs*
  —Review the signs and symptoms that should be reported to a physician or nurse.
- *Special instructions*
  —Discuss skin care.
  —Inspect the skin daily for redness, blistering, or cuts that are not healing.
  —Use mild, unperfumed lotions for dry skin.
  —Do not use heating pads or hot water bottles, which could burn the patient.

—Avoid restrictive clothing that could interfere with circulation to the affected areas.

—Keep the skin warm and dry. Do not expose the skin to cold. Avoid temperature extremes. Suggest wearing warm, loose-fitting socks at night.

—Avoid applying adhesive tape directly to the skin.

—Demonstrate proper care of skin ulcerations; advise on how and where to obtain necessary supplies.

—Discuss foot care.

Inspect feet and toes daily for cuts, bruises, calluses, and corns.

Wash with mild soap and warm water, rinse well, and pat dry. Check water temperature to avoid burns. Dry feet well, especially between toes.

Apply mild, nonperfumed lotion for dry skin. Permit foot to dry completely before putting shoes and socks on.

Cut toenails straight using clippers. If nails become thick or brittle, refer to a podiatrist; instruct patient not to cut corns or calluses, but to rub gently or see a podiatrist.

Protect feet from injury: use a night light to avoid hitting toes or shins; never go barefoot; wear cotton socks and comfortable, proper-fitting shoes.

—Offer techniques for dealing with chronic pain, such as visualization, guided imagery, meditation, and biofeedback.

• *Medications*

—Explain the purpose, dosage, schedule, and route of administration of any prescribed drugs, as well as side effects to report to the physician or nurse.

• *Activity*

—Discuss a planned exercise program.

Explain the importance of daily exercises to prevent further occlusion and to promote development of collateral circulation.

Review the types of exercises permitted: walking, swimming, bicycling.

Explain that progressive exercise can reduce the severity of claudication and increase the distance that the patient may walk. For example, the patient may begin by walking until claudication occurs, then stop and rest, then begin again when pain stops. Distance can be increased gradually.

Emphasize that for any type of exercise or activity, the patient should stop when pain occurs, rest, and resume activity when pain subsides.

—Instruct the patient to avoid vigorous exercise of the affected limb, since this can increase oxygen demand and increase pain.

—Instruct the patient on techniques that can increase circulation to the lower extremities, such as sleeping in an upright position and dangling the lower extremities over the side of the bed to relieve persistent leg pain.

—Advise the patient that if pain occurs at night, use blocks to raise the head of the bed 6 to 10 inches.

—Instruct the patient to avoid sitting or standing for prolonged periods, to keep legs elevated while sitting, and to avoid crossing the knees.

—Instruct the patient to notify the physician for prolonged pain, tingling or numbness, or inability to move the foot.

• *Diet*

—Stress the importance of developing a lifestyle that will decrease the risk of advancing the disease process: weight control, diet low in fats and cholesterol.

FOLLOW-UP CARE AND REFERRALS

• Stress the importance of regular follow-up visits. Make sure the patient has the necessary names and telephone numbers.

• Stress the importance of not smoking. Provide information on and referral to smoking cessation programs as necessary; provide literature and discuss nicotine's effect on circulation.

Arterial Revascularization

—Arterial revascularization: surgical procedure that increases arterial blood flow by bypassing a stenosed or occluded artery. Grafting material for bypass surgeries may be constructed from an autologous vein (e.g., saphenous vein) or a synthetic graft (Dacron).

TYPES OF BYPASS PROCEDURE

- Aortofemoral bypass graft: graft runs from the abdominal aorta to the external iliac or femoral arteries, increasing arterial blood flow to the lower extremities
- Aortoiliac bypass graft: graft runs from the abdominal aorta down to the iliac or femoral artery(ies)
- Axillofemoral bypass: graft runs from the axillary artery down alongside the artery in a tunnel created under the skin to the femoral artery(ies)
- Femoropopliteal bypass
- Femorotibial bypass

INDICATIONS

- Arterial insufficiency
  —Acute
    Embolism
    Thrombosis
    Trauma
  —Chronic
    Arteriosclerosis obliterans
    Arterial insufficiency
    Buerger's disease

PREPROCEDURAL TEACHING

- Review the physician's explanation of the procedure and the reason for it; encourage the patient to ask questions and to discuss fears or anxieties.

Review of Preprocedural Care

- Discuss the number of incisions that will be performed (e.g., for aortofemoral bypass there may be two or three incisions: one midline abdominal and one groin site for each femoral graft done) and the type of anesthesia to be used.
- Instruct the patient to discontinue any anticoagulant or antiplatelet medications 1 week before surgery; ask the patient to check with the physician or nurse about any other medications, including cardiac, birth control, and hormone drugs.

Review of Postprocedural Care

- Axillofemoral bypass
  —Instruct the patient not to lie on the same side as the graft, since this could cause graft occlusion, and to avoid reaching

high overhead or lifting anything heavy, which could dislodge the graft from the donor site.

—Discuss and demonstrate passive range-of-motion exercises to the affected limb.

• Femoral-popliteal-tibial grafts

—Explain that the patient may have an indwelling catheter and that surgery will be done under general anesthesia.

—Inform the patient that walking will be permitted 1 to 3 days after surgery, that ambulation will progress gradually, and that a cane or walker may be required for a few days.

—Discuss the importance of not bending the knee and hip of the affected limb and of not sitting or standing for prolonged periods, which could lead to graft occlusion.

—Inform the patient that a heat cradle may be used to avoid pressure on the affected limb.

• Review postoperative medications.

—Anticoagulants or aspirin: to keep graft open

—Antibiotics: to prevent infection

—Vasodilators: to promote circulation to the lower extremities

COMPLICATIONS

• Hematoma
• Graft thrombosis
• Infection of the entire graft
• Embolization to kidneys and bowel
  —Renal failure
  —Bowel ischemia

HOME CARE

• Give both the patient and the caregiver *verbal* and *written* instructions. Provide them with the name and telephone number of a physician or nurse to call if questions arise.

• *Warning signs*

—Review the signs and symptoms that should be reported to a physician or nurse.

  Infection: fever; incision sites that drain, are warm or hot to touch, or become red or more painful

  Thrombosis: pain in the surgical area or legs when the patient is at rest; abdominal bloating or tenderness

  Intermittent claudication: muscle cramping or burning that occurs with exercise and is relieved by rest

- *Special instructions*
  —Teach the patient to use antiembolic stockings, if prescribed.
  —For axillofemoral bypass graft: instruct the patient to avoid forceful use of the affected side, not to wear tight or restrictive garments (belt, suspenders) over graft site, to check graft pulse and notify physician or nurse if pulse is not felt.
- *Medications*
  —Explain the purpose, dosage, schedule, and route of administration of any prescribed drugs, as well as side effects to report to the physician or nurse.
- *Activity*
  —During the 6- to 8-week healing period:
  The patient should avoid sitting for prolonged periods, keep legs elevated while sitting, avoid crossing knees, and avoid vacuuming, lawn mowing, or lifting >25 pounds.
  The patient should walk every day, in a progressive program that begins slowly and increases in distance as directed.
  Rest periods should be scheduled during the day.
  —Long-term: To preserve the benefits of the surgery, the patient should follow habits that improve circulation and prevent further acceleration of atherosclerosis: careful diabetic control, control of blood pressure, regular exercise to promote circulation, avoidance of prolonged squatting.
- *Diet*
  —The patient should eat a balanced low-fat diet that includes protein to help tissues heal and fruits and vegetables to prevent constipation.
  —Alcohol use should be limited or avoided completely if the patient is taking medications that enhance its effects.

PSYCHOSOCIAL CARE

- Discuss the effects of stress on circulation. Review stress reduction (e.g., by relaxation, exercise).

FOLLOW-UP CARE AND REFERRALS

- Stress the importance of regular follow-up visits. Make sure the patient has the necessary names and telephone numbers.
- Emphasize the importance of not smoking. Refer the patient to smoking cessation programs, if necessary. Provide literature on smoking and discuss the effect nicotine has on circulation.

Arthritis

—**Rheumatoid arthritis (RA):** a chronic, systemic, autoimmune disease of unknown origin affecting primarily the synovial joints. RA is characterized by remissions and exacerbations of inflammation of the connective tissues throughout the body, leading eventually to destruction of joint cartilage and subsequent deformities. The most commonly affected joints are the hands, wrists, shoulders, elbows, feet, ankles, hips, and knees. Susceptibility is genetically determined. RA is a common condition with a prevalence of 1% to 2% in the general population. Females outnumber males 3:1. RA usually develops between 25 and 55 years of age, although juvenile RA or Sill's disease develops between 8 and 15 years of age.

—**Osteoarthritis (degenerative joint disease):** a chronic, progressive disease characterized by increasing pain, deformity, and loss of function caused by degenerative changes in the cartilage covering the ends of bones, primarily in the major weight-bearing joints: hip, knee, and spinal column. The joints of the fingers, elbows, wrists, and ankles are affected to a lesser degree. Osteoarthritis is a disease of older persons, affecting nearly everyone over 75 years of age. Women are affected more often than men, and the incidence increases after menopause. More than 50 million Americans have osteoarthritis.

CONTRIBUTING FACTORS
- For osteoarthritis (secondary osteoarthritis)
  —Obesity
  —Overuse of joints
  —Trauma

SIGNS/SYMPTOMS
- General
  —Joint involvement
    Stiffness (especially early morning)
    Pain (worsens with activity and is relieved by rest)

A

Swelling and deformity
Instability and impaired function
Decreased range of motion
Bony enlargements in affected joints
- Rheumatoid arthritis
  —Local warmth, redness
  —Anemia
  —Malaise, weight loss, fever
  —Red, blue, or white color of fingers and toes
  —Multiple joint involvement
  —Subcutaneous rheumatoid nodules over bony prominences (hands, elbows, knees)
  —Shiny, taut skin over impaired joint
  —Numbness, tingling in hands and feet

COMPLICATIONS

- General
  —Avascular necrosis of hip joint
  —Contractures
  —Loss of range of motion of joints (ankylosing of joints)
  —Muscle wasting
  —Loss of sensation and decreased mobility
- Rheumatoid arthritis
  —Cardiac degenerative conditions: cardiomyopathy, congestive heart failure, pericarditis
  —Chronic renal failure
  —Chronic obstructive pulmonary disease
  —Septic arthritis
  —Tenosynovitis
  —Pneumonitis
  —Fibrosis
  —Ankylosis of joints

DIAGNOSTIC TESTS

- Describe each procedure, its purpose, and the normal feelings or sensations that are likely, as well as any preprocedural and postprocedural care.
  —Laboratory tests
     Complete blood cell count
     White blood cell count
     Erythrocyte sedimentation rate

Synovial fluid analysis and tissue biopsy
For RA:
○ Antistreptolysin O (ASO) titer
○ Rheumatoid factor: positive in RA
○ C-reactive protein: present in acute episode of RA
○ γ-Globulins, immunoglobulin (Ig) M, IgG
○ Serum complement: decreased in acute episodes of RA
—Radiologic studies: to confirm diagnosis by showing narrowing of joint spaces
—Magnetic resonance imaging/computed tomography: to show changes before x-ray studies detect them
—Gait analysis: to show leg length discrepancy
—Muscle testing: to detect weakness of muscles supporting joints
—Bone scan

TREATMENT
Medical

• Therapy
—Physical therapy
Paraffin glow: to provide heat to affected small joints (hands and feet)
Whirlpool
Thermotherapy: moist heat, application of cold or heat to relieve pain and improve joint flexibility
Joint exercise: passive and active range-of-motion exercises to strengthen the muscles and tissues supporting the joint and to maintain as much joint mobility as possible
—Orthotics: splints, braces, etc. to maintain proper joint position and support and to rest the joint
—Use of ambulatory adjuncts: crutches, cane, walker, wheelchair, etc. to protect joints from stress
—Assistive devices
Stocking helpers
Builtup eating utensils
Pick-up sticks
Raised toilet seats
—Diet: weight reduction
• Drugs
—General
Salicylate medications, usually aspirin

A

Nonsteroidal antiinflammatory agents (NSAIDs)
Tranquilizers, antidepressants
Analgesics
Muscle relaxants
Intraarticular steroid injections
—Rheumatoid arthritis
Antirheumatic agents
Corticosteroids
Immunosuppressive agents
Antimalarials

Surgical

- Synovectomy: removal of the inflamed synovium
- Arthroplasty: repair of weakened joint
- Osteotomy: to correct bony malalignments
- Implant arthroplasty: repair of joint with prosthesis to increase functional capability
- Arthroscopy: for diagnosis and treatment (removal of foreign bodies, redundant tissue, and cartilage abraded through arthroscope)
- Arthrodesis: joint fusion to produce stability and reduce pain in severely affected joints
- Total joint replacement: see Hip Replacement (p. 356), Replacement of Knee or Shoulder (p. 547)
- Carpal tunnel release, tarsal tunnel release, ganglionectomy, tendon repair, and removal of Baker's cyst: to correct concurrent connective tissue defects

HOME CARE

- Give both the patient and the caregiver *verbal* and *written* instructions. Provide them with the name and telephone number of a physician or nurse to call if questions arise.
- *General information*
  —Explain and discuss type of arthritis, contributing factors, and signs and symptoms associated with the disease process. Discuss the progressive nature of the disease, explaining that the effects of arthritis can change daily and that the patient will have good and bad days. Discuss the importance of maintaining the prescribed medication and activity program to slow disease progression.

- *Warning signs*
  —Review the signs and symptoms that should be reported to a physician or nurse.

    Exacerbation ("flare-up") of symptoms
    Increased, uncontrolled pain
    Redness
    Swelling
    Inability to move joint
    Fatigue

- *Special instructions*
  —Discuss the importance of maintaining a safe home environment.

    Removal of small rugs
    Handrails in shower, tub, or toilet
    Raised toilet seat
    Rubber-tipped walker, cane, crutches
    Raised chair
    Wheelchair in locked position when stationary
    Wearing of well-fitting, sturdy shoes

  —Discuss pain management: applying heat or cold to a painful joint for temporary relief; avoiding temperature extremes, since decreased sensitivity to temperature can result in injury; maintaining proper body alignment to reduce pain.

    Extend joints as tolerated.
    Avoid external rotation of extremities.
    Avoid use of pillow under knee.
    Avoid flexion of neck.
    Avoid sitting for extended periods.

- *Medications*
  —Explain the purpose, dosage, schedule, and route of administration of any prescribed drugs, as well as side effects to report to the physician or nurse.

    Aspirin, NSAIDs: nausea, vomiting, gastrointestinal burning, blood in stool or sputum, headache, bleeding gums, ringing in ears

- *Activity*
  —Discuss the importance of alternating activities with rest periods and of getting 8 to 10 hours of sleep at night.
  —Emphasize that the patient should maintain a regular exercise program that includes such activities as walking and swimming to provide stretching and joint mobility. Daily

exercise can relieve soreness caused by stiff, unused muscles and helps maintain joint range of motion.

—Discuss the importance of coordinating pain medication with activities.

—Reinforce the need for range-of-motion exercises to prevent stiffening of joints and to avoid overworking that can cause stress to joints.

—Discuss the importance of using splints and braces to support affected joints.

—Explain the use of ambulatory aids such as crutches or a cane to lessen joint stress. Assist the patient in obtaining such equipment.

—Discuss the importance of physical therapy exercises to maintain strength and function.

—Encourage the patient to discuss allowances and limitations with respect to occupation, recreational sports, and activities.

—Remind the patient to dress warmly and wear gloves in cold, damp weather.

• *Diet*

—Encourage the intake of iron-rich foods (dried fruits, green vegetables) to combat anemia.

—Stress the importance of a well-balanced diet.

—Instruct the patient to reduce caloric and fat intake for weight reduction because increased weight or obesity increases joint stress.

PSYCHOSOCIAL CARE

• Discuss the role that emotions such as stress and depression play in disease progression. Encourage participation in support groups as needed; provide phone numbers for referral.

FOLLOW-UP CARE

• Stress the importance of regular follow-up visits: medical, laboratory examinations, and physical therapy. Make sure the patient has the necessary names and telephone numbers.

REFERRALS

• Advise the patient on community resources and encourage participation in support programs such as the Arthritis Foundation.

• Provide referrals for home health care and social service as indicated.

Arthroscopy

—Arthroscopy: the examination of joint tissues with a fiberoptic endoscope (arthroscope) or laser athroscopy, which allows direct visualization of the interior of a joint. Arthroscopy can be performed on any joint (wrist, elbow, shoulder, ankle, hip), but it is most frequently done for the diagnosis and treatment of knee injuries.

—Diagnostic arthropathy: reveals the condition of internal joint tissues, the existence of loose bodies, the presence of tears in cartilage or ligaments, or the condition of synovial tissues.

—Therapeutic, surgical arthropathy: removal (excision), repair, or reconstruction of loose bodies and torn cartilage; biopsy of tissues through an arthroscope.

INDICATIONS
- Meniscus injuries: removal or repair of meniscus
- Ligament tears: reconstruction
- Damage to cartilage: removal or shaving of rough cartilage
- Patella injury: realignment or shaving

PREPROCEDURAL TEACHING
- Review the physician's explanation of the procedure and the reason for it; encourage the patient to ask questions and to discuss any fears or anxieties.
- Explain that the procedure may take anywhere from ½ hour to several hours.
- Discuss the need for written consent for surgery and anesthesia.
- Explain that hospital admission may be on the day of surgery but that an overnight hospital stay may be necessary.

Review of Preprocedural Care
- The patient is NPO from midnight of the night before surgery.
- Skin preparation includes a shower with bactericidal soap and shaving of the incision site.
- Routine preoperative blood and urine tests will be conducted.
- Describe the procedure.

—Depending on the joint, the procedure will be done under local anesthesia, regional block, or general anesthesia.

—Tell the patient that the scope may be inserted in more than one area to visualize all areas of the joint and that two or three incisions (portals) may be needed.

Review of Postprocedural Care

• If surgery is done on an outpatient basis, the patient is discharged in the evening.

• The joint will be elevated with a compression dressing and ice bags to lessen swelling and pain.

• Vital signs are checked every 15 minutes for the first hour, then with decreasing frequency.

• Neurovascular status is checked every hour for 24 hours.

• Bed rest is needed until the patient is fully alert; then the patient can be up with crutches as tolerated.

• Moving the extremities is important to improve circulation and keep the joint mobile (e.g., move the feet after knee arthroscopy).

• After knee arthroscopy the patient will need external knee support by an elastic wrap or a knee immobilizer. Crutches may be ordered.

SIDE EFFECTS/COMPLICATIONS

• Infection
• Bleeding/hemorrhage
• Phlebitis/thrombus formation
• Posttraumatic degeneration and arthritis
• Instrument breakage in joint
• Effects of anesthesia

HOME CARE

• Give both the patient and the caregiver *verbal* and *written* instructions. Provide them with the name and telephone number of a physician or nurse to call if questions arise.

• *Wound/incision care*

—Keep the dressing clean and dry.

—Serosanguineous drainage should be scant; report any increase in drainage or signs of new bleeding to the physician or nurse.

—Do not remove the dressing until directed by the physician.

—Avoid bathing until able to stand for 10 to 15 minutes; then showering with the extremity covered by a plastic bag may be permitted. Check with the physician or nurse before resuming showers.

- *Warning signs*
  —Review the signs and symptoms that should be reported to a physician or nurse.
    Excess bleeding
    Infection: persistent or worsening pain, swelling, discoloration of skin at incision site, fever, joint immobility, purulent discharge
    Neurovascular impairment of joint and extremity: fingers and toes cold and discolored; increasing pain with joint movement; numbness or tingling of extremity (stress the importance of reporting these symptoms immediately)
    Phlebitis: swollen, painful, reddened, warm extremity

- *Special instructions*
  —Discuss the importance of keeping the extremity elevated above heart level on firm pillows and the need for applying ice bags to the surgical site to control swelling and relieve pain. Caution the patient not to apply the ice pack directly to the skin, but to wrap the ice bag in a small towel. The use of hot tubs, whirlpool baths, and heating pads should be avoided.
  —Discuss the importance of moving the extremities (fingers, toes, feet) to improve circulation and prevent blood clots. For example, after knee arthroscopy the patient should wiggle the toes every few minutes for the first week.

- *Medications*
  —Explain the purpose, dosage, schedule, and route of administration of any prescribed drugs, as well as side effects to report to a physician or nurse.

- *Activity*
  —The patient may ambulate as tolerated with an assistive device. Refer to physical therapy as indicated.
  —Following knee arthroscopy, instruct the patient in the proper use of crutches. Review physical therapy exercises needed for a gradual increase in strength and mobility.
  —Encourage the patient to discuss allowances and limitations with respect to occupation and resumption of recreational sports and activities.

- *Diet*
  —Encourage a light diet and fluids, progressing to a regular diet as ordered.

FOLLOW-UP CARE

- Stress the importance of regular follow-up visits. Make sure the patient has the necessary names and telephone numbers.

Asthma

—Asthma: a chronic respiratory disorder characterized by episodes of sudden, acute attacks of dyspnea, wheezing caused by airway narrowing (bronchospasm), and mucosal swelling that leads to mucus production. An attack may last minutes to hours and may resolve spontaneously or in response to medication and treatment. Although the exact cause is unknown, obstruction of the airways may occur as a result of spasms of the bronchial muscles caused by an irritant or inflammation of the airways, which causes swelling of the mucous membranes and overproduction of mucus.

CONTRIBUTING FACTORS

Bronchial irritants that can trigger asthmatic attacks include:
- Environmental allergens
  —Foods: shellfish, eggs, nuts, chocolate
  —Pollens: trees, flowers and ragweed, spores
  —Feathers: pillows, down comforters, wool
  —Animal dander: dogs, cats, rabbits, chickens
  —Dust: from carpets, brooms, dusters, dirty filters on furnaces and air conditioners
  —Household products: polishes, cleaning solvents, paint thinners, paint, room deodorizers
  —Weather and temperature: air pollution, extreme heat or cold, seasonal changes, excessive humidity or dryness
  —Industrial pollutants: wood vapors or smoke from fireplaces, dust, or fumes; metals; cotton
  —Other: powders, perfumes, tobacco smoking (cigarettes, cigars, pipes), hairspray, mold

- Intrinsic factors
  - —Respiratory infections: cold, flu, viruses
  - —Fatigue, overexertion
  - —Emotions: anxiety, stress

SIGNS/SYMPTOMS

- Wheezing
- Prolonged expiration
- Dyspnea; feeling of not being able to catch one's breath
- Physical exhaustion
- Anxiety, irritability, and restlessness
- Thick, tenacious mucus
- Tachypnea
- Labored respirations
- Chest tightness
- Cough

COMPLICATIONS

- Status asthmaticus
- Pneumonia
- Respiratory arrest

DIAGNOSTIC TESTS

- Describe each procedure, its purpose, and the normal feelings or sensations that are likely, as well as any preprocedural and postprocedural care.
  - —Serum studies: white blood cell count to identify infections, arterial blood gases to determine oxygen content of blood and evaluate acid-base status (elimination of carbon dioxide); blood drawn for theophylline until therapeutic levels (10 to 20 μg/ml) are achieved
  - —Sputum studies: to evaluate increase in viscosity or presence of mucus plugs; culture and sensitivity to detect infection
  - —Pulmonary function: to evaluate degree of obstruction and narrowing of the airways
  - —Chest x-ray

TREATMENT
Medical

- Therapy
  - —Oxygen therapy

of adminis-
e effects to

dose when

er allergy

lerance
during

ues to

mall
y of

he

maintain adequate dehydration

haled beta-2-agonists and anticho-
bronchospasm
mmatory response
x smooth muscle
ion

process. Give both the patient and the
d *written* instructions. Provide them with the
he number of a physician or nurse to call if
Jse visual aids to assist in instruction.

ation

tient identify irritants that trigger an asthmatic
discuss the importance of avoiding them or
them from the patient's environment. Advise
a diary of activities, foods, or irritants present before

n that devices that filter particles from the air may be
l in reducing asthma attacks.

ng signs

view the signs and symptoms that should be reported to a
hysician or nurse.

ecial instructions

—Review the purpose and demonstrate proper use of oral
inhaler, home nebulizer, humidifier, peak flow meter, home
oxygen, or incentive spirometer as ordered.

—Discuss the importance of avoiding smoking or being in a
smoke-filled room. Refer the patient to smoking cessation
programs as needed.

—Discuss the importance of emotions and their role in
triggering attacks. Review the need to learn to modify or deal
with stressful events using deep muscle relaxation techniques
or pursed-lip breathing techniques to prevent an attack.

—Discuss the importance of preventing respiratory infections;
avoid persons with infections and check with the physician
about annual flu and pneumococcal vaccinations.

- *Medications*
  —Explain the purpose, dosage, schedule, and rout[e of adminis]
  tration of any prescribed drugs, as well as sid[e effects to]
  report to the physician or nurse.
  —Warn against stopping or decreasing medication[s when]
  feeling better without checking with physician.
  —Discuss the importance of not using over-the-coun[ter]
  drugs when taking prescribed drugs.
- *Activity*
  —Emphasize the importance of regular exercise to t[olerance]
  and of avoiding or curtailing activities when fatigued[, during]
  extremes of weather, and on smoggy days.
  —Instruct patient on the use of adaptive breathing techni[ques to]
  prolong expiratory time.
- *Diet*
  —Instruct the patient to maintain a well-balanced diet, eat s[mall,]
  frequent meals during and after attacks, and drink plent[y of]
  fluids (2 to 3 liters per day) to keep mucus thin.

FOLLOW-UP CARE

- Stress the importance of regular follow-up visits. Make sure t[he]
  patient has the necessary names and telephone numbers.
- Encourage or assist patient to obtain a MedicAlert bracele[t]
  listing diagnosis and medications.
- Stress the need for follow-up if patient was seen in the
  emergency room or hospitalized after an exacerbation.

REFERRALS

- Refer the patient to the American Lung Association for a
  support group and further information.
- Assist the patient to identify community-based resources and
  emergency numbers.
- Provide referrals for home care services, supplies, and
  equipment as indicated.

A

—Nebulizer
—Nutritious, well-balanced diet
—Oral or parenteral fluids to maintain adequate dehydration
• Drugs
—Bronchodilators such as inhaled beta-2-agonists and anticho-linergic agents: to relieve bronchospasm
—Steroids: to relieve inflammatory response
—Aminophylline: to relax smooth muscle
—Antibiotics: for infection

🏠 HOME CARE

• Review the disease process. Give both the patient and the caregiver *verbal* and *written* instructions. Provide them with the name and telephone number of a physician or nurse to call if questions arise. Use visual aids to assist in instruction.
• *General information*
—Help the patient identify irritants that trigger an asthmatic attack and discuss the importance of avoiding them or removing them from the patient's environment. Advise keeping a diary of activities, foods, or irritants present before attacks.
—Explain that devices that filter particles from the air may be useful in reducing asthma attacks.
• *Warning signs*
—Review the signs and symptoms that should be reported to a physician or nurse.
• *Special instructions*
—Review the purpose and demonstrate proper use of oral inhaler, home nebulizer, humidifier, peak flow meter, home oxygen, or incentive spirometer as ordered.
—Discuss the importance of avoiding smoking or being in a smoke-filled room. Refer the patient to smoking cessation programs as needed.
—Discuss the importance of emotions and their role in triggering attacks. Review the need to learn to modify or deal with stressful events using deep muscle relaxation techniques or pursed-lip breathing techniques to prevent an attack.
—Discuss the importance of preventing respiratory infections; avoid persons with infections and check with the physician about annual flu and pneumococcal vaccinations.

- *Medications*
  - —Explain the purpose, dosage, schedule, and route of administration of any prescribed drugs, as well as side effects to report to the physician or nurse.
  - —Warn against stopping or decreasing medication dose when feeling better without checking with physician.
  - —Discuss the importance of not using over-the-counter allergy drugs when taking prescribed drugs.
- *Activity*
  - —Emphasize the importance of regular exercise to tolerance and of avoiding or curtailing activities when fatigued, during extremes of weather, and on smoggy days.
  - —Instruct patient on the use of adaptive breathing techniques to prolong expiratory time.
- *Diet*
  - —Instruct the patient to maintain a well-balanced diet, eat small frequent meals during and after attacks, and drink plenty of fluids (2 to 3 liters per day) to keep mucus thin.

FOLLOW-UP CARE

- Stress the importance of regular follow-up visits. Make sure the patient has the necessary names and telephone numbers.
- Encourage or assist patient to obtain a MedicAlert bracelet listing diagnosis and medications.
- Stress the need for follow-up if patient was seen in the emergency room or hospitalized after an exacerbation.

REFERRALS

- Refer the patient to the American Lung Association for a support group and further information.
- Assist the patient to identify community-based resources and emergency numbers.
- Provide referrals for home care services, supplies, and equipment as indicated.

Atelectasis

—Atelectasis: collapse of alveoli or airless condition of lung.

CAUSES/CONTRIBUTING FACTORS

- Mucus plugs
- Excessive secretions
- Compression of lung tissue by tumors, effusions, pneumothorax, or shallow breathing
- Anesthesia, sedation, and decreased mobility related to major abdominal or thoracic surgery

SIGNS/SYMPTOMS

- Elevated temperature
- Labored breathing
- Shortness of breath
- Nasal flaring
- Tachypnea
- Anxiety
- Restlessness
- Tachycardia
- Absent or decreased breath sounds over affected area

COMPLICATIONS

- Pneumonia
- Pneumothorax

DIAGNOSTIC TESTS

- Describe each procedure, its purpose, and the normal feelings or sensations that are likely, as well as any preprocedural and postprocedural care.
    - Chest x-ray: to define collapsed areas of the lung
    - Arterial blood gases: to detect hypoxia
    - Bronchoscopy: insertion of a fiberoptic scope into the airways for direct visualization and possible obtaining of specimens

TREATMENT
Medical

- Therapy
  —Oxygen therapy
  —Chest physiotherapy
  —Intermittent positive-pressure breathing (IPPB)/incentive spirometry
  —Bronchoscopy
  —Bronchodilators
  —Early ambulation

Surgical

- Excision of tumor

 HOME CARE

- Give both the patient and the caregiver *verbal* and *written* instructions. Provide them with the name and telephone number of a physician or nurse to call if questions arise.
- *General information*
  —Explain the underlying cause or contributing factors.
- *Warning signs*
  —Review the signs and symptoms that should be reported to a physician or nurse.
    Upper respiratory infection
    Flu
    Difficulty breathing
    Persistent cough
    Elevated temperature
- *Special instructions*
  —Discuss the importance of preventing respiratory infections by avoiding persons with infections.
  —Demonstrate the use of an incentive spirometer and discuss how frequently to use it.
  —Instruct the patient in coughing and deep breathing techniques. Demonstrate how to splint the chest when coughing.
- *Medications*
  —Explain the purpose, dosage, schedule, and route of administration of any prescribed drugs, as well as side effects to report to the physician or nurse.
    Explain the need to avoid taking over-the-counter medications without checking with a physician.

Caution the patient to avoid the use of respiratory depressants.

B

- *Activity*
  —Emphasize the importance of exercising to tolerance. Stress the need to avoid fatigue and to plan rest periods.
  —Explain the need for early and frequent ambulation.
- *Diet*
  —Instruct the patient to maintain a regular diet. Encourage the intake of fluids unless contraindicated by underlying condition.

FOLLOW-UP CARE

- Stress the importance of regular follow-up visits. Make sure the patient has the necessary names and telephone numbers.
- Stress the importance of not smoking or using tobacco products. Tobacco smoking increases the risk of respiratory infection because of cumulative damage to lung structures. Provide information about smoking cessation programs and offer a referral.

Back Pain

—Back pain: one of the most common health problems in the United States, affecting people of all ages and from all walks of life, from heavy laborers to those who lead sedentary lives. Persons with back pain may be in good health or have significant disease. The majority of back injuries occur in the lumbar (L) and lumbosacral spine, a portion of the spinal column that provides the flexibility necessary for movement and thus is especially vulnerable to strain and injury. The most commonly affected areas are the cervical spine (neck), C5-6 and C6-7, in which osteophyte formation causes nerve compression. Low back pain (LBP) is caused by a herniated nucleus pulposus, also known as a slipped disk or a herniated disk.

CAUSES/CONTRIBUTING FACTORS

- Ligament strain and fatigue
- Muscle strain or spasm
- Disk injury/trauma
- Disease: arthritis, ruptured disk, osteoporosis, congenital deformities
- Intervertebral degeneration (in elderly)
- Poor posture: slouching, swayback
- Lack of exercise: weak abdominal and back muscles
- Obesity, especially abdominal obesity
- Infection
- Spinal tumors

SIGNS/SYMPTOMS

- Muscle spasm
- Pain radiating down arm or leg
- Tenderness of back and involved extremity
- Lumbago: painful catches in lower back
- Sciatica: sharp pain in back of leg and buttocks
- Soreness, stiffness, achiness
- Neck stiffness, headache, dizziness, shoulder and arm pain (with cervical involvement)
- Paresthesia, numbness

COMPLICATIONS

- Paresis
- Motor weakness
- Sensory changes
- Footdrop
- Loss of bowel or bladder control

DIAGNOSTIC TESTS

- Describe each procedure, its purpose, and the normal feelings or sensations that are likely, as well as any preprocedural and postprocedural care.
  —Back x-rays: may show narrowing of intervertebral spaces, loss of curvature of the spine
  —Myelogram: to document level of disk involvement
  —Computed tomography: to identify disk protrusion or evaluate any bone or soft tissue involvement
  —Magnetic resonance imaging: to confirm rupture of disk and identify any disk compression on the spinal column

—Electromyography: to determine level of spinal injury
—Diskogram: to differentiate between disk infection and rupture

TREATMENT
Medical

• Therapy
  —Lower back
      Bed rest on firm mattress in position of comfort during acute pain: side-lying or recumbent position with pillow under knees
      Ice massage to lumbosacral area; hydrotherapy
      Back support or brace
      Exercise regimen to strengthen back and abdominal muscles (see Back Exercises, p. 97)
      Traction: skin traction with pelvic belt, bilateral Buck's traction, hanging traction
  —Cervical spine
      Head Holter traction
      Skeletal (halo) traction
  —General
      Ultrasound diathermy with back massage
      Heating pad to back to relieve stiffness; use for short intervals only (15 to 30 minutes)
      Transcutaneous electrical nerve stimulation
      Steroid injections: trigger point, epidural, selective nerve blocks
• Drugs
  —Analgesic-antipyretic agents
  —Muscle relaxants
  —Nonsteroidal antiinflammatory agents
  —Narcotic analgesics for severe pain uncontrolled by the above medications
  —Corticosteroids to reduce edema
  —Laxatives/stool softeners to prevent constipation or straining that can aggravate pain
  —Antianxiety agents

Surgical

• Surgery is considered only after conservative management has failed to relieve symptoms or if there are signs of spinal cord compression such as motor or sensory loss or loss of sphincter control.

- Laminectomy
  —Diskectomy: to remove one or more vertebrae
  —Spinal fusion: to stabilize spine
- Microdiskectomy: removal of affected disk using microscopic surgery performed through a 1-inch incision
- Percutaneous lateral diskectomy: removal of disk performed by insertion of metal cannula under fluoroscopy; requires 2 or 3 days in hospital
- Chemonucleolysis: injection of enzymes directly into affected disk to dissolve fibrocartilage causing compression on the spinal cord; rarely done
- Foramenotomy: to open nerve root exit sites
- Intradiskal electrothermal therapy (IDET): metal wire probe placed into disk under fluoroscopy to heat up and shrink bulging disc; outpatient procedure

HOME CARE

- Give both the paient and the caregiver *verbal* and *written* instructions. Provide them with the name and telephone number of a physician or nurse to call if questions arise.
- *General information*
  —Discuss the disorder and contributing factors.
  —Avoid lifting/stooping.
  —Avoid or stop smoking (nicotine decreases diskal circulation).
- *Warning signs*
  —Review the signs and symptoms that should be reported to a physician or nurse.
    Increased sensory loss (numbness, tingling)
    Increased motor loss/weakness (paralysis)
    Loss of bowel and bladder function
- *Medications*
  —Explain the purpose, dosage, schedule, and route of administration of any prescribed drugs, as well as side effects to report to the physician or nurse.
    Nonsteroidal antiiflammatory agents: warn the patient not to take over-the-counter analgesics or muscle relaxants without checking with a physician.

- *Activity*
  —Advise the patient to avoid factors that enhance muscle spasm, such as staying in one position too long, fatigue, chilling, and anxiety.
  —Explain the importance of resting when tired or stressed and of not exercising when in pain.
  —Discuss the importance of maintaining good body mechanics to relieve back strain.

  Standing:

  ○ Explain that standing erect or bent over for long periods increases pressure on the spine and causes the lower back and hips to sag forward. Therefore instruct the patient to stand with hips flexed and with one foot on a stool or a step.
  ○ Women should avoid wearing high heels, which can lead to swayback.

  Sitting: to avoid increasing the sway in the lower back, teach the patient to sit in the correct position:

  ○ Do not slouch.
  ○ Sit in a relaxed position.
  ○ Do not twist in the chair.
  ○ The back of the chair should support the back.
  ○ Place feet firmly on the floor.
  ○ Make sure the chair is firm, not soft.
  ○ Do not sit with head and neck thrust forward.
  ○ When driving, do not sit with the car seat too far back.

  Sleeping: explain that serious strains to the back occur during sleeping. To avoid this strain, advise the patient to:

  ○ Sleep on a firm mattress.
  ○ Place a piece of plywood between the mattress and springs.
  ○ Sleep on the floor if away from home or in a motel where the mattress is too soft.
  ○ Never sleep on the abdomen.

  Lifting, stooping, stretching: straining or injuring the back is common when performing ordinary activities. To minimize the chance of this:

  ○ Never lean forward without bending the knees.
  ○ Always bend the knees when lifting an object.
  ○ Always carry objects close to the body. Never lift anything above the level of the elbows.

○ When reaching or stretching upward, make sure there is a wide base of support and do not twist or rotate the body.

○ Never lie flat on the back with legs and hips stretched straight out.

○ Do not lie on the back with a high pillow under head or neck.

○ Lie on the side with hips and knees bent.

○ Lie on the back with a lift under the legs to relieve swayback.

○ Place an 8- to 10-inch support under the knees to relieve swayback and prevent sleeping on the abdomen.

At rest: maintain a position that will relieve back tension and pain (by straightening the spine):

○ Assume a squatting position.

○ Sit in a chair, lean forward, and lower the head to the knees.

○ Lie with the back flat on the floor and place legs on a chair.

○ Stand upright and place hands in the small of the back; bend forward slowly.

—Encourage general exercise such as daily walks, which provide strengthening and stretching of the back and thigh muscles and help with weight control.

—Remind the patient to wear comfortable, well-cushioned support shoes and to avoid shoes with more than half-inch heels.

• *Diet*

—Advise the patient to maintain a weight appropriate for age, sex, and height. If the patient is overweight, explain that excess body weight aggravates the strain on the spine. Refer the patient to a dietitian for a weight reduction diet.

FOLLOW-UP CARE

• Stress the importance of regular follow-up visits. Make sure the patient has the necessary names and telephone numbers.

B

BACK EXERCISES

Explain that to strengthen the back, the patient must have strong abdominal muscles to support the spinal column. Weak abdominal muscles allow the spinal column to sag forward, causing swayback. This places pressure on the cartilage disks between the vertebrae and on the nerves. Explain that the only way to build strength in the back is through regular exercise.

Stress the importance of obtaining the advice of the physician before beginning any exercise program.

Discuss the importance of doing all exercises slowly, faithfully, and exactly as directed by the physician or physical therapist. Remind the patient that exercises done occasionally will not help at all.

The following exercises should be done by those who have just recovered from a period of severe back pain. Review them with the patient and provide a demonstration.

Knee-to-chest lift (to stretch hip, buttocks, lower back muscles)
- Lie on back on floor with knees bent and feet flat on floor.
- Draw both knees up to chest.
- Place both hands around knees and pull them firmly against chest. Hold for 30 seconds.
- Lower legs and return to starting position.
- Repeat 5 to 10 times.

Simple leg lift
- Lie flat on back on floor with left knee bent and left foot flat on floor.
- Raise right leg as high as comfortably possible.
- Hold for 5 counts.
- Slowly return leg to floor.
- Bend right knee and put right foot flat on floor.
- Raise left leg and hold for 5 counts.
- Repeat 5 to 10 times for each leg.

Continued

BACK EXERCISES—cont'd

Double leg lift
- Lie flat on back.
- Slowly lift legs until feet are 12 inches from the floor.
- Keep legs straight and hold this position for 10 counts.
- Lower legs to floor.
- Repeat 5 times.

Pelvic tilt
- Lie flat on back on floor with knees bent and feet flat on the floor.
- Firmly tighten your buttock muscles.
- Hold for 5 counts.
- Relax buttocks.
- Repeat 5 to 10 times.
- Be sure to keep lower back flat against floor.

Half sit-ups (to strengthen abdominal muscles)
- Lie flat on floor on back with knees bent, feet flat on floor, and hands on chest.
- Slowly raise head and neck to top of chest.
- Reach both hands forward and place them on knees.
- Hold for 5 counts.
- Return to starting position.
- Repeat 5 to 10 times.

Elbow props (to extend lower back)
- Lie face down with your arms beside your body and your head turned to one side.
- Stay in this position for 2 to 5 minutes, making sure that you relax completely.
- Remain face down and prop yourself on your elbows.
- Hold this position for 2 to 3 minutes.
- Return to starting position and relax for 1 minute.
- Repeat 5 to 10 times.

Continued

B

BACK EXERCISES—cont'd

Hip tilts
- Lie flat on back with knees bent.
- Slowly bend legs and hips to one side as far as possible.
- Bend to other side.
- Repeat 5 times.

Toe touches
- Stand straight and relaxed.
- Lower head and body and try to touch floor with fingertips.
- Keep knees straight.
- Do not jerk or lunge toward floor.
- Bend only as far as you can.
- Repeat 5 times.

Bladder Cancer

—**Bladder cancer: the bladder is the most common site of urinary tract cancer. Types of cancer include transitional cell carcinomas, squamous cell carcinomas, and adenocarcinomas. The cancer spreads by local invasion into the bladder muscle, by regional spread into surrounding lymph nodes, the pelvis, and other pelvic structures, and via the blood to the lungs, bones, and liver. The bladder may also be invaded by cancer from other structures, such as the uterine body and cervix, prostate, sigmoid colon, and rectum.**

RISK FACTORS
- Occupational exposure to dust or fume of dyes, rubber, leather and its products, paint, and organic chemicals such as benzidine
- Cigarette smoking

SIGNS/SYMPTOMS
- Hematuria

- Marked urgency, dysuria, and frequency with small volumes of urine
- Low back pain, which may indicate sacral or lumbar metastases
- Pelvic pain or leg edema related to lymphatic or venous obstruction

DIAGNOSTIC TESTS

- Describe each procedure, its purpose, and the normal feelings or sensations that are likely, as well as any preprocedural and postprocedural care.
  —Urine culture and urinalysis: to determine presence of infection and hematuria
  —Excretory urography: to detect ureteral or urethral obstruction
  —Cystoscopy with biopsy and cytology: to see tumor and determine presence of malignant cells
  —Cystoscopic retrograde ureteropyelography: to see tumor and determine presence of obstruction
  —Renal arteriography and ultrasound: to determine extent of tumor, vessels, obstruction
  —Computed tomography and magnetic resonance imaging of abdomen and pelvis: to determine extent of lymph node involvement
  —Chest and skeletal x-rays, bone scan, liver function studies: to determine extent of metastatic disease

TREATMENT
Medical

- Therapy
  —Radiation therapy: external beam for palliation of hemorrhage and bony metastases
  —Photodynamic therapy
  —Chemotherapy
    For noninvasive bladder cancer: intravesical instillation with bacillus Calmette-Guérin (BCG); other drugs such as thiotepa, doxorubicin, mitomycin-C, interferons
    For invasive bladder cancer: CMDV (cisplatin, methotrexate, doxorubicin, vinblastine); MVC (methotrexate, vinblastine, cisplatin); single agents (methotrexate with or without leucovorin, doxorubicin, vinblastine)

Surgical

- For noninvasive bladder cancer: endoscopic resection and fulguration; laser therapy
- For invasive bladder cancer: radical cystectomy with urinary diversion
    —Complications: ureterocutaneous fistula, wound dehiscence, partial small bowel obstruction, wound infection, small bowel fistula

HOME CARE

- Give both the patient and the caregiver *verbal* and *written* instructions. Provide them with the name and telephone number of a physician or nurse to call if questions arise.
- *General information*
    —Discuss the disease, causes, and contributing factors.
- *Warning signs*
    —Review the signs and symptoms that should be reported to a physician or nurse.
        Infection: cloudy, odorous urine; frequency, urgency, burning
        Ileal conduit complications: stomal stenosis with pain, stones; ureteral reflux
        Kock pouch complications: leakage at stoma, difficult catheterization, stones
- *Special instructions*
    —Assist the patient to obtain appropriate and adequate supplies for care of a urinary diversion (see p. 740).
    —Teach the female patient to reduce the incidence of urinary tract infections by voiding after sexual intercourse, avoiding bubble baths, and wearing cotton undergarments.
    —Provide information about pain management as needed (see Pain Management, p. 708).
- *Activity*
    —Emphasize the importance of exercise and adequate rest.
- *Diet*
    —Stress the importance of adequate fluid intake.
    —Advise the patient to choose fluids and foods that cause alkaline urine, such as fruits, vegetables, and milk.
    —Advise the patient to avoid fluids and foods that irritate the bladder, such as alcohol, tea, and spices.

PSYCHOSOCIAL CARE

- Encourage verbalization regarding fears and concerns about disease and prognosis.
- Encourage expressions of feelings of frustration and grief.
- Provide information to patient and family/caretaker regarding counseling and support groups.

FOLLOW-UP CARE

- Stress the importance of regular follow-up visits. Make sure the patient has the necessary names and telephone numbers.
- Advise the patient to avoid using tobacco.

REFERRALS

- Assist the patient to obtain referral services such as sperm banking, sexual counseling, and reconstructive or implant surgery.

Blindness
(Visual Impairment)

—Blindness: diminished visual acuity ranging from low vision (partial vision) to total blindness; may involve one or both eyes. Types of blindness include color blindness (inability to distinguish certain colors), legal blindness (maximum acuity 20/200 with optimum correction and or visual field reduced to range of 20 degrees [normal is 180 degrees]), loss of peripheral vision, and loss of central vision.

CAUSES/CONTRIBUTING FACTORS

- Retinal detachment/degeneration
- Glaucoma
- Cataract
- Amblyopia
- Diabetes
- Stroke
- Aneurysm

- Brain tumor
- Trachoma (chronic conjunctivitis)
- Leprosy
- Onchocerciasis (river blindness caused by blackfly bites)
- Xerophthalmia (dry eye)
- Corneal diseases
- Herpes simplex virus
- Trauma

SIGNS/SYMPTOMS

- The following signs and symptoms necessitate evaluation to prevent permanent visual loss.
  - —Blurred vision
  - —Double vision
  - —Sudden loss of vision
  - —Alternating dimming and clearing of vision
  - —Eye pain
  - —Red eye
  - —Traumatized eye
  - —Loss of side vision
  - —Halos (colored rays or circles around lights)
  - —Flashes or streaks of light
  - —Turned or wandering eye
  - —Twitching or shaking eye
  - —Floaters (dots, streaks, or strands)
  - —Pressure or pulling within the eye
  - —Discharge, crusting, excessive tearing
  - —Swelling in eye
  - —Bulging of one or both eyes
  - —Unequal pupil size

HOME CARE

- Give both the patient and the caregiver *verbal* and *written* instructions. Provide them with the name and telephone number of a physician or nurse to call if questions arise.
- *General information*
  - —Reinforce the physician's explanation for the type and cause of blindness (disease process or trauma). Stress the importance of notifying the physician of any changes in the condition.

—Clarify the prognosis, explaining whether the visual impairment is temporary or progressive.

- *Warning signs*
  —Review the signs and symptoms that should be reported to a physician or nurse.

  > Pain
  > Itching
  > Redness
  > Swelling
  > Discharge

- *Special instructions*
  —Provide instruction and assist the patient to develop skills needed to maximize self-care and promote independence.

  > Explore and map out furniture, steps, and doorways in the home through guidance and touch.
  > Use another's arm as guide when walking.
  > Trace the wall or rail with the hand to orient to perimeters of room when walking.
  > When walking alone, use cane or walking stick to identify obstacles.
  > Touch food, containers, liquids, and utensils before eating.
  > Feel chairs and toilet before turning to sit.
  > Organize clothing and shoes to facilitate selection.
  > Place articles for grooming and hygiene in the same position.

  —Discuss home care with patient and caregiver, stressing the need to avoid hazards.

  > Living quarters should not be rearranged once the patient is familiar with the placement of furniture and furnishings.
  > Encourage the patient to move slowly and to have assistance when exploring living arrangements.
  > Ensure that living quarters are free of clutter (remove loose throw rugs, articles on floor or stairs, electrical cords).
  > Encourage the patient to explore outdoors slowly and with assistance to avoid falls on uneven ground, steps, loose gravel, and icy patches.
  > Encourage the patient to explore the community slowly and with assistance.
  > Encourage self-care, discussing the need to avoid being overprotective.

—Provide instruction on caring for the eyes.

> Review the method for administering eyedrops or ointment.
>
> Advise the patient of the importance of keeping the eyes free of infection: keeping the eye dropper clean, using a clean tissue or cloth to wipe eyes, wiping eyes from inner to outer lid.

- *Medications*
  —Explain the purpose, dosage, schedule, and route of administration of any prescribed drugs, as well as side effects to report to the physician or nurse.
  —Avoid over-the-counter medications, eyedrops, or ointments unless their use has been discussed with the physician.

FOLLOW-UP CARE

- Stress the importance of regular follow-up visits. Make sure the patient has the necessary names and telephone numbers.
- Encourage or assist the patient to obtain a MedicAlert bracelet and identification card listing the diagnosis and medication.

REFERRALS

- Encourage or assist the patient and family to seek additional support from community and health agencies for the visually impaired (e.g., state agency for the blind), which can provide early assistance with computer-assisted reading, talking books, time and temperature devices, rehabilitation for future employment, and acquisition of new skills.
- Initiate referral to medical social services for financial needs and to home health care for assistance with activities of daily living (ADLs).

Bone Cancer

—Bone cancer: primary bone cancers are uncommon, accounting for 0.2% of all malignancies in the United States. Peak incidence is between 15 and 19 years of age and after 65 years. Types include osseous (classic or periosteal osteosarcoma), cartilaginous (primary or secondary chondrosarcoma), fibrous (fibrosarcoma, malignant fibrous histiocytoma), and reticuloendothelial (Ewing's sarcoma, multiple myeloma).

RISK FACTORS

- Paget's disease
- Fibrous dysplasia
- Enchondromatosis
- Bone infarction
- Prior exposure to radiation

SIGNS/SYMPTOMS

- Osteosarcoma: complaints of pain or swelling in the affected extremity, usually worse at night and increasing as the tumor expands; severe, unremitting pain and pathologic fracture seen in the presence of Paget's disease
- Chondrosarcoma: persistent, dull, aching pain; firm, swollen area over the tumor site
- Fibrosarcoma: pain and swelling of the affected area
- Ewing's sarcoma: progressive pain and swelling of the affected area; anemia; leukocytosis; elevated erythrocyte sedimentation rate

DIAGNOSTIC TESTS

- Describe each procedure, its purpose, and the normal feelings or sensations that are likely, as well as any preprocedural and postprocedural care.
  —Computed tomography and magnetic resonance imaging: to define location and extent of tumor
  —X-ray: to define location, extent, and type of destruction and amount of reactive bone formed
  —Bone scans: to detect multiple areas of disease, extent of local disease, tumor activity, skeletal metastases
  —Biopsy: to determine type, stage, and grade of tumor
  —Chest x-ray: to detect pulmonary metastases

TREATMENT
Medical

- Therapy
  —Radiation therapy: external beam

—Chemotherapy
  For osteogenic sarcoma
  ○ Doxorubicin
  ○ Cisplatin
  ○ High-dose methotrexate
  ○ Ifosfamide
  ○ Dactinomycin
  ○ Cyclophosphamide
  For Ewing's sarcoma
  ○ Combinations of vincristine, actinomycin D, doxorubi-
    cin, and cyclophosphamide; ifosfamide and etoposide

Surgical

- Wide excision with limb salvage
- En bloc resection: wide excision of normal tissue around tumor, removal of entire muscle bundles at points of origin and insertion, resection of involved bone as well as vascular structures
  —Complications: long operating time, lengthy anesthesia, extensive blood loss
- Amputation (see Amputation, p. 32)
- Reconstruction: allograft, autograft, vascularized graft
- Prosthesis

HOME CARE

- Give both the patient and the caregiver *verbal* and *written* instructions. Provide them with the name and telephone number of a physician or nurse to call if questions arise.
- *General information*
  —Explain to a patient who has undergone limb salvage that he or she will not regain preoperative gait and will be partially disabled.
  —Reinforce the physician's explanation of the type of cancer and prescribed treatment (see Chemotherapy, p. 667; Radiation Therapy, p. 721; Amputation, p. 32).

Bone Marrow Harvest

—Bone marrow harvest: removal of bone marrow from a donor for purposes of transplanting into a patient.

PREPROCEDURAL TEACHING

- Review the physician's explanation of the procedure and the reason for it; encourage the patient to ask questions and to discuss any fears or anxieties.

Review of Preprocedural Care

- Review the need for written consent and explain that the hospital stay will be from 1 to 3 days.
- Review preprocedural tests: blood tests to ensure the donor's bone marrow matches the recipient's, physical examination, chest x-ray, electrocardiogram, urinalysis.
- Explain that the evening before the harvest the donor will take a shower with an antiseptic solution and should have nothing by mouth (NPO) from midnight on.
- Describe what will happen on the day of the procedure.
    - —A nurse will insert an IV line and administer a sedative and anesthetic agents to make the donor relaxed and drowsy.
    - —The bone marrow will be harvested from the donor's hip. The physician will insert a needle several times into the rear portion of the hip bones and withdraw a total of 1 to 2 quarts of bone marrow and blood.
    - —A pressure dressing will be applied over the harvest sites to prevent bleeding.
    - —The entire procedure will take about 2 to 3 hours.

Review of Postprocedural Care

- The patient will awaken in the recovery room after the anesthetic has worn off.
- A nurse will check on the donor every 15 minutes to record vital signs (pulse, blood pressure, temperature, and respirations) and ensure that no bleeding is occurring from the harvest sites. Blood transfusions may be given to make up for the loss of blood.

- Explain that if the marrow is for the donor's future use, it will be frozen until needed. If it is for another recipient, it will be given immediately to the recipient through an IV transfusion.
- Within a day the donor will be able to eat solid food and begin walking around. The pressure dressing will be removed and replaced by a bandage. If the donor has pain, the physician can prescribe medication to relieve it.
- The donor will be able to leave the hospital after 1 or 2 days and to resume normal activities soon after.

HOME CARE

- Give both the patient and the caregiver *verbal* and *written* instructions. Provide them with the name and telephone number of a physician or nurse to call if questions arise.
- *General information*
  —Explain the need to keep the harvest sites clean and covered with a bandage for 3 days.
- *Warning signs*
  —Review the signs and symptoms that should be reported to a physician or nurse.
  - Bleeding
  - Pain
  - Swelling at site

Bone Marrow Suppression

—Bone marrow suppression: depression of the bone marrow causing a depression of the immune system caused by cancer and cancer treatment. As a result, the patient is made more susceptible to infection, bleeding, and anemia.

INFECTION

- The sites of infection most commonly associated with bone marrow suppression are the bladder and urinary tract, skin, lungs, and blood.

SIGNS/SYMPTOMS

- Fever over 100° F
- Redness, swelling, or pain around or in any wound
- Coughing, sore throat, stuffy or runny nose
- Nausea, vomiting, or diarrhea
- Chest pain or shortness of breath
- Burning or frequency of urination; change in color or odor of urine
- Sores or white patches in mouth

Prevention

- Advise the patient of ways to prevent infection.
    —Eat healthy meals, drink plenty of fluids, get enough rest, and avoid stress as much as possible.
    —Keep mouth, teeth, and gums clean; use a soft-bristled toothbrush and saltwater rinse.
    —Wash hands often with soap and water, especially before eating and after using the toilet.
    —Shower rather than taking a bath.
    —Cleanse perianal area after each bowel movement.
    —For women, avoid bubble baths, douches, and feminine hygiene products such as tampons. Change sanitary napkins frequently.
    —Use a commercial lubricant during sexual intercourse.
    —Urinate before and after intercourse.
    —Avoid the following:
        People who are sick
        People recently vaccinated with a live virus
        Crowded places (waiting rooms, malls)
        Raw fruits and vegetables, raw eggs, and raw milk; eat only cooked food and pasteurized milk and milk products
        Sources of stagnant water (water in flower vases, pitchers, denture cups, humidifiers, and breathing equipment); water in these containers should be changed daily; preferably such items should not be in patient's room
        Dog, cat, and bird feces; bird cages or litter boxes should not be in patient's room; if they are, someone else should change them

BLEEDING

- Bleeding, especially from the skin or mucous membranes or internally, occurs because the bone marrow is not producing enough platelets (special blood cells that cause the blood to clot) or because the platelets already in the blood are being destroyed. The cancer, allergic reactions to medications, radiation therapy, or chemotherapy can cause bleeding.

Prevention

- Check the skin each day for bruises and call the physician if bruises get larger after first being noticed.
- Report to a physician any bleeding that does not stop after 5 minutes.
- Bleeding from the skin
  —Avoid physical activities that could cause injury, such as contact sports.
  —Shave with an electric razor.
  —Keep nails short; file rough edges.
  —Draw a circle around the perimeter of a bruise to measure an increase in size.
- Bleeding from the mucous membranes of the mouth, nose, gastrointestinal system, and genitourinary tract
  —Brush with a soft-bristled toothbrush. If gums still bleed, use sponge-tipped applicators or a WaterPik. Do not floss. Keep lips moist with petroleum jelly. Check with physician before having dental work done.
  —Avoid hot foods that might burn the mouth.
  —Blow nose gently. Humidify the house if the air is too dry. If nose bleeds, pinch nostrils shut for a few minutes. If bleeding persists, put an ice bag on the back of the neck.
  —Use stool softeners and drink plenty of water if constipated. Do not use enemas or suppositories. Take acetaminophen (e.g., Tylenol) or ibuprofen rather than aspirin, which can cause stomach bleeding. Avoid douches and vaginal supposi-tories. Use a lubricating jelly before sexual intercourse.
- Internal bleeding
  —Arrange furniture to avoid bumping into it. Keep clutter and loose rugs off floor.
  —Avoid tight-fitting clothing and any buttons or ornaments that could bruise or chafe skin.
  —Do not lift heavy objects.

ANEMIA

- Anemia is caused by a destruction or reduction of red blood cells to carry oxygen to the cells and take away carbon dioxide. Patients may tire easily and need to rest more often or decrease their physical activities.

Signs/Symptoms to Report

- Fatigue
- Pallor
- Dizziness
- Ringing in the ears
- Chest pain
- Shortness of breath

Special Instructions

- Schedule frequent rest periods during activities.
- Eat a high-protein diet.
- Take a multivitamin supplement with minerals.

Therapy

- Epoetin alfa
- Blood transfusions

Bone Marrow Transplantation

—Bone marrow transplantation (BMT): destruction of the patient's bone marrow with high doses of cancer chemotherapy or radiation and replacement with healthy bone marrow. The transplanted marrow begins making new blood cells within 10 to 14 days after the transplantation. BMT is a treatment for some cancers. The procedure involves intravenous infusion of bone marrow into the patient to replace the defective hematopoietic system with healthy stem cells. Types of BMT include autologous (harvesting of patient's marrow after treatment with cytoreductive therapy and sometimes cancer chemotherapy), syngeneic (using an identical twin as donor), and allogeneic (donation by a family member, usually a sibling, or by an unrelated donor with compatible human leukocyte antigen [HLA] and mixed lymphocyte culture [MLC]). The type selected depends on the disease or disorder, the availability of histocompatible donors, and the health status of potential donors.

INDICATIONS

- Leukemias
- Non-Hodgkin's lymphoma
- Burkitt's lymphoma
- Multiple myeloma
- Osteosarcoma
- Breast cancer

PREPROCEDURAL TEACHING

- Review the physician's explanation of the procedure and the reason for it; encourage the patient to ask questions and to discuss any fears or anxieties.

Review of Preprocedural Care

- For donor selection and bone marrow harvest, see Bone Marrow Harvest, p. 108.
- Discuss the need for placement of a central line.
- Explain that the hospital stay will last from 1½ to 2 months if there are no serious complications.
- Discuss the use of high-dose chemotherapy, either alone or with total body irradiation, as preparation for transplantation.
  —May take as long as 10 days
  —Common side effects: nausea, vomiting, anorexia, mucositis, parotitis, xerostomia, excessive salivation, diarrhea, low-grade fever, alopecia, electrolyte imbalance, aplasia
  —Life-threatening effects: severe thrombocytopenia, syndrome of inappropriate antidiuretic hormone, renal failure, sepsis, venous occlusive disease, capillary leak syndrome
- Describe the BMT procedure, discussing the following:
  —The patient is alone in a room with constant monitoring.
  —The patient is hydrated with bicarbonate solution to force brisk alkaline urine flow to prevent red blood cell (RBC) hemolysis.
  —Emergency drugs for anaphylactic reactions are kept at the bedside.
  —Bone marrow is infused via central line without a filter over a 1- to 4-hour period.

Review of Postprocedural Care

- Explain that after BMT the recipient progresses through stages of aplasia, lingering side effects of preparatory therapy, and finally engraftment of the donor marrow.
- Review self-care procedures that the patient will need to do while in the hospital: handwashing techniques, mouth care, skin care, measuring intake and output, use of incentive spirometer.
- Discuss activity allowances, limitations, and use of an exercise bicycle.
- Explain dietary procedures, use of total parenteral nutrition, and restrictions, such as food allowances.
- Explain posttransplant medications, their expected side effects, and the use of an indwelling catheter for administration.
- Discuss complications and measures that will be taken to prevent or treat them.
  —Infection: patient will be placed in protective isolation or laminar airflow rooms; prophylactic systemic antibiotics and antiviral agents; routine cultures of blood, urine, throat, stool
  —Acute graft-versus-host disease: usually appears within 2 weeks to 3 months after BMT; may cause erythema, maculopapular rash, blistering and desquamation, liver failure, diarrhea, abdominal pain, denuding of gastrointestinal (GI) tract; mild cases usually self-limiting; severe cases require treatment with agents such as high-dose steroids, antithymocyte globulin, monoclonal antibody, OKT-3
  —Chronic graft-versus-host disease: occurs 3 months to 1 year after BMT; manifested as scleroderma-like changes in skin, GI tract, and liver; immune deficiency; marrow suppression; changes in respiratory and musculoskeletal function; treated with prednisone and azathioprine
  —Potential long-term problems: neurologic damage; cataract formation; endocrine problems; changes in skin, eyes, mouth, and GI tract

SIDE EFFECTS/COMPLICATIONS

- Acute
  —Mucositis
  —Viral infection
  —Bacterial and fungal sepsis
  —Renal failure
  —Interstitial pneumonia

—Venoocclusive disease
—Graft-versus-host disease
- Common
    —Anemia
    —Bleeding stomatitis
    —Skin changes
    —Nausea
    —Vomiting
    —Diarrhea

🏠 HOME CARE

- Give both the patient and the caregiver *verbal* and *written* instructions. Provide them with the name and telephone number of a physician or nurse to call if questions arise.
- *General information*
    —Explain measures for preventing complications (see also Bone Marrow Suppression, p. 109).
    Infection
    ○ Precautions are more rigid during the first 3 months after BMT and become more relaxed as the year progresses.
    ○ Wear a face mask when outside the home in public.
    ○ Avoid contact with persons who may be infectious, young children attending school, or persons recently vaccinated.
    ○ Avoid crowds and trips to grocery stores, theaters, and restaurants.
    ○ Avoid having multiple sexual partners.
    ○ Wash hands before eating and after using the toilet.
    ○ Avoid contact with pets for the first 3 months after BMT. Do not clean litter boxes or come in contact with animal feces.
    ○ Avoid contact with plants and flowers.
    ○ Do not swim in private or public pools.
    Bleeding
    ○ Discuss emergency procedures to follow if spontaneous hemorrhage occurs. The patient or caregiver should have emergency numbers on hand. Teach methods for applying pressure to the bleeding site.
    ○ Review measures to prevent bleeding: maintain a safe, clutter-free environment; remove loose scatter rugs; avoid using sharp objects; use electric razors; wear

protective gloves when gardening; avoid going barefoot; use soft-bristled toothbrush; use soft sponge with mouthwash if gums are sensitive and bleeding.

○ Inform dentist and other medical personnel about BMT before any procedures are performed.

Stomatitis

○ Discuss the importance of routine oral hygiene in the morning, after meals, and at bedtime.

○ Discuss the need to avoid putting objects into the mouth.

○ Instruct the patient to avoid using mouthwash containing alcohol.

○ Discuss the need to avoid irritating foods such as citrus fruits and spicy or hard fruits and vegetables.

○ Instruct the patient on the use of any prescribed mouthwashes, sprays, or anesthetics.

○ Plan with the patient or caregiver for necessary changes in activities of daily living (see Bone Marrow Suppression, p. 109).

- *Warning signs*
  —Review the signs and symptoms that should be reported to a physician or nurse.

  Fever

  Rash

  Change in color or consistency of stool, urine

  Nausea or vomiting

  Pain

  Dryness of mouth, difficulty swallowing

  Change in skin color

  Cough or shortness of breath

- *Special instructions*
  —Teach self-care procedures as indicated.

  Central venous access device (see p. 665)

  Administration of total parenteral nutrition

  Use of volumetric pump

  Use of incentive spirometer

  Taking and recording of temperature; intake and output; urine and stool testing for blood

  —Discuss preparation of home environment.

  Advise patient on obtaining necessary equipment and supplies.

  Instruct patient's caregiver to have house cleaned and dusted before arrival of patient, to remove all plants and flowers, and to board pet away from home for the first 100 days or as ordered.

- *Medications*
  —Explain the purpose, dosage, schedule, and route of administration of any prescribed drugs, as well as side effects to report to the physician or nurse.
  —Emphasize the importance of not taking over-the-counter medications without checking with a physician or nurse.
- *Diet*
  —Explain the need to maintain diet as ordered.
  —Suggest a high-protein, high-caloric diet.
  —Encourage frequent small, light meals.
  —Maintain hydration.

PSYCHOSOCIAL CARE

- Encourage verbalization regarding concerns about different phases of procedure.
- Encourage expressions of feelings, fears regarding potential of or actual complications associated with procedure.

FOLLOW-UP CARE

- Stress the importance of regular medical and laboratory follow-up visits. Make sure the patient has the necessary names and telephone numbers.

REFERRALS

- Assist the patient to obtain referral services for home care supplies and psychologic support.

Bowel Obstruction and Resection with Anastomosis

—Bowel obstruction and resection with anastomosis: surgical resection of diseased intestinal tissue and anastomosis of the remaining healthy bowel segments. The surgical incision site depends on the location of the diseased intestinal tissue. The bowel resection may result in an end-to-end anastomosis or a side-to-side anastomosis. (If temporary ostomy is required, see Ostomy, p. 694.)

INDICATIONS

- Localized obstructive intestinal disorders, such as diverticulitis, intestinal polyps, adhesions, malignant or benign intestinal lesions
- Localized bowel cancer

PREPROCEDURAL TEACHING

- Review the physician's explanation of the procedure and the reason for it; encourage the patient to ask questions and to discuss any fears or anxieties.

Review of Preprocedural Care

- Review the need for informed consent and anesthesia.
- Discuss the administration of antibiotics, laxatives, and enemas.

Review of Postprocedural Care

- Discuss anticipated postoperative care, including nasogastric tube, IVs for fluid replacement, abdominal drains, and ambulation.
- Warn patient against manipulating or repositioning the nasogastric tube.
- Stress the importance of turning, coughing, deep breathing, and incisional splinting.
- Discuss the purpose of the incentive spirometer and demonstrate its use.

SIDE EFFECTS/COMPLICATIONS

- Bleeding
- Leakage from the anastomosis site
- Peritonitis
- Sepsis
- Postresection obstruction

 HOME CARE

- Give both the patient and the caregiver *verbal* and *written* instructions. Provide them with the name and telephone number of a physician or nurse to call if questions arise.

B

- *General information*
  —Review any explanation about the surgery and follow-up care.
  —Demonstrate proper wound management and dressing changes: procedure and frequency of dressing changes and inspection of the incision with each dressing change.
  —Advise the patient to dispose of soiled dressings in a plastic bag and thoroughly wash hands.
  —Instruct the patient to note and record the frequency and amount of bowel movements and the characteristics of the stool.
- *Warning signs*
  —Review the signs and symptoms that should be reported to a physician or nurse.
    Infection: fever, malaise, leakage of bowel contents, purulent drainage, foul odor, redness, tenderness at incision
    Abdominal distention, increased abdominal pain, bloody stools, leakage of bowel contents, abdominal rigidity
    Changes in frequency and amount of bowel movements or the characteristics of the stool
- *Special instructions*
  —Advise the patient where to obtain appropriate supplies, such as sterile dressings.
- *Medications*
  —Explain the purpose, dosage, schedule, and route of administration of stool softeners and analgesics, as well as side effects to report to the physician or nurse.
  —Advise the patient against using laxatives without consulting the physician.
- *Activity*
  —Encourage the patient to discuss allowances and limitations with respect to occupation, recreation, or activities.
  —Instruct the patient to avoid abdominal straining, such as during defecation, and heavy lifting until the sutures are completely healed or until advised by a physician.
- *Diet*
  —Advise a semibland diet until the bowel is completely healed, usually 4 to 8 weeks.
  —Advise the patient to drink plenty of fluids.

—Advise the patient to avoid carbonated beverages and gas-producing foods.
—Provide the patient with a list of specific gas-producing foods.

FOLLOW-UP CARE

• Stress the importance of regular follow-up visits. Make sure the patient has the necessary names and telephone numbers.

REFERRALS

• If appropriate, assist the patient to obtain a referral to the American Cancer Society and community-based support groups.
• Assist the patient to obtain referrals for home health care services, supplies, and medical social services as indicated.

Brain Tumors

—Brain tumors: space-occupying lesions that compress, invade, or destroy surrounding brain tissue and nerve structures. Brain tumors can occur at any age. In adults the incidence is highest between 40 and 60 years of age. In children most brain tumors occur before age 1 or between ages 2 and 12. Tumors are classified by histologic features and grade of malignancy. Tumors may have primary, metastatic, or developmental origins.

CAUSES/CONTRIBUTING FACTORS

• The cause of brain tumors is unknown. Some theories include genetic, hormonal, or angiogenesis factors, chemicals, radiation, trauma, viruses, or diet.

SIGNS/SYMPTOMS

The onset of signs and symptoms is insidious. Findings are specific to the type of tumor, its location, and the degree of invasion.

• Headache: localized or generalized

B

- Seizures
- Mental, behavioral, and personality changes: disorientation; inability to follow commands; irritability; forgetfulness; memory loss; impaired judgment
- Decreased level of consciousness, stupor, or coma
- Vomiting with or without nausea
- Dizziness occurring with position changes; vertigo
- Visual changes: double vision, decreased visual acuity; visual field defects
- Decreased motor strength; hemiparesis; hemiplegia
- Aphasia
- Gait disturbances; impaired balance; incoordination
- Auditory disturbances
- Sensory disturbances: hyperesthesia, paresthesia, astereognosis, agnosia, apraxia, agraphia
- Cranial nerve dysfunction

COMPLICATIONS

- Cerebral edema
- Compression of the brain, cranial nerves, and cerebral vessels
- Intracranial pressure
- Seizures
- Neurologic defects: mild to severe
- Hydrocephalus
- Hormonal changes
- Altered level of consciousness
- Alteration in respiratory function
- Brain herniation

DIAGNOSTIC TESTS

- Describe each procedure, its purpose, and the normal feelings or sensations that are likely, as well as any preprocedural and postprocedural care.
  - Skull x-rays: to locate the tumor and any calcified areas
  - Computed tomography brain scan: to locate the tumor, determine its size, and detect the presence of cerebral edema
  - Cerebral angiography: to assess the vascularity of tumor and the surrounding vessels
  - Magnetic resonance imaging: to assess tumor location, size, vascularity, and cerebral edema

—Stereotaxic biopsy: to assess histologic type and grading of tumors

—Intracranial pressure monitoring

TREATMENT

• Specific treatments vary with tumor histologic type, location, accessibility, and radiosensitivity.

Medical

• Therapy
  —Radiation therapy
  —Chemotherapy
• Drugs
  —Corticosteroids such as dexamethasone (Decadron): to control cerebral edema and decrease intracranial pressure
  —Osmotic diuretics: to decrease cerebral edema
  —Anticonvulsants such as phenytoin (Dilantin): to prevent seizures
  —H_2 blockers such as cimetidine (Tagamet) or ranitidine (Zantac): to prevent stress ulcers
  —Antacids
  —Analgesics: to relieve headaches
  —Antiemetics: to minimize nausea and vomiting
  —Fluid restriction: to prevent cerebral edema

Surgical

• Surgical resection
• Laser surgery
• Microsurgery
• Ventriculoatrial or ventriculoperitoneal shunting of cerebrospinal fluid

HOME CARE

• Give both the patient and the caregiver *verbal* and *written* instructions. Provide them with the name and telephone number of a physician or nurse to call if questions arise.
• *General information*
  —Reinforce the explanation of brain tumor type, its causes, and contributing factors.
  —Patient education is individualized, depending on the location, the type of tumor, its malignancy, and the prescribed treatment.

- *Warning signs*
  —Review the signs and symptoms that should be reported to a physician or nurse.
    Seizure activity
    Behavioral or neurologic changes
    Altered level of consciousness
    Changes in respiration
    Infection, including fever
    Bleeding
    Stress ulcers: abdominal distention, pain, vomiting, tarry stools
- *Special instructions*
  —Discuss with the family any residual deficits and physical limitations.
  —Assist the patient in obtaining appropriate adaptive devices for self-care, rehabilitation, mobilization, and sensory function, such as hearing aids or eyeglasses.
  —Assist the caregiver in identifying and correcting hazards in the home if the patient develops deficits.
  —Teach the patient and caregiver seizure precautions (see p. 567).
- *Medications*
  —Explain the purpose, dosage, schedule, and route of administration of any prescribed drugs, as well as side effects to report to the physician or nurse.
  —Explain the adverse effects of chemotherapy (see p. 667) and radiation therapy (see p. 721), if appropriate. Explain actions the patient can take to alleviate them.
- *Activity*
  —Identify and discuss limitations imposed by changes in neurologic function.
- *Diet*
  —Explain that the diet should be regular or as prescribed by a physician.

PSYCHOSOCIAL CARE

- Encourage verbalization of feelings, fears, and concerns about prognosis and body image changes.
- Discuss with the caregiver the need to maintain the patient's independence and avoid overprotection.
- Assist the caregiver to use resources to assist in developing a home care plan.

- Encourage the patient to continue to function in usual roles (occupational and social) as much as possible and to avoid sensory deprivation and social isolation.
- Encourage the patient to seek assistance to perform activities as needed.

FOLLOW-UP CARE

- Stress the importance of regular follow-up visits. Make sure the patient has the necessary names and telephone numbers.

REFERRALS

- Refer the patient to occupational and physical therapists to begin a rehabilitation program. If appropriate, refer the patient to a speech pathologist.
- Refer the patient for a dietary consultation to ensure adequate nutrition during chemotherapy and radiation therapy.
- Refer the patient to support groups, the American Cancer Society, and home health support services.
- Assist the caregiver to obtain referrals for a skilled nursing facility or social services as indicated.

Breast Cancer

—Breast cancer: cancer of the breast, the most common malignancy among American women. One of nine women will have breast cancer in her lifetime. Breast cancer is believed to be a systemic disease, with the possibility of occult distant metastases occurring early in the disease with or without lymph node involvement.

RISK FACTORS

- Family history of breast cancer: sister, mother, grand-mother, aunt
- Menarche before age 12
- Menopause after 55 years
- No children or first child after 30 years of age
- Exposure to excessive radiation, especially before age 35

- Fibrocystic change (atypical epithelial hyperplasia)
- Previous history of breast cancer
- Personal history of other cancers (endometrial, ovarian, colon, or thyroid types)

SIGNS/SYMPTOMS

- Painless mass or thickening in breast most common
- Nipple discharge: spontaneous, unilateral, from single duct, watery and clear, serosanguineous, bloody in color
- Advanced disease: skin or nipple dimpling; puckering or retraction; changes in breast size, shape, or contour; skin edema; discoloration; dilated superficial blood vessels; frank skin ulcerations; hard, fixed mass in axilla

COMPLICATIONS

- Metastases, most commonly to lungs, liver, bone
- Hypercalcemia
- Spinal cord compression
- Brachial plexopathy
- Pleural effusion
- Pathologic fracture

DIAGNOSTIC TESTS

- Describe each procedure, its purpose, and the normal feelings or sensations that are likely, as well as any preprocedural and postprocedural care.
  —Clinical examination: palpation of breasts and axillae
  —Mammogram and/or ultrasound: to determine shape, size, and location of tumor
  —Biopsy: to identify type of malignant cells
  —Estrogen and progestin receptors: to determine tumor response to hormones

TREATMENT
Medical

- Therapy
  —Radiation therapy
    Bradytherapy
    External beam
    Regional node irradiation
- Drugs (as adjuvant therapy for radiation)

—Combination chemotherapy: CMF (cyclophosphamide, methotrexate, 5-fluorouracil); CMFVP (CMF with vincristine and prednisone); CA (cyclophosphamide and doxorubicin); CAF (cyclophosphamide, doxorubicin, 5-fluorouracil)
—Antiestrogen therapy (ablative): tamoxifen citrate
—Estrogens (additive): diethylstilbestrol, ethinyl estradiol
—Androgens (additive): fluoxymesterone, testosterone, methyltestosterone
—Progestins (additive): megestrol acetate, medroxyprogesterone

Surgical

- Lumpectomy: wide excision and removal of tumor and margin of healthy tissue
- Partial mastectomy: simple excision of tumor and wider margin of healthy tissue
- Mastectomy
  —Subcutaneous: removal of all breast tissue, preserving overlying skin and nipple-areolar complex
  —Total (simple): complete removal of breast tissue and skin from clavicle to costal margin and from midline to the latissimus dorsi; axillary nodes not removed
  —Modified radical: removal of breast and axillary lymph nodes
  —Radical: removal of breast, underlying pectoral muscles, and axillary nodes
  —Extended or super radical: removal of internal mammary lymphatic chain with breast, pectoral muscles, and axillary nodes
- Breast reconstruction
- Bone marrow transplantation (see Bone Marrow Transplantation, p. 112)

HOME CARE

- Give both the patient and the caregiver *verbal* and *written* instructions. Provide them with the name and telephone number of a physician or nurse to call if questions arise.
- *General information*
  —Review explanation of the disease, the prescribed surgical procedure, and adjuvant therapy to be carried out. Explain that the decision is based on the stage of breast cancer, age, menopausal state, hormonal receptor status, and patient preference.

- *Special instructions*
  —Encourage discussion of feelings and emotions regarding impending surgery, adjuvant therapies, and prognosis. Clarify any misconceptions.

PSYCHOSOCIAL CARE

- Encourage discussion about side effects of radiation and chemotherapy and interventions available for treatment.
- Stress the importance of verbalizing feelings about the impact that losing a body part will have on lifestyle, sexuality, and relationships.
- Encourage the patient and partner to seek counseling to provide support.

FOLLOW-UP CARE

- Stress the importance of regular follow-up visits. Make sure the patient has the necessary names and telephone numbers.

REFERRALS

- Encourage the patient to visit or talk with another cancer survivor; contact the American Cancer Society's Reach for Recovery for volunteer.

Breast Surgery
(Mastectomy, Lumpectomy)

—Breast surgery: surgical treatment for breast cancer, determined by the size of the tumor, whether it has spread, the woman's age and physical condition, and her preference. Types of breast surgery include lumpectomy (the removal of the lump and a margin of healthy tissue surrounding it) and mastectomy, which may be as simple as removing all breast tissue while preserving the overlying skin and nipple-areolar complex or may involve radical removal of the internal mammary lymphatic chain with the breast, pectoral muscles, and axillary lymph nodes.

PREPROCEDURAL TEACHING

- Review the physician's explanation of the procedure and the reason for it; encourage the patient to ask questions and to discuss any fears or anxieties.

Review of Preprocedural Care

- Review the need for written consent for surgery and anesthesia.
- Explain that the skin will be cleansed with bactericidal soap or antiseptic solutions to remove bacteria.
- Discuss the complete blood count and urinalysis to check for infection and bleeding.
- Explain that the patient will be NPO from midnight of the evening before surgery.
- Describe the types of dressings and equipment that will be used postoperatively. If lymph node dissection is performed, one or two drains will be inserted around the incision site.
- Instruct the patient in exercises, hand and arm care, and drainage tube management.
- Encourage questions and the verbalization of fears, anxieties, and grieving for a change in body image.
- Encourage a preoperative visit by a Reach to Recovery volunteer for psychologic support when possible.

Review of Postprocedural Care

- Provide written information to supplement verbal instructions.
- Instruct the patient to report any unusual pain or swelling in the operative area or the arm on the operative side, as well as signs of infection (redness, pain, swelling, feeling of tenderness, fever, nonserous drainage, or odor).
- For modified radical or partial mastectomy with axillary node dissection, explain that the patient may be discharged with one or more drains in place.
- Review hand and arm care instructions (see box on p. 130).
- Teach arm exercises as prescribed.
- Alert the patient to a possible phantom breast experience; sensation usually consists of twinges or itching of the total breast or nipple.

SIDE EFFECTS/COMPLICATIONS

- Side effects are uncommon in all but radical procedures, which are done less frequently.
  —Infection in the incision line

—Seroma
—Lymphedema
—Impaired shoulder mobility
—Nerve injury

HOME CARE

- Give both the patient and the caregiver *verbal* and *written* instructions. Provide them with the name and telephone number of a physician or nurse to call if questions arise. Use visual aids to assist in instruction.
- *General information*
  —Review explanation of the disease, the prescribed surgical procedure, and adjuvant therapy to be carried out.
  —Explain that if the axillary nodes are removed, the affected arm may swell and is less able to fight infection. Discuss measures to prevent lymphedema:
    Daily arm exercises (see box on p. 130)
    Report loss of shoulder or joint mobility
    When healing is complete, begin strengthening and stretching exercises.
- *Wound/incision care*
  —Teach the patient how to care for the skin at the site of surgery, as well as the arm on the affected side.
  —For modified radical or partial mastectomy:
    Teach the patient to change the dressing, assess appearance of the incision and drain site, empty the drainage container, and record the amount and character of drainage.
    Caution the patient not to abduct the affected arm or raise the arm or elbow above the shoulder until drains are removed.
    Instruct the patient to report any redness or drainage around the drain.
  —Instruct the patient to avoid use of deodorants or antiperspirants until stitches and drains have been removed from the axilla and the wound has healed. If no drain is present, the patient may shower.
  —Caution the patient not to allow injections, placing of intravenous lines, drawing of blood, or taking of blood pressure in the affected arm.
  —Instruct the patient to avoid wearing constricting clothing or jewelry on the affected arm and to carry her handbag on the unaffected arm.

HAND AND ARM CARE INSTRUCTIONS

- While the patient is in bed, position the affected arm on one small and one large pillow so that the wrist is slightly higher than the elbow, and the elbow is slightly higher than the shoulder.
- The patient should get out of bed on the unaffected side.
- Encourage the patient to perform ball-squeezing and range-of-motion exercises as instructed by the physical therapist.
- Have the patient avoid using deodorants or antiperspirants until the stitches have been removed from the axilla and the wound has healed.
- Encourage the patient to perform activities of daily living (ADLs) as tolerated with the following precautions:
  —Wear canvas gloves when gardening.
  —Wear a long, padded glove on the affected arm when reaching into an oven.
  —Wear a thimble when sewing.
  —Wear rubber gloves when using harsh detergents or steel wool.
  —Apply hand lotion to prevent dry skin.
  —Use an electric razor for underarm shaving to avoid nicking the skin.
  —Do not allow injections, intravenous lines, blood to be drawn, or blood pressure to be taken on the affected arm.
  —Use insect repellent to avoid insect bites.
  —Avoid using constricting jewelry or clothing on the affected arm.
  —Use a sunscreen (SPF of 15 or greater), and avoid overexposure to the sun.
  —Use cuticle cream and a nail file to trim fingernails.

Continued

B

HAND AND ARM CARE
INSTRUCTIONS—cont'd

—If the affected arm is burned, apply ice and leave it exposed to the air until the blister breaks. Then wash with soap and water, apply an antiseptic solution (e.g., iodine), and cover the area with a bandage. Notify the health care provider if the area does not heal.

—If the affected arm is cut, wash the area with soap and water, apply an antiseptic (e.g., iodine), and cover the area with a bandage. Notify the health care provider if the area does not heal.

—Call the health care provider if redness, pain, or increased swelling develops.

From Belcher AE: *Cancer nursing,* St Louis, 1992, Mosby.

—Discuss the types of temporary and permanent prostheses available; assist with referral as needed. Advise the patient not to use an external prosthesis or bra pad until swelling has subsided and healing of the incision is complete. Tell her to check with a physician or nurse before using a prosthesis.

—Discuss the types of reconstruction available.

—Stress the importance of continuing breast self-examination and mammography of the unaffected breast.

• *Warning signs*

—Review the signs and symptoms that should be reported to a physician or nurse.

　　Swelling of arm

　　Drainage from incision, excessive drainage or blood in Hemovac, difficulty keeping container flat

　　Infection: redness, purulent drainage, pain, incision warm to touch

• *Medications*

—Explain the purpose, dosage, schedule, and route of administration of any prescribed drugs, as well as side effects to report to a physician or nurse.

—Provide pain management, offering alternative methods to deal with postoperative pain: visualization, guided imagery, meditation, relaxation, biofeedback.

- *Activity*
  —Discuss the need to continue postmastectomy exercises to regain full range of motion.
  —Encourage discussion of allowances and limitations with respect to occupation, recreational sports, or activities.
  —Encourage resumption of self-care activities (feeding, combing hair) and activities of daily living as tolerated.
  —Explain that sexual activity may be resumed when desired. The partner should use a position that does not place pressure on the chest wall.

PSYCHOSOCIAL CARE

- Encourage verbalization about fears over actual and perceived changes in body image and sexuality.
- Encourage consultation with mental health counselor for further support. Provide a referral number.

FOLLOW-UP CARE

- Stress the importance of regular follow-up visits. Make sure the patient has the necessary names and telephone numbers.
- Prepare the patient for adjuvant therapies: hormone therapy, chemotherapy, radiation therapy.

REFERRALS

- Provide referrals for home health services and social services as indicated.
- Assist the patient to obtain referral services and contact support groups such as the American Cancer Society's Reach to Recovery and Lymphoma International Network programs to cope with alterations in body image and other concerns.

Bronchitis

—Bronchitis: inflammation of the large airways (bronchi) and their branches (tracheobronchial tree) that results in production of mucus. Chronic bronchitis results from repeated exposure to irritants that cause tissue irritation, swelling

B

(hypertrophy) of mucus-producing cells in bronchi, and mucus secretion. Long-term exposure to irritants such as cigarette smoke, air pollutants, and toxic industrial gases or fumes is known to cause hypertrophy of mucus-producing cells.

SIGNS/SYMPTOMS

- Cough that is persistent and productive
- Sputum: clear and copious in the morning; thick, tenacious, and purulent during acute attack
- Wheezing and bronchospasm
- Duskiness or cyanosis
- Fever

COMPLICATIONS

- Emphysema
- Respiratory infections
- Respiratory failure

DIAGNOSTIC TESTS

- Describe each procedure, its purpose, and the normal feelings or sensations that are likely, as well as any preprocedural and postprocedural care.
  —Serum studies: complete blood count: to evaluate presence of elevated hemoglobin (polycythemia), presence of infections with increased white blood cells
  —Arterial blood gases: to evaluate presence of hypoxemia and acid-base abnormalities
  —Chest x-ray: to detect changes in chest (anterior-posterior) diameter
  —Sputum culture: to detect presence of infection
  —Pulmonary function: to evaluate degree of impaired respiratory function (reduced vital capacity, increased residual volume due to air trapping)

TREATMENT
Medical

- Therapy
  —Rest
  —Chest physiotherapy: to loosen and mobilize secretions
  —Oxygen therapy: low flow rate (1 to 2 liters) to treat hypoxemia

—Well-balanced diet; increased caloric intake if the patient begins to experience weight loss due to anorexia

—Oral or IV fluids: to maintain adequate hydration

- Drugs
  —Bronchodilators: to relieve bronchospasm
  —Sympathomimetics
  —Antibiotics: for infections
  —Diuretics: to reduce fluid retention in the presence of cardiac complications such as heart failure
  —Corticosteroids

▣ HOME CARE

- Give both the patient and the caregiver *verbal* and *written* instructions. Provide them with the name and telephone number of a physician or nurse to call if questions arise. Use visual aids to assist in instruction.
- *Warning signs*
  —Review the signs and symptoms that should be reported to a physician or nurse.
- *Special instructions*
  —Review the purpose and demonstrate the proper use of all equipment to be used at home, including the oral inhaler and oxygen therapy equipment. For the latter, include discussion of when to use it, the importance of not increasing the flow rate without checking with a physician or home health nurse, and the procedure for ordering replacements.
- Instruct the patient on adaptive breathing techniques to decrease the work of breathing.
- Stress the importance of not smoking.
- *Medications*
  —Explain the purpose, dosage, schedule, and route of administration of any prescribed drugs, as well as side effects to report to a physician or nurse.
- *Activity*
  —Encourage regular exercise to tolerance; avoid or curtail activities when fatigued, during weather extremes, or on smoggy days.
- *Diet*
  —Instruct the patient to eat a well-balanced diet. As the patient becomes more dyspneic, frequent small feedings may be needed to maintain adequate caloric intake.

—Encourage fluid intake to keep secretions moist (1 liter per day unless contraindicated).

REFERRALS

• Provide referral to smoking cessation programs in the community.

Bronchoscopy

—**Bronchoscopy: direct visual examination of the trachea and tracheobronchial tree with a flexible fiberoptic tube.**

INDICATIONS

• To determine the cause of respiratory symptoms
• To obtain a tissue specimen for analysis of lung diseases, infections, and bronchogenic cancers
• To remove foreign bodies, mucus plugs, or excessive secretions from the airway
• To prevent or treat collapsed lung tissue

PREPROCEDURAL TEACHING

• Review the physician's explanation of the procedure and the reason for it; encourage the patient to ask questions and to discuss any fears or anxieties.

Review of Preprocedural Care

• Discuss who will perform the procedure and where it will take place.
• Instruct the patient to have someone available after the procedure to drive the patient home.
• Instruct the patient not to eat or drink fluids for 6 to 12 hours before the test.
• Describe the procedure.
  —It is usually done on an outpatient basis and takes 45 to 60 minutes.
  —The patient is given medications before the procedure: atropine to decrease secretions and a barbiturate or narcotic for sedation.

—Any dental prostheses should be removed.

—The patient is usually placed in a supine position (alternative position is sitting upright) with the neck hyperextended. The patient is instructed to breathe through the nose.

—The physician sprays a local anesthetic in the patient's throat and nasal cavity to anesthetize the vocal cords and suppress the gag reflex. The anesthetic may cause a cold, unpleasant sensation in the throat.

—The lubricated bronchoscope is inserted through the nose or mouth. Explain that the patient will be able to breathe through and around the tube. The tube is advanced into the trachea and bronchi.

—Once the examination is completed and/or the specimens are obtained, the bronchoscope is removed.

Review of Postprocedural Care

• After the procedure the patient is moved to a recovery area where vital signs are monitored frequently. The patient remains NPO until the gag reflex returns.

• Explain that the patient may experience temporary hoarseness and a sore throat. Lozenges and throat gargles can be provided after the gag reflex returns.

▨ HOME CARE

• Give both the patient and the caregiver *verbal* and *written* instructions. Provide them with the name and telephone number of a physician or nurse to call if questions arise.

• *Warning signs*
  —Review the signs and symptoms that should be reported to a physician or nurse.
  > Difficulty breathing
  > Chest pain
  > Inability to swallow
  > Bloody mucus

• *Medications*
  —Explain the purpose, dosage, schedule, and route of administration of any prescribed drugs, as well as side effects to report to a physician or nurse.

• *Diet*
  —Inform the patient that a soft or liquid diet is needed for the first day or until throat pain disappears.

—Explain that extremely hot foods or liquids should be avoided.

—Encourage fluid intake unless contraindicated.

FOLLOW-UP CARE

- Stress the importance of regular follow-up visits. Make sure the patient has the necessary names and telephone numbers.
- Discuss the importance of not smoking.

Buerger's Disease

—Buerger's disease: a rare arterial vascular disease characterized by acute inflammatory lesions and occlusive thrombosis of the small and medium arteries and veins. The legs, feet, upper limbs, and viscera are most frequently affected. The arteries most commonly involved are the anterior and posterior tibial, plantar, digital, radial, ulnar, and palmar.

CAUSES/CONTRIBUTING FACTORS

- Hypersensitivity to nicotine
- Autoimmune disorder
- Male, age 20 to 40 years
- Heavy smokers
- Genetic predisposition
- Jewish ancestry
- Persons living in India and other Asian countries

SIGNS/SYMPTOMS

- Pain
- Intermittent claudication of the instep of the foot, cyanosis, and numbness of feet when exposed to cold, changing later to red, hot, tingly feet
- Ulcerated, painful fingertips, with associated impairment of peripheral pulses and thrombophlebitis
- Changes in the appearance of the nails or skin
- Edema of the legs
- Gangrene with involvement of the lower leg and in patients with diabetes

COMPLICATIONS

- Ulcerations
- Gangrene
- Muscle atrophy
- Infection

DIAGNOSTIC TESTS

- Describe each procedure, its purpose, and the normal feelings or sensations that are likely, as well as any preprocedural and postprocedural care.
  —Arteriography: to locate lesions and rule out atherosclerosis
  —Skin temperature determination
  —Blood studies
  —Chest x-rays
  —Doppler ultrasound: to show diminished circulation in the peripheral vessels
  —Plethysmography: to help detect decreased circulation in the peripheral vessels

TREATMENT
Medical

- The goal of medical treatment is to arrest the progress of the disease.
- Drugs
  —Vasodilators: to promote circulation, relieve pain, and provide emotional support

Surgical

- Regional sympathetic block or ganglionectomy: to produce vasodilation
- Amputation: for cases of severe infection or toxicity and to relieve extreme pain in severe cases of gangrene

HOME CARE

- Give both the patient and the caregiver *verbal* and *written* instructions. Provide them with the name and telephone number of a physician or nurse to call if questions arise.
- *General information*
  —Review explanation of the disease, underlying causes, and precipitating factors.

—Discuss the role nicotine plays in advancing the disease; stress the importance of not smoking or using tobacco.

• *Warning signs*
    —Review the signs and symptoms that should be reported to a physician or nurse.
        Intermittent claudication
        Coldness and numbness of extremities
        Ulcerations or sores that will not heal

• *Special instructions*
    —Caution the patient to avoid precipitating factors.
        Extreme temperatures or prolonged exposure
        Injuries to the feet
        Emotional stress
    —Sitting or standing in one position for long periods of time
    —Discuss measures to prevent complications.
    —Provide instruction on daily foot care.
        Wear well-fitted shoes; avoid going barefoot.
        Use cotton or wool socks.
        Inspect feet daily for cuts, abrasions, and sores and report any found to the physician or nurse.
        Keep feet clean and dry.
    —Instruct the patient on treating ulcers or gangrene.
        Maintain bed rest, using a padded footboard or heat cradle to avoid pressure from bed linens.
        Wash ulcers with mild soap and tepid water; avoid vigorous rubbing. Rinse thoroughly and dry well.
        Apply cotton padding over the area for protection or as directed.
        If there are sores between the toes, separate the toes with cotton to promote healing.
    —Caution the patient to avoid use of heating pads and hot water bottles.

• *Medications*
    —Explain the purpose, dosage, schedule, and route of administration of any prescribed drugs, as well as side effects to report to a physician or nurse.

• *Activity*
    —Encourage the discussion of allowances and limitations with regard to exercise and activities.

FOLLOW-UP CARE AND REFERRALS

- Stress the importance of regular follow-up visits. Make sure the patient has the necessary names and telephone numbers.
- Provide information and referrals for smoking cessation programs.

Bunion
(Hallux Valgus)

—Bunion: bony prominence of the first metatarsal head and enlarged bursa that develops as a result of the hallux valgus deformity. Bunions form because of pressure and inflammation in almost all cases of hallux valgus.

—Hallux valgus: lateral deviation (outward bending) of the great toe, away from the midline.

— Hallux valgus deformity: angulation of the great toe away from the midline toward the second and other toes. In some cases the great toe deviates over or under one or more of the toes. The deformity is common in women in their sixties with a strong familial tendency and in adolescent girls.

CAUSES/CONTRIBUTING FACTORS

- Prolonged pressure aggravated by wearing narrow-toed shoes that do not fit properly, are high heeled, or do not adequately support the feet
- Tendon and ligament degeneration because of increasing weight and weight-bearing activities
- Degenerative conditions: rheumatoid arthritis, osteoarthritis, diabetes mellitus
- Congenital hallux valgus

SIGNS/SYMPTOMS

- Valgus (away from midline) deformity with altered gait
- Inflammation of the bursa (bunion): redness, swelling, warmth, tenderness, pain

- Great difficulty in fitting shoes
- Deformity and crowding of second toe
- Splayfoot (spreading out of foot)

COMPLICATIONS

- Development of bunion
- Stress fracture
- Degenerative joint disease

DIAGNOSTIC TESTS

- Describe each procedure, its purpose, and the normal feelings or sensations that are likely, as well as any preprocedural and postprocedural care.
  - —X-rays: to show displacement of the great toe, degenerative arthritic joint changes

TREATMENT
Medical

- Therapy
  - —Appropriately fitted or molded footwear to accommodate the deformity
  - —Form-fitting insole in shoe to cushion foot
  - —Night splints to decrease discomfort
  - —Felt ring pads or covering cap around bunion to relieve pressure
  - —Application of moist compresses to bursitis area
  - —Application of ice to site of bunion to lessen pain and inflammation
  - —Foot exercises and metatarsal arch support to lessen splayfoot

Surgical

- Bunionectomy and arthroplasty
- Arthrodesis
- Osteotomy to realign bones

HOME CARE

- Give both the patient and the caregiver *verbal* and *written* instructions. Provide them with the name and telephone number of a physician or nurse to call if questions arise.
- *General information*
  - —Review explanation of the disease and contributing factors.

- *Special instructions*
    —Discuss the importance of and give examples of proper footware and its role in prevention and progression of bunion formation.
    —Provide instruction in the proper application of felt rings or pads and other orthoses to prevent the progression of deformities.
- *Medications*
    —Explain the purpose, dosage, schedule, and route of administration of any prescribed drugs, as well as side effects to report to a physician or nurse.
        Analgesics
        Antipyretics
        Antiinflammatory medications
- *Activity*
    —Instruct the patient in exercises to strengthen foot muscles, such as standing at the edge of a step on the heel and then raising and inverting the top of the foot.

Bunionectomy

—Bunionectomy: surgical procedure to correct hallux valgus, performed when the patient has significant pain and alterations in ambulation. This surgery involves removal of the projecting metatarsal head as well as excision of the proximal part of the proximal phalanx. Depending on the extent of involvement of the joint and surrounding soft tissues, a number of other procedures may be included in the operative procedure. The addition of these procedures will affect the length of recovery and rehabilitation:

- Arthroplasty: removal of part of the bone and realignment to permit rebuilding of the joints
- Osteotomy: cutting of the bone and resetting it using a pin or pins to maintain proper alignment

- Soft tissue reconstruction: realignment of the toes where the soft tissue, tendons, and muscles of the foot have become stretched or contracted
- Prosthetic implant: removal of part of the joint and replacement with an implant

INDICATIONS

- Severe deformity and pain of hallux valgus

PREPROCEDURAL TEACHING

- Review the physician's explanation of the procedure and the reason for it; encourage the patient to ask questions and to discuss any fears or anxieties.

Review of Preprocedural Care

- Explain that the procedure is usually done on an outpatient basis.
- Discuss preoperative tests: blood tests, chest x-ray, electro-cardiogram.
- Discuss skin preparation: the patient should shower with bactericidal soap the night before; the skin at the operative site will be shaved.
- Explain that the patient is NPO from midnight of the night before surgery.

Review of Postprocedural Care

- Discuss the need to immobilize the affected foot with a short leg cast, slipper cast, or bunion boot (to immobilize the great toe).
- Discuss the need to maintain complete bed rest for 12 to 24 hours, then up with crutches without weight bearing as prescribed by the physician.
- Explain the need to elevate the extremity on firm pillows to lessen swelling.
- Explain that ice bags will be placed on the operative site to reduce swelling for 24 to 72 hours.
- Inform the patient that vital signs and neurovascular status will be checked every 15 minutes for the first hour and then with decreasing frequency.

SIDE EFFECTS/COMPLICATIONS

- Excessive scarring or recurrence of bunion
- Weakening of foot joint

- Infection
- Neurovascular damage

🏠 HOME CARE

- Give both the patient and the caregiver *verbal* and *written* instructions. Provide them with the name and telephone number of a physician or nurse to call if questions arise.
- *Warning signs*
  —Review the signs and symptoms that should be reported to a physician or nurse.

  > Neurovascular impairment of affected extremity: persistent changes in color (pallor, cyanosis, redness), coolness, paresthesias (numbness, tingling)

  > Infection: increased redness, swelling at incision, purulent drainage from wound, foul odor from cast or dressing, fever, increasing pain

- *Special instructions*
  —Discuss the importance of wearing an immobilization device (cast or bunion boot) for 3 to 6 weeks after surgery.
  —Instruct the patient on caring for the extremity in the cast (or the dressed foot) (see Cast Care, p. 656).
  —Advise the patient to wear flat, wide-toed shoes and sandals after the dressing or cast is removed.
  —Discuss principles and examples of proper footwear.
  —Instruct the patient to elevate the feet whenever pain or swelling of the feet is experienced and to report to the physician if pain and swelling do not subside.
  —Explain that friction and pressure of light shoes can cause recurrence.
- *Medications*
  —Explain the purpose, dosage, schedule, and route of administration of any prescribed drugs, as well as side effects to report to a physician or nurse.
- *Activity*
  —Inform the patient of the importance of limiting activity and resting frequently with feet elevated.
  —Discuss the importance of using crutches without weight bearing as prescribed by the physician. Refer the patient to physical therapy for instruction.
  —Review safety precautions to be taken when ambulating with crutches (see Crutch Walking, p. 671).

FOLLOW-UP CARE

- Stress the importance of regular follow-up visits. Make sure the patient has the necessary names and telephone numbers.

Burns

—Burn: injury to the skin and epithelial tissues that results from direct contact or exposure to temperature extremes or electrical, chemical, or radiation sources.

CLASSIFICATION OF BURNS

- Superficial (first degree): epidermal layer involvement only; epidermis is red with no blister formation
    —Signs/symptoms
        Pain
        Redness
        Blanching with pressure
        Normal texture
- Partial thickness (second degree): destruction of epidermal and dermal layers, which are blistered, with subcutaneous edema and pain
    —Signs/symptoms
        Pain
        Blisters
        Redness
        Blanching with pressure
        Firm texture
- Full thickness (third and fourth degree): all layers of skin destroyed; fat, muscle, nerves, blood supply, and bone may be affected
    —Signs/symptoms
        Dryness
        Pale, white, brown, or red color
        Charring
        No capillary refill
        No pain
        Firm, leathery skin texture

CAUSES

- Thermal burns: exposure to flames, hot liquids, radiation
- Chemical burns: contact, ingestion, inhalation, or injection of acids, alkalies, or vesicants
- Electrical burns: electrical current passing through the body to the ground

COMPLICATIONS

- Dehydration
- Hypoxia
- Circulatory collapse
- Hematuria, oliguria
- Anemia
- Adult respiratory distress syndrome
- Septic shock
- Emotional shock
- Curling's ulcer
- Gastric atony
- Disseminated intravascular coagulation
- Disuse atrophy, contractures
- Infection
- Stress diabetes

DIAGNOSTIC TESTS

- Describe each procedure, its purpose, and the normal feelings or sensations that are likely, as well as any preprocedural and postprocedural care.
  - —Laboratory studies
    - Complete blood count
    - Electrolytes
    - Blood urea nitrogen, creatinine
    - Arterial carboxyhemoglobin
    - Arterial blood gases
    - Bilirubin
    - Phosphorus
    - Alkaline phosphatase
    - Urine for myoglobin and hemoglobin tests
    - Clotting studies
  - —Bronchoscopy: to determine upper airway injury
  - —Lung scan: to determine small airway burns

TREATMENT
Immediate Treatment of Major Burns
Medical

- Therapy
    —NPO for first 12 to 24 hours; total parenteral nutrition
    —Airway maintenance
    —Humidification with 10% oxygen for inhalation injuries
    —Fluid replacement
    —Urethral catheterization
    —Nasogastric tube insertion
    —Wound cleansing with bactericidal solution
    —Central venous line insertion
    —Swan-Ganz catheter to monitor pulmonary arterial and capillary wedge pressures
- Drugs
    —Narcotic analgesics
    —Sedatives
    —Tetanus immunization
    —Diphtheria-tetanus vaccine

Surgical

- Escharotomy
- Fasciotomy

Long-Term Treatment of Major Burns
Medical

- Therapy
    —Hydrotherapy: 1 to 2 times daily to remove dressings and debride wounds
    —Dressings: wet to dry or dry
    —Hyperalimentation if necessary; high-calorie, high-protein diet with vitamin and iron supplement
- Drugs
    —Antibiotics: topical sterile application
    —Narcotic analgesics

Surgical

- Skin grafts
- Amputation if limb severely injured
- Wound debridement

Minor Burns
Medical

- Therapy
  —Wound cleansing with bactericidal solution
  —Wound debridement
  —Dressing changes: nonadherent multilayered dressings changed 1 to 2 times daily; polyurethane, hydrocolloid, silver sulfadiazine dressings left on for several days to 1 week
- Drugs
  —Tetanus vaccine
  —Diphtheria-tetanus vaccine
  —Topical antibiotics
  —Narcotic analgesics
  —Analgesic-antipyretics

🏠 HOME CARE

- Give both the patient and the caregiver *verbal* and *written* instructions. Provide them with the name and telephone number of a physician or nurse to call if questions arise.
- *General information*
  —Review the explanation of the type of burn and the extent of damage.
  —Discuss and prepare the patient for transfer to rehabilitation or long-term facility as ordered.
- *Wound/incision care*
  —Instruct the patient in wound care and dressing changes (for minor burns).
     Inspect wound for signs of infection.
     Cleanse wound with half-strength Betadine using sterile gauze; rub gently to remove existing topical agent.
     Apply topical antibiotic thickly enough to cover wound to provide healing and prevent dressing from adhering.
     Apply nonadherent fine-mesh gauze, then fluffed bulky coarse gauze to absorb drainage. Hold in place with semielastic net to exert even pressure.
  —Discuss the importance of avoiding contamination. Explain how to dispose of soiled dressings.
  —Discuss that the healing process with new skin development is expected in 6 weeks with mature healing within 6 to 12 months, depending on the extent of injury.

—Review the care of healed burns.

Wash skin gently, rinse well, dry thoroughly, and apply cream.

Avoid exposure to direct sunlight, harsh detergent, fabric softeners, and irritation by rubbing of clothing.

Use moisturizers and sunscreens to decrease irritation.

- *Warning signs*
  —Review the signs and symptoms that should be reported to a physician or nurse.

  Fever, malaise

  Redness, swelling, pain from burn area

  Bleeding, odor, drainage from burn area

- *Special instructions*
  —Advise the patient to avoid contact with persons with infections, especially upper respiratory infections.

  —Advise and assist the patient in obtaining medical supplies for dressings and any special assistive devices for home care management.

  —Inform the patient that cosmetic or reconstructive surgery may be required for extensive burns.

- *Medications*
  —Explain the purpose, dosage, schedule, and route of administration of any prescribed drugs, as well as side effects to report to a physician or nurse.

  —Caution the patient to avoid using over-the-counter medications unless approved by a physician.

- *Activity*
  —Explain the importance of planning rest periods.

  —Discuss maintaining normal activity as tolerated.

  —Encourage active and passive range-of-motion exercises of affected limbs to prevent muscle wasting and contractures.

  —Instruct the patient on the use of any assistive-adaptive or positioning devices as ordered.

  —Explain the importance of physiotherapy to assist in the exercise regimen.

  —Encourage water exercises to maintain limb mobility.

  —Encourage discussion of allowances and limitations with regard to occupation, recreational sports, and activities.

- *Diet*
  —Emphasize the importance of a diet high in calories, protein, and vitamins to maintain weight and aid in healing. Refer the

patient to the dietary department for assistance in meal planning.
—Encourage adequate fluid intake.

PSYCHOSOCIAL CARE

- Encourage verbalization of fears, concerns, and grief over disfigurement and loss of any function.
- Promote self-care activities as soon as possible.

FOLLOW-UP CARE

- Stress the importance of regular medical, laboratory, and physical therapy follow-up until recovery is complete. Make sure the patient has the necessary names and telephone numbers.

REFERRALS

- Advise about and refer the patient to support groups and community resources to assist in the resumption of usual activities and relationships.
- Provide referrals for medical social services, home health care assistance, and rehabilitation.

Cancer

—Cancer: the most common cause of death in the United States, cancer is a universal disease that affects people without regard to race, gender, socioeconomic status, or culture. However, different forms of cancer strike specific age, ethnic, and gender groups with varying frequency and severity. The most common sites of fatal cancer in men are the lungs, prostate, colon, and rectum; in women they are the lungs, breasts, colon, and rectum. Some cancers, such as those of the stomach, breast, colon, rectum, uterus, and lung, occur in a familial pattern. Certain diseases, such as multiple familial polyposis and Gardner's syndrome, are premalignant. Other possible causes of cancer include immunosuppressive drugs and viruses (adenoviruses, papovaviruses, herpes viruses, human T-cell lymphoma-leukemia virus, Epstein-Barr virus, and hepatitis B virus).

PREVENTION

- Assess the patient's level of knowledge about risk factors, preventive measures, and signs and symptoms of specific types of cancer that should be reported to a physician or nurse. Clarify any fears or misconceptions.
- Review primary prevention guidelines.
  —Smoking: do not smoke; stop smoking if already a habit; avoid use of tobacco products such as cigarettes, cigars, snuff, chewing tobacco, and pipe tobacco.
  —Sunlight: avoid exposure to sunlight; use a sunscreen if being in the sun is necessary; wear protective clothing, especially a cover for the face and head.
  —Radiation: avoid excessive exposure to ionizing radiation and radon.
  —Occupational hazards: avoid exposure to industrial agents such as asbestos.
  —Alcohol: limit consumption of alcohol.
  —Nutrition: eat high-fiber foods, low-fat foods, and vegetables and fruits rich in vitamins A and C; avoid salt-cured, smoked, and nitrite-cured foods; maintain proper weight for age, sex, and body frame.
- For female patients review specific *preventive measures* for women.
  —Breast
    Perform monthly self-breast examinations (SBE), preferably after the menstrual period.
    Have regular clinical breast examinations: every 3 years for women ages 20 to 39, every year for women 40 and older.
    Have mammography: baseline examination between the ages of 35 and 39, every 1 to 2 years for ages 40 to 49, every year for ages 50 and older.
  —Cervix
    Have a Papanicolaou (Pap) test and pelvic examination every year if sexually active or age 18 and older.
    Use caution with estrogen replacement therapy to control symptoms of menopause.
    Avoid prolonged use of estrogen birth control pills.

Cancer staging using TNM classification*

Stage	T	N	M	Survival	Comments
I	1	0	0	70%-90%	Operable and resectable
II	2	1	0	±50%	Operable but uncertainty of total resection
III	3	2	0	±20%	Operable but not resectable
IV	4	3	+	<5%	Distant metastases; inoperable

T, Primary tumor; T_1, T_2, T_3, T_4, progressive increase in tumor size or involvement; *N*, regional lymph nodes; N_1, N_2, N_3, increasing degree of abnormal regional lymph nodes; *M*, metastasis present; M_0, absence; M_+, presence.

*Survival rates and comments may vary with type and location of primary tumor, nodes, and metastases.

- For male patients review specific preventive measures for men.
  —Perform testicular self-examination every month after age 15.
  —Have regular physical examinations for prostate cancer: yearly for men younger than 50 years, every 6 months for men 50 years and older.
  —Obtain prostate specific antigen (PSA) assay for men aged 50 years and older.

STAGING AND GRADING OF CANCER

The purpose of cancer staging and grading is to describe the extent of the malignant tumor so that the physician can plan treatment, determine the prognosis, and evaluate the results. Staging should be done during the pretreatment phase of disease and after surgery if that is one of the prescribed treatments. It is also done if the disease recurs after a disease-free interval.

Clinical staging includes physical examination and evaluation of biopsy specimens (tumor and lymph nodes). The generally used staging system (TNM) is based on measurement of primary tumor (size, depth of penetration, invasion of adjacent structures); lymph node involvement (presence, extent, and location); and metastatic spread (presence of distant metastases) (see table on opposite page).

Grading is histologic classification of a tumor, which is useful in determining prognosis. Cancers are usually classified as 1 (well differentiated) to 4 (poorly differentiated). The more poorly

Differences between benign and malignant tumors

Characteristic	Benign tumor	Malignant tumor
Structure and differentiation	Typical of tissue origin	Atypical of tissue origin
Rate of growth	Usually slow	May be slow, rapid, or very rapid
Progression	Slowly progressive (may remain stationary; may regress); rarely fatal if treated	Usually progressive; almost always fatal if untreated
Mode of growth	Expansion (encapsulated)	Infiltration and/or metastasis
Tissue destruction	No	Common (ulceration and necrosis)
Recurrence	Rare	Common
Prognosis	May be fatal if inaccessible	Fatal if uncontrolled

From Belcher AE: *Cancer nursing*, St Louis, 1992, Mosby.

differentiated a tumor is, the less it looks like normal cells and the poorer the prognosis.

TERMINOLOGY

- Benign versus malignant: see table above.
- Doubling time: mean length of time for division of all tumor cells present; it has been calculated that approximately 30 doubling times are required for a tumor to reach 1 centimeter in diameter.
- Direct invasion of contiguous organs or local spread: tumor cells can invade a structure such as the uterus; spread from one organ to another, such as from the colon to the liver; or implant in surrounding serous cavities such as cancer of the ovary that spreads to the peritoneal surface (also called seeding).
- Metastasis: spread of cancer from a primary site of origin to distant organs by lymphatics or blood vessels, such as the spread of lung cancer to the brain; common sites of metastasis are the lungs, liver, bones, and brain.

- Types of cancer:
  - —Carcinomas: cancers of epithelial cells
  - —Sarcomas: cancers of bone, muscle, or connective tissue
  - —Leukemias: cancers of blood-forming organs
  - —Lymphomas: cancers of infection-fighting organs

Cardiac Catheterization

—**Cardiac catheterization: an invasive procedure used to visualize the heart's chambers, valves, great vessels, and coronary arteries.**

INDICATIONS

- To evaluate heart muscle and valve function
- To evaluate coronary arteries
- To diagnose valve abnormalities (insufficiency and stenosis)
- To identify and diagnose congenital heart anomalies
- To obtain an endomyocardial biopsy to evaluate for rejection of cardiac transplant.
- Used in diagnostic and therapeutic procedures: electrophysiologic studies, hemodynamic monitoring, percutaneous transluminal angioplasty (PTA), intracoronary stenting, rotational atherectomy of thrombus, intracoronary injection of medications to dissolve clot, palliative procedures for congenital heart defects

PROCEDURE

The procedure, which uses a flexible radiopaque catheter, may involve one or all of the following:
- Right-sided catheterization: performed to evaluate the function of the right side of the heart, including pressures and cardiac output. This technique is also used for continuous hemodynamic monitoring at the bedside. Catheter insertion is through the arm, neck (basilic or subclavian vein), or leg (femoral vein). The catheter is then guided into the chambers of the right side of the heart and the pulmonary artery.

- Left-sided catheterization: performed to evaluate function and pressures of the aorta and left side of the heart. Information about muscle function and the mitral and aortic valves can be obtained. Catheter insertion is usually via an artery in the arm (brachial) or leg (femoral). The catheter is guided up to the aorta and then into the left ventricle across the aortic valve. The route of entry for either left or right catheterization is by cut-down or more commonly percutaneously.
- Angiography: performed during left-sided catheterization, angiography involves injection of radiopaque contrast material through a cardiac catheter to obtain sequential films that selectively visualize the coronary blood vessels or heart chambers. There are two filming methods: cineangiography, a technique that produces a motion picture film of the fluoroscopic images, and serial angiography, which produces a series of x-ray (roentgenographic) films.

Other techniques that are available to evaluate heart function include the following:

- Coronary arteriography: shows abnormalities in the coronary arteries
- Ventriculography of the right or left ventricle: demonstrates chamber volume, wall thickness, and wall motion and detects abnormalities of contraction and atrioventricular valve regurgitation

PREPROCEDURAL TEACHING

- Review the physician's explanation of the procedure and the reason for it; encourage the patient to ask questions and to discuss any fears or anxieties. Explain the need to obtain informed consent.

Review of Preprocedural Care

- Determine whether the patient has any allergies to shellfish or iodine.
- Explain that the procedure is usually done on an outpatient basis and that no food or fluids are permitted for 6 to 12 hours beforehand.
- Inform the patient that routine medications must be withheld as directed by the physician.
- Explain that the skin at the insertion site will be shaved and cleansed.

- Inform the patient that light sedation will be given before the procedure.
- Describe the procedure.
  —The patient is taken to a special laboratory room and placed on a padded surgical table.
  —Depending on the type of catheterization to be performed, the procedure takes 1 to 3 hours.
  —The selected site is again cleansed and sterilized.
  —A local anesthetic is injected into a selected site (groin, inside of right arm, right side of neck).
  —A catheter is inserted and threaded up through the vein or artery. Once it is in place, the physician injects a contrast dye through it.
- Inform the patient that he or she will be required to lie flat for the procedure.
- Review sensations likely to be experienced during the procedure: palpitations; warm, flushed feeling; nausea or chest pain during insertion of the dye. Assure the patient that the sensations will pass quickly. Instruct the patient to follow directions to cough or breathe deeply.

Review of Postprocedural Care

- Explain that after the procedure is completed, the catheter is removed and a pressure dressing is applied to the site to control bleeding. The site is checked frequently for bleeding. For certain procedures (e.g., PTA), the catheter may be left in place. If the procedure is being done for diagnostic reasons, the patient is returned to a recovery room. If it is done for therapeutic reasons, the patient may be transferred to a special care unit.
- Discuss the sensations that may be felt: soreness at the insertion site, possible backache from lying on a table for 1 to 3 hours.
- Inform the patient of the need to maintain complete bed rest with the head slightly (20 to 30 degrees) elevated.
- Stress the importance of keeping the extremity straight and immobile for 2 to 4 hours after the procedure or as ordered.
- Inform the patient that vital signs, including peripheral pulses, will be checked every 15 minutes for the first hour, then with decreasing frequency.
- Tell the patient that diet and fluids will be resumed after return to the recovery area. Fluids are encouraged.

SIDE EFFECTS/COMPLICATIONS

- Ventricular dysrhythmias
- Allergic reaction to dye
- Nausea and vomiting
- Hypotension
- Bleeding at insertion site
- Thrombus (pain) at insertion site
- Local infection
- Cardiac perforation
- Myocardial ischemia
- Cardiac tamponade
- Renal insufficiency or failure

HOME CARE

- Give both the patient and the caregiver *verbal* and *written* instructions. Provide them with the name and telephone number of a physician or nurse to call if questions arise.
- *General information*
  —Review the procedure, answering any questions about the purpose or the physician's explanation of the findings.
- *Wound/incision care*
  —Provide instruction on care of the puncture site.
  —Inform the patient that bruising of and around the insertion site is normal.
- *Warning signs*
  —Review the signs and symptoms that should be reported to a physician or nurse.
      Pain, swelling, bleeding, or discoloration of puncture site
      Chest pain
      Elevated temperature
- *Activity*
  —Unless otherwise instructed, the patient may resume all normal activities within 1 week. Showers may be resumed within 48 hours or as ordered. Strenuous activities such as running, biking, or heavy lifting should be avoided for 5 to 7 days after the procedure.

FOLLOW-UP CARE

- Stress the importance of regular follow-up visits. Make sure the patient has the necessary names and telephone numbers.

Carotid Endarterectomy

—**Carotid endarterectomy: surgical removal of atherosclerotic plaque or thrombus from the carotid artery to increase blood flow through the carotid arteries to the brain.**

INDICATIONS

- Transient ischemic attacks
- Syncope
- Dizziness
- Asymptomatic high-grade carotid lesions

PREPROCEDURAL TEACHING

- Review the physician's explanation of the procedure and the reason for it; encourage the patient to ask questions and to discuss any fears or anxieties. Review the location of the lesion. Explain the need for written consent.

Review of Preprocedural Care

- Explain that the operation may be performed under local (cervical block) or general anesthesia. An incision is made on the side of the neck where the diseased artery is located. The incision extends down from the jawline to the base of the neck. Explain that the patient may experience transient numbness in the earlobe after surgery.
- Review diagnostic tests that will be done to confirm the diagnosis: cerebral angiography, carotid ultrasound, and photo-angiography.
- Discuss preoperative laboratory tests: blood and urine test, chest x-ray, electrocardiogram.
- Explain the need for the patient to have nothing by mouth (NPO) for 12 to 24 hours before the operation.
- Explain that the patient may be admitted to the hospital on the day of surgery.
- Tell the patient that the operative site will be cleansed and shaved.

Review of Postprocedural Care

- Inform the patient that ambulation will be permitted on the day of surgery if there are no complications.

- Explain that the patient may remain in the intensive care unit for 24 hours after surgery for monitoring and then transferred to a regular room.

SIDE EFFECTS/COMPLICATIONS

- Stroke
- Heart attack
- Transient episodes of postoperative hypertension and hypotension
- Cranial nerve injuries
- Wound hematoma
- Infection
- Shock
- Seizure activity

HOME CARE

- Give both the patient and the caregiver *verbal* and *written* instructions. Provide them with the name and telephone number of a physician or nurse to call if questions arise.
- *Wound/incision care*
  —Provide instruction regarding daily care of the surgical incision and dressing changes.
- *Warning signs*
  —Review the signs and symptoms that should be reported to a physician or nurse.
      Unusual pain or swelling in the operative area
      Signs of infection: redness, pain, swelling, soreness, feeling of tenderness, drainage
      Sudden changes in vision, gait, or muscle strength
      Dizziness, numbness, or weakness on one side of the body
- *Special instructions*
  —Describe the atherosclerotic process and discuss the importance of risk factor modification to reduce the chance of future plaque buildup in the carotid and other arteries (see Coronary Artery Disease, p. 209).
  —For any neurologic deficit or stroke complications, see p. 593.
- *Medications*
  —Explain the purpose, dosage, schedule, and route of administration of any prescribed drugs, as well as side effects to report to a physician or nurse.

- *Activity*
    —Tell the patient to exercise to tolerance but to avoid bending from the waist or lifting and straining.

FOLLOW-UP CARE

- Stress the importance of regular follow-up visits. Make sure the patient has the necessary names and telephone numbers.

Carpal Tunnel Release

—Carpal tunnel release: surgical decompression of the nerve by releasing the carpal ligament to restore sensation and mobility to the hand.

INDICATIONS

- Persistent or progressive signs and symptoms of carpal tunnel syndrome, unrelieved by conservative treatment

PREPROCEDURAL TEACHING

- Review the physician's explanation of the procedure and the reason for it; encourage the patient to ask questions and to discuss any fears or anxieties. Discuss the need for written consent for the surgery and local anesthesia.

Review of Preprocedural Care

- Explain the need for the patient to be NPO from midnight of the night before surgery.
- Discuss the preoperative blood and urine tests.
- Inform the patient about the skin preparation: arm, wrist, and hand shaved and cleansed with bactericidal soap.
- Explain that hospital admission may be on the day of surgery.
- Explain that the procedure takes about 45 minutes and is done under local anesthesia.

Review of Postprocedural Care

- Explain that the hand will be bandaged and the arm will be elevated in a cast or splint.

- Inform the patient that vital signs and neurovascular status will be checked every 15 minutes for the first hour and then at increasing intervals.
- Discuss the need to move all fingers of the affected hand frequently to improve circulation.

SIDE EFFECTS/COMPLICATIONS

- Infection
- Neurovascular injury
- Keloid formation

HOME CARE

- Give both the patient and the caregiver *verbal* and *written* instructions. Provide them with the name and telephone number of a physician or nurse to call if questions arise.
- *General information*
  —Review any explanation about the procedure and specific follow-up care.
- *Wound/incision care*
  —Instruct the patient on care of the hand and dressing: to keep the arm and hand elevated above heart level to reduce swelling and promote healing.
  —Tell the patient to check the dressing daily for signs of increased bleeding or drainage. Discuss the need to keep the dressing clean, dry, and intact. Explain that when bathing is permitted (usually as soon as the patient feels strong), the patient should shower with the dressing covered by a plastic bag.
- *Warning signs*
  —Review the signs and symptoms that should be reported to a physician or nurse.
    Neurovascular impairment: burning, tingling sensation of fingers; increased pain or throbbing in fingers unrelieved by prescribed analgesics; inability to move fingers; discoloration of fingers; fingers that are cool and do not warm up after being covered
    Infection: fever >101° F, malaise, increased pain, foul odor from dressing
- *Medications*
  —Explain the purpose, dosage, schedule, and route of administration of any prescribed drugs, as well as side effects to report to a physician or nurse.

- *Activity*
  —Review activity allowances and limitation. Encourage discussion regarding return to work, recreational sports, and activities.
  —Discuss any prescribed exercises to maintain circulation and improve range of motion, such as sponge squeezing.

FOLLOW-UP CARE

- Stress the importance of regular follow-up visits. Make sure the patient has the necessary names and telephone numbers.

Carpal Tunnel Syndrome

—**Carpal tunnel syndrome: a combination of symptoms affecting the functioning of the wrist, hand, and fingers. Carpal tunnel syndrome occurs when inflammation and fibrosis of the tendon sheaths that pass through the carpal tunnel structures of the hand cause swelling and compression of the median nerve at the wrist, resulting in pain and numbness. Carpal tunnel syndome is one of the most common industrial or work-related conditions. It occurs most frequently in women between 30 and 60 years of age.**

CAUSES/CONTRIBUTING FACTORS

- Trauma, injury: wrist fractures, dislocation, sprains (but may occur with no prior history of trauma)
- Repetitive hand or wrist movement such as wrist twisting, turning, or pounding as occurs in some occupations (e.g., painters, computer users, jackhammer operators)
- Chronic medical disorders: rheumatoid arthritis, renal failure, Raynaud's disease
- Pregnancy: last trimester because of fluid retention and edema
- Menopause

SIGNS/SYMPTOMS

Signs and symptoms may affect one or both hands. They are worse in the morning or at night and may awaken the patient.

They may occur while the patient is holding the hand in one position, such as while driving or typing.

- Pain, numbness, tingling
- Grip strength loss, inability to make a fist
- Muscle weakness
- Wrist swelling
- Burning
- Palmar thenar (base of thumb) atrophy
- Comparative sensations loss over palmar thumb, index, middle, and radial half of ring finger

COMPLICATIONS

- Prolonged muscle weakness and atrophy
- Rupture of tendon sheath from inadvertent injection of corticosteroids

DIAGNOSTIC TESTS

- Describe each procedure, its purpose, and the normal feelings or sensations that are likely, as well as any preprocedural and postprocedural care.
  —Compression tests of the median nerve
    Positive Tinel's sign: tingling over the median nerve with a light tapping over the tendon sheath on the ventral (inner) surface of the wrist
    Positive Phalen's test: appearance of symptoms with the forearm in vertical position and wrist held in complete flexion for 1 minute
    Positive compression test: pain, numbness, and tingling provoked when a blood pressure cuff is inflated above systolic pressure on the forearm for 1 to 2 minutes
  —Electroconductive tests
    Electromyogram: detects denervation of thenar muscles (base of thumb)
    Nerve conduction velocity study: measures speed of electricity along nerve; may show delayed nerve response
  —X-ray: may show bony pressure on tunnel area; rules out fractures, arthritis

TREATMENT
Medical

- Therapy
  —Conservative treatment usually tried first if symptoms have been present for less than 2 months
  —Wrist immobilization:
    Splint to relieve pressure and decrease wrist flexion
    Ice application to volar (ventral) wrist
    Elevation to decrease edema
    Restriction of twisting and turning of wrist
- Drugs
  —Local injection of hydrocortisone (into tendon sheath) to relieve inflammation
  —Antiinflammatory agents

Surgical

- Carpal tunnel release

HOME CARE

- Give both the patient and the caregiver *verbal* and *written* instructions. Provide them with the name and telephone number of a physician or nurse to call if questions arise.
- *General information*
  —Describe the disorder, causes, and contributing factors.
- *Warning signs*
  —Review the signs and symptoms that should be reported to a physician or nurse. Sensory changes are indicative of increased compression of the median nerve.
    Increased burning, tingling of fingers
    Increased pain
    Numbness
    Discoloration of fingers (i.e., red, blue, or white rather than pink)
- *Medications*
  —Explain the purpose, dosage, schedule, and route of administration of any prescribed drugs, as well as side effects to report to a physician or nurse.
- *Activity*
  —Instruct the patient to avoid activities that increase stress on inflamed tissues (grasping and gripping action of hand and

wrist); to keep the wrist in neutral position; to avoid using the wrist in a bent (flexed), twisted, turned position; and to minimize repetitive movements, including holding an object for extended periods of time. Advise the patient to wear a wrist splint to help keep the wrist in neutral position.

—Discuss the role prevention plays in controlling carpal tunnel syndrome; review preventive measures.

> Use the whole hand and all fingers to grasp an object versus using the thumb and index finger, which will put stress on the wrist.
>
> Limit wrist movement as flexion increases compression and tension of the inflamed nerve.
>
> Instruct the patient how and when to apply a night or occupational wrist splint, explaining that its purpose is to decrease wrist flexion and movement, especially at night or when engaging in repetitive wrist movement. Advise patient where to obtain splints.
>
> Rest the hands periodically.
>
> Reduce speed in doing forceful and repetitive movements.

—Elevate the hand above heart level to decrease swelling.

—Apply ice to the wrist to decrease swelling.

—Teach the patient range-of-motion exercises and explain their importance for maintaining strength of muscles. If the patient is wearing a splint, tell the patient to remove it to perform daily exercises.

FOLLOW-UP CARE

• Stress the importance of regular follow-up visits. Make sure the patient has the necessary names and telephone numbers.

Cataract and Cataract Surgery

—**Cataract: growing opacity of the lens and lens capsule usually associated with aging, although it can be congenital or caused by trauma, heat, toxins, intraocular inflammation, or chronic disease.**

RISK FACTORS

- Women older than 65 years of age
- Residence in warm, sunny climate
- High-dose radiation
- Long-term use of drugs such as corticosteroids, phenothiazines, chemotherapy agents
- Diabetes
- High blood pressure
- Blunt trauma
- Maternal rubella in first trimester
- Down syndrome

SIGNS/SYMPTOMS

- Painless, gradual blurring
- Decreased peripheral vision
- Photophobia, glare, especially at night
- Milky white appearance of pupil
- Poor reading vision

DIAGNOSTIC TESTS

- Ophthalmoscopy with dilatation
- Slit lamp examination

TREATMENT
Surgical

- Cataract surgery if patient has diminished visual acuity or cataracts that may cause eye damage
- Cataract extraction: surgical extraction of the defective lens
  —Intracapsular: most common procedure; removal of the entire lens, including surrounding capsule
  —Extracapsular: removal of the anterior portion of the capsule and lens, leaving the posterior capsule intact; done on children and adults
  —Phacoemulsion: breaking the lens into fragments and particles using ultrasonic vibrations and removing them by suction; performed on patients younger than 30 years
  —Lens implantation: insertion of an intraocular lens implant following cataract excision; done to avoid the need to wear cataract glasses or contact lenses postoperatively; used for the following indications:
      Patients with good vision in the unoperated eye

Patients who are unable to manage self-care and insertion or removal of contact lenses (e.g., mentally impaired or with limited manual dexterity)

Patients who cannot wear a contact lens (dry eyes, severe allergies, severe astigmatism)

Adverse work environment (presence of dust or fumes)

Only one eye affected

PREPROCEDURAL TEACHING

- Review the physician's explanation of the procedure and the reason for it; encourage the patient to ask questions and to discuss any fears or anxieties.

Review of Preprocedural Care

- Explain that the procedure is done as same-day surgery.
- Explain the need for the patient to be NPO from midnight of the night before surgery.
- Discuss routine preoperative laboratory tests: blood and urine.
- Discuss preoperative medications.
  —Topical antiinfective agents, usually prescribed 1 week before surgery
  —Mydriatic-cycloplegic agents, usually prescribed 2 hours before surgery
  —Hyperosmotic agents
  —Sedatives/hypnotics

Review of Postprocedural Care

- Discuss the necessity of wearing an eye patch postoperatively for 24 to 72 hours.
- Discuss the need to wear a protective eye shield at night.
- Discuss postoperative medications.
  —Mydriatic-cycloplegic agents (not used in patients with lens implants)
  —Antiinfective eyedrops and ointments
  —Corticosteroids
  —Antiemetics
  —Analgesics
- Explain that medication will be administered to prevent nausea, vomiting, and straining with elimination to avoid increasing ocular pressure as indicated.

SIDE EFFECTS/COMPLICATIONS

- Cataract
  —Glaucoma
  —Blindness
- Cataract surgery
  —Wound rupture (from sutures loosening)
  —Hyphema
  —Hemorrhage
  —Prolapse of the iris into the anterior chamber
  —Loss of vitreous
  —Adhesions
  —Infection
  —Retinal detachment
  —Corneal edema
  —Lens displacement (if lens implant performed)

HOME CARE

- Give both the patient and the caregiver *verbal* and *written* instructions. Provide them with the name and telephone number of a physician or nurse to call if questions arise.
- Advise the patient to avoid squeezing the eyelids shut or touching the eyes postoperatively; encourage elderly patients to wear glasses during the day to avoid rubbing the eyes.
- *Warning signs*
  —Review the signs and symptoms that should be reported to a physician or nurse.
      Increased intraocular pressure: sudden onset of eye pain, photophobia, sudden decrease in vision, sudden severe headache
      Infection: redness and watering of eyes, swelling, blurred vision, pain
- *Special instructions*
  —Discuss the need to wear an eye shield at night for 2 to 6 weeks to avoid eye injury.
  —Warn that depth perception may be lost and that 50% of peripheral vision will be lost because of the eye patch. Review safety precautions.
      Instruct the patient to avoid falls by turning the head fully to the affected side to view objects.
      Advise the patient to use up-and-down head movements to judge stairs and oncoming objects and to move slowly.

Discuss the need to wear dark glasses during the day to avoid pupil constriction and glare, since the eye is sensitive to light after surgery.

—If the patient had cataract surgery without a lens implant, warn that vision will be diminished in one or both eyes until prescription eyeglasses or contact lenses are obtained (in about 4 to 8 weeks).

—If the patient is receiving eyeglasses, explain that images will be magnified 30%, peripheral vision will be impaired and distorted, and lenses will be bifocal or trifocal. Review safety precautions.

Turn head side to side to see peripherally.

Judge distances when descending stairs or viewing oncoming objects.

—If the patient is receiving contact lenses, explain that images will be magnified 7% to 10%, peripheral vision will be intact, and reading glasses may also be prescribed.

—Review the care, insertion, and removal of lenses. Advise the patient of the importance of routine appointments with the physician for removal, cleansing, and reinsertion of extended-wear lenses.

—If the patient is receiving an intraocular lens implant, explain that the lens implant aids in focusing but that glasses will be prescribed for close vision in 8 to 12 weeks; there will be no loss in depth perception.

• *Medications*

—Explain the purpose, dosage, schedule, and route of administration of any prescribed drugs, as well as side effects to report to a physician or nurse.

—Review the correct procedure for instilling eyedrops and ointments and applying an eye shield (without touching or applying pressure on the eyeball) to avoid self-inflicted injury.

—Advise the patient to avoid over-the-counter medications, eyedrops, or ointments without checking with the physician.

• *Activity*

—Explain the need to avoid activities that can increase intraocular pressure: heavy lifting, straining with elimination, bending over at the waist, coughing, vomiting.

—Instruct the patient to take medications for nausea and constipation as ordered.

—Instruct the patient to avoid sleeping on the operative side.
—Explain the need to avoid any strenuous exercise for 6 weeks; tell the patient to check with the physician before resuming occupational or recreational activities.
—Explain that it will be necessary to adjust to mild magnification when performing daily activities.

FOLLOW-UP CARE

- Stress the importance of regular follow-up visits. Make sure the patient has the necessary names and telephone numbers.

Cellulitis

—**Cellulitis: a suppurative inflammation of the dermis and subcutaneous tissue, usually from bacterial invasion through a broken area of the skin. Cellulitis may occur without an evident site of entry and spreads throughout the tissue spaces. Lymphangitis may occur. *Streptococcus pyogenes* and *Staphylococcus aureus* are the most common infecting organisms.**

CAUSES/CONTRIBUTING FACTORS

- Skin trauma
- Ulceration of skin
- Lymphedema

SIGNS/SYMPTOMS

- Localized pain, redness, swelling, skin tenderness
- "Peau d'orange": skin resembling that of an orange
- Lymphangitic streaks: red streaks on skin
- Pitting of skin with pressure
- Fever, chills, malaise
- Headache
- Characteristic lesion or open wound
- Purulent discharge from wound

C

COMPLICATIONS

- Abscesses
- Sepsis
- Gangrene
- Necrotizing subcutaneous infection
- Damage to lymphatic system

DIAGNOSTIC TESTS

- Describe each procedure, its purpose, and the normal feelings or sensations that are likely, as well as any preprocedural and postprocedural care.
    —Tests to identify causative organism: group A beta-hemolytic *Streptococcus* or *Staphylococcus aureus*
    —Culture of skin lesion
    —Blood culture
    —Blood tests
        Complete blood count and white blood cell count: to detect inflammatory process
        Erythrocyte sedimentation rate: will be elevated

TREATMENT
Medical

- Therapy
    —Intravenous antibiotic therapy for severe infection requiring hospitalization, usually about 2 days
    —Immobilization and elevation of the affected limb to reduce edema
    —Cool compresses for discomfort alternating with warm compresses or soaks to increase circulation to promote wound healing
- Drugs
    —Analgesics and antipyretics (aspirin or Tylenol)

Surgical

- Incision and drainage for formation that is unresponsive to treatment or in which tissue damage has occurred
- Debridement of devitalized structures: to remove damaged tissues

⌂ HOME CARE

- Give both the patient and the caregiver *verbal* and *written* instructions. Provide them with the name and telephone number of a physician or nurse to call if questions arise.
- *General information*
  —Explain the disorder and contributing causes.
- *Warning signs*
  —Review the signs and symptoms that should be reported to a physician or nurse.
    Headache, fever, chills
    Pain, redness, swelling, heat
    Purulent discharge
    Odor from dressing
- *Special instructions*
  —Explain the importance of elevation and immobilization of the affected limb for at least 2 to 3 days or until redness and swelling have subsided.
  —Instruct the patient in wound care and dressing changes.
    Explain how to wash an open wound or draining wound gently with a clean washcloth and soap and water and how to apply dressings using aseptic technique.
    Instruct the patient to wash hands before and after changing dressings and explain how to dispose of dirty dressings.
    Advise the patient on handling soiled linens and clothing; washing them separately in hot water prevents spread of infection.
  —Demonstrate how to apply cool compresses for discomfort, alternating with a warm compress or warm soak to increase circulation to the affected area.
- *Medications*
  —Explain the purpose, dosage, schedule, and route of administration of any prescribed drugs, as well as side effects to report to a physician or nurse.
  —Explain the need to take oral antibiotics for 1 week after infection has cleared. Tell the patient that it may be necessary to prolong the treatment for several weeks, depending on the severity of infection.
- *Activity*
  —Inform the patient that activity to tolerance using supportive devices (e.g., sling, crutches) is permitted. Instruct in the use of ambulatory aids as needed.

FOLLOW-UP CARE

- Stress the importance of regular follow-up visits. Make sure the patient has the necessary names and telephone numbers.

Cervical Cancer

—Cervical cancer: cancer of the cervix, the second most common cancer in women. The incidence is greater among women of lower socioeconomic status. Cervical cancers are classified as preinvasive and invasive. Preinvasive cancers are limited to the cervix and are curable in 75% to 90% of patients. Invasive cancers involve the cervix and other pelvic structures. The incidence of invasive cervical cancer is decreasing, but premalignant changes, referred to as "carcinoma in situ," are increasing, especially in young women. Cervical cancers are predominantly of the squamous cell type. Some are adenocarcinomas; the clear cell type is seen most commonly in younger women, and its incidence is increasing. The term "cervical intraepithelial neoplasia" is used to describe the malignant changes in the squamocolumnar junction that progress to involve full thickness. Cervical cancer spreads by direct extension and via the lymphatics and blood. Seventy-five percent of recurrence is local; 25% is distant metastases to the liver, bones, and mediastinal and supraclavicular nodes.

RISK FACTORS

- Initial intercourse at an early age, especially between 15 and 17 years of age
- Multiple sex partners
- Sexually transmitted diseases (particularly human papillomavirus, possibly herpes simplex virus)
- Pregnancies in the teen years
- History of smoking
- Long-term use of hormones such as progestin

SIGNS/SYMPTOMS

- Abnormal vaginal bleeding: painless, thin, watery, blood-tinged vaginal discharge that progresses to spotting and frank bleeding
- Prolonged menstrual period or intermittent periods
- "Contact" bleeding after intercourse
- Anemia caused by chronic blood loss
- Advanced disease: vaginal discharge becomes dark and foul smelling; pain in lower back, legs, and groin (pelvis); leg edema; difficulty voiding, urgency, and hematuria; rectal tenesmus and bleeding

DIAGNOSTIC TESTS

- Describe each procedure, its purpose, and the normal feelings or sensations that are likely, as well as any preprocedural and postprocedural care.
  - —Cervical examination and biopsy via colposcopy: to detect mass or malignant cells or both
  - —Computed tomography of abdomen: to determine retroperitoneal lymph node involvement
  - —Magnetic resonance imaging: to estimate tumor volume
  - —Lymphangiography: to determine lymph system involvement
  - —Chest x-ray, excretory urography, cystoscopy, proctosigmoidoscopy: to detect evidence of tumor spread

TREATMENT
Medical

- Therapy
  - —Cryotherapy (freezing of malignant lesion with portable cautery) or laser ablation
    - Complications: immediate: hemorrhage, uterine perforation; delayed: cervical stenosis, infertility, cervical incompetence, increased incidence of preterm (low-birth-weight) delivery
  - —Radiation therapy: external beam, intracavity
  - —Chemotherapy
    - Cisplatin
    - Carboplatin
    - Cyclophosphamide
    - Melphalan
    - 5-Fluorouracil

Vincristine

Methotrexate

Hydroxyurea

Surgical

- Conization: to treat carcinoma in situ in women of childbearing age
- Abdominal or vaginal radical hysterectomy and pelvic node dissection
  —Complications: ureteral fistulas, bladder dysfunction, pulmonary embolus, pelvic infection, bowel obstruction, rectovaginal fistulas, hemorrhage
- Pelvic exenteration: nodal dissection and removal of bladder, urethra, uterus, cervix, vagina, rectum, and all lateral supporting tissues; patient will have permanent fecal stoma and urinary diversion
  —Complications: pulmonary embolus or edema, cerebrovascular accident, hemorrhage, myocardial infarction, sepsis, small bowel obstruction

PREPROCEDURAL TEACHING

- Review the physician's explanation of the procedure, the reason for it, and any specific preprocedural or postprocedural care; encourage the patient to ask questions and to discuss any fears or anxieties, especially about changes in body image and function, fertility, and sexual function.

Review of Preprocedural Care

- For radiation therapy, explain that therapy induces menopause.
- For conization, tell the patient to expect spotting and bleeding for as long as a week after the procedure. Explain that cramping may occur.
- For hysterectomy and pelvic exenteration, see general preprocedural teaching for Abdominal Surgery, p. 6.
- For pelvic exenteration, encourage a preoperative visit by a rehabilitated person who has undergone similar surgery, including vaginal reconstruction when appropriate. The visitor may be from the United Ostomy Association. Offer to make referral to a sexual counselor.

Review of Postprocedural Care

- Encourage the patient to turn, cough, and deep breathe at regular intervals.
- Prepare the patient for the presence of bulky dressings on the surgical site, urethral catheters, and colostomy or ileostomy depending on the type of surgical procedure.
- Explain that the dressing will be inspected frequently and changed as needed.
- Encourage early ambulation.

HOME CARE

- Give both the patient and the caregiver *verbal* and *written* instructions. Provide them with the name and telephone number of a physician or nurse to call if questions arise.
- Review the explanation of the type of cancer and the therapeutic or surgical procedures to be performed. For radiation treatment see p. 721; for chemotherapy see p. 667.

Patient Undergoing Surgery

- *General information*
  —See Abdominal Surgery, p. 6.
- *Warning signs*
  —Review the signs and symptoms that should be reported to a physician or nurse.
  Infection: redness, edema, drainage, warmth, fever, pain at incision site
- *Activity*
  —Explain that the patient should avoid coitus and douching for 2 to 6 weeks after surgery as indicated by physician.
  —Stress the importance of walking at regular intervals and not sitting for long periods.
  —Avoid heavy lifting and vigorous activity for 6 to 8 weeks after surgery.

Patient Undergoing Cryosurgery/Laser Therapy

- *Special instructions*
  —Explain that perineal drainage is clear and watery initially, progressing to a foul-smelling discharge that contains dead cells. Report drainage that lasts longer than 8 weeks.

—Review perineal care and hygiene. Advise the patient that showers and sponge baths are permitted but that tub baths and sitz baths should be avoided.

—Discuss the need for regular Papanicolaou smears and pelvic examinations because of the high percentage of recurrence.

Patient Undergoing Pelvic Exenteration

• *Special instructions*

—Assist patient to obtain appropriate supplies for ostomy care (see Ostomy, p. 694).

—Provide instruction on perineal care. Explain that drainage may continue for several months and that the patient should take sitz baths as directed. Demonstrate wound irrigation procedures and application of sanitary pads as needed.

—Tell the patient to avoid prolonged sitting.

PSYCHOSOCIAL CARE

• Encourage expression of feelings, frustration, anger.
• Encourage questions and provide information.
• Provide referrals for counseling with psychologist as indicated.
• Encourage the patient to express feelings of loss of sexuality and body image.

FOLLOW-UP CARE

• Stress the importance of regular follow-up visits. Make sure the patient has the necessary names and telephone numbers.

REFERRALS

• Assist the patient to obtain services as needed for support groups and sexual and fertility counseling.

Charcot's Syndrome
(Neurogenic Arthropathy)

—Charcot's syndrome: a progressive degenerative disease of the stress-bearing portion of joints caused by impaired sensory nerve innervation. The resulting loss of sensation to the joints permits further destruction from trauma or from the underlying disease, which leads to laxity of supporting ligaments and disintegration of the affected joints. The weight-bearing joints are most commonly affected: knees, hips, ankles, and lower spine. The condition is most common in men over 40 years of age.

CAUSES/CONTRIBUTING FACTORS

- Diabetes mellitus: affects joints of feet
- Tabes dorsalis: degeneration of dorsal vertebrae affecting the large weight-bearing joints (knee, hip, ankle, lower spine)
- Syringomyelia: affects shoulder and upper extremity joints
- Charcot-Marie-Tooth disease: progressive atrophy of the peroneal nerve
- Intraarticular injection of corticosteroids: affects hip or knee joint
- Spinal cord trauma
- Paraplegia
- Peripheral nerve injury
- Myelomeningocele in children
- Leprosy
- Pernicious anemia

SIGNS/SYMPTOMS

- Neuropathy: loss of sensation in affected area
- In affected joint
  —Swelling
  —Warmth
  —Increased mobility
  —Instability
  —Deformity
  —Backache (if vertebral joints are affected)

COMPLICATIONS

- Joint subluxation or dislocation
- Articular (joint) fractures
- Pathologic fractures
- Amputation

DIAGNOSTIC TESTS

- Describe each procedure, its purpose, and the normal feelings or sensations that are likely, as well as any preprocedural and postprocedural care.
    - —X-rays: to confirm the diagnosis and assess the severity of joint damage
    - —Vertebral examination: to document narrowing of the disk spaces and vertebral deterioration
    - —Synovial biopsy: to detect bony fragments and bits of calcified cartilage
    - —Neuromuscular test: to look for sensory or motor defects

TREATMENT
Medical

- Therapy
    - —Immobilization: to protect the joint from stress and injury
        - Crutches, braces, splints
        - Restriction from weight bearing
        - Wheelchair
    - —Protective footwear
- Drugs
    - —Analgesics

Surgical

- Arthrodesis (joint fusion) for immobilization
- Amputation

HOME CARE

- Give both the patient and the caregiver *verbal* and *written* instructions. Provide them with the name and telephone number of a physician or nurse to call if questions arise.
- *General information*
    - —Explain the causes or contributory factors of the disorder and identify affected joints.
    - —Assist the patient to become familiar with his or her own pain pattern and sensory perceptions so that a baseline can be established against which to measure changes and responses to medication and treatment.
    - —Caution the patient that because of loss of sensation (neuropathy), injury can occur without causing pain or discomfort.

- *Warning signs*
  —Review the signs and symptoms that should be reported to a physician or nurse.
     Increasing joint pain, swelling, or instability
- *Special instructions*
  —Explain how to apply warm compresses to relieve local joint pain and tenderness.
  —Instruct the patient to inspect the skin of affected joints daily, checking for abrasions, cuts, or ulcers, and to report any lesions that do not heal. Alert the patient to the need to check water temperature to avoid burns.
  —Provide instruction in the proper technique for crutches or other immobilization devices. Refer the patient to the physical therapy department for proper fitting and the readjustment of devices.
  —Advise the patient to wear prescribed protective footwear and to avoid tight-fitting shoes and heels higher than 1 inch.
- *Medications*
  —Explain the purpose, dosage, schedule, and route of administration of any prescribed drugs, as well as side effects to report to a physician or nurse.
- *Activity*
  —Explain the importance of developing lifestyle techniques to protect the joints.
     Avoid fatigue.
     Pace daily activities and plan regular rest periods even when not feeling tired.
     Avoid physical activities that may cause pathologic fractures, such as walking and running.
     Take safety precautions at home to avoid falls or other injuries: remove throw rugs and keep passageways clear of clutter.
  —Encourage the discussion of allowances and limitations with regard to exercise, occupation, and recreation.

FOLLOW-UP CARE

- Stress the importance of regular follow-up visits. Make sure the patient has the necessary names and telephone numbers.

REFERRALS

- Provide referral for home health care as indicated.

Chest Trauma
(Flail Chest)

C

—Chest trauma: chest cage injury causing multiple fractures of ribs. Types of chest injury include penetrating (e.g., bullet and knife wounds, impaled objects) and nonpenetrating (e.g., falls, blunt trauma, deceleration injuries from automobile accident).

CAUSES/CONTRIBUTING FACTORS
- Automobile accidents
- Assaults
- Explosions
- Other types of accidents

SIGNS/SYMPTOMS
- Sharp chest pain
- Difficulty in breathing
- Shallow, rapid respirations
- Uneven chest wall movement
- Tachycardia
- Cyanosis
- Copious, blood-tinged sputum

COMPLICATIONS
- Tension pneumothorax
- Hemothorax
- Pulmonary edema
- Cardiac tamponade
- Respiratory arrest
- Shock

DIAGNOSTIC TESTS
- Explain that the following diagnostic procedures help confirm the diagnosis. Describe each procedure, its purpose, and the normal feelings or sensations that are likely, as well as any preprocedural and postprocedural care.
    —Chest x-ray: to examine for atelectasis, pneumothorax, evidence of fractured ribs

—Arterial blood gases: to monitor for hypoxemia (decreased Pao_2) and hypercapnia (increased $Paco_2$)

—Pulmonary function tests: performed by measuring the volume of air moving in and out of the lungs and then calculating lung capacities

TREATMENT
Medical

- Therapy
  —Oxygen therapy
  —Chest tube insertion
  —Intubation and mechanical ventilation
  —Pain management
- Drugs
  —Antibiotics
  —Neuromuscular blocking agents

HOME CARE

- Give both the patient and the caregiver *verbal* and *written* instructions. Provide them with the name and telephone number of a physician or nurse to call if questions arise.
- *General information*
  —Explain the underlying cause or contributing factors.
  —Show how to splint the chest when coughing to avoid pain.
- *Warning signs*
  —Review the signs and symptoms that should be reported to a physician or nurse.
     Upper respiratory infection
     Shortness of breath
     Persistent cough
     Persistent chest pain
- *Medications*
  —Explain the purpose, dosage, schedule, and route of administration of any prescribed drugs, as well as side effects to report to a physician or nurse. Explain the need to avoid taking over-the-counter medication without checking with a physician.
- *Activity*
  —Advise the patient of the importance of exercising to tolerance and the need to avoid overexertion and excessive participation in sports and activities.

FOLLOW-UP CARE

- Stress the importance of regular follow-up visits. Make sure the patient has the necessary names and telephone numbers.

C

Cholecystectomy

—Cholecystectomy: removal of the gallbladder for gallstones or because of inflammation to restore flow of bile from the liver to the small intestine. The procedure may be done as abdominal surgery (open cholecystectomy) or as a laparoscopic procedure.

PREPROCEDURAL TEACHING

- Review the physician's explanation of the procedure and the reason for it; encourage the patient to ask questions and to discuss any fears or anxieties.

Review of Preprocedural Care

- Review the physician's explanation of the procedure. Explain the need for consent forms and signature for surgery, anesthesia, blood transfusions, and photographs, if needed.
- Inform the patient that admission is usually on the day of surgery and that the procedure is performed under general anesthesia.
- Review routine preprocedure tests: complete blood count, urinalysis, chest x-ray, and electrocardiogram.
- Tell the patient that NPO status must be maintained from the night before surgery.
- Review skin preparation; the patient will shower with bactericidal soap (e.g., Safeguard, Dial, Hibiclens).
- Inform the patient that a small cleansing enema (e.g., Fleet) is necessary the night before the procedure.
- For open cholecystectomy:
  - Explain that an incision will be made below the right rib cage.
  - Explain that the procedure may take 2 to 4 hours if x-rays are done during surgery.

- For laparoscopy:
  —Tell the patient that NPO status must be maintained from the night before surgery.
  —Explain that the procedure usually takes 2 to 3 hours.
  —Inform the patient that the largest incision will be 2 to 4 inches below the umbilicus (for removal of the gallbladder) and that three or four punctures will be made in the abdomen to insert other scopes (to inject gas into the abdominal cavity, which makes vision and maneuvering easier), to hold, and to cut.

Review of Postprocedural Care

- For open cholecystectomy:
  —See Abdominal Surgery (p. 6).
  —Inform the patient that the hospital stay will be 4 days or more.
  —Explain that drainage tubes will be inserted: nasogastric tube, T-tube for bile drainage, possibly Penrose or Jackson-Pratt drain.
- For laparoscopy:
  —Tell the patient that fluids will be permitted on the evening of surgery if the patient is not nauseated.
  —Explain that the patient will be encouraged to get out of bed and walk.
  —Inform the patient that the abdomen will be distended from gas.
  —Tell the patient what analgesics will be provided for pain.
  —Explain that the patient will be discharged the day after surgery.

SIDE EFFECTS/COMPLICATIONS

- Hemorrhage
- Shock
- Paralytic ileus
- Peritonitis
- Electrolyte imbalance
- Wound infection
- Pulmonary problems
- Postcholecystectomy syndrome (fever, jaundice, pain)
- From laparoscopy:
  —Bleeding

—Wound infection
—Abdominal cramps and shoulder pain
—Sepsis
—Biliary peritonitis

▦ HOME CARE

- Give both the patient and the caregiver *verbal* and *written* instructions. Provide them with the name and telephone number of a physician or nurse to call if questions arise.
- *Wound/incision care*
  - —Explain any specific care of the surgical incision and dressing changes as indicated.
  - —Teach the patient how to care for the T-tube and drainage bag.
    - Secure the tube by taping it to the body.
    - Keep the tube and bag level with the abdomen when lying flat to prevent excessive drainage.
    - Do not disconnect the tube and drainage bag.
    - Avoid kinks in the tubing.
    - When emptying the bag: wash hands, wipe the connection with alcohol, disconnect and drain into a receptacle, reconnect and wipe connection if drainage is apparent, measure drainage, record the amount, discard drainage into the toilet, rinse receptacle.
    - Inspect the insertion site daily for leakage, redness, tenderness, or swelling. Wash with soap and water and replace dressing.
    - Clamp the T-tube 1 hour before and after eating (unless instructed otherwise).
- *Warning signs*
  - —Review the signs and symptoms that should be reported to a physician or nurse.
    - Wound infection: redness, tenderness, swelling
    - Biliary obstruction: persistent pain, jaundice, itching (pruritus); lack of bowel movements or clay-colored stools; dark urine
    - Fever, chills
    - Nausea, vomiting
- *Medications*
  - —Explain the purpose, dosage, schedule, and route of administration of any prescribed drugs, as well as side effects to report to a physician or nurse.

- *Activity*
  —For laparoscopy:
    Encourage the patient to increase mobility to reduce abdominal distention.
    Explain that normal activities are usually possible in 2 days.
    Explain that the patient should avoid heavy lifting (>10 pounds) or strenuous work or sports for 1 week or longer as prescribed by the physician.
  —For open cholecystectomy:
    Avoid heavy lifting (>10 pounds) for the first 4 to 6 weeks.
    Gradually increase activity and allow for maximum rest.
- *Diet*
  —Tell the patient that a low-fat (for 6 weeks, and then fat may be increased gradually), high-carbohydrate, high-protein diet is needed. Encourage frequent, small meals.
  —Inform the patient that alcohol should be avoided for the first 2 months after surgery to minimize the risk of pancreatic involvement.

FOLLOW-UP CARE

- Stress the importance of regular follow-up visits. Make sure the patient has the necessary names and telephone numbers.

Cholelithiasis, Cholecystitis

—Cholelithiasis: abnormal formation of stones in the gallbladder. Incidence increases with age; it is estimated that 1 in 3 persons aged 75 years will have gallstones.

—Cholecystitis: acute or chronic inflammation of the gallbladder most commonly caused by blockage of the cystic duct by gallstones.

CAUSES/CONTRIBUTING FACTORS

- Familial tendencies
- Diet: high fat, high calorie

- Obesity
- Diabetes
- Liver disease
- Pancreatitis
- In women: elevated estrogen levels, oral contraceptives, hormone replacement therapy, pregnancy
- Use of clofibrate (anticholesterol drug)

SIGNS/SYMPTOMS

- After fatty snacks or meals: indigestion, belching, flatulence, nausea, vomiting
- Pain: acute and colicky; midepigastric area, may spread to back and between shoulder blades or right shoulder
- Fever: low grade or high with chills
- Jaundice
- Pruritus (severe itching)
- Dark, concentrated urine
- Clay-colored stools

COMPLICATIONS

- Jaundice
- Infection
- Electrolyte imbalance
- Bowel obstruction
- Peritonitis
- Bleeding tendencies (lack of vitamin K)
- Pancreatitis

DIAGNOSTIC TESTS

- Describe each procedure, its purpose, and the normal feelings or sensations that are likely, as well as any preprocedural and postprocedural care.
    —Radiographic tests: cholecystography, x-rays
    —Ultrasound: to differentiate location and size of stones
    —Blood studies: to show increase in certain enzymes (serum bilirubin, serum amylase)
    —White blood cell count: to check for infection
    —Percutaneous transhepatic cholangiography: to confirm the presence of stones or obstruction
    —Endoscopic retrograde cholangiopancreatography: to visualize and evaluate the biliary tree or pancreatic duct

TREATMENT
Medical

- Therapy
  —Hydration (parenteral fluids with electrolytes)
  —Gallstone dissolution therapy (bile acid therapy): to dissolve certain types of stones; indicated for small stones
  —Percutaneous transhepatic biliary catheterization: to remove gallstones; catheter is inserted through small abdominal incision under fluoroscopy; catheter may remain temporarily and drain into small external bag; procedure done on outpatient basis under local anesthesia
  —Endoscopic retrograde sphincterotomy: flexible endoscopic tube inserted through mouth to stomach and through to the common bile duct to permit stones to pass; done on an outpatient basis with local anesthesia to throat
  —Endoscopic retrograde cholangiopancreatography: flexible endoscopic tube passed as above but used to remove stones
  —Extracorporeal shock wave lithotripsy: use of high-energy shock waves to break up stones without damaging surrounding tissue (see p. 631)
- Drugs
  —Analgesics
  —Antibiotics
  —Antiemetics
  —Bile sequestrant therapy: given to bind with bile salts and facilitate excretion
  —Anticholinergics
  —Vitamin K

Surgical

- Cholecystectomy: surgical removal of the gallbladder

🏠 HOME CARE

- Give both the patient and the caregiver *verbal* and *written* instructions. Provide them with the name and telephone number of a physician or nurse to call if questions arise. Explain the disease, causes, and contributing factors.
- *Warning signs*
  —Review the signs and symptoms that should be reported to a physician or nurse.
     Biliary colic: severe pain, tachycardia, pallor, diaphoresis

- *Special instructions*
  —Review the explanation for prescribed medical therapies (see p. 188).

  Describe the procedure and its purpose, reviewing any specific preprocedural preparation.

  After the procedure, provide instruction on postprocedural care.

  Review catheter care if a catheter is present.

  ○ Explain that the catheter is to remain taped securely in place. Teach the patient how to empty the bag.

  ○ Review the signs and symptoms that should be reported to a physician or nurse: no drainage coming out of the tube, signs of infection (redness, swelling, tenderness around site, fever, chills).

  —Review the explanation of surgery if prescribed.

- *Medications*
  —Explain the purpose, dosage, schedule, and route of administration of any prescribed drugs, as well as side effects to report to a physician or nurse.

- *Diet*
  —Explain that the patient should follow a low-fat diet and take vitamin supplements (A, D, E, and K); refer the patient to the dietary department for specific instructions.

  —Discuss the need to decrease dietary fat and cholesterol. Explain the role diet plays in controlling biliary colic.

  —Discuss the need to maintain weight control. Advise weight reduction as necessary.

FOLLOW-UP CARE AND REFERRALS

- Stress the importance of regular follow-up visits. Make sure the patient has the necessary names and telephone numbers.
- Provide referrals for home care services if indicated.

Cirrhosis

—**Cirrhosis: chronic, progressive liver disease characterized by diffuse destruction and fibrotic regeneration of hepatic cells, resulting in changes in liver structure and portal blood flow.**

CAUSES/CONTRIBUTING FACTORS/RISK FACTORS

- Chronic alcoholism (accounts for 50% of cases)
- Viral hepatitis
- Exposure to industrial and chemical toxins, such as arsenic, carbon tetrachloride, phosphorus
- Biliary obstruction or inflammation
- Right-sided congestive heart failure
- Genetic factors

SIGNS/SYMPTOMS

- Fatigue
- Weakness
- Anorexia
- Weight loss or gain
- Abdominal pain or tenderness
- Diarrhea or constipation
- Nausea and vomiting
- Dyspepsia
- Pruritus
- Petechiae, ecchymosis, bleeding tendencies
- Palmar erythema
- Spider angioma
- Edema of extremities
- Ascites
- Jaundice
- Umbilical hernia
- Distended abdominal veins
- Fetor hepaticus: fruity, musty breath odor
- Asterixis: coarse tremors of the hands
- Changes in reproductive system: amenorrhea, testicular atrophy, gynecomastia, impotence

COMPLICATIONS

- Portal hypertension
- Bleeding, esophageal varices
- Hepatic encephalopathy
- Hepatorenal syndrome
- Death

DIAGNOSTIC TESTS

- Describe each procedure, its purpose, and the normal feelings or sensations that are likely, as well as any preprocedural and postprocedural care.
  - —Blood studies: liver enzymes, bilirubin levels, total serum albumin, serum protein, prothrombin time, complete blood count, serum electrolytes
  - —Urine and stool studies: to measure urobilinogen levels
  - —Abdominal x-rays: to detect liver size, cysts, calcification, ascites
  - —Liver biopsy: to detect hepatic tissue destruction and fibrosis
  - —Computed tomography of liver: to determine liver size, identify masses, and visualize hepatic blood flow
  - —Esophagogastroduodenoscopy: to detect esophageal varices, duodenal bleeding, irritation, ulceration
  - —Angiographic studies: to establish patency of the portal vein and to determine the cause of effective treatment for variceal bleeding.

TREATMENT

Treatment goals are to alleviate the underlying cause for cirrhosis, prevent further hepatic damage, and prevent or treat complications.

Medical

- Therapy
  - —Gastric intubation: to assess bleeding
  - —Esophageal balloon tamponade: to control bleeding esophageal varices
  - —Sclerotherapy: to control hemorrhage by inducing sclerosis in the bleeding tissues
  - —Low-sodium, low-protein diet
  - —Fluid restriction
  - —Vitamin supplements
  - —Total parenteral nutrition
- Drugs
  - —Diuretics
  - —Vasopressin
  - —Neomycin
  - —Lactulose
  - —Propranolol

—Hematinics (iron)
—Laxatives and stool softeners

Surgical

- Peritoneovenous shunt: to drain ascites into the venous circulation, decreasing portal hypertension
- Portal-systemic shunt: to divert portal venous blood flow, decreasing portal hypertension
- Paracentesis: to relieve abdominal pressure
- Liver transplantation

 HOME CARE

- Give both the patient and the caregiver *verbal* and *written* instructions. Provide them with the name and telephone number of a physician or nurse to call if questions arise.
- *General information*
  —Explain cirrhosis, its causes, and contributing factors. Patient education is individualized, depending on the cause of the disease.
- *Warning signs*
  —Review the signs and symptoms that should be reported to a physician or nurse.
    Changes in weight, edema, abdominal girth
    Behavioral or neurologic changes: stupor, lethargy, restlessness, hallucinations, neuromuscular function
    Excessive bleeding, bloody vomitus or stools
- *Special instructions*
  —Advise the patient to avoid using soap. Suggest the use of emollients and antipruritic lotions. Emphasize the importance of maintaining skin integrity.
  —Instruct the patient to weigh self daily and to record daily weights and abdominal girth measurements.
  —Instruct the patient to minimize the risk of bleeding by not straining during defecation, blowing the nose forcefully, or using razor blades or hard-bristled toothbrushes.
- *Medications*
  —Explain the purpose, dosage, schedule, and route of administration of any prescribed drugs, as well as side effects to report to a physician or nurse.
  —Stress the importance of avoiding over-the-counter medications.

- *Activity*
  —Encourage the patient to discuss allowances and limitations with respect to occupation, recreation, and activities.
  —Instruct the patient to alternate periods of rest or activity.
  —Instruct the patient in energy conservation methods in activities of daily living.
- *Diet*
  —Stress the importance of abstaining from alcohol.
  —Advise the patient to eat small, frequent meals.
  —Assist the patient to plan a diet low in sodium and high in carbohydrates, protein, vitamins, and calories. For advanced-stage disease or encephalopathy, tell the patient to limit protein intake.
  —Instruct the patient and caregiver in total parenteral nutrition, if appropriate.

FOLLOW-UP CARE

- Stress the importance of regular follow-up visits. Make sure the patient has the necessary names and telephone numbers.
- Encourage the patient to obtain a MedicAlert bracelet and identification card listing the diagnosis, medications, and treatment.

REFERRALS

- Assist the patient to obtain referral to home health services.
- Assist the patient and caregiver to participate in Alcoholics Anonymous, if appropriate.

Colorectal Cancer

—Colorectal cancer: cancer of the colon and rectum. Colorectal cancer occurs more frequently in the elderly; prognosis in the young is very poor. Ninety-five percent of tumors begin with the development of a benign, adenomatous polyp in the large bowel or rectum. Most colon and rectal tumors are adenocarcinomas; others are carcinoid tumors, leiomyosarcomas, and lymphomas.

RISK FACTORS

- Age older than 40 years
- Diet heavy in fats and refined carbohydrates
- Family history of colorectal cancer
- Past history of colorectal adenocarcinoma or cancer; breast cancer, endometrial cancer
- Ulcerative colitis
- Familial polyposis
- Exposure to asbestos
- Member of higher socioeconomic group and urban population

SIGNS/SYMPTOMS

- Rectal bleeding
- Sudden changes in bowel pattern (constipation or diarrhea)
- Excessive flatus
- Distention
- Cramps
- Unexplained anemia
- Altered bowel habits caused by left-sided colonic lesions: decreased stool caliber (pencil like), urgency to defecate, vague abdominal pain, hemorrhoids
- Unexplained iron deficiency, anemia, and gastrointestinal tract bleeding caused by right-sided lesions
- Obstruction owing to napkin ring growth of tumors of sigmoid colon
- Gross rectal blood and tenesmus with feeling of incomplete evacuation caused by rectal tumors

COMPLICATIONS

- Infection
- Paralytic ileus
- Leak of anastomosis with possible fistula formation

DIAGNOSTIC TESTS

- Describe each procedure, its purpose, and the normal feelings or sensations that are likely, as well as any preprocedural and postprocedural care.
    - —Hematocrit: to detect blood loss
    - —Occult fecal blood test: to detect blood loss
    - —Digital rectal examination: to determine presence of lesion

—Colonic visualization (barium enema, colonoscopy): to determine size, shape, and location of lesion
—Biopsy: to determine type of malignant cells
—Carcinoembryonic antigen (CEA): nonspecific tumor marker elevated in presence of colorectal tumor

TREATMENT
Medical

- Therapy
  —Radiation therapy
      Intraoperative radiation therapy
      Radiation seeds
      External beam for inoperable obstructing rectal rumors
      Transanal irradiation
  —Postoperative adjuvant therapy with radiation sensitizers for tumors dissecting bowel wall or with positive lymph nodes
  —Endoscopic laser for inoperable obstructing rectal tumors
  —Chemotherapy
      Adjuvant regimen of 5-fluorouracil (5-FU) with levamisole
      Radiation sensitizers with 5-FU and metronidazole
      Camptothecins

Surgical

- Local excision of well-defined rectal tumors
- Resection of primary colon lesion with mesentery (containing lymph nodes to which tumor is likely to spread) and end-to-end anastomosis
- En bloc resection of colon, small bowel, bladder, uterus, ovaries
- Surgical bypass for inoperable obstructing tumors, with creation of fecal stoma

PREPROCEDURAL TEACHING FOR SURGERY

- Review the physician's explanation of the procedure and the reason for it; encourage the patient to ask questions and to discuss any fears or anxieties.
- For general preprocedural and postprocedural teaching, see Abdominal Surgery (p. 6).
- Review bowel preparation: liquid diet 2 to 3 days before surgery, laxatives, enemas, and antibiotics to cleanse and sterilize bowel.

- If a stoma is expected, arrange to meet with the enterostomal therapist before surgery to mark the site of the stoma. The stoma should avoid the waistline and skin folds and should be located where the patient can see and reach the pouch easily.
- Provide emotional support. Encourage questions and discussion to correct any misconception and alleviate fears and concerns regarding changes in body image and lifestyle.

🏠 HOME CARE

- Give both the patient and the caregiver *verbal* and *written* instructions. Provide them with the name and telephone number of a physician or nurse to call if questions arise. Use visual aids to assist in instruction.
- *General information*
  —Review the disease process and the type of surgical procedure performed or scheduled. Discuss follow-up care.
- *Warning signs*
  —Review the signs and symptoms that should be reported to a physician or nurse.
    Infection: purulent drainage, pain, incision warm to the touch, fever, redness
    Paralytic ileus: inability to defecate, distention, abdominal pain and swelling
    Leak at site of anastomosis: increased drainage around the surgical site
    Stoma retraction or prolapse
    Rectal bleeding
    Intestinal obstruction
- *Special instructions*
  —Review the care of the surgical dressing, explaining how to inspect the incision.
  —For the patient with a colostomy, explain how to care for the ostomy (see Ostomy, p. 694).
  —Review prevention and detection procedures to avoid recurrence.
    Maintenance of regular bowel movements: eat a high-fiber, low-fat diet; drink up to 8 glasses of fluids per day unless contraindicated; avoid constipation; check with physician or nurse regarding use of laxatives and enemas.

Inspect stools regularly and report any signs of bleeding. Show the patient how to perform a Hemoccult test procedure.

FOLLOW-UP CARE

- Stress the importance of regular follow-up visits. Because of the high recurrence rate, discuss the importance of having yearly screening (rectal examination, stool test for occult blood and sigmoidoscopy) as ordered. Make sure the patient has the necessary names and telephone numbers.

Compartment Syndrome

—Compartment syndrome: increased pressure within anatomic compartments caused by constriction of edematous tissues, leading to progressive degeneration of muscle, impaired circulation, nerve damage, and tissue necrosis. The elbow, wrist, knee, and ankle are the most commonly affected areas. The cause of constriction is unyielding fascial coverings over muscles. When an injury, such as a fracture, frostbite, or burn, causes swelling, there may be no room for edema within the muscle group or compartment. Thus blood flow is interrupted, causing damage to the blood vessels, nerves, and muscles within this limited space.

CAUSES/CONTRIBUTING FACTORS

- Trauma or surgery
- Bleeding disorders (e.g., hemophilia)
- Major vascular surgery
- Thermal injury: burns, frostbite
- Snakebite
- Intravenous infiltration
- Tight casts or dressings

SIGNS/SYMPTOMS

- Pain: in compartment area; increasing, unrelenting, and unrelieved by narcotics

- Paresthesia: of hand or foot; numbness, decreased sensation or burning
- Pallor: caused by decreased circulation in the compartment
- Polar (coolness): from decreased circulation
- Swelling and localized redness
- Progressive loss of motor function
- Paralysis
- Pulselessness: absence of pulse below level of compartment

COMPLICATIONS

- Ischemic contractures
- Neurovascular dysfunction of extremity
- Muscle weakness
- Infection
- Tissue necrosis
- Gangrene
- Chronic infection, osteomyelitis
- Amputation
- Shock
- Renal failure

DIAGNOSTIC TESTS

- Describe each procedure, its purpose, and the normal feelings or sensations that are likely, as well as any preprocedural and postprocedural care.
  —Compartment pressure: measured by various methods, such as slit, wick, or large-bore catheter introduced into the compartment and attached to a saline-primed transducer
  —Arteriogram/venogram: to rule out blood vessel blockage or damage
  —Doppler ultrasound: to assess peripheral circulation
  —Magnetic resonance imaging: to show muscle damage
  —Ankle or brachial index
  —Blood tests: complete blood count, prothrombin time

TREATMENT
Medical

- Therapy
  —Dressing removed; cast removed, bivalved, or windowed to limit the swelling

—Immobilization with posterior cast or splint if fracture is involved

—*Caution:* the extremity should *not* be iced and elevated, since this contributes to decreased blood flow to the affected area

—Continuous fascial pressure monitoring: normal 0 to 30 mm Hg; sustained pressure >30 mm Hg can damage blood vessels, nerves, and muscles

- Drugs
  —Analgesics: often larger than normal levels of narcotics are needed to control pain
  —Antibiotics

Surgical

- Fasciotomy: surgical incision of the fascia for the entire length of the involved compartment to remove restriction or swelling: before procedure, explain that it is necessary to control progressive symptoms of neurovascular compromise and that after several days the surgical incision will be closed or that a skin graft may be necessary
- Surgical repair of lacerated artery: for arterial injury
- Amputation: for severe tissue necrosis or infection

HOME CARE

- Give both the patient and the caregiver *verbal* and *written* instructions. Provide them with the name and telephone number of a physician or nurse to call if questions arise.
- *General information*
  —Describe the disorder, explaining causes or contributing factors.
- *Warning signs*
  —Review the signs and symptoms of recurrence of the syndrome that should be reported to a physician or nurse.
    Increasing pain
    Numbness, tingling
    Paralysis
    Changes in color: pallor, redness, cyanosis
    Coolness
- *Special instructions*
  —If fasciotomy was performed:
    Explain that there is an increased potential for infection.

Review the signs of infection to be reported immediately to the physician or nurse: increased temperature, increased pain, foul odor from wound.

Instruct the patient in the proper technique for care of the surgical incision and aseptic procedures for dressing changes; advise the patient how to dispose of soiled dressings.

Instruct the patient to inspect the wound daily to check for increased drainage.

—If vascular surgery to repair blood vessels was performed:

Review signs of vascular changes requiring attention: pallor, cyanosis, pulselessness, decreased or absent capillary refill (when extremity is pinched, it turns white; pink color returns in 4 to 6 seconds).

- *Medications*
  —Explain the purpose, dosage, schedule, and route of administration of any prescribed drugs, as well as side effects to report to a physician or nurse.
- *Activity*
  —Explain the need for rest and elevation of the extremity postoperatively.
  —Review the use of assistive devices and ambulatory aids as prescribed by the physician.

FOLLOW-UP CARE

- Stress the importance of regular follow-up visits. Make sure the patient has the necessary names and telephone numbers.

COPD: Chronic Obstructive Pulmonary Disease
(Chronic Obstructive Lung Disease)

—Chronic obstructive pulmonary disease: a progressive disorder of the lungs and airways. Chronic obstructive pulmonary disease (COPD) affects oxygen and carbon dioxide gas exchange and causes chronic inflammation and narrowing of the small airways, affecting air outflow. COPD includes such diseases as emphysema and chronic bronchitis.

C

—Emphysema: destruction of lung tissue, causing a reduced expiratory flow rate and overinflated alveoli (air sacs); a progressive disease that is irreversible.

—Chronic bronchitis: inflammation of the mucous membrane of the bronchus with excessive mucus secretion in the bronchial tree; occurs as a result of irritation to tissue that causes swelling and hypertrophy of the mucus-producing cells.

CONTRIBUTING FACTORS
- Cigarette smoking
- Exposure to pollutants: industrial, air
- Chronic respiratory infections

SIGNS/SYMPTOMS
- Dyspnea on exertion
- Shortness of breath
- Wheezing
- Thick mucus production
- Restlessness
- Fatigue
- Anorexia, weight loss
- Persistent cough: productive, nonproductive
- Malaise
- Somnolence
- Peripheral cyanosis with clubbing

COMPLICATIONS
- Cor pulmonale
- Acute respiratory failure
- Peptic and esophageal reflux
- Pneumonia
- Polycythemia
- Dysrhythmias
- Hepatomegaly

DIAGNOSTIC TESTS

- Describe each procedure, its purpose, and the normal feelings or sensations that are likely, as well as any preprocedural and postprocedural care.
  —Chest x-ray
  —Pulmonary function studies: to assess the presence and severity of disease in the large and small airways
  —Sputum specimen analysis
  —Laboratory tests: complete blood count, electrolytes, arterial blood gases
  —Electrocardiogram

TREATMENT
Medical

- Therapy
  —Oxygen therapy
  —Chest physiotherapy: postural drainage and chest percussion
  —Ultrasonic or mechanical nebulizer treatments
  —Physical training program
  —Adequate hydration
- Drugs
  —Bronchodilators
  —Antibiotics
  —Corticosteroids

Surgical

- Lung reduction surgery
- Lung transplantation

HOME CARE

- Give both the patient and the caregiver *verbal* and *written* instructions. Provide them with the name and telephone number of a physician or nurse to call if questions arise.
- *General information*
  —Explain the disease process and underlying cause. Assist the patient to identify individual factors that contribute to the disease process.
- *Warning signs*
  —Review the signs and symptoms that should be reported to a physician or nurse.
    Elevated temperature
    Sore throat

Increased sputum production

Change in color of sputum from clear white to yellow-green

Upper respiratory infection

Increased difficulty in breathing

Decreased activity tolerance

Decreased appetite

- *Special instructions*
  —Discuss the importance of avoiding bronchopulmonary irritants.

  Cigarette smoking

  Industrial air pollutants

  Dust

  Powders and perfumes

  Aerosol sprays

  Smoke

  —Demonstrate the use of bronchodilator nebulizers. Watch for side effects such as rapid heart rate. Avoid overuse.

  —Teach and demonstrate to the patient and caregiver adaptive breathing techniques, such as deep-breathing exercises, coughing techniques, pursed-lip breathing, abdominal breathing, and positions for postural drainage if needed.

  —Explain the need to avoid persons with infections, especially upper respiratory tract infections. Urge the patient to seek medical care at the beginning of infections.

  —Explain the importance of taking vaccines for influenza and pneumococcal pneumonia.

  —Instruct the patient and caregiver on cleaning of all home respiratory equipment (see Oxygen Therapy, p. 700).

  —Explain the importance of environmental control: avoid dry air by using a humidifier; provide a warm house (75° to 80° F [23.8° to 26.6° C]). Explain the need to keep warm and avoid chilling.

  —Explain the need to avoid going out in cold temperatures, which may cause bronchospasm.

  —Stress the importance of not smoking and of avoiding secondhand smoke. Explain that tobacco smoke is an irritant and can increase the risk of respiratory infection. Provide information about and referral to community-based smoking cessation programs and the local chapter of the American Lung Association.

—Suggest avoiding clothing that restricts chest or abdominal expansion.
- *Medications*
  —Explain the purpose, dosage, schedule, and route of administration of any prescribed drugs, as well as side effects to report to a physician or nurse.
  > Bronchodilators: to open the airways and make breathing easier
  >
  > Antibiotics: to prevent or treat respiratory infections
  >
  > Corticosteroids: to reduce swelling in bronchi and bronchioles
  —Explain the need to avoid taking over-the-counter medications without checking with the physician. Avoid sedatives and narcotics, which can depress respiration.
  —Emphasize the importance of not stopping medication unless instructed by the physician.
- *Activity*
  —Advise the patient to exercise to tolerance and to avoid fatigue by planning rest periods during the day.
  —Explain the need to limit activity on days of high air pollution.
  —Instruct the patient to breathe deeply and slowly during periods of activity.
  —Discuss energy conservation techniques (e.g., perform such activities as bathing and shaving in a seated position or place frequently used items in easy-to-reach areas to avoid reaching or bending).
  —Teach the patient and caregiver to watch for signs of extreme fatigue, chest pain, or diaphoresis during and after activity.
  —Instruct the patient to avoid emotional stress. Teach and demonstrate stress reduction techniques.
  —Explain the need to avoid constipation and straining at stool.
  —Instruct the patient on the use of oxygen during mealtimes and sexual activity.
- *Diet*
  —Explain the need to maintain high-calorie diet as indicated.
  —Encourage fluid intake of 2000 to 3000 ml/day, unless contraindicated, to keep secretions thin.
  —Suggest that the patient rest before and after meals if shortness of breath increases at mealtime.
  —Suggest small, frequent meals to avoid abdominal distention.
  —Avoid gas-producing foods.

FOLLOW-UP CARE

- Stress the importance of regular follow-up visits. Make sure the patient has the necessary names and telephone numbers.
- Discuss the need to wear a MedicAlert band.

REFERRALS

- Provide referral to a pulmonary rehabilitation program.
- Provide referral to pulmonary support groups.
- Suggest that the patient apply for handicapped parking permits to conserve energy when traveling.

Coronary Artery Bypass Graft Surgery

—**Coronary artery bypass graft surgery: a surgical procedure that increases blood flow to the heart muscle. Increasing the supply of oxygen and nutrient to the myocardium prevents myocardial infarction. Coronary artery bypass grafting (CABG) is an open heart procedure that requires cardiopulmonary bypass, is performed under general anesthesia, and generally involves two incisions. A leg (calf or thigh) incision is made to remove a segment of the saphenous vein, and a second incision is made in the chest (sternum) to allow one end of the vein to be connected to the aorta and the other to be connected to the affected coronary artery below the level of blockage. Multiple vein grafts can be done. Alternatively, a segment of the internal mammary artery may be used.**

INDICATIONS

- Acute or chronic ischemic heart disease

PREPROCEDURAL TEACHING

- Review the physician's explanation of the procedure and the reason for it; encourage the patient to ask questions and to discuss any fears or anxieties. Discuss the need to obtain written consent.

Review of Preprocedural Care

- Review preparation of the skin of the chest and leg: the patient is shaved from chin to toes and takes an antiseptic shower or bath.
- Explain that a sedative will be given the night before and the morning of surgery.
- Inform the patient that an anesthesiologist and respiratory therapist will visit the patient before surgery.

Review of Postprocedural Care

- Explain that the patient will be taken to the surgical intensive care unit right after the procedure; the usual stay in the unit is 1 to 2 days.
- Describe the unit, the noises the patient may hear, visiting privileges, the pain the patient will feel, and the medications that will be provided.
- Discuss the number of tubes (nasogastric tube, endotracheal tube, chest tube, Foley catheter) and the intravenous and arterial lines. Explain that they will be removed as the patient's condition is stabilized.
- Explain the method of communication that will be used after the operation while the patient is intubated.
- Inform the patient about routine care: frequent turning, coughing, deep breathing, and monitoring of vital signs.
- Emphasize the importance of coughing, deep breathing, and using the incentive spirometer; permit time for practice.
- Tell the patient that dangling at the side of the bed and sitting in a chair may be permitted as early as the evening of surgery.
- Explain that the patient may be disoriented because of medications or lack of sleep and that sedation is used to keep the patient comfortable.

SIDE EFFECTS/COMPLICATIONS

- Stroke
- Arrhythmias
- Bleeding or hemorrhage
- Hypotension/hypertension
- Cardiac tamponade
- Perioperative myocardial infarction
- Intraoperative myocardial infarction (2.5% to 5% of patients)
- Pericarditis

- Postpericardiectomy syndrome
- Shock
- Postpump psychosis

🏠 HOME CARE

- Give both the patient and the caregiver *verbal* and *written* instructions. Provide them with the name and telephone number of a physician or nurse to call if questions arise.
- *General information*
  —Review the operative procedure, discussing any specific precautions and complications associated with the surgery and what to expect with recovery.
  —Explain that complete healing and recovery take 8 to 12 weeks.
  —Inform the patient that the sternum was wired together and that a feeling of movement or a clicking sound is normal during the healing period.
  —Tell the patient that mild itching, redness, numbness, soreness, swelling, or a drawing feeling is normal during the healing period.
- *Wound/incision care*
  —Inform the patient that showers are allowed within a few days after surgery. The patient should use warm water and wash the incision gently.
  —Explain that most sutures dissolve slowly and do not require removal by a medical team.
  —Suggest that the patient wear loose, comfortable clothing. Women who have a submammary incision should not wear a bra for the first few days. When a bra can be worn again, it should not be an underwire bra, which could cause irritation.
- *Warning signs*
  —Review the signs and symptoms that should be reported to a physician or nurse.
     Wound infection: swelling, drainage, redness, pain
     Swelling of hands, legs; weight gain; shortness of breath
     Fever, rapid pulse, night sweats, chills
     Chest pain with inspiration or exertion
- *Medications*
  —Explain the purpose, dosage, schedule, and route of administration of any prescribed drugs, as well as side effects to report to a physician or nurse.

- *Activity*
  —Discuss activity limitations and allowances.
  > Instruct the patient to increase activities gradually and to begin a daily exercise program such as walking. Review guidelines provided by a hospital cardiac exercise program (see table on p. 216).
  > Advise the patient to avoid fatigue by alternating activity with rest.
  > Tell the patient to avoid prolonged standing or sitting. When sitting, the patient should not cross the legs or elevate the leg with the incision.
  > Caution the patient to avoid lifting or carrying heavy objects or performing isometric activities. Driving should be restricted for the first few weeks or as ordered.
  —Encourage questions about when specific activities can be resumed, for example:
  > Sexual activity when the patient and partner feel comfortable
  > Sports such as swimming, golf, and tennis at 6 weeks
  > Vacuuming, snow blowing, and moving furniture at 6 weeks
  > Return to work usually at 4 to 6 weeks; depends on occupation
  —Explain that CABG does not cure coronary artery disease. Emphasize the importance of lifestyle changes to prevent the recurrence of obstructions (see Coronary Artery Disease, p. 209).
- *Diet*
  —Explain that the diet should be low fat or as ordered and that salt intake should be restricted.

PSYCHOSOCIAL CARE

- Explain that emotions, irritability, and depression are commonly associated with recovery. Reassure the patient that they are temporary.

FOLLOW-UP CARE

- Stress the importance of regular follow-up visits. Make sure the patient has the necessary names and telephone numbers.

REFERRALS

- Refer the patient to local and national support groups, such as the Mended Hearts Club.
- Refer the patient to a hospital- or community-based exercise program.
- Provide referrals for home care or social services as indicated.

Coronary Artery Disease

—Coronary artery disease: a progressive disease process characterized by narrowing or blockage of the coronary arteries resulting in decreased blood flow to the heart muscle. Coronary artery disease (CAD) results from atherosclerosis, the buildup of fatty plaques (made up of cholesterol) and lipids on the inside walls of the arteries. Restriction of blood flow deprives the heart muscle of oxygen and nutrients, causing tissue damage. Chest pain occurs when the demand for oxygen by the heart muscle is greater than can be delivered by the blood vessels. CAD can present itself as angina pectoris or as myocardial infarction. Symptomatic CAD is also referred to as ischemic heart disease.

CAUSES/CONTRIBUTING FACTORS OF ATHEROSCLEROSIS

- Family history
- Gender and age: males aged 35 to 55, females older than 50 or postmenopausal
- Hyperlipidemia
- Hypertension
- Diabetes
- Cigarette smoking
- Physical inactivity; sedentary lifestyle
- Obesity: body mass index, weight circumference
- Personality traits:
  —Hostility
  —Competitiveness

SYMPTOMS OF HEART DISEASE IN WOMEN

- Chest pain (angina): Pain in center of the chest that is described as pressure, tightness, sometimes radiating down the left arm or jaw; often mistaken for indigestion
- Breathlessness: shortness of breath; may wake up at night having a hard time catching breath
- Unexplained fatigue
- Unexplained lightheadedness, dizziness, nausea
- Palpitations, cold sweat

    —Aggression
    —Anger
- Homocysteine levels >15 μmol/liter
- In premenopausal females:
  - Severe hypertension
  - Use of estrogen oral contraceptives
  - Smoking history

ANGINA

Angina is chest pain that typically occurs during periods of exertion or emotion but is relieved by rest or nitroglycerin. It is caused by an imbalance in the supply and demand of oxygen-rich blood to the heart muscle resulting from a narrowed coronary artery, which is usually more than 70% blocked. Types of angina include stable, which comes on with effort and is relieved by rest and nitroglycerin; unstable, which can increase in frequency, duration, and severity even when little effort is expended; Prinzmetal's (variant angina), which is unrelated to exercise and occurs at rest and is usually caused by coronary artery spasm; and intractable, which is frequent or continuous pain unrelieved by therapy. Complications of angina include myocardial infarction (heart attack), arrhythmias, sudden death, and heart failure.

A woman's risk profile

Cholesterol levels (mg/dL)	Desirable (low risk)	Borderline-high risk	High risk
Total cholesterol	Less than 200	200-239	240 or higher
LDL ("bad") cholesterol	Less than 130*	130-159†	160 or higher
HDL ("good") cholesterol	35 or higher	Less than 35	Less than 35

mg/dL = milligrams per deciliter of blood.

*LDL 100 mg/dL or less is optimal in women who already have heart or blood vessel disease.

†LDL greater than 100 mg/dL is higher than optimal in women who already have heart or blood vessel disease.

Blood pressure (mm Hg)	Optimal	Normal	High normal	Hyper-tension
Systolic (top number)	Less than 120	Less than 130	130-139	140 or higher
Diastolic (bottom number)	Less than 80	Less than 85	85-89	90 or higher

mm Hg = millimeters of mercury.

From American Heart Association: *Take care: A woman's guide to fighting heart disease,* 1998.

MYOCARDIAL INFARCTION

Myocardial infarction, or heart attack, is the death of myocardial tissue from lack of oxygen, caused by severe or complete occlusion of a coronary artery. The area of dead tissue is eventually replaced by scar tissue. Types of myocardial infarction and the associated blocked arteries are anterior wall (left anterior descending artery), anteroseptal (left anterior descending artery septal perforator), anterolateral (left anterior descending artery diagonal branch), inferior wall (right coronary artery in 90% of cases, circumflex artery in 10%), and lateral wall (circumflex artery).

SIGNS/SYMPTOMS

- Chest pain and discomfort, such as tightness, pressure, squeezing, aching, burning
- Indigestion above the waist
- Aching in the neck, jaw, throat, shoulder, or back (between the shoulder blades), may radiate down one arm
- Breathlessness, weakness, sweating, dizziness
- Diaphoresis or nausea associated with the above symptoms
- Anxiety
- Nausea and vomiting

COMPLICATIONS

- Arrhythmias
- Heart failure
- Cardiogenic shock
- Arterial embolism
- Phlebothrombosis and pulmonary embolism
- Pericarditis
- Left ventricular aneurysm
- Cardiac rupture
- Ventricular septal defect
- Dressler's syndrome
- Valvular dysfunction
- Sudden death

DIAGNOSTIC TESTS

- Describe each procedure, its purpose, and the normal feelings or sensations that are likely, as well as any preprocedural and postprocedural care.
  - —Electrocardiogram: to identify ischemic or infarcted area
  - —Chest x-ray: to visualize enlarged heart and signs of left ventricular failure
  - —Echocardiography: to detect abnormalities of left ventricular wall motion and mechanical defects
  - —Coronary arteriography
  - —Blood tests
    - Serum lipids: high-density lipoprotein, cholesterol, triglycerides, low-density lipoprotein
    - Homocysteine levels
    - Cardiac enzymes: to determine amount of heart muscle damage

Troponin levels: to confirm myocardial damage

Complete blood count, erythrocyte sedimentation rate, and white blood cell count: to detect an inflammatory process

—Indium-111 antimycin antibody imaging: to detect infarcted cells and tissue

—Graded exercise test: to determine the amount of exercise that causes angina, detect lack of blood supply to the tissues during exercise, and assess the risk to heart muscle

—Radionuclide studies

Thallium treadmill: to determine if areas of the heart muscle are receiving inadequate circulation during exercise

Technetium scan: to determine the amount of damage to the heart muscle

—Multigated acquisition scan: to evaluate ventricular function and detect aneurysms and wall motion abnormalities

TREATMENT
General
Medical

- Therapy
  —Control of hypertension and diabetes
  —Stress management
  —Reduction of cholesterol and lipid levels
  —Weight reduction
  —Exercise
  —Smoking cessation
  —Dietary modification

Angina
Medical

- Drugs
  —Nitrates: to improve circulation to the heart muscle
  —Beta blockers: to decrease heart rate, blood pressure, and force of contraction of the heart muscle and prevent cardiac arrhythmias
  —Calcium channel blockers, such as nifedipine, verapamil, diltiazem: to decrease coronary artery vasospasm
  —Antiplatelets (aspirin): to reduce the risk of clot formation
  —Antilipidemic agents

Surgical

- Percutaneous balloon coronary angioplasty
- Coronary atherectomy

Myocardial Infarction
Medical

- Drugs
    —Nitrates: to increase circulation to the muscles
    —Beta blockers: to decrease heart rate, blood pressure, and force of contraction of the heart muscle and prevent cardiac arrhythmias
    —Antiplatelets (aspirin): to reduce clot formation
    —Angiotensin-converting enzyme (ACE) inhibitors: to improve the healing of heart muscle by reducing its work and provide protective effects
    —Thrombolytic therapy: to restore circulation and prevent further damage that begins within 4 to 6 hours of the onset of chest pain
    —Antilipidemic agents
    —Low molecular weight heparin: for subendocardial ischemia

Surgical

- Coronary artery bypass surgery

🏠 HOME CARE

- Give both the patient and the caregiver *verbal* and *written* instructions. Provide them with the name and telephone number of a physician or nurse to call if questions arise.
- Use a heart model or other visual aids to help the patient understand coronary anatomy. Discuss the atherosclerosis process, plaque formation, the role of lipids (high-density versus low-density lipoprotein) and cholesterol in plaque formation, and the various manifestations of coronary artery disease.

Coronary Artery Disease

- *General information*
    —Review ischemic heart disease, discussing the differences between angina and myocardial infarction. Angina is a temporary lack of blood supply, whereas myocardial

infarction is a complete blockage that results in heart muscle damage. Damaged tissue heals into a scar in 6 to 8 weeks.

—Review the physician's explanation of the patient's form of coronary artery disease and the recommended treatment. Point out the location of the patient's coronary lesion.

—Discuss the importance of controlling any coexisting disease such as hypertension, diabetes, or hyperlipidemia.

—Discuss risk factors, assist the patient to identify his or her risk factors, and outline a plan for risk factor modification.

- *Medications*
  —Explain the purpose, dosage, schedule, and route of administration of any prescribed drugs, as well as side effects to report to a physician or nurse.

- *Special instructions*
  —Stress the importance of not smoking or using tobacco products. Explain the effect nicotine has on the cardiac system: causing the heart to work faster, constricting blood vessels, decreasing the amount of oxygen delivered to the heart, and in the presence of coronary artery disease, increasing the likelihood of chest pain. Refer the patient to a community-based smoking cessation program.

  —Discuss the role that stress plays in aggravating coronary artery disease. Help the patient to identify stress-producing factors and discuss methods of stress management. Discuss the need to recognize and deal with feelings of denial, anger, and depression. Provide the patient with a referral to psychologic and support groups to contact as needed.

- *Activity*
  —Discuss the benefits of exercise: increase in high-density lipoproteins, which lowers blood pressure; weight loss; improved cardiovascular status.

  —Encourage a regular home exercise program that includes aerobic activities: walking, jogging, swimming, bicycling (see table on p. 216). Refer the patient to community-based cardiac fitness programs.

- *Diet*
  —Explain how the diet can modify cholesterol and lipid levels.

  —Discuss dietary modifications: limit intake of eggs, saturated fats (e.g., butter and cream), foods high in animal fat (e.g., bacon, red meat, luncheon meat); use monounsaturated fats

Postdischarge exercise program

Week after discharge	Total distance (miles)	Time (minutes)
1	0.25	8-10
2	0.25	5
3	0.5	15
4	1.0	30

Instruct patient to take pulse (resting heart rate) before and immediately after exercise activity, noting rate and rhythm.

Adjust speed and time to maintain heart rate at <100 beats/minute.

Instruct patient to report heart rate increase of >20 to 25 beats/minute.

Modified from Tucker SM, Canobbio MM, Paquette E, et al: *Patient care standards,* ed 7, St Louis, 2000, Mosby.

(e.g., canola oils) for cooking; restrict table salt and sodium intake.

—Explain the importance of controlling weight and avoiding obesity. Inform the patient of the appropriate weight range for age, sex, and body composition (see Appendix A).

Angina Pectoris

* *Warning signs*
  —Review signs and symptoms that should be reported.
  —Assist patient to review and identify anginal pain.
  —Explain to women that symptoms may be atypical (see box on p. 210).
* *Activity*
  —Assist the patient to identify and avoid physical and emotional factors that precipitate pain.
  —Tell the patient to avoid exercise in extremes of weather (hot or cold days), after heavy meals, when emotionally upset, and on smoggy days.
  —Caution the patient to reduce the intensity and effort of activities such as shoveling snow; work slower and in as easy a manner as possible.
  —Inform the patient that sexual activity should be avoided when fatigued and 2 to 3 hours after a meal. If chest pain occurs during sexual activity, the patient should stop and take nitrate if ordered. If pain persists or extreme fatigue occurs, the patient should notify the physician or nurse.

—Discuss self-management during episodes of chest pain: stop activity and rest; take nitrates as ordered (e.g., place a nitroglycerin tablet under the tongue and wait; pain will subside within 20 seconds); seek medical attention if pain persists longer than 20 minutes or diaphoresis and shortness of breath appear.

—Instruct the patient to carry nitroglycerin at all times.

- *Diet*

—Tell the patient to avoid eating heavy meals and exercising after eating.

—Explain that caffeine and heavy alcohol intake should be avoided.

Myocardial Infarction

- *General information*

—Review the physician's explanation of infarction and associated complications.

- *Warning signs*

—Review the signs and symptoms of escalation of angina to myocardial infarction that should be reported to a physician. Angina is chest pain or pressure that is associated with physical or emotional strain and is usually relieved by rest or vasodilators. Myocardial infarction is chest pain or discomfort that is not necessarily associated with physical exertion and is unrelieved by medication or rest. Stress the importance of seeking medical attention if chest pain lasts longer than 20 minutes or is associated with other symptoms.

—Instruct the patient to take baby aspirin daily if ordered.

- *Activity*

—Discuss activity limitations during recovery.

The patient should have 1 to 2 weeks of relative rest with short periods of activity, followed by 2 to 3 weeks of slowly increasing activity, such as walking and stair climbing, then several weeks of progressive activity before returning to work. Refer the patient to a cardiac rehabilitation program as indicated.

The physician should be consulted for specific exercise limitations. Encourage questions about resumption of work and recreational or sports activities.

The patient should avoid or modify activities after heavy meals or alcohol intake and during periods of emotional stress and temperature extremes.

—Discuss long-term modification of activity.

> The patient should begin a lifelong aerobic exercise program.
>
> Sexual activity can be resumed when the patient can climb two flights of stairs without shortness of breath; inform male patients that beta blockers may cause erectile dysfunction.
>
> If symptoms occur, the patient should take nitroglycerin. If no relief occurs within 15 minutes, the patient should contact a physician or go to the nearest emergency room.
>
> Explain the importance of maintaining independence in self-care activities.
>
> Instruct the patient to carry nitroglycerin at all times.

PSYCHOSOCIAL CARE

- Encourage discussion about the need to deal with feelings about possible role changes. Discuss the importance of communication between the patient and the caregiver or significant others.

REFERRALS

- Provide information and referrals for community-based programs: cardiac rehabilitation, smoking cessation, social support.
- Provide referrals for home health care or medical social work services as indicated.

Craniotomy and Craniectomy

—Craniotomy: a surgical opening into the skull to provide access to intracranial structures for surgical revision, resection, or removal of abnormalities.

—Craniectomy: surgical removal of a portion of the skull.

INDICATIONS

- Removal of tumor or hematoma
- Repair of aneurysms
- Intracranial bleeding

- Relief of intracranial pressure
- Decompression

PREPROCEDURAL TEACHING

- Review the physician's explanation of the procedure and the reason for it; encourage the patient to ask questions and to discuss any fears or anxieties. Discuss the need to obtain written consent.

Review of Preprocedural Care

- Discuss the use of antiseptic shampoo, the administration of corticosteroids and anticonvulsants, and the need for a baseline neurologic assessment.

Review of Postprocedural Care

- Discuss the intensive care unit environment, intracranial pressure monitoring, ventilatory support, cardiac monitoring, intravenous lines, postoperative neurologic checks, fluid balance management, surgical drains, proper positioning, bed rest, and the potential for a cervical collar.
- Reassure the patient that precautions for seizures will be taken.
- Discuss anticipated body changes: loss of hair at the surgical site, head dressing, and the potential for and duration of periorbital and facial edema.
- Warn the patient against pulling or tugging at the head dressing and drains.
- Stress the importance of deep breathing and avoiding coughing and sneezing. Maintain NPO until otherwise indicated, then provide fluids and diet within restrictions as ordered. Assess for swallowing and chewing ability.

SIDE EFFECTS/COMPLICATIONS

- Increased intracranial pressure
- Seizures
- Meningitis
- Respiratory distress
- Cardiac dysrhythmias
- Wound infection
- Diabetes insipidus
- Hemorrhage: intracranial; gastrointestinal
- Thrombophlebitis, deep vein thrombosis (DVT)
- Visual disturbances

- Personality changes
- Motor and sensory disturbances
- Diminished gag and swallowing reflexes
- Communication deficits

🏠 HOME CARE

- Give both the patient and the caregiver *verbal* and *written* instructions. Provide them with the name and telephone number of a physician or nurse to call if questions arise.
- *General information*
  —Review the physician's explanation of the surgery and specific follow-up care.
  —Encourage the caregiver to verbalize anxieties related to the procedure, underlying conditions, and rehabilitative process.
- *Wound/incision care*
  —Demonstrate proper wound management and dressing changes: procedure, frequency of dressing change, and inspection of incision with each dressing change.
  —Instruct the patient to avoid scratching sutures and to keep the incision dry.
  —Advise the patient that hair may be shampooed when the sutures are removed but to avoid scrubbing around the suture line.
  —Advise the patient to avoid using a hair dryer until the hair grows back.
- *Warning signs*
  —Review the signs and symptoms that should be reported to a physician or nurse.
    Infection: fever, erythema, tenderness, pain, warmth, purulent drainage from the incision, seizures, lethargy, headache
    Meningitis: fever, chills, malaise, back stiffness and pain, nuchal rigidity, seizures, lethargy, headache
    Neurologic changes: behavioral, personality, motor, or sensory changes, lethargy
    Increased intracranial pressure: altered level of consciousness, nausea, vomiting, seizures, headache
    Leakage of cerebrospinal fluid: clear or bloody drainage from ear, nose, or throat; complaints of salty taste or frequent swallowing; presence of "halo ring" on pillowcase
    Increased urine output

- *Special instructions*
  —Teach the caregiver seizure precautions as indicated.
  - Try to prevent or break the fall.
  - Ease the patient onto the floor.
  - Support and protect the patient's head.
  - Turn the patient to one side.
  - Remove surrounding furniture and any hard or sharp objects.
  - Loosen constrictive clothing around the neck.
  - Stay with the patient and call the physician immediately.
  —Stress the importance of maintaining proper positioning and body mechanics as indicated by the surgical procedure.
  - Teach the patient to avoid bending from the waist: keep back straight, bend knees, and lower body to pick up objects.
  - Use straight, flat chairs; avoid soft-cushioned chairs.
  - Avoid crossing the knees.
  - Avoid lifting while the back is flexed or twisted.
  - Keep the head and neck in proper alignment with the cervical collar.
  - Avoid hyperextension of the spine: avoid sleeping in a prone or supine position; sleep on one side with knees and hips in flexion.
  —Teach the patient to avoid extreme hot and cold temperatures of the lower extremities because of possible sensory nerve loss.
  —Instruct the patient to avoid straining during defecation and to avoid constipation through the use of prescribed stool softeners and laxatives.
  —Instruct the patient to avoid coughing, sneezing, and nose blowing. If unavoidable, they must be done with an open mouth to control intracranial pressure.
- *Medications*
  —Explain the purpose, dosage, schedule, and route of administration of any prescribed drugs, as well as side effects to report to a physician or nurse.
  —Advise the patient against taking over-the-counter medications without consulting the physician.
- *Activity*
  —Encourage the patient to discuss allowances and limitations with respect to occupation, recreation, and activities.

—Encourage independent activities as the patient is able. Assist the patient and caregiver to identify and implement measures that assist with reorientation and communication, if indicated.

—Discuss safety measures specific for postoperative residual motor deficits, sensory deficits, cognitive deficits, and seizure activity. Assist the patient and caregiver to identify and correct hazards in the home.

FOLLOW-UP CARE

- Stress the importance of regular follow-up visits with the physician, physical therapist, occupational therapist, speech therapist, and rehabilitation therapist as indicated. Make sure the patient has the necessary names and telephone numbers.
- Assist the patient in obtaining a MedicAlert bracelet and identification card listing diagnosis and medications.

REFERRALS

- Refer the patient to local support groups available through the American Cancer Society, American Brain Tumor Association, Acoustic Neuroma Association, or home health support services.

Cushing's Disease and Cushing's Syndrome

—Cushing's disease and Cushing's syndrome: a condition resulting from the overproduction of adrenal steroid, particularly cortisol. The high levels of circulating glucocorticoids affect protein, carbohydrate, and lipid metabolism. The disease may occur as a primary disease or resulting from a pituitary tumor. It more commonly affects females.

CAUSES/CONTRIBUTING FACTORS
Cushing's Disease

- Hypersecretion of the pituitary gland, which secretes an excess of adrenocorticotropic hormone (ACTH) in the face of high levels of plasma cortisol

Cushing's Syndrome

- ACTH-secreting tumors of the adrenal glands
- Iatrogenic causes, such as excessive doses of cortisol or ACTH

SIGNS/SYMPTOMS

- Physical changes
  —Central obesity (large trunk, thin legs and arms)
  —Buffalo hump (supraclavicular fat pads)
  —Round face ("moonface")
- Other changes
  —Weight gain
  —Muscle weakness
  —Thin, transparent skin
  —Bruising
  —Impaired wound healing
  —Susceptibility to infections
  —Hypertension, fluid retention with pitting edema
  —Emotional and mental disturbances
  —Thirst and polyuria
  —Abdominal striae, with red and purple lines showing through
- Orthopedic changes
  —Kyphosis and back pain
  —Osteoporosis
  —Pathologic fractures
  —Aseptic necrosis (especially femoral head)
- In women
  —Masculinization
  —Menstrual changes
- In men
  —Feminization
  —Impotence
  —Decreased libido

COMPLICATIONS

- Pathologic fractures
- Congestive heart failure

- Peptic ulcers
- Diabetes insipidus: with adrenalectomy
- Diabetes mellitus

DIAGNOSTIC TESTS

- Describe each procedure, its purpose, and the normal feelings or sensations that are likely, as well as any preprocedural and postprocedural care.
    - —Computed tomography or magnetic resonance imaging: to identify causative tumor of the pituitary gland
    - —Serum tests
        Blood glucose: increased (tested after meals)
        Potassium: decreased
        Overnight dexamethasone suppression test: plasma cortisol levels decreased to 50% of baseline
    - —Urine tests
        24-Hour for free cortisol (17-ketosteroid and 17-hydroxycorticosteroid) levels: elevated

TREATMENT
Medical

- Therapy
    - —Irradiation of the pituitary gland: used for mild disease or poor surgical risk
- Drugs
    - —Adrenocortical inhibitors
        Metopirone
        Mitotane
        Aminoglutethimide
        Cyproheptadine
        Ketoconazole

Surgical

- Transsphenoidal pituitary surgery
- Adrenalectomy: unilateral or bilateral

 HOME CARE

- Give both the patient and the caregiver *verbal* and *written* instructions. Provide them with the name and telephone number of a physician or nurse to call if questions arise.

- *General information*
  —Review the physician's explanation of Cushing's disease and Cushing's syndrome, the causes, and contributing factors.
  —Review skin care, explaining the need to avoid bruising and cuts.

    Advise the patient to inspect the skin for reddened areas, signs of excoriation, and breakdown.

    Keep the skin clean and dry. Use moisturizing skin lotions.

    Advise the patient against using razor blades for shaving.
- *Warning signs*
  —Review the signs and symptoms that should be reported to a physician or nurse.

    Excessive adrenal hormone: weight gain, polydipsia, polyuria, easy bruising, and muscle weakness

    Insufficient adrenal hormone: easy fatigability, weight loss, abdominal pain

    Infection of upper respiratory tract, urinary tract, oral cavity: fever, cough, malodorous sputum; burning, frequency, urgency with urination, malodorous urine; red, swollen, bleeding, painful oral mucosa, painful mucosal lesions, painful teeth
- *Special instructions*
  —For patients with bilateral adrenalectomy: help the patient to organize or obtain an emergency kit including alcohol and prefilled syringes (hydrocortisone) for episodes of severe adrenal insufficiency (see p. 12).
  —Instruct the patient to self-monitor laboratory values and assist the patient to identify personal baseline levels.
  —Discuss the need to prevent injury associated with osteoporosis.

    Keep rooms free of throw rugs and hazardous furniture to prevent falls.

    Use ambulatory aids (e.g., walker, cane) as necessary.
- *Medications*
  —Explain the purpose, dosage, schedule, and route of administration of any prescribed drugs, as well as side effects to report to a physician or nurse.
  —Teach the patients with bilateral adrenalectomy about the need for lifelong hormonal therapy.
  —Discuss hormonal replacement (see Steroid Therapy, p. 590).
  —Discuss the need to avoid over-the-counter medications without first consulting the physician or nurse.

- *Activity*
  - —Encourage the patient to discuss allowances and limitations with respect to occupation, recreation, and activities.
  - —Encourage the patient to pace activites, allow for frequent rest periods, and avoid overexertion.
  - —Teach the importance of using protective devices (decubitus matrices, well-fitting shoes) and practices (changing position frequently, range-of-motion exercises) to avoid injury.
  - —Discuss the relationship between stress and cortisol levels. Teach stress reduction methods: imagery, progressive relaxation, breathing exercises, and meditation.
- *Diet*
  - —Discuss the importance of a well-balanced diet that is high in potassium and low in sodium, calories, and carbohydrates. High-potassium foods include avocadoes, apricots, bananas, meat, poultry, potatoes, and milk.

PSYCHOSOCIAL CARE

- Explain the effects of hormones on emotional status.
- Discuss methods for managing labile emotional states.
- Encourage open communication between the patient and caregivers.

FOLLOW-UP CARE

- Stress the importance of regular follow-up visits for medical and laboratory evaluation. Make sure the patient has the necessary names and telephone numbers.
- Emphasize the need to wear a MedicAlert bracelet and carry an identification card at all times.

Cystic Fibrosis

—**Cystic fibrosis: an autosomal recessive disorder of the exocrine (mucus-secreting) glands: respiratory, pancreatic, and sweat. Cystic fibrosis (CF) causes respiratory glands to produce and accumulate abnormally thick, tenacious secretions. Pancreatic function is affected by a deficiency of trypsin** and lipase, which prevents the absorption of fat and protein in the intestinal tract and interferes with the digestion of food. CF, a chronic, progressive, and incurable genetic disease, may manifest itself soon after birth or may take years to develop. Survival rates have been improving, with patients living into their thirties and forties.

SIGNS/SYMPTOMS

- Salty tasting skin
- Gastrointestinal system
  —Excessive appetite but poor weight gain
  —Thin extremities with abdominal distention
  —Stool (steatorrhea): frequency; large, bulky, frothy, greasy; float in toilet; foul smelling
  —Anorexia
- Pulmonary system
  —Dry, chronic cough followed by loose, productive cough
  —Thick, tenacious mucus
  —Shortness of breath with activity
  —Wheezing
  —Cyanosis, clubbed fingers
- Frequent upper respiratory infections (URIs)

COMPLICATIONS

- Respiratory
  —Severe atelectasis
  —Emphysema
  —Pneumonia
  —Pneumothorax
  —Cor pulmonale
  —Pulmonary hypertension
- Gastrointestinal
  —Intestinal obstruction
  —Esophageal varices
  —Portal hypertension
  —Cirrhosis
- Other
  —Dehydration
  —Arthralgia of distal long bones and associated joints (e.g., knees, ankles, wrists)

—Sterility: secondary amenorrhea in women, azoospermia (lack of sperm) in men

DIAGNOSTIC TESTS

- Describe each procedure, its purpose, and the normal feelings or sensations that are likely, as well as any preprocedural and postprocedural care.
    - —Sweat electrolytes: elevated sweat chloride level (>60 mEq/L)
    - —Pancreatic enzymes: decreased or absent trypsin, lipase, and amylase
    - —Stool examination: minimal or absent trypsin in stool, elevated fat in stool, and increased albumin (azotorrhea, >20 mg/dl)
    - —Chest x-ray: identifies pulmonary complications
    - —Pulmonary function tests

TREATMENT
Medical

- Therapy
    - —Respiratory management: pulmonary hygiene, oxygen therapy, postural drainage
- Drugs
    - —Bronchodilators, mucolytics, expectorants
    - —Antibiotics: to treat pulmonary infections
    - —Pancreatic enzyme replacement with meals and snacks
    - —Fat-soluble vitamins
    - —Daily iron supplements
    - —Salt tablet supplements during hot weather

Surgical

- Pulmonary lavage or bronchial washings
- Resection of blebs and pleural scars
- Lung transplantation

HOME CARE

- Give both the patient and the caregiver *verbal* and *written* instructions. Provide them with the name and telephone number of a physician or nurse to call if questions arise.
- *General information*
    - —Explain the disease process, causes, and prescribed treatments.

- *Warning signs*
    —Review the signs and symptoms that should be reported to a physician or nurse.

    Excessive number of large, bulky, foul-smelling stools

    Change in sputum characteristics or color (e.g., thickened and contains blood)

    Decreased activity tolerance

    Poor appetite

    Fatigue

    Weight loss

    Fever

    Stress symptoms

- *Special instructions*
    —Stress the importance of breathing exercises, percussion, and postural drainage techniques. Demonstrate and permit time to practice.
    —Teach the patient and family the use of the home nebulizer, metered-dose nebulizer, and other respiratory equipment necessary to loosen secretions and dilate the bronchi. Assist the patient to obtain equipment from a pharmacy or medical supply company.
    —Explain the need to avoid known respiratory irritants such as smoke and air pollutants and persons with upper respiratory infections.
    —Instruct the patient on methods of clearing secretions, such as coughing, positioning, or suctioning.
    —Instruct the patient on adaptive breathing techniques to decrease work of breathing.

- *Medications*
    —Explain the purpose, dosage, schedule, and route of administration of digestive agents, bronchodilators, and antibiotics, as well as side effects to report to a physician or nurse.
    —Demonstrate administration of aerosolized antibiotics, if ordered.
    —Advise the patient against taking over-the-counter medications without consulting the physician.
    —Explain indications and administration of oxygen, if ordered.

- *Activity*
    —Encourage the patient to participate in a program of aerobic exercise. Swimming helps strengthen the muscles of respiration and promotes good breathing habits.

—Tell the patient to perform respiratory treatment before participating in physical activity.

—Discuss modifications needed during warm days to prevent dehydration: avoid activities on hot and polluted days, drink plenty of fluid, and take salt supplements.

- *Diet*

  —Review the prescribed diet, which is high in calories and protein and low in fat.

  —Discuss the need to include vitamin supplements (A, D, E, K).

  —Encourage the patient to eat salty foods and add salt at the table.

  —Explain the need to mix supplemental pancreatic enzymes with carbohydrate foods such as applesauce. Protein foods cause enzymes to break down immediately. Instruct the patient to take supplements with snacks as well as meals and to adjust pancreatic enzyme replacement as necessary in accordance with food intake and stool patterns.

  —Tell the patient to avoid known dietary irritants.

  —Assist the patient and caregiver to consult a dietitian for special diet instructions and counseling, alternative ways to prepare foods, and modification of family recipes.

FOLLOW-UP CARE

- Stress the importance of regular follow-up visits. Make sure the patient has the necessary names and telephone numbers.
- Obtain influenza and pneumonia vaccines as recommended.

PSYCHOSOCIAL CARE

- Encourage the patient and caregiver to communicate feelings and concerns to health care professionals and each other. Encourage the caregiver and patient to talk with another family living with cystic fibrosis about its prognosis.
- Discuss with the caregiver the need for everyone to participate in the care of a family member with cystic fibrosis.

REFERRALS

- Provide referral for genetic counseling.
- Refer the patient to the Cystic Fibrosis Foundation.
- Provide referral for psychologic counseling if necessary.
- Assist the patient to obtain referrals for home care, equipment, supplies, and financial assistance as indicated.

Diabetes Insipidus

—Diabetes insipidus: a transient or permanent disturbance of water metabolism that results in the excretion of a large volume of dilute urine. The disease may be pituitary, nephrogenic, or psychogenic in nature.

CAUSES/CONTRIBUTING FACTORS
- Central (pituitary)
- Nephrogenic
- Psychogenic (polydipsia)

SIGNS/SYMPTOMS
- Excretion of large volumes of dilute urine (polyuria; 4 liters/day)
- Polydipsia, unquenchable thirst, preference for cold or iced water
- Low specific gravity (1.001 to 1.005)
- Poor skin turgor, dry skin, weight loss
- Constipation

DIAGNOSTIC TESTS
- Describe each procedure, its purpose, and the normal feelings or sensations that are likely, as well as any preprocedural and postprocedural care.
  - —Dehydration test
    - Central and nephrogenic: no change in urine concentration
    - Psychogenic: urine will become concentrated
  - —Administration of vasopressin following dehydration
    - Central: urine becomes concentrated
    - Nephrogenic and psychogenic: no change
  - —Visual field testing: defects suggest hypothalamic pituitary lesions
  - —Computed tomography scan: useful for detection of hypothalamic pituitary lesions

TREATMENT
Medical
- Drugs
  - —Pituitary hormones

Vasopressin (aqueous Pitressin): short acting, emergency and diagnostic use

Vasopressin (Pitressin tannate in oil): longer acting, chronic and diagnostic use

Lypressin nasal solution (Diapid nasal spray; synthetic lysine): may be used alone or with Pitressin tannate

Desmopressin (DDAVP; synthetic arginine, vasopressin): drug of choice for chronic treatment

Thiazide diuretics: block the ability of the kidneys to excrete free water

🏠 HOME CARE

- Give both the patient and the caregiver *verbal* and *written* instructions. Provide them with the name and telephone number of a physician or nurse to call if questions arise.
- *General information*
  —Explain and discuss with the patient diabetes insipidus, its specific causes, and contributing factors.
- *Warning signs*
  —Review the signs and symptoms that should be reported to a physician or nurse.
    Polydipsia
    Polyuria
    Dilute urine
    Weight loss or gain
- *Special instructions*
  —Show the patient how to measure and record intake and output, stressing that intake should equal output.
  —Demonstrate how to check the urine's specific gravity. Advise the patient where to obtain supplies.
  —Instruct the patient to weigh self daily at the same time with the same clothing and to record weight.
  —Advise the patient to avoid fluids that may have diuretic effect: coffee, tea, alcohol.
- *Medications*
  —Explain the purpose, dosage, schedule, and route of administration of any prescribed drugs, as well as side effects to report to a physician or nurse.
  —Demonstrate how to administer vasopressin. Discuss with the patient side effects or toxic effects to report to the physician and how to use urine volume and characteristics as parameters for the need for administration.

- *Activity*
  —Encourage the patient to discuss allowances and limitations with respect to occupation, recreation, or activities.
  —Discuss the need to plan rest periods and avoid overexertion.

FOLLOW-UP CARE

- Stress the importance of regular follow-up visits for medical and laboratory evaluation. Make sure the patient has the necessary names and telephone numbers.
- Discuss the importance of wearing a MedicAlert bracelet and having a disease identification card.

Diabetes Mellitus
(Ketoacidosis)

—Diabetes mellitus: a metabolic disorder characterized by glucose intolerance. It is a systemic disease caused by a relative or absolute lack of insulin, affecting carbohydrate, protein, and fat metabolism.

CAUSES/CONTRIBUTING FACTORS

- Primary
  —Insulin–dependent diabetes mellitus (IDDM) (type I, juvenile, brittle, labile)
  —Non-insulin–dependent diabetes mellitus (NIDDM) (type II, adult)
- Secondary
  —Impaired glucose tolerance
  —Gestational diabetes mellitus

RISK FACTORS

- Familial tendency (heredity)

SIGNS/SYMPTOMS

- Polyphagia
- Polydipsia
- Polyuria

- Weight loss or gain
- Blurred vision, headaches
- Lethargy
- Impotence, vaginal discharge, increased vaginal infections
- Increased wound healing time
- Orthostatic hypotension, decreased pedal pulses
- Paresthesias, decreased sensations (extremities)

COMPLICATIONS

- Diabetic neuropathies (loss of sensation in extremities)
- Charcot's syndrome
- Retinopathy, kidney failure
- Atherosclerosis of the heart and large vessels
- Amputation

DIAGNOSTIC TESTS

- Describe each procedure, its purpose, and the normal feelings or sensations that are likely, as well as any preprocedural and postprocedural care.
  —Serum
      Fasting blood sugar
      Glucose tolerance test
      Blood insulin levels
      Plasma proinsulin
      Plasma C-peptide
      Glycosylated hemoglobin
      Serum fructosamine

TREATMENT
Medical

- Therapy
  —American Diabetes Association (ADA) diet
  —Insulin infuser pens, open-loop infusion pumps, injection ports, jet injectors
  —Photocoagulation
- Drugs
  —Insulin preparations: human, pork, beef-pork
      Short acting: regular, semilente, Lispro (Humalog)
      Intermediate acting: NPH, lente
      Long acting: ultralente, protamine zinc
      Premixed insulins

—Oral hypoglycemic agents: sulfonylureas, biguanides

—First generation: tolbutamide (Orinase), chlorpropamide (Diabinese), acetohexamide (Dymelor), tolazamide (Tolinase)

—Second generation: glipizide (Glucotrol), glyburide (Diabeta, Micronase), metformin (Glucophage)

D

HOME CARE

- Give both the patient and the caregiver *verbal* and *written* instructions. Provide them with the name and telephone number of a physician or nurse to call if questions arise. Include visual aids and permit time before discharge for return demonstration.
- *General information*
  —Explain and discuss with the patient the specific type of diabetic disorder, the causes, and contributing factors.
- *Warning signs*
  —Review the signs and symptoms of hyperglycemia and hypoglycemia that should be reported to a physician or nurse.
    Polydipsia
    Polyuria
    Lethargy
    Shakiness
    Nausea
    Blood glucose >200 mg
  —Discuss complications associated with diabetes, their signs and symptoms, and measures to prevent them.
- *Special instructions*
  —Discuss blood glucose monitoring.
    Discuss when the test will take place, the technique, the desirable blood sugar range, how to read test results, what to do for abnormal results, the cleaning of equipment, and quality control measures (expiration of strips, calibration of equipment).
    Discuss the importance of washing the hands before using equipment.
  —Discuss self-care when the patient is sick.
    Monitoring is increased to every 4 hours when the patient is sick because illness or injury increases glucose demand. A change in food and medication also is usually required.
    Test results and symptoms should be reported to a physician: blood glucose level >300 mg, inability to take oral fluid and food, signs and symptoms of hyperglycemia.

The patient should keep a log of blood glucose results near the phone as a reference when talking to the physician.

Hydration should be maintained with broth, tea, non-dietetic soda, gelatin, or fluid with electrolytes.

Insulin administration should be based on test results and discussions with the physician.

—Discuss issues of safety and personal hygiene, stressing specifics related to dental, foot, and skin care.

Maintain meticulous dental hygiene to prevent infection.

Wear shoes or slippers at all times to prevent foot injury.

Inspect the feet daily with a handheld mirror to detect cuts, abrasion, and sores.

Visit a podiatrist to have nails, calluses, and corns trimmed.

Keep skin surfaces clean and dry to prevent injury and infection. Report any nonhealing lesions to the physician or nurse for follow-up.

Wear gloves while gardening.

—Advise a female patient to monitor for vaginal infections (fungal) and report them to a physician or nurse for follow-up.

—Discuss with the patient the need to carry fast-acting sugar (LifeSavers, sugar packets) for treatment of hypoglycemia.

—Advise the patient to obtain appropriate items, equipment, and assistive devices for various diabetic needs (glucose monitor, MedicAlert bracelet and identification card, protective shoes).

—Discuss the need to prepare for travel.

Inform the physician.

Obtain immunizations. Have duplicate prescriptions (medications, syringes, needles). Have a letter describing the condition. Obtain a MedicAlert bracelet.

Arrange for special meals en route.

Carry insulin and supplies in hand luggage to prevent loss or exposure to extreme temperature changes. Carry emergency medications to treat travel complications. Carry food.

Be aware of the need to adjust meal and medication schedules as time zones change.

Find out where to obtain emergency assistance if needed.

Travel with a companion if possible.

—For women of childbearing age:

Stress the importance of planning all pregnancies. Explain that pregnancy presents serious risks to the mother and infant.

Encourage the patient to discuss her particular risks with the physician or nurse.

- *Medications*

—Explain the purpose, dosage, schedule, and route of administration of any prescribed drugs, as well as side effects to report to a physician or nurse.

—Demonstrate insulin administration (see discussion of subcutaneous injection below). Review the following:

Peak action times

Insulin storage

Preparation and injection

Site selection and rotation

Techniques for self-injection

—Discuss the use and side effects of oral hypoglycemic agents.

—Tell the patient that new supplies and medication prescriptions should be refilled 1 to 2 weeks before stocks run out.

—Instruct the patient to keep a daily log of blood glucose and doses of insulin and oral hypoglycemics.

—Review subcutaneous insulin injection. Demonstrate and explain the following steps of the procedure, and permit sufficient time for the patient or caregiver to practice.

Rotate the injection sites weekly to prevent hypertrophy or lipoatrophy of the subcutaneous tissues.

Wash hands and use aseptic technique when holding the syringe and needle.

Mix insulin correctly (rolling, not shaking).

Withdraw the correct amount of insulin.

Select the injection site: use subcutaneous fatty tissue and avoid the area within 2 inches of the umbilicus.

Cleanse the skin with alcohol and allow to dry.

Hold the syringe filled with correct insulin dosage like a dart.

Pinch up the skin, forming a fat roll between the fingers.

Using a dartlike motion, quickly insert the needle up to the hub or syringe at a 45-degree angle into the subcutaneous tissue.

Inject the insulin. After completing the injection, pull the needle out quickly and cover the site with cotton. Apply slight pressure for 5 to 8 seconds. *Do not rub.* Rubbing can cause too rapid absorption.

Record the date, time, site, and dosage of each injection on the home record.

Dispose of needles/sharps in a stiff plastic container (gallon bleach container, sharps container). Tape lid or lock closed when two thirds full.

—Arrange to have the necessary equipment available at home.

• *Activity*

—Stress the importance of regular exercise and activity to control blood glucose level and weight.

—Tell the patient to carry simple carbohydrates (raisins, LifeSavers) while exercising in case of emergency.

—Encourage the patient to discuss allowances and limitations with respect to occupation, recreation, or activities.

—Explain that aerobic exercise such as walking, swimming, running, and cycling is preferable because it decreases glucose and benefits cardiovascular status.

• *Diet*

—Obtain a dietary consult and review the prescribed diet.

—Discuss with the patient the need to spread meals throughout the day and to eat meals and snacks at regular times and in prescribed amounts. ADA guidelines suggest 55% to 60% carbohydrates, 30% fat, and 12% to 20% protein.

—Instruct the patient in methods for adjusting the diet to meet a change in activity (greater caloric intake is required for prolonged or strenuous activity to prevent hypoglycemia).

PSYCHOSOCIAL CARE

• Discuss with the patient and significant others the need for support for required lifestyle changes.

• Encourage the patient to verbalize concerns and fears on how the disease may affect lifestyle and activities.

• Encourage the patient and caretaker to participate in planning home care.

FOLLOW-UP CARE

• Stress the importance of regular medical, podiatry, and laboratory follow-ups. Make sure the patient has the necessary names and telephone numbers.

REFERRALS

- Encourage participation in and provide information about local diabetes support groups, the ADA, and the Juvenile Diabetes Foundation.
- Assist the patient to identify community-based resources for education and supplies.
- Provide referrals for home health care and medical social work services as indicated.
- Refer the patient to a community-based exercise program such as those offered by the YMCA or YWCA.

Dilated Cardiomyopathy

—Dilated cardiomyopathy: cardiomyopathy is a heart muscle disorder resulting in impaired function of the heart's pumping action. Dilated cardiomyopathy, the most common form, results from damaged myocardial fibers. The heart takes on a globular shape and contracts poorly during systole.

CAUSES/CONTRIBUTING FACTORS

- Primary: idiopathic
- Secondary
    —Infection (e.g., viral, streptococcal)
    —Immunologic disorders (e.g., rheumatic heart disease, systemic lupus erythematosus, scleroderma)
    —Metabolic disorders (e.g., thyrotoxicosis, myxedema)
    —Toxic processes (alcohol, immunosuppressive drugs, cobalt, lead, mercury)
    —Nutritional: thiamine deficiency
    —Miscellaneous: pregnancy, postpartum, radiation

COMPLICATIONS

- Congestive heart failure
- Arrhythmias
- Emboli
- Pulmonary edema
- Cardiogenic shock

DIAGNOSTIC TESTS

- Describe each procedure, its purpose, and the normal feelings or sensations that are likely, as well as any preprocedural and postprocedural care.
  —Chest x-ray: to detect enlarged heart
  —Echocardiogram: to assess heart chamber size and function and valve function
  —Radionuclide studies: to assess ineffective wall motion and decreased cardiac output
  —Cardiac catheterization: to detect impaired heart function, such as coronary artery disease and valve abnormalities; findings may include impaired cardiac motion, decreased cardiac output, and increased ventricular pressures
  —Electrocardiogram: to detect enlarged heart muscle, rhythm disturbances, conduction disturbances, and evidence of previous heart muscle damage

TREATMENT
Medical

- Therapy
  —Correction of underlying cause
  —Bed or chair rest: to reduce the work of the heart
  —Oxygen: to improve the oxygen content of tissues
  —Diet: sodium restriction (2 g/day)
- Drugs
  —Angiotensin-converting enzyme (ACE) inhibitors: to reduce the work of the heart and myocardial oxygen demand
  —Digitalis: to strengthen the force of contraction by the heart muscle and regulate abnormal rhythms
  —Diuretics: to help the kidney eliminate extra salt and fluid
  —Vasodilators: to reduce the amount of blood coming into the heart and thus reduce the work of the heart
  —Anticoagulants (with prolonged bed rest): to prevent clots from forming
  —Beta blockers: to improve ventricular function

Surgical

- Heart transplant

⌂ HOME CARE

- Give both the patient and the caregiver *verbal* and *written* instructions. Provide them with the name and telephone number of a physician or nurse to call if questions arise.
- *General information*
  —Describe the type of cardiomyopathy and contributing causes.
  —Review the prognosis: in certain cases the prognosis is excellent if the cause is corrected (e.g., if the patient stops using alcohol or delivers a baby, or if toxic agents are removed).
  —For specific home care, see Heart Failure, p. 333.
- *Activity*
  —Explain any limitations imposed on the patient's lifestyle.

Diverticulosis and Diverticulitis

—**Diverticulosis: the development of small pockets along the mucosa of the colon, formed by herniation of mucosal and submucosal linings through the muscular layers of the large intestine. They can occur anywhere throughout the intestine but are most common in the sigmoid colon.**

—**Diverticulitis: the inflammatory process in which a diverticulum ruptures or feces become impacted in the diverticulum.**

CAUSES/CONTRIBUTING FACTORS

- Low-fiber diet
- Increased intracolonic pressures
- Weakened intestinal wall

SIGNS/SYMPTOMS

- Cramplike pain and tenderness in the left lower quadrant
- Anorexia
- Nausea and vomiting
- Fever
- Changes in bowel function: constipation or diarrhea

- Mucus or blood in stools
- Increased flatulence
- Abdominal distention

COMPLICATIONS

- Peritonitis
- Fistulas to the bladder, vagina, or abdominal wall
- Hemorrhage
- Intraabdominal abscesses
- Intestinal obstruction or perforation

DIAGNOSTIC TESTS

- Describe each procedure, its purpose, and the normal feelings or sensations that are likely, as well as any preprocedural and postprocedural care.
  —Water-soluble contrast enema: to locate abscess cavities, fistulas, sinus tracts
- Abdominal x-rays: to detect presence of free air and fluid, obstruction, or ileus
- Complete blood count with differential: to determine the presence of infection as reflected by a shift to the left
- Urinalysis: to rule out bladder involvement
- Computed tomography: to locate diverticula, abscesses, or fistulas
- Stool examination: to assess for occult blood
- Sigmoidoscopy, colonoscopy, or ultrasonography: to reveal the presence of diverticula

TREATMENT
Medical

- Therapy
  —Intravenous fluid replacement with electrolytes
  —Diet is nothing by mouth (NPO) for acute diverticulitis; when inflammation is resolved, progression to high-fiber diet
  —Nasogastric tube aspiration: to relieve nausea, vomiting, and abdominal distention
- Drugs
  —Antibiotics
  —Analgesics: meperidine (Demerol) the agent of choice, since it also decreases gastrointestinal motility and spasms
  —Hydrophilic colloid laxatives

Surgical

- Bowel resection with anastomosis
- Bowel resection with temporary colostomy

⊞:: HOME CARE

- Give both the patient and the caregiver *verbal* and *written* instructions. Provide them with the name and telephone number of a physician or nurse to call if questions arise. Use visual aids to assist in instruction.
- If a temporary colostomy is present, see also Ostomy, p. 694.
- *General information*
  —Explain and discuss the development of diverticulitis and diverticulosis, the causes or contributing factors, care, and treatment.
- *Warning signs*
  —Review the signs and symptoms that should be reported to a physician or nurse.
  > Fever
  > Nausea or vomiting
  > Cloudy or malodorous urine
  > Changes in bowel function: constipation or diarrhea
  > Wound infection: fever, incisional pain, redness, drainage, or swelling
  > For temporary colostomy: change in stoma color from the normal bright red or peristomal skin irritation
- *Special instructions*
  —Assist the patient in obtaining appropriate supplies, such as sterile dressings or ostomy devices, if indicated.
  —Demonstrate proper wound care or stoma management and dressing changes: procedure, frequency, and wound or stoma inspection.
  —Advise the patient to avoid straining during defecation, constipation, enemas, and harsh laxatives.
  —Stress the importance of establishing regular bowel habits.
- *Medications*
  —Explain the purpose, dosage, schedule, and route of administration of any prescribed drugs, as well as side effects to report to the physician or nurse.
  —Instruct the patient to take hydrophilic colloid laxatives as prescribed; advise against taking other laxatives without consulting a physician.

- *Activity*
  —Encourage the patient to discuss allowances and limitations with respect to occupation, recreation, or activities.
  —Instruct the patient to resume activities of daily living gradually but to avoid heavy lifting (>10 pounds), pushing, or pulling for 6 weeks to prevent herniation.
  —Advise that baths or showers may be taken when drains or sutures are removed.
- *Diet*
  —Explain the relationship between diet and diverticular disease. Review foods to eat and to avoid (see Appendix E).
  —Assist the patient to plan a home care diet that includes high fiber, fruits, vegetables, and bran. Provide a list of high-fiber foods and ways to make bran more palatable.
  —Instruct the patient to increase bran gradually because bran may cause abdominal distention and increased flatus.
  —Advise the patient to avoid large meals, alcohol, or extremely cold foods.
  —Advise the patient to drink plenty of fluids, up to 2 to 3 L/day, unless contraindicated.

PSYCHOSOCIAL CARE

- Discuss pain management techniques for dealing with chronic pain: visualization, guided imagery, meditation, relaxation, biofeedback, or back rubs.

FOLLOW-UP CARE

- Stress the importance of regular follow-up visits with the physician and enterostomal therapy (ET) nurse (if indicated). Make sure the patient has the necessary names and telephone numbers.

REFERRALS

- Assist the patient to obtain referral for home health support services and an ET nurse, as indicated.

Dysrhythmia
(Arrhythmia)

D

—Dysrhythmia: disturbance of the normal heart rhythm. Normal heart rhythm begins at the sinus node and follows a normal sequence through the heart's electrical system. Normal resting heart rate is 60 to 100 times/minute. A heartbeat that is too slow (bradycardia) or too fast (tachycardia) can interfere with normal heart function and produce symptoms that can be minor or life threatening. Interruption of the electrical impulse is termed heart block. The heart rate is governed by emotions (nervous system), activities, exercise or rest, drugs, and other stimulants, such as caffeine, tobacco, and electrolytes (body chemicals). Dysrhythmias can be classified by the area where they originate:

—Atrial dysrhythmias: above the atrioventricular node originating in the upper heart chambers (right and left atrium)

—Supraventricular dysrhythmias: involving the upper chamber and atrioventricular node

—Ventricular dysrhythmias: involving primarily the lower heart chambers (right and left ventricles)

SINUS BRADYCARDIA

Sinus bradycardia is a sinus rhythm of <60 beats/minute. The rhythm is normal. Sinus bradycardia can be normal in well-conditioned athletes; it may occur in response to drugs or increased vagal tone. Slowing heart rates are often found in the elderly.

Causes/Contributing Factors

- Increased intracranial pressure
- Increased vagal tone (bowel straining or vomiting)
- Hypothyroidism
- Sick sinus syndrome

- Medications (beta blockers and calcium channel blockers: digoxin, quinidine, propranolol, procainamide)
- Diminished blood flow to the sinoatrial node

Signs/Symptoms

- Usually asymptomatic
- Dizziness
- Weakness
- Altered level of consciousness
- Low blood pressure
- Chest pain
- Fatigue
- Shortness of breath

Complications

- Syncope

Treatment
Medical (necessary only if symptomatic)

- Therapy
  —Correction of underlying cause
  —Pacemaker: temporary or permanent
- Drugs
  —Atropine: as emergency measure to increase heart rate

HEART BLOCK

Heart block (first-, second-, or third-degree) is a conduction disturbance that results in a slow heart rate with partial or complete electrical dissociation between the atria and ventricles. In complete, or third-degree, heart block the ventricles function independently, resulting in decreased efficiency of the heart.

Causes/Contributing Factors

- Lack of blood supply to the electrical system of the heart
- Ischemic heart disease
- Myocardial infarction
- Hypothyroidism
- Congenital heart disease
- Digitalis toxicity

Signs/Symptoms

- Dizziness
- Lightheadedness
- Loss of consciousness
- Low blood pressure
- Weakness
- Difficulty breathing (signs of congestive heart failure)
- Chest pain

Complications

- Syncope (loss of consciousness)
- Heart failure
- Asystole (heart stops beating)

Treatment
Medical

- Therapy
  —Observation: heart block associated with myocardial infarction; usually corrects itself with time
  —Pacemaker: temporary or permanent
- Drugs
  —Discontinuation of causative drug
  —Atropine
  —Isoproterenol

JUNCTIONAL RHYTHM

Junctional rhythm originates in the atrioventricular node or junction. The rate is usually 40 to 60 beats/minute. Atrial activity (corresponding to the P-wave on the electrocardiogram) either is absent or occurs simultaneously with or after the ventricular activity (corresponding to the QRS on the electrocardiogram).

Causes/Contributing Factors

- Digitalis toxicity
- Inferior wall myocardial infarction or ischemia (inadequate blood supply to the sinus node)
- Hypoxia
- Vagal stimulation
- Acute rheumatic fever
- Valve surgery

Signs/Symptoms

- Asymptomatic
- Dizziness
- Weakness
- Altered level of consciousness

Treatment
Medical

- Therapy
  —Observation: junctional rhythm is not usually permanent
  —Treatment of underlying cause
  —Permanent pacemaker
- Drugs
  —Atropine: to block effects of vagal stimulation
  —Isoproterenol

SINUS TACHYCARDIA

Sinus tachycardia is sinus rhythm that is >100 beats/minute. The origin of the beat and the transmission of the electrical impulse are normal. Rhythm is regular.

Causes/Contributing Factors

- Fever
- Exercise
- Anxiety
- Pain
- Dehydration
- Heart disease
- Hyperthyroidism
- Hypovolemia
- Hypoxia
- Drugs affecting the autonomic nervous system (e.g., caffeine, alcohol)

Signs/Symptoms

- Shortness of breath (depending on underlying cause)
- Palpitations
- Fatigue

Complications

- Hypotension
- Dizziness
- Syncope

Treatment
Medical

- Therapy
  —Treatment of underlying cause

ATRIAL FLUTTER

Atrial flutter is a rapid, regular rhythm disturbance that starts in the right atrium. The atrial rate is 200 to 300 beats/minute. The electrical impulses are transmitted to the atrioventricular node. Usually the node is blocked so that not all electrical impulses get through to the ventricles. The ventricular rate is 100 to 150 beats/minute.

Causes/Contributing Factors

- Heart failure
- Valvular heart disease
- Congenital heart disease
- Pulmonary embolism
- Digitalis toxicity
- Coronary artery bypass surgery
- Ischemic heart disease

Complications

- Heart failure (shortness of breath)
- Low cardiac output
- Coronary insufficiency
- Embolization

Treatment
Medical

- Therapy
  —Treatment of the underlying cause
  —Synchronized cardioversion: to restore normal sinus rhythm
  —Atrial pacemaker: to restore heart rhythm
  —Vagal stimulation: to slow heart rate

- Drugs
  —Digitalis (unless dysrhythmia is due to digitalis toxicity)
  —Propranolol: to decrease heart rate (blocks catecholamine stimulation)
  —Quinidine: to decrease heart rate by blocking conduction through the atrioventricular node
  —Procainamide: to block abnormal excitation from abnormal focuses in the heart muscle
  —Verapamil: to slow conduction through the atrioventricular node and decrease heart tone as a vasodilator
  —Antiarrhythmic agents
      Amiodarone: to prolong cardiac action
      Setalol (Beta Pace): has beta-blocking and antiarrhythmic properties
      Propafenone (Rhythmol): to stabilize heart muscle; has local anesthetic effects

ATRIAL FIBRILLATION

Atrial fibrillation is rapid irregular rhythm disturbances that originate in the atrium. The atrial rate is greater than 400 beats/minute and is irregular and chaotic. The atrial impulses (electrical) are transmitted to the atrioventricular node. The node is blocked so that not all electrical impulses get through to the ventricle. Ventricular rate varies (90 to 100 beats/minute), and P-waves are not visible on the electrocardiogram. The condition is common in the elderly.

Causes/Contributing Factors

- Heart failure
- Chronic obstructive pulmonary disease
- Hyperthyroidism
- Sepsis
- Pulmonary embolism
- Mitral stenosis
- Atrial irritation
- Coronary bypass surgery
- Valve surgery

Complications

- Embolization
- Heart failure
- Low cardiac output

Treatment
Medical

- Therapy
  —Treatment of underlying condition
  —Cardioversion
- Drugs
  —Antiarrhythmics
  —Anticoagulants
  —Beta blockers, calcium channel blockers, digitalis: to control rate

VENTRICULAR TACHYCARDIA

Ventricular tachycardia is an abnormally rapid (usually regular) rhythm that originates in the ventricles. Atrial activity is usually unrelated to ventricular activity (dissociated) during ventricular tachycardia. The rate can vary from 120 to 250 beats/minute. Ventricular tachycardia usually occurs in patients who have had underlying heart disease but rarely may occur in individuals without heart disease, in which case it is usually drug related. Because ventricular tachycardia is usually a precursor to ventricular fibrillation, it is treated as a serious dysrhythmia.

Causes/Contributing Factors

- Heart disease
  —Myocardial ischemia
  —Myocardial infarction
  —Congenital heart disease
  —Ventricular aneurysm
  —Left ventricular dysfunction
- Digitalis or quinidine toxicity
- Low potassium and magnesium levels
- High calcium levels

Signs/Symptoms

- Chest pain
- Anxiety
- Palpitations
- Dyspnea
- Low blood pressure
- Loss of consciousness

Complications/Contributing Factors

- Ventricular fibrillation/cardiac arrest
- Shock

Treatment
Medical

- Therapy
  —Treatment of underlying condition
  —Catheter ablation
  —DC cardioversion
  —Implantable defibrillator
- Drugs
  —Antiarrhythmics

VENTRICULAR FIBRILLATION

Ventricular fibrillation is an abnormally rapid, irregular rhythm that originates in the ventricles. Atrial activity is unrelated to ventricular activity. The heart rhythm becomes so rapid and chaotic that the heart becomes totally ineffective as a pump. Blood no longer flows forward, there is no blood pressure, and the patient loses consciousness. If the fibrillation is untreated, the patient will die within minutes.

Causes/Contributing Factors

- Acute or chronic heart disease
- Untreated ventricular tachycardia
- Electrolyte imbalances, such as sodium, potassium, calcium
- Digitalis or quinidine toxicity
- Electric shock (electrocution)
- Hypothermia

Signs/Symptoms

- Loss of consciousness
- Possible seizures
- Sudden death

Treatment
Medical

- Therapy
  —Emergency measures

      Cardiopulmonary resuscitation (CPR): to maintain circulation

      Electrical defibrillation

—Ongoing treatment to prevent recurrence

      Catheter ablation

      Implantable defibrillator

- Drugs
  —Emergency measures
        Epinephrine
        Lidocaine

DIAGNOSTIC TESTS

- Describe each procedure, its purpose, and the normal feelings or sensations that are likely, as well as any preprocedural and postprocedural care.
- Inform the patient that several diagnostic procedures may be performed to aid in the diagnosis of the dysrhythmia.
  —12-Lead electrocardiogram: to detect dysrhythmias and identify possible causes
  —Echocardiogram: to rule out thrombi and to assess left ventricular function
  —Serum electrolyte levels: to assess sodium, potassium, calcium, and magnesium levels that might be abnormally high or low
  —Drug levels: to identify toxicities that can precipitate dysrhythmias
  —Ambulatory monitoring (24-hour Holter monitor or cardiac event recorder): to identify dysrhythmias and associated abnormal rhythms to the patient's symptoms
  —Signal-averaging electrocardiogram: computerized electrocardiogram used to detect areas of slow electrical conduction that are associated with certain rhythm disturbances
  —Event recorder: 30-day recording device activated during symptoms to correlate symptoms with electrocardiographic rhythm changes
  —Electrophysiologic study: to determine origin of dysrhythmia and inducibility and effectiveness of drug therapy in dysrhythmia suppression
  —Exercise stress testing: to assess cardiac response to an increase in workload that can precipitate rhythm abnormali-

ties, such as premature ventricular contractions caused by lack of blood supply to the heart muscle, and to guide therapy

—Arterial blood gases: to identify lack of oxygen in the blood, caused by a compromise in the heart function and circulation in the presence of dysrhythmias

HOME CARE

- Give both the patient and the caregiver *verbal* and *written* instructions. Provide them with the name and telephone number of a physician or nurse to call if questions arise. Use heart models, diagrams of the conduction system, and other visual aids to assist in instruction.

- *General information*
  —Explain what the particular rhythm disturbance is and the identified or suspected cause.
  —Emphasize the importance of not smoking or using tobacco products. Discuss how nicotine can cause dysrhythmias.
  —For a patient receiving an implantable defibrillator, see p. 387.

- *Warning signs*
  —Review the signs and symptoms that should be reported to a physician or nurse.
    Palpitations
    Chest pain
    Shortness of breath
    Rapid pulse
    Dizziness
    Syncope

- *Special instructions*
  —Teach the patient how to take the pulse for a full minute (see Pulse Taking, p. 719).
  —Explain the importance of leading a normal, productive life in the patient's present condition.
  —Help the patient understand what precautions to take at work and at home and how to prepare for vacations.
  —For patients with chronic or serious dysrhythmias, explain the need to identify a health care facility near home and work and to have emergency numbers at hand.

- *Medications*
  —Explain the purpose, dosage, schedule, and route of administration of any prescribed drugs, as well as side effects to report to the physician or nurse.

—Instruct the patient not to stop taking medications abruptly, because of side effects, but to notify the physician so a plan for changing medications can be developed.

—Explain the need for continued follow-up to assess the effectiveness of the medications and to alter treatment if necessary.

—Stress the importance of reordering medications before they run out and ordering enough medication when planning a vacation or travel.

—Discuss the need to avoid taking over-the-counter drugs.

- *Activity*

—Advise the patient to avoid strenuous activity and overexertion. Warn the patient to stop exercise or activity immediately if experiencing dizziness, lightheadedness, or chest pain.

—Encourage questions about allowances and limitations with respect to occupation, recreation, and activities.

- *Diet*

—Advise the patient to eliminate or reduce intake of products containing caffeine, such as coffee, chocolate, tea, colas, and alcohol.

PSYCHOSOCIAL CARE

- Explain the psychologic implications of the presence of cardiac disease and life-threatening arrhythmias: loss of control over lifestyle, anxiety and fear associated with death, possible nightmares or other sleep disturbances, denial, depression, and anger.

- Advise the patient to use relaxation techniques to reduce stress and prevent dysrhythmias by preventing the release of hormones, such as adrenaline, that stimulate the heart rate.

FOLLOW-UP CARE AND REFERRALS

- Stress the importance of regular follow-up visits. Make sure the patient has the necessary names and telephone numbers.

- Discuss the importance of carrying a MedicAlert bracelet and a card listing all medications.

- If telephone monitoring service is available, provide a referral.

Electrophysiology Study
(Cardiac Mapping)

—Electrophysiology study: an invasive procedure used to detect, induce, and treat dysrhythmias. By use of an electrode catheter that is placed through a peripheral vein into the right atrium or ventricle, the heart can be stimulated to recreate and locate the origins of the abnormal heart rhythm, as well as determine the effectiveness of antiarrhythmia therapy.

CONTRAINDICATIONS

- Acute myocardial infarction

PREPROCEDURAL TEACHING

- Review the physician's explanation of the procedure and the reason for it; encourage the patient to ask questions and to discuss any fears or anxieties. Explain that the procedure can be done on an outpatient basis and requires informed consent.

Review of Preprocedural Care

- Instruct the patient not to eat for 6 to 12 hours before the procedure. Fluids may be permitted until 3 hours before the test.
- Explain what will happen during the procedure.
  —Medications are given before the procedure.
  —A peripheral intravenous infusion is started, and oxygen may be administered.
  —The site of the catheter insertion is shaved and cleansed.
  —Dentures and eyewear are removed.
  —The patient is taken to a special laboratory room and placed on a padded surgical table. The procedure takes about 2 to 4 hours.
- Review the sensations to be expected during the procedure.
  —Pressure or discomfort in the groin during the catheter insertion; local anesthesia is used to decrease pain and discomfort
  —Discomfort associated with electrical cardioversion; patient is sedated and usually does not remember the discomfort

- Explain that the patient is sleepy and unaware of surroundings, but is arousable and able to communicate with the physician if necessary.
- Instruct the patient to report any feelings of pain, nausea, dizziness, or palpitations felt during or after the procedure.
- Review the procedure.
  —Electrocardiographic leads are attached for continuous cardiac monitoring.
  —Special patches are applied to the chest to be used for defibrillation, if needed.
  —The groin is cleansed and draped.
  —Several catheters are inserted under fluoroscopy, threaded through the vein or artery in the groin, and positioned in the heart.
  —The patient is heavily sedated.
  —Various parts of the heart's electroconduction system are stimulated by atrial or ventricular pacing. The electroconduction system and its defects are mapped, and dysrhythmias are identified.
  —Antiarrhythmic medications are given to see if they are effective in controlling the dysrhythmia. If the medication is effective, the abnormal rhythm can no longer be induced.
  —Dysrhythmias that do not stop spontaneously may be terminated by rapid overdrive pacing or electrical cardioversion.
  —When all necessary information has been obtained, catheters are removed. Pressure is applied to the sites for 10 minutes, and the patient is returned to his or her room.

Review of Postprocedural Care

- Explain that the patient remains on bed rest and is closely monitored for bleeding or rhythm disturbances. The leg is kept straight for 3 to 6 hours.

COMPLICATIONS

- Ventricular tachycardia or fibrillation
- Perforation of the myocardium
- Cardiac tamponade
- Catheter-induced embolic events (cerebrovascular accident, myocardial infarction)
- Phlebitis, thrombosis at venipuncture site
- Hemorrhage

🏠 HOME CARE

- Give both the patient and the caregiver *verbal* and *written* instructions. Provide them with the name and telephone number of a physician or nurse to call if questions arise.
- For specific home management, see Cardiac Catheterization (p. 154) and Dysrhythmia (p. 245).
- *General information*
  —Review the physician's explanation of electrophysiology study findings and explain recommended treatment.
- *Medications*
  —Explain the purpose, dosage, schedule, and route of administration of any prescribed drugs, as well as side effects to report to the physician or nurse.

PSYCHOSOCIAL CARE

- Encourage expression of fears and concerns regarding any identified dysrhythmias and prescribed treatment.

REFERRALS

- Provide the patient and caregiver with telephone numbers and names of people to contact with questions and concerns.
- Provide referrals for telephone monitoring if available.
- Assist the patient to identify and obtain emergency numbers and referrals.

Encephalitis and Meningitis

—Encephalitis and meningitis: inflammation of the tissues of the brain and spinal cord, resulting in altered function of various portions of these tissues. Encephalitis is frequently accompanied by signs of systemic infection. Encephalitis usually follows a systemic viral infection, mosquito exposure, or swimming or diving in fresh water (amebic). Meningitis may result from a direct invasion of the meninges by bacterial, viral, fungal, or parasitic agents or from the iatrogenic introduction of irritating substances. Meningitis usually follows a recent upper respiratory infection or ear infection or contact with infected persons.

CAUSES/CONTRIBUTING FACTORS

- Encephalitis
  - —Toxemia accompanying an infectious disease
  - —Allergic response
  - —Primary infection
    - Mosquito-borne viral encephalitides
    - Amebic meningoencephalitis
  - —Secondary infection
    - Viral: herpes zoster, herpes simplex, poliomyelitis
    - Toxic substances: lead, carbon monoxide
    - Post vaccination for measles, mumps, rubella
- Meningitis
  - —Meningococcal *(Neisseria meningitidis):* acute communicable
  - —*Haemophilus (Haemophilus influenzae):* acute communicable
  - —Pneumococcal *(Streptococcus pneumoniae):* high risk of fatality
  - —Viral (aseptic or serous): self-limiting and benign

SIGNS/SYMPTOMS

- Encephalitis
  - —Frontal headache, nausea, vomiting, dizziness, fever and chills
  - —Tachypnea, tachycardia
  - —Level of consciousness/behavioral changes
    - Mild listlessness progressing to eventual coma
    - Irritability, seizures, agitation, restlessness
  - —Neurologic: aphasia, olfactory hallucinations, nuchal rigidity, weakness, accentuated deep tendon reflexes, extensory plantar response, ataxia, spasticity, tremors, motor deficits, ocular paralysis
  - —Excess or deficient antidiuretic hormone secretion
- Meningitis
  - —Throbbing headache
  - —Muscle pains
  - —Stiff neck
  - —Backache
  - —Chills
  - —Irritability
  - —Fever (38° to 41° C)
  - —Flushed, hot, dry skin

—Increased blood pressure with increasing intracranial pressure

—Delirium progressing to deep coma

—Positive Brudzinski's sign (flexion of neck elicits flexion of knees and hips)

—Positive Kernig's sign (pain elicited in hamstring after straight leg lift in supine position)

—Generalized seizures

COMPLICATIONS

- Encephalitis
  - —Mental deterioration
  - —Paralysis
  - —Convulsive disorders
- Meningitis
  - —Bacterial: hydrocephalus, cranial nerve involvement (blindness and deafness), arthritis, myocarditis, pericarditis
  - —Aseptic: clinical encephalitis

DIAGNOSTIC TESTS

- Describe each procedure, its purpose, and the normal feelings or sensations that are likely, as well as any preprocedural and postprocedural care.
  - —Neurologic assessment and eye examination
  - —Culture and Gram's stain of blood, cerebrospinal fluid, and respiratory secretions: to identify causative organism
  - —Serologic tests of blood: to identify viral antibodies
  - —Lumbar puncture: to obtain spinal fluid for culture and microsopic examination
  - —Immunofluorescence staining of biopsy specimen of brain
  - —Petechial skin scrapings for Gram's stain

TREATMENT
Medical

- Therapy
  - —Fluid and electrolyte therapy
  - —Nasogastric tube feedings
  - —Ventilatory and oxygenation support
- Drugs
  - —Amebic meningoencephalitis
    - Antiinfective agents (amphotericin B [Fungizone], sulfadiazine, miconazole [Monistat], rifampin [Rifamycin])

—Mosquito-borne encephalitis
  No specific treatment
—Infectious viral encephalitides
  No specific treatment except for herpes infections: adenine arabinoside (vidarabine, ara-A) intravenously; acyclovir
—Meningitis
  Antiinfective agents: ampicillin, chloramphenicol
  Immunologic agents: meningococcal polysaccharide, pneumococcal polysaccharide, *H. influenzae* type B
—Encephalitis and meningitis
  Sedatives
  Antiepilepsy agents
  Glucorticorticoids
  Osmotic diuretics
  Analgesics
  Stool softeners and laxatives
  Antipyretics

🏠 HOME CARE

- Give both the patient and the caregiver *verbal* and *written* instructions. Provide them with the name and telephone number of a physician or nurse to call if questions arise.
- *General information*
  —Review the physician's explanation of the specific type of disorder, its causes, and contributing factors.
- *Warning signs*
  —Review the signs and symptoms of meningeal irritation that should be reported to a physician or nurse. Emphasize the importance of immediately reporting any exacerbation of symptoms.
    Throbbing frontal headache
    Stiff neck
    Any change in mental status
    Fever
    Nausea and vomiting
- *Special instructions*
  —Encourage the patient with encephalitis to swim only in chlorinated water to avoid amebic infection.
  —For bacterial meningitis:
    Encourage the patient to notify all contacts to be evaluated for detection and treatment.

Discuss prophylactic measures to prevent bacterial transmission; immunization may be indicated for close contacts.

- *Medications*
  —Explain the purpose, dosage, schedule, and route of administration of any prescribed drugs, as well as side effects to report to the physician or nurse.

  Acyclovir: teach the patient to monitor for side effects involving the kidney: weight gain, respiratory difficulty, imbalance between fluid intake and output, edema

- *Activity*
  —Encourage the patient to discuss allowances and limitations with respect to occupation, recreation, and activities.
  —Explain to the patient and significant others that convalescence is of variable duration, depending on the severity of the disease.
  —Tell the patient to allow adequate time for recovery before resuming full activities.
  —Explain that rest is needed to decrease stimulation of the irritated meninges.

FOLLOW-UP CARE

- Stress the importance of regular follow-up visits. Make sure the patient has the necessary names and telephone numbers.

Endocarditis

—**Endocarditis: an inflammatory process involving the lining of the heart that may involve the heart valves. Endocarditis results from an infectious process that leads to bacteremia. A number of organisms may cause bacteremia, the most common of which are staphylococci, streptococci, and *Escherichia coli.* Common portals of entry for bacteremias are the mouth, urinary tract, and gastrointestinal tract. While infective endocarditis generally occurs in patients with preexisting heart disease, it can occur in patients with normal heart valves.**

RISK FACTORS

- Preexisting heart disease
  —Valvular heart disesase
  —Congenital heart disease
- Invasive diagnostic and therapeutic procedures
- Intravenous drug use
- Immunosuppression
- Old age

E

SIGNS/SYMPTOMS

- Fatigue
- Elevated temperature
- Chills, night sweating
- Joint aches and pains
- Weight loss
- Loss of appetite
- Just not feeling well

COMPLICATIONS

- Cardiac
  —Abscesses
  —Valvular heart disease
  —Heart failure
  —Myocarditis
- Systemic embolization: cerebral, renal, splenic, coronary
- Other
  —Pulmonary embolism
  —Stroke

DIAGNOSTIC TESTS

- Describe each procedure, its purpose, and the normal feelings or sensations that are likely, as well as any preprocedural and postprocedural care.
  —Blood tests: to identify the causative organism and look for damage to other organs, including the heart and kidneys
     Blood cultures: to detect causative organism
     Complete blood count: to detect inflammatory process and anemia
     Rheumatoid factor
     Erythrocyte sedimentation rate

—Echocardiography: to identify any vegetations or abscesses on the heart valves; to evaluate ventricular function
—Electrocardiogram: to identify any irregular heart rhythms that may result from damage to the heart
—Radionuclide studies: to identify damage to heart structures and function
—Other: blood chemistry analysis, special blood studies (e.g., serum assays), chest x-ray

TREATMENT
Medical

- Drugs
  —Intravenous antibiotics: therapy may last 4 to 6 weeks depending on the infecting organism and heart involvement
  —Antipyretics (aspirin)
  —Anticoagulants if patient has vegetations on valves and develops atrial fibrillation

Surgical

- Generally not indicated, but may be considered in the presence of acute infection with abscess that is unresponsive to intravenous therapy

HOME CARE

- Give both the patient and the caregiver *verbal* and *written* instructions. Provide them with the name and telephone number of a physician or nurse to call if questions arise.
- *General information*
  —Review the physician's explanation of the disease, its causes, and contributing factors.
- *Warning signs*
  —Review the signs and symptoms that should be reported to a physician or nurse.
    Persistent temperature
    Chills alternating with diaphoresis
    Fatigue
- *Special instructions*
  —Review factors that can lead to bacteremia and reinfection: poor oral hygiene, dental work (cleaning, gum treatment, extractions), gastrointestinal or genitourinary procedures, vaginal deliveries, furuncles, staphylococcal infections, surgical procedures.

 —Explain the importance of notifying all physicians and dentists of endocarditis risk before having any procedures performed.

 —Explain the need for good oral hygiene and regular dental care. Stress the importance of notifying the dentist at the first sign of oral infection or gum disease.

- *Medications*
  —Explain the purpose, dosage, schedule, and route of administration of any prescribed drugs, as well as side effects to report to the physician or nurse.
  —Explain the need for antibiotic prophylaxis before a procedure that may cause bacteremia.

- *Activity*
  —Explain the need to avoid fatigue and schedule regular rest periods.

FOLLOW-UP CARE AND REFERRALS

- Stress the importance of regular follow-up visits. Make sure the patient has the necessary names and telephone numbers.

- Provide information and referral for rehabilitation for IV drug abusers.

Endometrial Cancer
(Uterine Cancer)

 —Endometrial cancer: cancer of the uterus, the most common gynecologic malignancy. A slow-growing tumor, endometrial cancer is found primarily in postmenopausal women. Most endometrial cancers are adenocarcinomas. Others are adeno-acanthomas, clear cell tumors, and squamous cell tumors (these are rare but aggressive and affect younger women). Metastatic spread is most commonly to the pelvic and paraaortic lymph nodes. Bloodborne metastases are most commonly to the lungs, liver, bone, and brain.

RISK FACTORS

- Obesity (>15% over normal weight)
- Nulliparity (never having had a child)
- Endometrial hyperplasia
- Polycystic ovarian disease
- Late menopause (after age 52)
- History of irregular menses
- Failure of ovulation
- History of breast, colon, or ovarian cancer
- Diabetes
- Hypertension
- Prolonged use of exogenous estrogen therapy (unopposed)
- Incidence higher among urban, white, and Jewish women

SIGNS/SYMPTOMS

- Postmenopausal bleeding
- Pain in lumbosacral, hypogastric, and pelvic areas
- Advanced disease: bowel obstruction, jaundice, ascites, respiratory difficulty

DIAGNOSTIC TESTS

- Describe each procedure, its purpose, and the normal feelings or sensations that are likely, as well as any preprocedural and postprocedural care.
  —Papanicolaou (Pap) smear: to detect malignant cells
  —Endometrial biopsy or fractional dilation and curettage: to detect malignant cells
  —Laparotomy with sampling of peritoneal fluid or washings: to detect malignant cells

TREATMENT
Medical

- Therapy
  —Radiation therapy
    Preoperative: intracavity radiation therapy
    Postoperative: external beam
  —Chemotherapy
    Progesterone (Megace), hydroxyprogesterone, or medroxyprogesterone acetate
    Single-agent chemotherapy: cisplatin, doxorubicin, hexamethylmelamine, cyclophosphamide

Surgical

- Stage I tumors
  —Total abdominal hysterectomy with bilateral salpingo-oophorectomy and pelvic and paraaortic lymph node biopsies
- Stage II tumors
  —Radical hysterectomy

🏠 HOME CARE

- Give both the patient and the caregiver *verbal* and *written* instructions. Provide them with the name and telephone number of a physician or nurse to call if questions arise. Use visual aids to assist in instruction.
- *General information*
  —Review the physician's explanation of the disease, its causes, and contributing factors.
  —Provide pain management (see Pain Management, p. 708).
  —Prepare the patient for intracavity radiation therapy (see Radiation Therapy, p. 721).
  —Prepare the patient for hysterectomy (see Hysterectomy, p. 384).
- *Warning signs*
  —Review the signs and symptoms that should be reported to a physician or nurse.
  > Infection: redness, drainage, pain, warmth, fever
  > Bleeding: evidence of vaginal or incisional bleeding
  > Fluid volume deficit: decreased urinary output, concentrated urine, weakness, change in mental status

PSYCHOSOCIAL CARE

- Encourage verbalizations and questions regarding prognosis and treatment options.
- Encourage the patient to seek a mental health counselor for support.

FOLLOW-UP CARE

- Stress the importance of regular follow-up visits. Make sure the patient has the necessary names and telephone numbers.

REFERRALS

- Assist the patient to obtain referral services for sexual counseling and support groups.

Endometriosis

—Endometriosis: abnormal growth of endometrial tissue outside the uterus, commonly on the ovaries, peritoneal cul-de-sac (pouch of Douglas), uterosacral ligaments, and peritoneal surface of the uterus. The ectopic tissue is also responsive to the hormonal changes of the menstrual cycle. A benign disease of unknown cause, endometriosis possesses the ability to infiltrate and spread. It commonly occurs in nulliparous women 30 to 40 years of age and in older women who delay childbearing.

CAUSES/CONTRIBUTING FACTORS/RISK FACTORS

- Congenital obstruction of the vagina or cervix associated with reflux menstruation
- Hormonal or inflammatory factors

SIGNS/SYMPTOMS

- Changes in menstrual bleeding pattern: excessive, prolonged, frequent
- Dysmenorrhea: pain with menstruation
- Pain with defecation
- Vague aching or cramping in pelvic or sacral regions
- Dyspareunia: pain with sexual intercourse

COMPLICATIONS

- Infertility
- Decreased fertility
- Spontaneous abortion

DIAGNOSTIC TESTS

- Describe each procedure, its purpose, and the normal feelings or sensations that are likely, as well as any preprocedural and postprocedural care.
  - Laparoscopy: to visualize lesions or adhesions; to perform biopsy of lesions

TREATMENT
Medical

- Therapy
  —Pregnancy for women wishing to have children
- Drugs
  —Gonadotropin-releasing hormone agonists
  —Antigonadotropic agents
  —Progestins

Surgical

  —Laparoscopic removal, laser therapy, or cauterization of endometrial implants and lysis of adhesions
  —Total abdominal hysterectomy with bilateral salpingo-oophorectomy: to remove the organs producing hormones that influence disease
  —Resection or cautery: for destruction of visible lesions

HOME CARE

- Give both the patient and the caregiver *verbal* and *written* instructions. Provide them with the name and telephone number of a physician or nurse to call if questions arise.
- *General information*
  —Review the physician's explanation of the disease, its causes and contributing factors, care, and treatment.
  —Prepare the patient for hysterectomy (see Hysterectomy, p. 384).
- *Warning signs*
  —Review the signs and symptoms that should be reported to a physician or nurse.
    Fever
    Vaginal bleeding and discharge
    Abdominal pain and distention
- *Special instructions*
  —Provide pain management, offering alternative methods to deal with chronic pain: visualization, guided imagery, meditation, relaxation, biofeedback.

PSYCHOSOCIAL CARE

- Encourage the patient and partner to explore and share feelings, fears, and anxiety about potential infertility, changes in body image, and changes in sexual function.

- Advise the patient and partner not to postpone childbearing, since infertility is a complication.

FOLLOW-UP CARE

- Stress the importance of regular follow-up visits, including pelvic examinations. Make sure the patient has the necessary names and telephone numbers.

REFERRALS

- Assist the patient to obtain referral to community groups, such as RESOLVE, or to a counselor for further support.
- Assist the patient and partner to obtain referral to infertility specialists, if desired.

Endoscopy

—**Endoscopy: visualization of the lining of the digestive tract, used to detect sources of bleeding; to identify abnormalities such as ulcers, tumors, polyps, or inflammation; and to obtain tissue samples (biopsy) for laboratory analysis. Types and organs imaged include gastroscopy (stomach), duodenoscopy (duodenum), gastroduodenoscopy (stomach and duodenum), and esophagogastroduodenoscopy (esophagus, stomach, and duodenum).**

INDICATIONS

- Achalasia
- Cancer of the oral cavity or esophagus
- Esophagitis and esophageal varices
- Mallory-Weiss syndrome
- Acute or chronic gastritis
- Gastric and duodenal ulcers
- Gastric cancer

PREPROCEDURAL TEACHING

- Review the physician's explanation of the procedure and the reason for it; encourage the patient to ask questions and to discuss any fears or anxieties. Explain that the procedure takes 15 to 30 minutes, is usually done on an outpatient basis, and involves passage of a long, flexible, lighted tube with an optical head for direct visualization. Explain the need to obtain informed consent.

Review of Preprocedural Care

- Allow the patient to verbalize fears and concerns about the procedure.
- Explain that the patient will have nothing by mouth (NPO) for 6 to 12 hours before the procedure.
- Review the procedure.
  —If the procedure is done on an emergency basis, a nasogastric tube is inserted to aspirate gastric contents.
  —An intravenous line or heparin lock is inserted.
  —Dentures and partial plates are removed.
  —Sedatives and analgesics are given.
  —Atropine is given to decrease gastrointestinal motility and prevent aspiration.
  —A local anesthetic is sprayed into the mouth and throat to ease the passage of the endoscope. Explain that the mouth and throat will feel swollen and it will be difficult to swallow. Instruct the patient to allow saliva to drain from the side of the mouth into an emesis basin.

Review of Postprocedural Care

- Explain what will happen after the procedure.
  —The patient is NPO until the gag reflex returns, about 2 to 4 hours.
  —Throat lozenges and analgesics are prescribed for throat soreness.
  —The patient is monitored for signs and symptoms of complications.
- Advise the patient to have someone available to drive him or her home because of the effects of sedation.

COMPLICATIONS

- Hemorrhage
- Esophageal or gastric perforation
- Difficult or painful swallowing
- Fever

- Hematemesis
- Respiratory and hemodynamic instability

HOME CARE

- Give both the patient and the caregiver *verbal* and *written* instructions. Provide them with the name and telephone number of a physician or nurse to call if questions arise.
- *General information*
  —Review the physician's explanation of the procedure, findings, and specific follow-up care.
- *Warning signs*
  —Review the signs and symptoms that should be reported to a physician or nurse.
      Persistent difficulty in swallowing
      Increased pain
      Bleeding: bloody emesis, black stools
      Respiratory distress
- *Special instructions*
  —Advise the patient that a sore throat or burping may continue for 3 days after the procedure.
  —Suggest throat lozenges or warm saline gargles to ease throat discomfort.
- *Diet*
  —Instruct the patient to resume a regular diet or a diet prescribed for the underlying condition when gag and swallowing reflexes return, in 2 to 4 hours.
  —Suggest beginning with soft, bland foods until soreness subsides.

FOLLOW-UP CARE

- Stress the importance of regular follow-up visits. Make sure the patient has the necessary names and telephone numbers.

Enucleation

—Enucleation: surgical removal of the eyeball, performed when other treatment of the eyeball is insufficient to prevent pain, disfigurement, or spread of malignant disease.

There are two procedures: evisceration, in which the eyeball and cornea are removed but the sclera remains, and exenteration, in which the eyelids, eyeball, and orbital contents are removed. This radical procedure is usually done for malignancies.

INDICATIONS

- Severe infections
- Malignancies (melanoma, retinoblastoma)
- Large, infiltrating tumors
- Extensive trauma
- Blindness with severe eye pain
- End-stage glaucoma
- Prophylaxis in sympathetic ophthalmia

PREPROCEDURAL TEACHING

- Review the physician's explanation of the procedure and the reason for it; encourage the patient to ask questions and to discuss any fears or anxieties. Explain the need for informed consent for surgery and general or local anesthesia.
- Explain that the procedure may be done under local or general anesthesia.

Review of Preprocedural Care

- Review preprocedural tests.
  —Blood tests: to determine the status of electrolytes and show the presence of infection
  —Urine tests: to determine the presence of infection
  —Chest x-ray and electrocardiogram if indicated by age: to provide baseline and detect potential problems
- Inform the patient of the need to be NPO from the night before surgery.
- Discuss the need for a shower and shampoo with bactericidal soap the night before surgery.

Review of Postprocedural Care

- Explain that the physician will implant a temporary artificial globe (conformer) made of Teflon or plastic, which is inserted to maintain orbit shape until a permanent ocular prosthesis can be made (usually 10 to 14 days after enucleation).
- Discuss the need for a pressure dressing for 2 to 3 days postoperatively to minimize swelling and prevent bleeding.

- Explain that diet and activity will be progressed as tolerated after the first postoperative day.
- Explain that touching and rubbing the orbit or tightly squeezing the eyelid is to be avoided because these actions can cause injury and infection.
- Explain that some pain is normal after surgery and will be controlled with analgesics. However, advise the patient to report the presence of headache or sharp pain, which could indicate hemorrhage, infection, or broken sutures.
- Tell the patient not to lie on the operative side but rather to lie supine or with head elevated 30 degrees to minimize intraorbital pressure.
- Advise the patient to avoid stooping, bending, lifting heavy objects, straining with bowel movements, and coughing or sneezing with a closed mouth, since these may cause bleeding.

SIDE EFFECTS/COMPLICATIONS
- Hemorrhage
- Shock
- Infection
- Abscess formation
- Meningitis

HOME CARE
- Give both the patient and the caregiver *verbal* and *written* instructions. Provide them with the name and telephone number of a physician or nurse to call if questions arise.
- *Warning signs*
  —Review the signs and symptoms that should be reported to a physician or nurse.
  - Purulent drainage or bleeding
  - Swelling of the orbit
  - Pain
  - Persistent orbital redness
  - Fever
- *Special instructions*
  —Explain the importance of not rubbing, touching, or bumping the orbit or wearing eye makeup without the consent of the physician.
  —Discuss the need for cleaning the lid, and demonstrate how to remove drainage by gently sweeping the cotton ball from the inner to the outer aspect of the lid, using a new cotton

ball with each sweeping motion. Permit time for a return demonstration.

—Review care of the eye socket. Discuss how to care for, insert, and remove an artificial eye if used.

—Explain the need to wear an eye shield or patch to keep the socket clean until the prosthesis is fitted. Demonstrate application of the shield.

—Discuss the need to protect the vision in the remaining eye. Advise the patient to wear safety glasses for protection and to have regular follow-up eye examinations.

—Explain that the conformer for the eyeball may become dislodged but that this is not a serious problem and that the conformer need not be reinserted.

- *Medications*

—Explain the purpose, dosage, schedule, and route of administration of any prescribed drugs, as well as side effects to report to the physician or nurse.

—Explain the importance of good handwashing before administering ophthalmic medications.

—Explain proper storage of each drug (some eye drops require refrigeration).

- *Activity*

—Remind the patient that with the loss of one eye, the field of vision is limited and depth perception changes. Discuss the need to exaggerate head movement to attain a full visual field. Advise using caution during activities until the patient adjusts to the loss.

FOLLOW-UP CARE

- Stress the importance of regular follow-up visits to the physician and ocular prosthetist. Make sure the patient has the necessary names and telephone numbers.

- Discuss the importance of wearing a MedicAlert band and carrying an information card that identifies the presence of an ocular prosthesis.

Epididymitis

—Epididymitis: inflammation of the epididymis, which may be caused by infection of the prostate, chemicals, or trauma. It may also result from long-term indwelling catheters or prostate surgery. Epididymitis usually affects only one side of the scrotum but may affect both. It is sometimes confused with torsion of the testis.

CAUSES/CONTRIBUTING FACTORS

- Men younger than 35 years
  —Sexually transmitted diseases such as gonorrhea, syphilis, *Chlamydia* infection
- Men older than 35 years
  —Abnormality of the urinary tract
  —Straining to urinate
  —After urologic procedures
  —Strenuous exercise
  —Mumps

SIGNS/SYMPTOMS

- Early
  —Heavy feeling in the scrotum
  —Painful urination
  —Scrotal pain and swelling
- Acute stage
  —Scrotum reddened, warm to touch, swollen (one side or both)
  —Extreme pain that may radiate to the groin or flank
  —Nausea, vomiting
  —Fever
  —Possible urethral discharge

COMPLICATIONS

- Hydrocele
- Orchitis, prostatitis, urethritis, cystitis
- Fibrosis of area
- Sterility

DIAGNOSTIC TESTS

- Describe each procedure, its purpose, and the normal feelings or sensations that are likely, as well as any preprocedural and postprocedural care.
  - —Blood studies
    - White blood cell count: to check for infection
  - —Urine studies

    - Urinalysis: to check for infection
    - Culture: to identify bacteria
    - Culture of urethral discharge: to check for sexually transmitted diseases
  - —Testicular radionuclide scan: to rule out torsion of the testis
  - —Doppler stethoscope: to rule out torsion of the testis

TREATMENT
Medical

- Therapy
  - —Bed rest with elevation of the scrotum and application of ice packs to decrease swelling
- Drugs
  - —Antibiotics
  - —Analgesics
  - —Spermatic cord block for extreme pain

HOME CARE

- Give both the patient and the caregiver *verbal* and *written* instructions. Provide them with the name and telephone number of a physician or nurse to call if questions arise.
- *General information*
  - —Review the disease, discussing causes and contributing factors.
- *Warning signs*
  - —Review the signs and symptoms that should be reported to a physician or nurse.
    - Increasing pain
    - Swelling
    - Scrotal area hot to touch
    - Urethral discharge
- *Special instructions*
  - —Advise the use of comfort measures: ice packs; elevation of scrotum; loose, lightweight clothing; scrotal support while walking.

—Stress the importance of notifying all sexual partners if the inflammation is due to sexually transmitted disease.

- *Medications*
  —Explain the purpose, dosage, schedule, and route of administration of any prescribed drugs, as well as side effects to report to the physician or nurse.
- *Activity*
  —Discuss the need to maintain rest and to avoid exercise, sexual activity, or other strenuous activity during a period of inflammation and swelling.

FOLLOW-UP CARE

- Stress the importance of regular follow-up visits to the physician and for laboratory examinations. Make sure the patient has the necessary names and telephone numbers.

REFERRALS

- Refer the patient to appropriate supportive services if sterility is suspected.

Erectile Dysfunction
(Impotence)

—**Erectile dysfunction: inability to produce an erection of the penis of sufficient duration and rigidity to engage in intercourse.**

CONTRIBUTING FACTORS/RISK FACTORS

- Endocrine problems (diabetes mellitus)
- Congenital problems (e.g., Klinefelter's syndrome)
- Chronic heart disease
- Drugs (immunosuppressants associated with transplants)
- Chronic renal insufficiency
- Chronic renal failure
- Neurologic conditions or injury (multiple sclerosis, trauma, epilepsy)

- Arteriosclerosis
- Surgical procedures (prostatectomy, ileostomy, colostomy)
- Mechanical defects (priapism [painful erection], abnormal lateral curvature)
- Reversible risk factors
  —Medications: antihypertensives, antidepressants, alpha and beta blockers, some heart medications such as digoxin, diuretics, immunosuppressants, weight reduction drugs, anabolic steroids
  —Recreational drugs: cocaine, marijuana, amphetamines, opiates
  —Alcohol

SIGNS/SYMPTOMS

- Inability to initiate erection
- Inability to attain erection
- Inability to sustain erection

COMPLICATIONS

- Psychosocial implications (depression, marital problems)
- Following penile implants
  —Infection
  —Rejection of penile implant
  —Mechanical failure
  —Seepage of fluid from balloon (inflatable device) into surrounding tissue
  —Erosion of glans and urethra
  —Persistent penile pain (after 4 weeks)

DIAGNOSTIC TESTS

- Describe each procedure, its purpose, and the normal feelings or sensations that are likely, as well as any preprocedural and postprocedural care.
  —Endocrine blood studies: to evaluate presence of hormones or glucose
  —Nocturnal penile tumescence
  —Snap-gauge testing: to check for nocturnal erections; a pressure-sensitive rubber band around the penis will break under the pressure
  —Penile blood pressure
  —Penile pulse recording

—Dynamic infusion cavernosometry and cavernosography: to check blood flow in the blood vessels necessary for erection

TREATMENT
Medical

- Therapy
  —Mechanical devices: vacuum pump (Erect-Aid or Correct-Aid)
- Drugs
  —Hormones: to stabilize the endocrine condition
  —Intracavernosal injection therapy, vasodilator injection (papaverine, prostaglandin E, phentolamine): to correct vascular impotence
  —Sildenafil (Viagra)

Surgical

- Prosthetic device
- Penile prosthesis implantation: semirigid or flexible rods
- Inflatable prosthetic device
- Revascularization of blood vessels
- Corrective surgery for mechanical defects

PREPROCEDURAL TEACHING

- Review the physician's explanation of prosthetic implantation and the reason for it; encourage the patient to ask questions and to discuss any fears or anxieties.
- Discuss postoperative care after a prosthetic implantation.
  —Explain the possible need for a temporary urinary drainage tube and restrictive dressing.
  —Discuss the reason for elevating the scrotum and applying cold packs.
  —Stress the need to avoid erections.

⊞ HOME CARE

- Give both the patient and the caregiver *verbal* and *written* instructions. Provide them with the name and telephone number of a physician or nurse to call if questions arise.
- *General information*
  —Explain the patient's particular disorder, contributing causes, and type of prescribed treatment.

—Review the types of sexual dysfunction associated with prostate or testicular cancer and following bilateral orchiectomy or chemotherapy, radiation therapy, and hormonal therapy: reduced fertility, ejaculatory and erectile dysfunction.

—Discuss actual or potential dysfunctional problems the patient may encounter. Explain that some problems may be reversible; for example, hormonal therapy in prostate cancer may affect libido and erectile function but changes may be reversible once treatment is complete, or sperm production may be decreased for an extended time after chemotherapy. Discuss possible strategies to deal with problems; for example, for permanent infertility, strategies include banking sperm before therapy is begun or using alternative fertilization procedures such as artificial insemination through donor sperm, electroejaculation stimulation with intrauterine insemination, or in vitro fertilization.

—Discuss alternative expressions of sexuality: physical intimacy, hugging, kissing, massage.

—Review the written protocol for the prescribed prosthetic device or therapy (prosthetic implantation, vascular therapy, mechanical device) as provided by the nurse specialist or physician.

- *Vasodilating injections*
  —Teach the patient to perform self-injections, stressing the importance of using the correct dosage.
  —Review injection sites, frequency, and potential side effects such as priapism.

- *Prosthetic implantation*
  —Explain the name and type of prosthesis implanted.
  —Review the signs and symptoms of problems with the prosthetic implant that should be reported to a physician or nurse.

    Infection: redness, swelling, warm to touch, tenderness, drainage

    Persistent penile pain

    Inability to urinate

    Any mechanical failure of the pump (no erection after pumping)

    Painful intercourse

    Urinary tract infection (see Pyelonephritis, p. 535)

Erosion of glans of penis: painful sexual intercourse, reddened area over implant and tender to touch, thinning area over implant area or visibility of implant

—Advise how and where to obtain supplies.

—Explain the need to keep the incision clean and dry.

—Explain the allowable time frame for the inability to urinate.

—Discuss the need to avoid the use of tight or restrictive clothing initially.

—Encourage the use of jockey briefs or loose-fitting trousers if the patient is bothered with an aroused penis.

- *Vascular therapy*
  —Discuss care associated with vascular therapy.

  Stress the importance of condoms if performing self-injection therapy and having intercourse with multiple partners. Discuss and provide instructions on safe sex practices.

  Demonstrate and explain how and where to inject drugs, such as papaverine.

  Explain the need to report priapism (painful, sustained erection) to the physician or nurse.

- *Mechanical devices*
  —Discuss care associated with mechanical devices.

  Reinforce the physician's or nurse specialist's explanation and demonstrate the external vacuum device operation.

  For a patient with an internal inflatable pump device, explain when to start inflating and the length of time to keep inflated. Reinforce the need to inflate the device (as instructed) before actual use to encourage fibrous formation around the sheath.

  For a patient using a vacuum erection device, explain that he must remove the restriction device promptly after intercourse is completed to prevent ischemia.

  Encourage questions regarding devices; permit time and privacy to practice activating devices.

- *Medications*
  —Explain the purpose, dosage, schedule, and route of administration of any prescribed drugs, as well as side effects to report to the physician or nurse.

  Amyl nitrate ampoules: to suppress penile erections after surgery

Papaverine: injected into the base of the penis to produce erection

Stress the importance of the amount to be used and the frequency (as prescribed). Explain that certain medications (heart medications or antihypertensives) cannot be stopped without consulting a physician.

Sildenafil: contraindicated in men taking nitrates (e.g., nitroglycerin) and with conditions causing sustained erections (e.g., sickle cell anemia, leukemia).

- *Activity*
  —Advise the patient to avoid sitting for long periods (more than 2 hours).
  —Explain the need to avoid strenuous exercise, jogging, or sports for about 3 weeks or as ordered.
  —Tell the patient to avoid lifting anything >10 pounds.
  —Advise the patient to avoid intercourse until all pain and swelling are gone, the incision is completely healed, or the physician gives approval (approximately 6 weeks).
- *Diet*
  —Explain that a regular diet or one prescribed by the physician should be followed.

PSYCHOSOCIAL CARE

- Encourage verbalization of fears and anxiety regarding sexuality and body image change. Encourage questions from the patient and partner.
- Encourage the patient to seek counseling and support.

FOLLOW-UP CARE

- Stress the importance of regular follow-up visits with the physician, physical therapist, or rehabilitation therapist. Make sure the patient has the necessary names and telephone numbers.

REFERRALS

- Provide referrals for sexual counseling and supportive counseling, including family planning and urology, as needed.

Fixator Devices

—Fixator devices: use of fixation devices to immobilize and repair damaged bones and joints and treat musculoskeletal conditions.

—External fixation: surgical procedure used to immobilize and reduce complicated fractures and nonunion fractures. External fixation is also used in maintaining bones, in limb-lengthening procedures such as the Ilizarov method, and in the treatment of other musculoskeletal disorders such as osteomyelitis. Stabilizing pins or wires are inserted into and through the bone and attached to an external metal frame. Fixation may be applied to the jaw, arm, leg, ribs, pelvis, fingers, or toes. External fixator devices are also used to increase use of the joint while maintaining immobilization of bone. Thus they permit earlier discharge to home because they hold unstable fractures in place while permitting the patient to ambulate.

—Internal fixation: surgical implantation of metallic pins, nails, screws, plates, rods, and other devices for immobilizing or repairing traumatized or damaged bones and joints. Open reduction with internal fixation can be performed on most bones except the skull and facial bones. Bones most frequently treated with this type of procedure include the arms, legs, forearms, thighs, and vertebral column. Internal fixation is used most frequently to repair fractured bones. Similar to external fixation, it permits the patient to be ambulatory, to be discharged earlier, and to regain independence relatively quickly.

PREPROCEDURAL TEACHING

• Review the physician's explanation of the procedure and the reason for it; encourage the patient to ask questions and to discuss any fears or anxieties. Discuss the need for informed consent for surgery and anesthesia.

Review of Preprocedural Care

- Review care before external fixation.
  —The skin of the affected extremity or operative site will be cleansed with bactericidal soap.
  —X-rays will be taken to determine the location of the repair.
  —Prophylactic antibiotic therapy will be prescribed.
- Review care before internal fixation.
  —The physican may order skin or skeletal traction before surgery to lessen muscle spasm.
  —Routine diagnostic studies will be ordered: complete blood count, urinalysis, chest x-ray, electrocardiogram, and x-rays to determine location of repair.
  —Bowel preparation with an enema may be ordered the night before.
  —The skin will be cleansed with bactericidal soap.
  —Nothing by mouth (NPO) status will be maintained from midnight the night before.
  —Intravenous therapy is initiated.
  —An indwelling catheter may be ordered before surgery.
  —Type and crossmatch for blood transfusion may be ordered.

Review of Postprocedural Care

- Review postprocedural care for external fixation.
  —The patient will remain in the hospital 2 to 3 days.
  —Routine postoperative procedures will be performed: frequent checks of neurovascular status and peripheral pulses, decreasing in frequency; application of ice to the incision site; elevation of the extremity on pillows; upper extremity in a sling; for lower extremity, patient instructed to use crutches with no weight bearing; the nuts on the fixator will be turned and tightened.
  —Stress the importance of range-of-motion exercises, quadriceps setting, and gluteal contractions according to the location of the fracture.
  —Explain that the fixator causes little pain and permits early ambulation.
  —Instruct the patient in proper use of ambulatory aids (crutches, cane, walker).
  —Inform the patient of the need to monitor the neurovascular status of the affected extremity: color, sensation, mobility, peripheral pulse, temperature.

- Advise the patient of the need to turn nuts every 6 hours if ordered by the physician.
- Instruct the patient in pin care: cleanse around each pin with hydrogen peroxide and rinse with normal saline, then dry; apply antibacterial agent around each pin.
- Review postprocedural care for internal fixation.
  —The length of hospital stay varies with the specific operation.
  —Routine postoperative procedures will be performed: frequent checks of vital signs, neurovascular status, and peripheral pulses in the first hour, decreasing in frequency thereafter; dressing and wound checks; possible presence of drainage tube in the wound.
  —The patient will be instructed in the proper use of a cane, crutches, or walker with the ordered amount of weight bearing.
  —The signs of neurovascular impairment of the affected extremity will be reviewed: persistent changes in color (pallor, cyanosis, redness), coolness, delayed capillary refill, paresthesia (numbness, tingling), inability to move distal areas.
  —The patient will be taught range-of-motion exercises for the unaffected joints.

SIDE EFFECTS/COMPLICATIONS

- External fixation
  —Infection
  —Delayed healing because of torque and twist
  —Refracture after pin removal
  —Nonunion
  —Muscle or nerve damage or injury
  —Deep vein thrombosis
  —Compartment syndrome
  —Fat embolism
- Internal fixation
  —Infection
  —Hemorrhage
  —Loss of reduction or dislocation
  —Pneumonia
  —Thrombophlebitis
  —Nonunion
  —Refracture

🏠 HOME CARE

- Give both the patient and the caregiver *verbal* and *written* instructions. Provide them with the name and telephone number of a physician or nurse to call if questions arise.
- *General information*
  —Review the specific type of device ordered and specific care.
- *Warning signs*
  —Review the signs and symptoms of problems after external fixation that should be reported to a physician or nurse.

  Infection
  ○ Fever
  ○ Chills
  ○ Redness
  ○ Swelling
  ○ Purulent drainage at pin sites
  Pin migration: tenting of the skin on the pin, which signals movement of the pin or infection
  Neurovascular impairment: pallor, cyanosis, coolness, tingling, numbness

  —Review the signs and symptoms of problems after internal fixation that should be reported to a physician or nurse.

  Infection: persistent redness, swelling, increasing pain, wound drainage, local warmth, foul odor from cast, sensation of burning within cast, drainage from cast, fever
  Neurovascular impairment: pallor, cyanosis, coolness, tingling, numbness

- *Special instructions*
  —External fixation
  Provide instruction on pin and fixator care: cleanse fixator with sterile water and cover each pin head with cork or rubber tip to prevent injury.
  —Internal fixation
  Explain that presence of the internal fixator poses a risk for refracture and review preventive measures: safety in crutch walking, no weight bearing until ordered by the physician.
  Inform the patient that some nails, rods, or large plates may be removed within a year.

- *Medications*
  —Explain the purpose, dosage, schedule, and route of administration of any prescribed drugs, as well as side effects to report to the physician or nurse.

- *Activity*
  - —Remind the patient to plan frequent rest periods.
  - —Review special instructions for a patient who has undergone external fixation.

    Stress the need to increase movements and weight bearing slowly to lessen tenderness and to permit muscles to regain strength. Instruct the patient not to use the external fixator as a handle or support for the extremity but to support the extremity with pillows, two hands, or a sling to prevent excessive stress on the pins.

    Advise the patient to elevate the extremity when sitting or lying down.

    Stress the importance of not changing or adjusting the fixator bars, since this can cause misalignment.

    Explain that showering is permitted but that swimming should be avoided because chlorine and salt can corrode metal.

- *Diet*
  - —Discuss the importance of eating a well-balanced diet and drinking plenty of fluids for healing, circulation, and elimination.

FOLLOW-UP CARE AND REFERRALS

- Stress the importance of regular follow-up visits to ensure that the device is functioning properly and to maintain adequate immobilization of the fracture(s) (for external fixation). Maintain appointments with the physician for physical therapy until recovery is complete (for internal fixation). Make sure the patient has the necessary names and telephone numbers.

Fractures

—Fracture: a discontinuity or break in bone. Fractures occur when stress placed on the bone exceeds the bone's loading capacity. The majority of fractures occur as a result of trauma. Pathologic (spontaneous) fractures, which occur with minimal stress or trauma, affect bones weakened by disease (e.g., osteoporosis, cancer, Paget's disease). Fractures are described according to a number of characteristics, including the extent of soft tissue damage:

—Closed: the skin is intact

—Open: the skin is pierced

—Transverse, oblique, spiral, or linear: describes the line of the fracture

—Compression: describes the force of the fracture

—Comminuted: describes the number of pieces

—Displaced, angulated: describes the anatomic position of the distal fragment

—Intraarticular, extraarticular: describes whether the fracture involves the joint

SIGNS/SYMPTOMS

- Fracture site
  —Pain, tenderness, edema
  —Skin open or closed
  —Pallor, coolness of surrounding tissues
  —Numbness, tingling
  —Restricted or limited mobility, decreased range of motion
  —Abnormal position of extremity; deformity
  —Limb shortening
  —Crepitus (movement of parts not normally movable)
  —Bleeding, hematoma
  —Bruising, blisters

COMPLICATIONS

- Malunion, delayed union, or nonunion of fracture
- Thrombophlebitis
- Fat embolism
- Compartment syndrome
- Infection
- Nerve compression

- Pseudoarthrosis
- Avascular necrosis
- Limb length discrepancy

DIAGNOSTIC TESTS

- Describe each procedure, its purpose, and the normal feelings or sensations that are likely, as well as any preprocedural and postprocedural care.
  —X-rays of the fracture
  —Magnetic resonance imaging: to evaluate complicated fractures
  —Arthroscopy: to identify intraarticular fractures
  —Bone scans
  —Computed tomography
  —Blood tests: complete blood count, electrolytes

TREATMENT
Medical

- Therapy
  —Immobilization of bone
  —Closed reduction
  —Electrical bone stimulation
  —Bed rest
  —No weight bearing on affected bone (use of crutches, cane, walker)
  —Ice applications
  —Antiembolic stockings
  —Application of cast, splint, traction, sling
- Drugs
  —Analgesics
  —Antibiotics for open fractures
  —Muscle relaxants
  —Sedatives

Surgical

- Open reduction with internal fixation
- Arthroplasty with replacement with prosthesis
- Total joint replacement for crush injuries
- Amputation for severe crush injuries
- Application of external fixator, such as Hoffman, Ilizarov, or Ace-Fischer device

- Microvascular surgery, such as replantation of an amputated body part and revascularization of crush, avulsion, and other soft-tissue injuries

 HOME CARE

- Give both the patient and the caregiver *verbal* and *written* instructions. Provide them with the name and telephone number of a physician or nurse to call if questions arise.
- Provide instruction regarding specific treatments: cast care (see Cast Care, p. 656) and external fixator (see Fixator Devices, p. 284).
- *General information*
  —Discuss and review the type of fracture, causes or contributing factors, and prescribed treatment.
  —Explain the bone healing process.
- *Warning signs*
  —Review the signs and symptoms that should be reported to a physician or nurse.
    Neurovascular impairment of affected extremity: numbness, tingling, decreased movement, coolness, pallor, redness, blueness, decreased capillary refill
    Infection: fever, increased pain, swelling at fracture site, purulent drainage from cast or dressing, foul odor from cast or dressing
    Fat embolism: chest pain; fever; rash on abdomen, neck, arms, or axillae; anxiety
- *Special instructions*
  —Stress the importance of turning and moving frequently to avoid skin breakdown; advise the patient to handle injured tissues gently by supporting the joint above and below the site.
  —Review and demonstrate wound care.
- *Medications*
  —Explain the purpose, dosage, schedule, and route of administration of any prescribed drugs, as well as side effects to report to the physician or nurse.
- *Activity*
  —Explain the importance of maintaining immobility and not bearing weight on the injured limb as prescribed by the physician.
  —Explain that the recovery program takes twice the amount of time spent immobilized, so it will take that amount of time to

use the fractured limb or bear weight on it again (i.e., if 6 weeks was spent in a cast, it will take 6 more weeks to recover fully).
—Instruct the patient to elevate the extremity and apply ice bags as indicated.
—Instruct the patient in the use of ambulatory aids (crutch walking, cane, walker).
—Explain the importance of range-of-motion exercises to maintain function of unaffected joints. Teach exercises to maintain strength and facilitate resolution of inflammation: quadriceps, buttocks, and triceps setting exercises.

• *Diet*
—Emphasize the importance of a well-balanced diet high in vitamins, proteins, carbohydrates, and minerals to promote healing and prevent weight loss.
—Stress the need to eat foods high in calcium and vitamins A, B, C, and D to promote bone healing and avoid hypocalcemia.
—Encourage fluids to avoid constipation and maintain skin turgor (8 to 10 glasses/day).

FOLLOW-UP CARE AND REFERRALS

• Stress the importance of regular follow-up visits with the physician, physical therapist, or rehabilitation therapist. Make sure the patient has the necessary names and telephone numbers.

Frostbite

—**Frostbite: a localized injury to tissues and blood vessels caused by exposure to cold or freezing temperatures. Individuals at risk include the elderly, the homeless, infants and small children, debilitated and immobile patients, and patients with chronic illnesses (e.g., cardiac disease, diabetes, vascular disease). Frostbite is classified as either superficial (affecting skin and subcutaneous tissue, especially of the face, ears, and other exposed body parts) or deep (affecting the** skin, subcutaneous tissue, muscle, tendon, and neurovascular structures).

CAUSES/CONTRIBUTING FACTORS

- Lack of insulating body fat
- Lack of acclimatization to cold temperatures
- Wet or inadequate clothing
- Drug abuse
- Smoking
- Hunger, fatigue
- Fear
- Excessive alcohol intake

SIGNS/SYMPTOMS

- Superficial frostbite
  —Burning
  —Tingling
  —Numbness
  —Skin waxy and soft
  —White or grayish skin color
  —Absence of capillary refill
- With thawing, area becomes:
  —Flushed
  —Edematous
  —Painful
  —Purplish
  —Mottled
  —Blistered within 24 hours
- Deep frostbite
  —Hard and solid
  —Cold
  —Mottled
  —Blue or gray after thawing
  —Swelling of entire limb
  —Blisters after several weeks

COMPLICATIONS

- Vasospasm
- Hyperesthesia
- Infection
- Gangrene
- Amputation

TREATMENT
Medical

- Therapy
  —Rapid rewarming via immersion in water at 38° to 41° C (100° to 106° F)
  —Protective isolation
  —Whirlpool baths three times a day at 32° to 37° C (90° to 98° F)
- Drugs
  —Immunologic agents (tetanus)
  —Plasma expanders
  —Antibiotics
  —Analgesics

Surgical

- Escharotomy: removal of dead tissue
- Sympathectomy: for severe vasospasm and pain
- Debridement: after retraction of viable tissue, done 13 weeks to 4 months after injury
- Fasciotomy: to decrease tissue swelling, thereby increasing circulation
- Amputation of nonviable extremity: may be done several months after injury

▦ HOME CARE

- Give both the patient and the caregiver *verbal* and *written* instructions. Provide them with the name and telephone number of a physician or nurse to call if questions arise.
- *General information*
  —Explain the disorder and factors that contributed to the problem.
  —Prepare the patient for amputation if indicated (see p. 32).
- *Warning signs*
  —Review the signs and symptoms that should be reported to a physician or nurse.
  Persistent increasing pain
  Foul-smelling drainage
  Fever
  Swelling area
- *Special instructions*
  —Provide instruction and demonstrate the application of dry, sterile dressings to small, open areas.

—Discuss the importance of protecting the extremity from temperature extremes and rapid changes in temperature because the tissue is sensitive to temperature changes and refreezing causes tissue loss.

—Instruct the patient to avoid tight, constrictive clothing or pressure to an area that might decrease circulation.

—Discuss preventive measures to avoid future episodes or reinjury of the frostbitten part: protective, multilayered, warm, nonconstrictive clothing; avoidance of cold temperatures, fatigue, and hunger.

—Emphasize the importance of not smoking or using alcohol when exposed to cold.

—Advise the patient that there may be long-term residual effects: increased sensitivity to cold, burning and tingling, and increased sweating.

- *Medications*

—Explain the purpose, dosage, schedule, and route of administration of any prescribed drugs, as well as side effects to report to the physician or nurse.

- *Activity*

—If lower extremities are affected, advise the patient to avoid weight bearing and provide instruction in the use of ambulatory aids.

—Stress the importance of elevating the affected extremity.

—Instruct the patient in range-of-motion exercises to prevent contractures.

- *Diet*

—Avoid drinks that contain caffeine, which causes vasoconstriction: coffee, tea, cola.

FOLLOW-UP CARE AND REFERRALS

- Stress the importance of regular follow-up visits with the physician, physical therapist, or rehabilitation therapist. Make sure the patient has the necessary names and telephone numbers.

Gangrene

—Gangrene: tissue necrosis or death usually resulting from decreased blood supply (ischemia), bacterial infection, and subsequent putrefaction. The extremities are most often affected, but gangrene can occur internally (e.g., in the intestines or gallbladder). Gangrene may be a complication of strangulated hernia, appendicitis, thrombosis, mesenteric arteries, infection, or diabetes mellitus. Gangrene may also follow a crush injury or acute obstruction of blood flow (e.g., vascular disease, tourniquet, or embolism). Gas gangrene is necrosis accompanied by gas bubbles in soft tissue. It is caused by the anaerobic, spore-forming, gram-positive rod *Clostridium perfringens* or another clostridial species and usually follows trauma or surgery.

SIGNS/SYMPTOMS
- Dry gangrene
  —Affected extremity cold, dry, shriveled, black
- Moist gangrene
  —Affected extremity or wound necrotic, putrid
- Gas gangrene
  —Crepitation caused by carbon dioxide and hydrogen accumulation in necrotic tissues
  —Severe localized pain, swelling, and discoloration
  —Tissue necrosis and rupture
  —Foul-smelling discharge
  —Tachycardia, tachypnea, hypotension
  —Fever
  —Delirium

COMPLICATIONS
- Amputation
- Gas gangrene: rapidly fatal
- Moist gangrene: death if untreated

DIAGNOSTIC TESTS
- Describe each procedure, its purpose, and the normal feelings or sensations that are likely, as well as any preprocedural and postprocedural care.

—Laboratory studies

Blood tests: white and red blood cell counts to show infectious process and hemolysis

Anaerobic wound cultures and Gram's stain of wound drainage: to identify *C. perfringens*

—X-rays: to document the presence of gas in tissues

TREATMENT
Medical (for gas gangrene)

- Therapy
  —Hyperbaric oxygenation: to prevent multiplication of anaerobic bacteria
- Drugs
  —Intravenous antibiotics, usually high doses of penicillin
  —Antipyretics
  —Analgesics

Surgical

- Debridement of affected tissues and necrotic muscle
- Amputation

HOME CARE

- Give both the patient and the caregiver *verbal* and *written* instructions. Provide them with the name and telephone number of a physician or nurse to call if questions arise.
- *General information*
  —Explain the disorder and contributing factors.
  —Prepare the patient for amputation if indicated (see p. 32).
- *Warning signs*
  —Review the signs and symptoms that should be reported to a physician or nurse.
    Recurrence of infection
    Vascular impairment (ischemia) of surrounding area: cool skin, pallor, blueness of skin, sudden swelling or severe pain
- *Special instructions*
  —Prepare the patient for debridement and discuss the reason for the procedure.
  —After debridement, discuss wound care and dressing changes.
    Inspect the wound daily.
    Use aseptic technique.
    Perform meticulous wound cleansing.

- *Medications*
  —Explain the purpose, dosage, schedule, and route of administration of any prescribed drugs, as well as side effects to report to the physician or nurse.
- *Activity*
  —Explain the need for rest to conserve energy, promote healing, and lessen stress on involved tissues.
  —Stress the importance of immobilizing the affected extremity to decrease the spread of purulent drainage.
  —Instruct the patient in range-of-motion exercises to maintain strength of muscles and joints and to prevent atrophy of tissues.
  —Teach the use of ambulatory aids when the patient is allowed out of bed.
- *Diet*
  —Avoid drinks containing caffeine such as cola, coffee, and tea, since they cause vasoconstriction.
  —Encourage the patient to eat foods high in protein to aid in healing.

FOLLOW-UP CARE AND REFERRALS

- Stress the importance of regular follow-up visits with the physician, physical therapist, or rehabilitation therapist. Make sure the patient has the necessary names and telephone numbers.
- Emphasize the importance of not smoking or using alcohol when exposed to cold.

Gastrectomy and Gastrostomy

—Gastrectomy: surgical removal of the entire or a portion of the stomach with anastomosis to the small intestine.

—Gastrostomy: surgically constructed stoma (ostomy) in the stomach for the insertion of a catheter for tube feedings, decompression, or drainage.

INDICATIONS
- Hemorrhage
- Intractable ulcers
- Esophageal disorders: carcinoma, stricture, atresia, trauma, dysphagia
- Perforation
- Gastritis
- Stomach cancer

PREPROCEDURAL TEACHING
- See also Abdominal Surgery, p. 6.
- Review the physician's explanation of the procedure and the reason for it; encourage the patient to ask questions and to discuss any fears or anxieties. Explain the need for informed consent.

Review of Preprocedural Care
- Explain and enforce nothing by mouth (NPO) status before and after the procedure.

Review of Postprocedural Care
- Review anticipated postoperative care, including the nasogastric tube, incisions, intravenous fluid and electrolyte therapy, and indwelling urethral catheter.
- Discuss anticipated postoperative body changes: gastrostomy and presence of gastrostomy tube.
- Discuss anticipated lifestyle modifications: eating pattern, altered feeding methods, diet modifications, and symptomatic relief of dumping syndrome.
- Demonstrate coughing, deep breathing, and splinting incision.
- Discuss the purpose of and demonstrate the use of the incentive spirometer.
- Encourage early ambulation.
- Provide explanation of stoma or catheter care, the initiation of tube feedings, or diet modifications.

COMPLICATIONS/SIDE EFFECTS
- Dehydration
- Electrolyte imbalance
- Aspiration pneumonia
- Wound infection

- Hemorrhage or shock
- Atelectasis

⊞ HOME CARE

- Give both the patient and the caregiver *verbal* and *written* instructions. Provide them with the name and telephone number of a physician or nurse to call if questions arise.
- *General information*
  —Review the explanation of the procedure and specific follow-up care.
  —Explain and discuss the relationships among the underlying disease, the need for gastrectomy or gastrostomy, contributing factors (e.g., smoking, alcohol, irritating foods or drugs, or stress), care, and treatment. Stress the importance of eliminating causative factors.
- *Wound/incision care*
  —Discuss and demonstrate proper wound management, dressing changes, and ostomy care: procedure, frequency, and inspection of skin integrity and stoma site.
- *Warning signs*
  —Review the signs and symptoms that should be reported to a physician or nurse.
    Retention and bowel obstruction: nausea, vomiting, abdominal distention, abdominal pain, abdominal rigidity
    Infection: fever, erythema, pain, tenderness, purulent drainage, foul odor, warmth at the site
    Weight loss or failure to gain weight
    Diarrhea
    Dumping syndrome: abdominal fullness, cramping, nausea, vomiting, diarrhea, diaphoresis, fatigue, tachycardia, dizziness, palpitations
    For gastrostomy: change in color of stoma from normal bright red, change in color, consistency, or amount of gastric drainage; peristomal skin irritation
- *Special instructions*
  —Assist the patient in obtaining appropriate devices, such as ostomy appliances, sterile dressings, and tube feedings and feeding pump.
  —For patient with gastrectomy, discuss symptomatic relief of dumping syndrome.
    Assist the patient to plan a low-carbohydrate, high-fat, high-protein diet.

Instruct the patient to eat small, frequent meals and to avoid taking liquids with meals.

Instruct the patient to asssume a recumbent position after meals.

—After gastrostomy, discuss and demonstrate the preparation and administration of tube feedings, including amount and frequency.

Instruct the patient to sit upright during feeding and for 1 hour after feeding to prevent reflux into the esophagus or backflow into the gastrostomy tube.

For continuous tube feedings, see p. 734.

—Teach care of the gastrostomy tube and provide written instructions.

Wash area gently with soap and water. Use cotton tip applicators to clean around the stoma site.

Rinse well and pat dry.

Apply skin barrier as needed.

Reapply dressings and appliance. Avoid dressings, if possible.

Securely tape gastrostomy tube to the skin to prevent stress and accidental dislodgment.

Change the tube every 2 to 3 days.

If a gastrostomy tube is permanent, explain that it may eventually be removed and inserted only for feedings; tell the patient to protect the stoma with a small gauze pad.

- *Medications*
  —Explain the purpose, dosage, schedule, and route of administration of any prescribed drugs, as well as side effects to report to the physician or nurse.
  —Stress the importance of taking iron supplements as ordered for the treatment of iron deficiency anemia.
  —Explain and demonstrate vitamin B_{12} injections for the treatment of pernicious anemia, if ordered. Demonstrate medication preparation and administration via the gastrostomy tube.
- *Activity*
  —Encourage the patient to discuss allowances and limitations with respect to occupation, recreation, and activities.
  —Instruct the patient to gradually resume activities of daily living but to avoid heavy lifting (>10 pounds), pushing, or pulling.

—Instruct the patient to weigh and record weight every 2 to 3 days.
- *Diet*
  —Refer the patient for a dietary consultation.
  —Provide the patient with a list of irritating foods and drugs to avoid, including coffee, caffeine, spicy food, alcohol, aspirin, and ibuprofen.
  —Emphasize the importance of not using alcohol or taking gastric-irritating drugs.

PSYCHOSOCIAL CARE

- Encourage the patient to verbalize psychosocial concerns regarding body image, inability to consume food and drink orally, social value of mealtime, altered feeding methods, and lifestyle implications.
- Assist the patient and family to integrate the patient's altered feeding methods into social patterns of mealtime to prevent isolation.
- Encourage stress reduction techniques.

FOLLOW-UP CARE

- Stress the importance of regular follow-up visits with the physician, dietitian, and enterostomal nurse. Make sure the patient has the necessary names and telephone numbers.
- Provide strategies for smoking cessation. Refer the patient to community resources for smoking cessation, if appropriate.

REFERRALS

- Refer the patient to a social worker for psychosocial support, assistance with financial concerns over long-term feedings, and home health care support services.
- Refer the patient to support services such as Alcoholics Anonymous, if appropriate.

Gastroenteritis

—Gastroenteritis: inflammation of the stomach and small intestine, characterized by vomiting and severe diarrhea, leading to depletion of intracellular fluids. Gastroenteritis can occur in persons of all ages but is particularly dangerous in children, the elderly, and debilitated patients.

CAUSES/CONTRIBUTING FACTORS/RISK FACTORS

- Ingestion of contaminated food and water: bacteria *(Staphylococcus aureus, Salmonella, Shigella, Escherichia coli),* viruses, or parasites
- Allergy or intolerance of specific foods; drug reactions
- Direct or indirect fecal-oral transmission from an infected person
- Poor sanitation conditions
- Crowded living conditions
- Travel to a foreign country
- Ingestion of toxins, such as poisonous plants, arsenic, lead, and mercury

SIGNS/SYMPTOMS

- Frequent diarrhea: may be mucoid or bloody
- Abdominal pain or cramping
- Nausea and vomiting
- Weight loss or failure to gain weight
- Anorexia
- Abdominal distention
- Fever
- Irritability
- Lethargy
- Dehydration: change in level of consciousness; loss of skin turgor; oliguria; dark, concentrated urine; dry mucous membranes; sunken eyes; no tears with crying; depressed anterior fontanels

COMPLICATIONS

- Dehydration
- Electrolyte imbalance
- Hypovolemia or septic shock
- Death

DIAGNOSTIC TESTS

- Describe each procedure, its purpose, and the normal feelings or sensations that are likely, as well as any preprocedural and postprocedural care.

—Complete blood count with differential
—Stool cultures: to detect pathogenic organisms, occult blood, mucus, or reducing substance
—Serum antibody titers
—Serum electrolytes
—Blood cultures
—Direct swab rectal cultures

TREATMENT
Medical

• Therapy
  —Intravenous fluids and electrolyte therapy
  —NPO until rehydrated, then small, frequent amounts of clear liquids
• Drugs
  —Antibiotics

🏠 HOME CARE

• Give both the patient and the caregiver *verbal* and *written* instructions. Provide them with the name and telephone number of a physician or nurse to call if questions arise.
• *General information*
  —Explain and discuss gastroenteritis, causes and contributing factors, care and treatment, and prevention.
• *Warning signs*
  —Review the signs and symptoms that should be reported to a physician or nurse.
      Dehydration: change in level of consciousness, loss of skin turgor, oliguria, dark concentrated urine, dry mucous membranes, sunken eyes, no tears with crying, depressed anterior fontanels
      Continued diarrhea
      Increase in abdominal pain
      Fever
• *Special instructions*
  —Assist the patient or caregiver in obtaining appropriate supplies, such as oral glucose electrolyte solutions.
  —Teach the patient preventive measures.
      Wash hands before eating and after toileting.
      Thoroughly cook all meats, especially pork, and avoid recontamination with kitchen utensils after cooking.

Refrigerate perishable foods: mayonnaise, potato or egg salad, cream-filled pastries.

Drink pasteurized milk and chlorinated water. When traveling to areas with unprotected or untreated water supply, boil all water used in cooking, drinking, or making ice.

Maintain foods at the appropriate hot or cold temperatures.

Protect foods from fly and roach contamination.

—Teach the patient that gastroenteritis is communicable while the organisms are present in the feces.

—Teach the patient and family that persons with *Shigella* infections should not handle food or provide child care until two successive fecal samples are free of the organism; instruct the patient to use disinfectant after toileting.

—Demonstrate proper disposal of contaminated materials.

—Discuss skin care for anal irritation.

Keep rectal area clean and dry.

Wash skin with mild soap and water after each stool, rinse well, and dry thoroughly.

Apply topical ointment as ordered.

Culture stool specimens from other family members and treat as appropriate.

• *Medications*

—Explain the purpose, dosage, schedule, and route of administration of any prescribed drugs, as well as side effects to report to the physician or nurse.

• *Diet*

—Instruct the patient to drink clear juices, bouillon, tea, and broth as tolerated.

—Advise the patient to advance the diet from clear liquids to a soft, bland diet that includes bananas, rice, applesauce, toast, clear soup, soda crackers, and dry cereals, avoiding milk products, and then to a regular diet as stools continue to firm.

FOLLOW-UP CARE

• Stress the importance of regular medical and laboratory follow-up visits. Make sure the patient has the necessary names and telephone numbers.

Gastrointestinal Bleeding
(Including Esophageal Bleeding)

—Gastrointestinal bleeding: a complication of various gastrointestinal disorders in which ulceration of the mucosa has progressed to the vasculature; bleeding may be acute or chronic.

CAUSES/CONTRIBUTING FACTORS/RISK FACTORS

- Peptic ulcer disease
- Erosive gastritis
- Esophageal varices
- Esophagitis
- Diverticular disease
- Cancer of the esophagus, stomach, or intestines
- Trauma
- Mallory-Weiss syndrome
- Blood dyscrasias

SIGNS/SYMPTOMS

- Hematemesis: bloody vomitus may appear red, dark red, brown, or black or have "coffee ground" characteristics
- Melena: black, tarry stools
- Hematochezia: passage of red blood through the rectum
- Occult blood in the stool
- Fatigue
- Pallor
- Nausea and vomiting
- Abdominal distention
- Abdominal cramping, tenderness, pain
- Diarrhea
- Fever, chills
- Dehydration
- With acute hemorrhage >500 ml, lightheadedness, syncope, diaphoresis, tachycardia, shock

COMPLICATIONS

- Hypovolemic shock
- Anemia
- Electrolyte imbalance
- Perforation
- Death

DIAGNOSTIC TESTS

- Describe each procedure, its purpose, and the normal feelings or sensations that are likely, as well as any preprocedural and postprocedural care.
  - —Hemoglobin and hematocrit: to measure circulating erythrocytes and assess blood loss
  - —Blood urea nitrogen: to detect digestion and absorption of blood proteins from the gastrointestinal tract
  - —Electrolytes
  - —Esophagogastroduodenoscopy: to identify the cause and site of the hemorrhage
  - —Upper gastrointestinal barium study: to identify the cause and site of hemorrhage
  - —Stool specimen: to detect occult blood

TREATMENT
Medical

- Therapy
  - —Whole blood or packed red blood cell transfusions
  - —Intravenous fluid replacement with normal saline and plasma expanders
  - —NPO until bleeding subsides
  - —Central venous pressure or Swan-Ganz catheter: to assess circulatory volume
  - —Nasogastric tube: to aspirate blood and gastric contents
  - —Gastric intubation with ice water or saline lavage: to control hemorrhage
  - —Angiography with vasopressin infusion: to localize hemorrhage and promote vasoconstriction
  - —Esophageal balloon tamponade: to help control hemorrhage
- Drugs
  - —Antacids
  - —Histamine receptor antagonists

—Antiulcer drugs
—Vasopressin
—Analgesics

Surgical

- For esophageal bleeding
  —Endoscopic sclerotherapy
  —Portocaval or splenorenal shunt: to divert blood flow from the liver and thus reduce pressure
  —Ligation of bleeding esophageal varices
  —Esophageal tamponade
- For gastric bleeding
  —Partial gastrectomy
  —Vagotomy, excision of ulcer, pyloroplasty
- For intestinal bleeding
  —Bowel resection with anastomosis
  —Bowel resection with temporary colostomy
  —Exploratory laparotomy if source of hemorrhage is unknown

HOME CARE

- Give both the patient and the caregiver *verbal* and *written* instructions. Provide them with the name and telephone number of a physician or nurse to call if questions arise.
- *General information*
  —Discuss the type of bleeding disorder, explaining the relationships among causative factors, disease process, care and treatment, and potential for recurrence.
  —Review the physician's explanation of scheduled medical procedures, permitting time to answer any questions.
  —Review the physician's explanation of surgical procedures as ordered: gastrectomy (see p. 298), bowel resection (see p. 117), and abdominal surgery (see p. 6).
- *Warning signs*
  —Review the signs and symptoms that should be reported to a physician or nurse.
  - Epigastric distress on an empty stomach
  - Pain with ingestion of food
  - Anorexia, nausea, hematemesis, abdominal distention, abdominal fullness
  - Weight loss
  - Black or bloody stools

- *Special instructions*
  —Teach the patient how to monitor stools for blood and demonstrate stool occult blood test, if indicated.
  —Provide pain management, offering alternatives to medications: visualization, guided imagery, meditation, relaxation, and biofeedback.
  —Stress the importance of smoking cessation and complete abstinence from alcohol.
  —Advise the patient to avoid coughing, sneezing, lifting, straining during defecation, or vomiting. Discuss the need to take stool softeners as prescribed to prevent constipation.
- *Medications*
  —Explain the purpose, dosage, schedule, and route of administration of any prescribed drugs, as well as side effects to report to the physician or nurse.
  —Specify whether medications should be taken with food or require an empty stomach.
  —Advise the patient to avoid use of aspirin-containing medications, ibuprofen, and other nonsteroidal antiinflammatory drugs (NSAIDs).
- *Diet*
  —Assist the patient to plan a diet high in vitamin K. Provide a list of specific foods high in vitamin K.
  —With associated advanced liver disease, advise the patient to plan a diet low in sodium, protein, and ammonia.
  —Instruct the patient to eat small, frequent meals, to chew food well, and to eat slowly.
  —Instruct the patient to drink water with meals.
  —Provide the patient with a list of irritating foods and drugs to avoid, including coffee, tea, caffeine, spicy foods, rough foods, citric acid juices, extremely hot foods or liquids, and alcohol.
  —Advise the patient to avoid milk because it sometimes contributes to increased gastric acid secretion.
  —Refer the patient to a dietitian for nutritional counseling.

FOLLOW-UP CARE

- Stress the importance of regular medical, surgical, and laboratory follow-up visits, even in the absence of overt symptoms. Make sure the patient has the necessary names and telephone numbers.

REFERRALS

- Refer the patient to Alcoholics Anonymous if appropriate.
- Refer the patient to community programs for alcohol and smoking cessation if appropriate.

Glaucoma

—Glaucoma: a disorder characterized by high intracellular pressure of the aqueous humor, leading to atrophy of the optic nerve (disc), visual field loss, death of the nerve fibers, and irreversible vision loss. Glaucoma results from the overproduction or inadequate drainage of aqueous fluid. With aqueous fluid buildup, increasing intraocular pressure blocks blood supply to the optic nerve and retina, causing tissues to become ischemic.

TYPES OF GLAUCOMA

- Primary glaucoma
  - —Open angle
    - Chronic, simple glaucoma
    - Most common form, affecting 90% of all people with glaucoma
    - May be familial, affects adults over 40 years of age
    - More common in persons with a history of myopia, diabetes, hypertension
    - Onset insidious and asymptomatic
    - Slow progression
  - —Closed angle
    - Acute: onset usually dramatic, rapid development of severe pain in eye(s)
    - Chronic: follows untreated acute attack of closed angle glaucoma; onset gradual and usually asymptomatic
- Secondary glaucoma
  - —Progressive blurring of vision
  - —Results from trauma, tumors, surgery, uveitis, drug therapy (e.g., corticosteroids)
- Congenital glaucoma
  - —Rapidly developing myopia

SIGNS/SYMPTOMS

- Open angle
  - Visual changes: decreased acuity especially at night, loss of peripheral vision, seeing halos
  - Mild aching in eyes
  - Dull headache in morning
- Closed angle
  - Severe pain
  - Visual changes: blurred vision, rainbows in artificial light, halos around lights
  - Headache
  - Nausea, vomiting
  - Dilated pupil(s)
- Congenital glaucoma
  - Decreased visual acuity
  - Excessive tearing
  - Photophobia

COMPLICATIONS

- Increased intraocular pressure
- Progressive visual impairment
- Blindness
- After surgery
  - Retinal detachment
  - Cataract development
  - Hemolytic glaucoma
  - Hemorrhage
  - Infection
  - Decreased visual acuity
  - Light sensitivity

DIAGNOSTIC TESTS

- Describe each procedure, its purpose, and the normal feelings or sensations that are likely, as well as any preprocedural and postprocedural care.
  - Tonometry: to measure intraocular pressure
  - Gonioscopy: to identify width of aqueous fluid drainage area, adhesions, trauma, and tumors; also differentiates open angle from closed angle glaucoma
  - Funduscopy: dilation of pupil to inspect the optic disc; identifies disc degeneration

—Ophthalmoscopic examination: to identify increased cupping of the disc

—Visual field studies: to identify blind spots and subsequent degeneration

—Tonography: to measure how well aqueous humor flows

TREATMENT
Open Angle Glaucoma
Medical

- Drugs: to reduce intraocular pressure by decreasing aqueous humor production or to reduce the volume of intraocular fluid
  —Miotics
  —Synthetic epinephrine
  —Beta blockers

Surgical

- Laser trabeculoplasty: to create an opening and thus increase outflow of aqueous humor; done under local anesthetic on an outpatient basis
- Trabeculectomy: surgical filtering procedure to build a new channel for the aqueous humor; done as an inpatient procedure under general anesthetic

Closed Angle Glaucoma (Acute)
Medical

- Drugs: to lower and control intraocular pressure so that surgery can be performed
  —Hyperosmotic agents
  —Carbonic anhydrase inhibitors (Diamox)
  —Narcotic analgesics
  —Miotics

Surgical

This is a medical emergency. If pressure is not relieved within a few hours, eye damage occurs. Surgery is performed once intraocular pressure is stabilized.

- Laser iridotomy: to create a channel for aqueous fluid flow; done on an outpatient basis
- Iridectomy: to create a fine hole in the periphery of the iris through which aqueous fluid can flow

Secondary Glaucoma

• Medications or surgery depending on causative factor

Congenital Glaucoma
Surgical

• Trabeculectomy
• Goniotomy: to ensure patency of the drainage system

HOME CARE

• Give both the patient and the caregiver *verbal* and *written* instructions. Provide them with the name and telephone number of a physician or nurse to call if questions arise.
• *General information*
    —Explain the type of glaucoma, causes or contributing factors, and prescribed medical or surgical therapy.
• *Warning signs*
    —Review the signs and symptoms that should be reported to a physician or nurse.
        Severe pain in eye(s)
        Blurred vision
        Headache
        Halos or rainbows
        Tearing
        Nausea, vomiting
• *Special instructions*
    —Review the factors that increase intraocular pressure and should be avoided:
        Constrictive clothing around the neck or torso
        Constipation (straining)
        Exertion or lifting heavy objects
        Bending at the waist
        Sneezing or coughing (upper respiratory infection)
        Nausea, vomiting
    —Review postoperative care.
        Inform the patient of the need to wear an eye patch or sunglasses to avoid discomfort associated with light exposure.
        Advise the patient of the importance of follow-up visits to check intraocular pressure, which may increase temporarily after surgery.

Explain the importance of not rubbing, squeezing, or touching the eye.

Discuss the procedure for cleansing the eye.

Review the signs and symptoms that may indicate infection or increasing inraocular pressure and should be reported to a physician: pain, redness, fever, drainage, decreased visual acuity, excessive lacrimation, marked photophobia, halos, sparks.

Explain the importance of using glaucoma medication in the unoperated eye.

Provide a detailed explanation of drug therapy, stressing the importance of compliance.

Discuss the consequences of noncompliance, including optic nerve damage and blindness.

—Review home safety precautions needed because of diminished peripheral vision.

Turn the head to visualize either side.

Use up-and-down head movements to judge stairs and oncoming objects and walk slowly.

Reduce clutter (e.g., loose rugs, electrical cords, items on floor) to prevent falls.

Be aware that seeing at night, in dim light, or at dusk will be difficult because in diminished light miotic pupils do not dilate to admit more light to the retina.

Provide extra lighting in darkened areas and use extra caution when driving at night.

• *Medications*

—Explain the purpose, dosage, schedule, and route of administration of any prescribed drugs, as well as side effects to report to the physician or nurse.

—Stress the importance of taking drugs on schedule.

—Teach the patient to label each eyedrop bottle and to write out schedules for administration (especially important for patients with minimal visual acuity, to whom all bottles look alike).

—Teach the proper technique for administration of eyedrops or ointment. Allow time for return demonstration and practice.

—Stress the importance of good handwashing technique before instilling drops or ointment to minimize risk of infection.

—Explain that medications do not cure glaucoma but can control it.

—Review side effects of medications to report:

Miotics: blurred vision, diarrhea

Timolol: fatigue, weakness, depression

Acetazolamide (Diamox): numbness, tingling of extremities and lips, decreased appetite, nausea, impotence

FOLLOW-UP CARE AND REFERRALS

• Stress the importance of regular follow-up visits. Make sure the patient has the necessary names and telephone numbers.

• Provide referrals for support services such as Glaucoma Foundation.

Glomerulonephritis and Nephrotic Syndrome

—**Glomerulonephritis: inflammatory process involving the glomerulus that causes a problem in filtration of urine. Glomerulonephritis may occur as an acute or a chronic disease.**

—**Nephrotic syndrome: disorder characterized by a high concentration of protein in the urine that is caused by a filtration problem of the glomeruli. Nephrotic syndrome may occur in a number of diseases such as diabetes mellitus, as a reaction to drugs and allergens, or during pregnancy. The majority of cases, however, result from primary glomerulonephritis.**

CAUSES/CONTRIBUTING FACTORS

• Immune system response

—Systemic lupus erythematosus

—Mixed connective tissue disease

—Polyarteritis nodosa

—Goodpasture's syndrome

• Diabetes mellitus

• Hepatitis B

- Polycystic kidneys
- Essential hypertension
- Tuberculosis
- Vascular disease (affects the renal vein)
- Infections and infectious processes
  —Bacterial: *Streptococcus, Staphylococcus*
  —Syphilis
  —Malaria
  —Schistosomiasis
  —Mediterranean fever

SIGNS/SYMPTOMS

- Urine: reddish brown, foamy
- Edema: extremities, periorbital, peritoneal, external genitalia
- Hypertension
- Shortness of breath on exertion, orthopnea
- Fatigue, malaise, lethargy
- Weight gain

COMPLICATIONS

- Renal failure
- Severe hypertension
- Renal vein thrombosis

DIAGNOSTIC TESTS

- Describe each procedure, its purpose, and the normal feelings or sensations that are likely, as well as any preprocedural and postprocedural care.
  —Blood studies: to evaluate kidney function
      Electrolytes
      Blood urea nitrogen
      Creatinine
      Protein
      Phosphates
      Cholesterol
      Albumin
  —Urine studies
      Urinalysis: to determine the presence of protein and blood
      Culture and sensitivity: to determine the presence and type of bacteria
      24-Hour study: to determine levels of creatinine and protein

—Radiographic tests: kidney-ureter-bladder (KUB)
—Ultrasound: to determine the size of the kidney
—Renal biopsy: to establish underlying disease

TREATMENT
Medical

- Therapy
  —Plasmapheresis: to remove immune complexes or antibodies
  —Dialysis: peritoneal or hemodialysis
  —Dietary: low sodium, low potassium, low protein (protein intake is based on glomerular filtration rate [GFR]; if GFR is decreased, protein intake is lowered; if GFR is normal, protein intake is increased)
- Drugs
  —Diuretics
  —Antihypertensives
  —Corticosteroids or cytotoxic agents
  —Immunosuppressants
  —Antineoplastics
  —Plasma expanders

Surgical

- Bilateral nephrectomy
- Kidney transplant

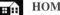 **HOME CARE**

- Give both the patient and the caregiver *verbal* and *written* instructions. Provide them with the name and telephone number of a physician or nurse to call if questions arise.
- *General information*
  —Explain the disease process and underlying cause.
- *Warning signs*
  —Review the signs and symptoms, including fluid and electrolyte imbalance, that should be reported to a physician or nurse.
     Weight increase: >2 pounds in one day
     Change in urine color, amount, or froth
     Progressive edema: puffy, swollen eyes
     Decreased urine output: <600 ml in 24 hours
     Increased blood pressure

Heart palpitations, muscle weakness, lethargy, light-headedness

Hypokalemia

Hyperkalemia: abdominal cramping, diarrhea

Uremia: anorexia, nausea, metallic taste in mouth, confusion, itching, lethargy

- *Special instructions*
  —Explain the importance of daily weights: same time, same clothing, after urination, and before eating.
  —Demonstrate blood pressure measurement and discuss how often to perform it. Advise the patient on obtaining supplies for home blood pressure monitoring.
  —Instruct the patient on maintaining a written daily log of weight, vital signs, and intake and output.
  —Discuss the need to maintain good skin care of edematous body areas to prevent excoriation and skin breakdown (see Pressure Ulcer Sores, p. 715).
  —Advise female patients to avoid pregnancy. Provide information on contraception.
- *Medications*
  —Explain the purpose, dosage, schedule, and route of administration of any prescribed drugs, as well as side effects to report to the physician or nurse.
  —If the patient is taking immunosuppressants, stress the importance of avoiding persons with infections and upper respiratory infections. Discuss the need to report signs of infection: fever, fatigue, malaise.
- *Activity*
  —Encourage the patient to discuss allowances and limitations with respect to occupation, recreation, or activities.
  —Discuss the need to avoid fatigue, exercise to tolerance, and plan frequent rest periods.
- *Diet*
  —Refer the patient to a dietitian for a specific diet plan. Review dietary restrictions and provide a list of foods to avoid (see Appendix C).
  —Explain how to read labels on cans and boxes for ingredients and sodium content. Instruct the patient to rinse canned foods in water to remove excess salt.
  —Discuss fluid restrictions. Explain that fluids may depend on how much urine is put out.

FOLLOW-UP CARE

- Stress the importance of regular follow-up visits, including blood pressure checks if the patient is not on a home monitoring program. Make sure the patient has the necessary names and telephone numbers.

REFERRALS

- Assist the patient to obtain referrals for home health care, social, and financial services.

G

Gout

—**Gout: a metabolic disorder in which urate salts are deposited in joints and other body tissues such as ear, cartilage, and kidneys. The urate crystals form masses called tophi, which are sharp and pointed and cause irritation and inflammation of the joints. While any joint may be affected, gout commonly (90%) affects the first metatarsal joint of the great toe, causing excruciating pain. The ankle, midfoot, and wrist are also frequently affected. Primary gout is a hereditary disease in which overproduction or decreased excretion of uric acid and urate salts leads to high levels of uric acid in the blood. Primary gout most commonly occurs in men older than 30 years of age. Secondary gout is associated with other conditions in which uric acid is overproduced or retained, such as lead poisoning, use of thiazide diuretics, alcohol abuse, chronic renal disease, psoriasis, and chemotherapy.**

SIGNS/SYMPTOMS

- Joints inflamed, edematous, shiny, hot, painful
- Malaise
- Headache
- Increased temperature
- Fever, chills
- Constipation
- Subcutaneous tophi: ear, joints, knuckles
- Limited motion of affected joints

COMPLICATIONS
- Renal calculi
- Gouty arthritis
- Hypertension
- Infection of ruptured deposits

DIAGNOSTIC TESTS
- Describe each procedure, its purpose, and the normal feelings or sensations that are likely, as well as any preprocedural and postprocedural care.
    —Laboratory tests
    > Blood tests: uric acid, white blood cells, erythrocyte sedimentation rate
    > Urine tests: uric acid levels to determine if the patient is an overexcretor or underexcretor of uric acid
    —Needle aspirations
    > Joint fluid: to detect presence of urate crystals
    > Tophaceous material: to identify urate crystals
    —X-rays: to document evidence of radiolucent tophi

TREATMENT
Medical
- Therapy
    —During acute phase
    > Joint rest
    > Complete bed rest with elevation of inflamed joint
    > Cold packs to the affected joint to decrease inflammation
    —Low-purine diet
    —Limitation of alcohol intake
    —Weight reduction
- Drugs
    —Nonsteroidal antiinflammatory drugs (NSAIDs)
    —Uricosuric agents (e.g., probenecid): to increase excretion of urate salts
    —Allopurinol: to decrease serum uric acid
    —Antiinflammatory agents (colchicine)
    —Corticosteroids, analgesics, antipyretics

Surgical
- Excision of gouty tophi when they erode through the skin or cause mechanical impairment
- Joint replacement

HOME CARE

- Give both the patient and the caregiver *verbal* and *written* instructions. Provide them with the name and telephone number of a physician or nurse to call if questions arise.
- *General information*
  —Describe the disease process, underlying causes, and contributing factors.
- *Warning signs*
  —Review the signs and symptoms of possible kidney stones that should be reported to a physician or nurse.
    Severe pain in the flank, side, lower back, suprapubic area, groin, labia, or scrotum
    Urinary retention
    Nausea
    Vomiting
- *Special instructions*
  —Instruct the patient in checking urine pH using a test tape; if pH is <6.0, advise the patient to increase fluid intake and avoid high-purine foods.
  —Describe home care of inflamed joints during an acute attack.
    Complete bed rest with elevation of the affected joint with pillows
    Ice applications to inflamed joints
    As inflammation subsides, need for rest periods to avoid fatigue
    Bed cradle to keep linens off joint; advise the patient where to obtain equipment
    Avoidance of weight bearing
  —Teach range-of-motion exercises of joints, and instruct the patient to increase these exercises as inflammation decreases to avoid disuse syndrome.
  —Explain that gout cannot be cured but can be controlled with medication.
- *Medications*
  —Explain the purpose, dosage, schedule, and route of administration of any prescribed drugs, as well as side effects to report to the physician or nurse.
  —Review specific drug therapies. Explain that the type of treatment depends on whether the patient overexcretes or underexcretes uric acid.
    Colchicine: instruct the patient to notify the physician or nurse when pain subsides or when nausea, vomiting,

abdominal cramping, or diarrhea occurs. Explain that the drug is usually stopped when symptoms occur

Uricosuric agents: stress the importance of drinking 2 to 3 liters of fluid per day unless contraindicated to prevent the development of kidney stones

Alkalinizing agents (sodium bicarbonate): to maintain urinary pH above 6.0 and thus prevent kidney stone formation

Allopurinol: caution patients of the potential for renal and hepatic complications

—Explain the need to avoid diuretics, low-dose aspirin, and nicotinic acid because these can increase serum uric acid.

- *Diet*
  —Discuss the need to restrict intake of purines, which are metabolic precursors to uric acid. Advise the patient about foods that are high in purine: anchovies, liver, sardines, kidneys, sweetbreads, lentils.
  —Instruct the patient to avoid alcoholic beverages, especially beer and wine.
  —Discuss the need to decrease weight if obese. Refer the patient to the dietitian for a low-calorie diet plan for weight reduction.

FOLLOW-UP CARE

- Stress the importance of regular follow-up visits. Make sure the patient has the necessary names and telephone numbers.

Guillain-Barré Syndrome

—Guillain-Barré syndrome: an acute syndrome characterized by widespread inflammation or demyelination of the peripheral nerves. Guillain-Barré syndrome is also known as acute idiopathic polyneuritis, acute polyradiculoneuropathy, and postinfectious polyneuritis. It is thought to be an autoimmune disease triggered by viral infection. Over half of affected persons have had a nonspecific infection (e.g., upper respiratory or gastrointestinal infection) 10 to 14 days before the onset of symptoms. The onset is rapid, and the symptoms are generally reversible.

CAUSES/CONTRIBUTING FACTORS

- Upper respiratory infection
- Infectious mononucleosis
- Cytomegalovirus infection
- Herpes zoster
- Influenza A
- *Mycoplasma* infection
- Mumps
- Acquired immune deficiency syndrome (AIDS)
- Lyme disease
- Lymphoma (especially Hodgkin's)
- Serum sickness
- Postsurgical
- Inoculation for swine flu

SIGNS/SYMPTOMS

- Symmetric muscle weakness beginning in the legs and ascending rapidly (in a few days) to the arms
- Weakness accompanied by paresthesia, pain
- Paralysis of upper extremities (partial or complete); quadriplegia
- Reduced reflexes, then loss of deep tendon reflexes
- Bilateral facial and oropharyngeal paresis
- Difficulty swallowing
- Urinary retention
- Respiratory muscle paralysis
- Respiratory insufficiency
- Blood pressure fluctuation
- Numbness (worse in toes)

COMPLICATIONS

- Aspiration, atelectasis
- Pneumonia
- Thrombophlebitis
- Pulmonary embolus
- Respiratory failure
- Ileus, gastric dilation
- Gastrointestinal bleeding
- Septicemia

- Autonomic dysfunction, arrhythmias, postural hypertension
- Chronic inflammatory demyelinating polyradiculoneuropathy
- Pressure ulcers

DIAGNOSTIC TESTS

- Describe each procedure, its purpose, and the normal feelings or sensations that are likely, as well as any preprocedural and postprocedural care.
  - —Cerebrospinal fluid sampling: protein initially decreased (15 to 45 mg), then increased as high as 600 mg
  - —Electromyography: reduced nerve conduction velocity at peak of illness
  - —Pulmonary function tests: decreased

TREATMENT
Medical

- Therapy
  - —Intensive care admission
    - Cardiac monitoring
    - Arterial blood gas monitoring
    - Mechanical ventilation and respiratory support
  - —Plasmapheresis (blood exchange)
  - —Chest physiotherapy
  - —Nutritional maintenance (intravenous or nasogastric feedings)
  - —Physical therapy

Surgical

- Tracheostomy for prolonged ventilatory support as indicated

HOME CARE

- Give both the patient and the caregiver *verbal* and *written* instructions. Provide them with the name and telephone number of a physician or nurse to call if questions arise.
- *General information*
  - —Review the explanation of the disorder, causes, and residual neurologic effects.
- *Warning signs*
  - —Review the signs and symptoms that should be reported to a physician or nurse.
    - Difficulty breathing
    - Increased weakness
    - Numbness

- *Special instructions*
  —Instruct the caregiver to inspect the patient's skin daily for signs of irritation or breakdown if the patient is on bed rest (see Pressure Ulcer Sores, p. 715).
  —Stress the importance of avoiding persons who have infections, especially upper respiratory infections.
  —Assist the patient to obtain any adaptive devices (e.g., splints, wheelchair, or walker) and provide instruction on use.
  —Demonstrate proper transferring technique from bed to chair and from chair to toilet.
- *Medications*
  —Explain the purpose, dosage, schedule, and route of administration of any prescribed drugs, as well as side effects to report to the physician or nurse.
  —Stress the need to check with a physician before taking any over-the-counter medications.
- *Activity*
  —Encourage the patient to discuss allowances and limitations with respect to resuming work, recreation, and other activities.
  —Explain the need to resume activities slowly, exercising to tolerance level and then stopping.
  —Explain the importance of maintaining planned rest periods.
  —Stress the need for independence and socialization; advise self-care and eating with the caregiver.
  —Explain the need for diversional activities (television, reading, listening to the radio).
  —Teach the patient and caregiver necessary exercises and ask for a return demonstration.
    Speech exercises
    Active or passive range-of-motion exercises with massage of all extremities
    Exercises that increase strength and mobility of fingers (squeeze toys, clay, balls)
  —Refer the patient for specific home therapy exercises.
  —Discuss the importance of warm baths to alleviate pain and stiffness.
- *Diet*
  —Advise a high-calorie, high-protein diet, cautioning the patient to progress from soft to solid food if facial weakness is present.

—Explain the need to have eating utensils and food arranged so the patient can manage them easily.

—Stress the importance of avoiding constipation.

Drink fluids to maintain intake at 2000 ml/day unless contraindicated.

Use stool softeners (as approved by physician).

Eat foods and fruits high in roughage.

PSYCHOSOCIAL CARE

• Encourage verbalization regarding fear of permanent disability, changes in body image, loss of function (temporary or permanent), and dying.

FOLLOW-UP CARE

• Stress the importance of regular follow-up visits with the physician, physical therapist, and occupational therapist. Make sure the patient has the necessary names and telephone numbers.

REFERRALS

• Provide the patient with the following address to obtain patient education materials: Guillain-Barré Syndrome Foundation International, P.O. Box 262, Wynnewood, PA 19096, (610) 667-0131.

Head Trauma

—Head trauma: any sudden impact, blow, or physical injury to the head that causes damage to brain tissue. Head injuries are categorized as open, or penetrating, and closed, or blunt. Types of injuries include scalp injuries (lacerations, abrasions, hematomas), skull fractures (linear, depressed, basilar), concussions (temporary loss of consciousness after the brain strikes the skull; may last for a few days), and contusions (bruising of the brain tissue, disrupting neural function).

CAUSES/CONTRIBUTING FACTORS/RISK FACTORS

• Trauma: motor vehicle accidents, falls
• Assaults: gunshot and stab wounds

SIGNS/SYMPTOMS

- Periods of consciousness followed by unconsciousness
- Concussion
  —Amnesia: anterograde, retrograde
  —Headache
  —Nausea, vomiting
  —Dizziness
- Contusion
  —Mental changes: confusion, agitation, restlessness, delirium, stupor, coma
  —Posturing: decorticate or decerebrate
  —Sensorimotor disturbances: unilateral or bilateral; paresis or paralysis
  —Unequal pupils and uncoordinated eye movements
- Skull fractures
  —Drainage from ears and nose
  —Localized headache
  —Bilateral periocular ecchymosis (raccoon's eyes)
  —Hearing impairment

COMPLICATIONS

- Cerebral edema
- Sensorimotor and neurologic deficits
- Increased intracranial pressure
- Intracranial hemorrhage
- Hematoma: subdural, epidural
- Brain herniation
- Seizures
- Brain damage
- Respiratory failure

DIAGNOSTIC TESTS

- Describe each procedure, its purpose, and the normal feelings or sensations that are likely, as well as any preprocedural and postprocedural care.
  —Skull x-rays: to visualize bone fragments and fractures
  —Cervical x-rays: to confirm or rule out cervical spinal injury
  —Computed tomography or magnetic resonance imaging: to assess hematoma or distortion of cerebral ventricles
  —Cerebrospinal fluid sampling: may be contraindicated with increased intracranial pressure

—Cerebral angiography: to locate hematomas and displacement of vessels

—Electroencephalogram: to assess for development of pathologic waves

—Pneumoencephalogram: to assess for cerebral ventricular shift, distortion, or dilation

—Cisternogram: to identify dural tear site with basal skull fractures

TREATMENT
Medical

- Therapy
  —Patent airway and adequate ventilation and oxygenation
  —Proper positioning with head of bed elevated to promote venous drainage and thus reduce intracranial pressure, cerebral edema, and congestion
  —Hypothermia blanket
  —Cervical collar
  —Cardiac monitoring
  —Hyperventilation
  —Rehabilitation
     Physical therapy
     Occupational therapy
     Speech therapy
     Bowel and bladder retraining
     Cognitive rehabilitation
  —Diet
     Immediate: nothing by mouth (NPO)
     Later, total parenteral nutrition, intralipids, tube feedings, or progressive diet, depending on the patient's level of consciousness, ability to swallow, and gastrointestinal tract functioning
     Fluid restriction to decrease cerebral edema
  —Intracranial pressure monitoring
  —Hemodynamic monitoring: to assess fluid volume status
  —Indwelling urinary catheter: to measure urinary output
  —Nasogastric tube: to aspirate gastric contents and free air
- Drugs
  —Antiepilepsy drugs
  —Glucocorticoids
  —Osmotic diuretics: mannitol

—Loop diuretics: furosemide (Lasix)
—Antibiotics
—Tetanus prophylaxis
—Antipyretics
—Analgesics
—Sedatives
—Antacids and H_2 blockers
—Stool softeners
—Neuromuscular blocking agents
—Barbiturate coma therapy

Surgical

- Suturing: to repair superficial lacerations
- Craniotomy, craniectomy: to evacuate hematomas, control hemorrhage, remove bone fragments or foreign objects, debride tissues, or elevate depressed fractures
- Trephination (burr holes): to evacuate hematoma or insert intracranial monitoring devices
- Cranioplasty: to repair traumatic defects in the skull
- Ventriculostomy: to remove excess cerebrospinal fluid
- Ventricular shunting procedures: to drain cerebrospinal fluid and reduce intracranial pressure

HOME CARE

- Give both the patient and the caregiver *verbal* and *written* instructions. Provide them with the name and telephone number of a physician or nurse to call if questions arise. Provide a head injury sheet to assist in instruction.
- *General information*
  —Explain and discuss types of head injuries, causes, contributing factors, care and treatment, residual effects, and prevention of further injury.
- *Wound/incision care*
  —Discuss and demonstrate the care of any lacerations or surgical incisions, if indicated.
  Wash area gently.
  Wear clean gloves and cover scalp wounds with gauze dressings.
- *Warning signs*
  —Review the signs and symptoms that should be reported to a physician or nurse.

Infection from surgical incision: fever, erythema, tenderness, pain, warmth, purulent drainage

Meningitis: fever, chills, malaise, back stiffness and pain, nuchal rigidity

Neurologic changes: behavioral and personality changes, irritability, confusion, slurred speech, lethargy

Sensorimotor changes: incoordination, weakness in extremities, difficulty walking

Increased intracranial pressure: altered level of consciousness, such as difficulty in waking patient or increased drowsiness; nausea and vomiting; seizures; worsening headache

Visual abnormalities: blurred vision; diplopia; changes in visual field, depth, or perception

Changes in cognitive ability, judgment, emotional control, orientation, memory, and concentration

Leakage of cerebrospinal fluid: clear or bloody drainage from ear, nose, or throat; complaints of salty taste or frequent swallowing; presence of "halo ring" on pillowcase

Respiratory distress

- *Special instructions*
  —If the patient is discharged home with a mild head injury for observation, instruct a responsible caregiver to stay with the patient for 24 to 48 hours. Tell the caregiver to awaken the patient every 2 hours the first night, asking name, where the patient is, and whether the patient can identify the caregiver. If unable to arouse the patient, the caregiver should notify the physician and return the patient to the hospital.
  —Teach seizure precautions, as indicated.
    Try to prevent or break a fall.
    Ease the patient onto the floor.
    Support and protect the patient's head.
    Turn the patient to one side.
    Remove surrounding furniture and any hard or sharp objects.
    Loosen constrictive clothing around the neck.
    Stay with the patient and call the physician immediately.
  —Explain that possible residual effects (postconcussion syndrome), such as dizziness, headaches, and memory loss, may persist for up to 3 to 4 months after trauma.

—Explain that the patient may experience changes in personality, inappropriate social behavior, inappropriate affect, hallucinations, and altered sleep patterns after head injury.

—Assist the patient in obtaining assistive devices for ambulation or activities of daily living, as indicated.

—For concussion, advise the patient to avoid Valsalva maneuvers such as straining during defecation, vigorous coughing, nose blowing, or sneezing.

—Offer methods other than medications for dealing with pain: visualization, guided imagery, meditation, relaxation, biofeedback.

• *Medications*

—Explain the purpose, dosage, schedule, and route of administration of any prescribed drugs, as well as side effects to report to the physician or nurse.

—Stress the importance of avoiding over-the-counter medications without consulting the physician. Tell the patient not to take aspirin because of the risk of bleeding.

• *Activity*

—Encourage the patient to discuss allowances and limitations with respect to resuming work, recreation, and other activities.

—Encourage the patient in self-care activities as tolerated.

—Encourage decision making by the patient.

—Provide structured daily activities and routines with planned rest periods.

—Advise the caregiver to avoid overprotection. Assist the family and caregiver to identify and correct hazards in the home to prevent falls and injuries.

Remove all hazardous objects.

Maintain clear pathways.

Provide good lighting.

Provide the patient with proper shoes and glasses. Place objects within the patient's visual field.

Install assistive and safety aids such as ramps, rails, and shower chairs.

—Instruct the family and caregivers to supervise or assist with ambulation.

—Teach the family range-of-motion exercises and involve them in the exercise program.

—Instruct the patient to avoid alcohol, driving, smoking, use of hazardous appliances and machinery, contact sports, tub baths, and swimming until advised by a physician.

- *Diet*
  —Advise the patient to chew food well and swallow slowly.
  —Provide supplemental feedings, if ordered.

PSYCHOSOCIAL CARE

- Encourage the patient and caregiver to verbalize fears and concerns regarding head injury, disability, body and functional changes, and adaptation to the patient's residual deficits and mental and emotional sequelae.
- Encourage participation in counseling.

FOLLOW-UP CARE

- Stress the importance of regular follow-up visits with the physician, physical therapist, occupational therapist, and speech therapist. Make sure the patient has the necessary names and telephone numbers.
- Encourage the patient to obtain a MedicAlert bracelet and identification card listing the diagnosis, medications, and treatment, if appropriate.

REFERRALS

- Refer the patient to a social worker for further support and counseling.
- Assist the patient and caregivers to obtain referral to support groups, community resources, and home health support services.
- Provide referral for support services (See Appendix F for listing of The Brain Injury Association and Head Injury Rehabilitation Services).

Heart Failure
(Congestive Heart Failure)

—Heart failure: inability of the heart muscle to pump with enough force to meet the body's metabolic demands. In this chronic and progressive syndrome, impairment of heart function or heart failure may involve the right or left side of the heart or both sides. Symptoms depend on which side of the heart is failing; right-sided failure usually follows left heart failure.

CAUSES/CONTRIBUTING FACTORS
- Coronary artery disease
- Myocardial infarction
- Valvular heart disease
- Congenital heart defects
- High blood pressure
- Cardiomyopathy
- Inflammatory heart disease
- Alcohol abuse
- Dysrhythmias
- Pregnancy
- Hyperthyroidism

SIGNS/SYMPTOMS
- Left-sided failure
  —Shortness of breath with exertion at rest or night
  —Orthopnea
  —Cough with blood-tinged sputum
  —Restlessness
  —Fatigue, weakness
  —Nocturia
- Right-sided failure
  —Dry cough
  —Edema: pretibial, ankle
  —Abdominal swelling (ascites)
  —Abdominal pain and fullness
  —Anorexia
  —Sudden weight gain

COMPLICATIONS

- Pulmonary edema
- Dysrhythmias
- Thromboembolism
- Venostasis
- Myocardial infarction

DIAGNOSTIC TESTS

- Inform the patient that several procedures may be done to aid in the diagnosis of this condition. Describe each procedure, its purpose, and the normal feelings or sensations that are likely, as well as any preprocedural and postprocedural care.
  —Blood tests: electrolytes, blood chemistry profile
  —Chest x-ray: to detect pulmonary congestion and an increase in heart size
  —Electrocardiogram
  —Echocardiogram
  —Multiple gated acquisition

TREATMENT
Medical

- Treat underlying cause
- Drugs
  —Digitalis
  —Diuretics
  —Angiotensin-converting enzyme (ACE) inhibitors
  —Beta blockers
  —Inotropic drugs
  —Vasodilators
  —Potassium replacements
  —Home oxygen therapy

Surgical

- Heart transplant for end-stage heart failure

▣ HOME CARE

- Give both the patient and the caregiver *verbal* and *written* instructions. Provide them with the name and telephone number of a physician or nurse to call if questions arise.
- *General information*
  —Explain the disease process, causes, and contributing factors.

- *Warning signs*
  —Review the signs and symptoms that should be reported to a physician or nurse.
  - Decreased exercise tolerance
  - Shortness of breath
  - Dyspnea on exertion
  - Paroxysmal nocturnal dyspnea
  - Persistent cough
  - Swelling of extremities
- *Special instructions*
  —Instruct the patient to take and record the pulse. Provide guidelines and rates to report.
  —Instruct the patient to weigh daily at the same time, using the same scale, and wearing the same clothing, and to report a weight gain of 2 to 3 pounds in one day or 5 pounds in a week.
  —Instruct the patient to avoid hot, humid weather, which can put extra demand on the heart.
  —Provide information and instruction for home oxygen therapy if ordered; refer to respiratory therapist as indicated.
- *Medications*
  —Explain the purpose, dosage, schedule, and route of administration of any prescribed drugs, as well as side effects to report to the physician or nurse.
  —Discuss the need to take potassium supplements if non-potassium-sparing diuretics (thiazides, furosemide) are prescribed.
  —Discuss the need to avoid over-the-counter medications such as laxatives and cough medications, which may contain sodium.
- *Activity*
  —Assist the patient to identify activities that elicit symptoms or cause fatigue or shortness of breath.
  —Encourage activity as tolerated, but advise the patient to avoid strenuous activity that will put undue burden on the heart, such as heavy lifting, prolonged walking, carrying heavy suitcases, shoveling snow, changing a tire, and mowing the lawn.
  —Suggest energy-saving devices and techniques for activities of daily living.
  —Tell the patient to space activities with periods of rest and to stop and rest when tired.

—Encourage questions regarding occupation or recreation.
—Explain the need to avoid extremes in temperature or activities during days with high pollution.
—Tell the patient to avoid situations that might cause colds, flu, or other infections.
• *Diet*
—Explain the importance of maintaining the prescribed diet and fluid restrictions.
—Discuss the need to avoid food high in sodium. A 3 g of sodium diet, or in severe cases a 2 g of sodium diet, may be prescribed. Explain the need to read food and drink labels for sodium content, to avoid commercially prepared or frozen foods, to wash all canned vegetables to remove sodium, and to eat foods high in potassium (bananas, orange juice) to replenish potassium lost from the use of diuretics.
—Encourage the use of herbs and spices for flavoring.
—Caution against use of certain salt substitutes because they may have a high potassium content.

PSYCHOSOCIAL CARE

• Provide an opportunity for the patient and caregiver to verbalize fears and concerns regarding home care, financial constraints, or support services available in the community.
• Encourage the patient and caregiver to participate in planning discharge care.
• Provide consultation and referral for mental health counseling as indicated.

FOLLOW-UP CARE

• Stress the importance of regular follow-up visits for medical and laboratory evaluation. Make sure the patient has the necessary names and telephone numbers.
• Emphasize the importance of not smoking, using tobacco products, or drinking alcohol.

REFERRALS

• Provide referrals for home health care, skilled nursing facility, and social services as indicated. Provide community-based supportive resources as needed.

Hemolytic Anemia

—Hemolytic anemia: a disorder in which the rate of erythrocyte destruction is greatly accelerated. Hemolytic anemia, which occurs as a result of an intracorpuscular (inherited) defect or extracorpuscular (acquired) factors, results in a shortened red blood cell life span. The bone marrow is unable to replace the destroyed red blood cells.

CAUSES/CONTRIBUTING FACTORS

- Intracorpuscular defects
  - —Deficiency in glucose 6-phosphate dehydrogenase
  - —Hereditary spherocytosis
- Extracorpuscular factors
  - —Trauma (burns, prosthetic valve replacement)
  - —Chemical agents/medications
  - —Immune response
  - —Infections
  - —Systemic diseases
  - —Hemolytic reactions (blood transfusion)
  - —Autoimmune disorders

SIGNS/SYMPTOMS

- Decreased urinary output
- Fluid loss or overload
- Nausea and vomiting
- Jaundice
- Fever and chills
- Weakness and fatigue
- Back or abdominal pain
- Headache

COMPLICATIONS

- Acute renal failure

DIAGNOSTIC TESTS

- Describe each procedure, its purpose, and the normal feelings or sensations that are likely, as well as any preprocedural and postprocedural care.

—Laboratory studies
   Red blood cell (RBC) count
   Reticulocyte count
   Red blood cell fragility
   Erythrocyte life span
   Fecal and urinary urobilinogen
—Bone marrow biopsy
—Ultrasound/gallbladder studies

TREATMENT
Medical

- Therapy
  —Blood component transfusion
  —Erythrocytopheresis (RBC exchange)
- Drugs
  —Corticosteroids
     Prednisone
  —Osmotic diuretics
  —Sodium bicarbonate or lactate
  —Folic acid

Surgical

- Splenectomy if steroids fail to arrest RBC destruction

🏠 HOME CARE

- Give both the patient and the caregiver *verbal* and *written* instructions. Provide them with the name and telephone number of a physician or nurse to call if questions arise.
- *General information*
  —Explain and discuss the type of hemolytic disorder, causes, and contributing factors if acquired. Explain the underlying condition and prescribed treatment.
- *Special instructions*
  —Teach the patient to rate pain on a scale of 1 to 10 and to monitor pain levels. Assist the patient to identify precipitating factors. Discuss methods of relieving pain or discomfort.
- *Warning signs*
  —Review the signs and symptoms of hemolytic crisis that should be reported to a physician or nurse.
     Jaundice
     Shortness of breath
     Joint or abdominal pain

Headache

Vertigo

—Stress the need to avoid factors that precipitate hemolytic crisis: infection, trauma, chemicals, toxic drug reactions.

- *Medications*
  —Explain the purpose, dosage, schedule, and route of administration of any prescribed drugs, as well as side effects to report to a physician or nurse.
  —Review the side effects of steroid therapy (see Steroid Therapy, p. 590).
- *Activity*
  —Encourage the patient to discuss allowances and limitations with respect to occupation, recreation, and activities.
  —Discuss the need to find a balance between activity and rest and to keep physical and emotional stress at a minimum.
  —Instruct the patient to decrease activities during crises or when symptoms appear.
- *Diet*
  —Discuss the need for a well-balanced diet that is rich in iron and protein.
  —Advise the patient to avoid fatty foods.
  —Teach the patient to take small, frequent meals.
  —Discuss methods to maintain hydration status; encourage daily fluids unless contraindicated. Instruct the patient to notify the physician or nurse if output decreases.

FOLLOW-UP CARE

- Stress the importance of regular follow-up visits for medical and laboratory evaluation. Make sure the patient has the necessary names and telephone numbers.
- Discuss the need to wear a MedicAlert bracelet and carry an information card if receiving long-term treatment.

Hemophilia

—**Hemophilia: a hereditary disorder characterized by impaired coagulability of the blood with a tendency to bleed. Hemophilia A (classic hemophilia) is caused by a deficiency of** factor VIII and affects 80% of hemophilia cases. Hemophilia B results from deficiency of factor IX and affects 5% of cases. Both types of hemophilia are sex-linked genetic disorders. The disease affects males. Females are asymptomatic carriers, with a mother having a 50% chance of transmitting the disease to her son.

SIGNS/SYMPTOMS

- Easy bruising
- Bleeding after minimal trauma
- Bleeding from mucous membranes, gastrointestinal tract, genitourinary tract
- Joint pain, swelling from bleeding into the joint (hemarthrosis)

COMPLICATIONS

- Joint deformity
- Hemorrhagic shock
- Intracranial hemorrhage
- Peripheral neuropathy

DIAGNOSTIC TESTS

- Describe each procedure, its purpose, and the normal feelings or sensations that are likely, as well as any preprocedural and postprocedural care.
    —Partial thromboplastin time
    —Bleeding time
    —Platelet count
    —Activated clotting time
    —Assays of factors VIII and IX
    —Fibrinogen level
    —Prothrombin time
    —Thrombin time
    —Prenatal fetal serum

TREATMENT
Medical

- Therapy
    —Factor transfusion (for hemophilia B)
    —Transfusion of fresh frozen plasma
    —Cryoprecipitate (for hemophilia A)

—Treatment for the development of antibody inhibitors against the specific coagulation factor
—Plasmapheresis to remove the inhibitor
—Prothrombin complexes to bypass inhibitors
- Drugs
—Agents such as desmopressin (DDAVP) and aminocaproic acid (Amicar)
—Immunosuppressive agents

HOME CARE

- Give both the patient and the caregiver *verbal* and *written* instructions. Provide them with the name and telephone number of a physician or nurse to call if questions arise.
- *General information*
—Explain and discuss with the patient the specific hemophilia disorder, its causes, and contributing factors.
- *Special instructions*
—Review the procedure in case of bleeding.
    Apply cold compresses and gentle direct pressure to the site.
    Elevate the affected part if possible.
    Seek medical attention promptly.
—Review precautions to prevent bleeding as appropriate.
    Use an electric razor.
    Avoid constipation.
    Use a soft-bristled toothbrush, and maintain good dental hygiene.
—Stress the importance of frequent assessment of joint function to allow rapid identification and treatment of hemophilic arthritis.
—Discuss the need to receive regular dental care.
—Stress the importance of informing all physicians and dentists of the bleeding disorder.
—Stress the importance of notifying the physician immediately of any injury to the head or the abdomen for evaluation and treatment of internal bleeding.
- *Medications*
—Explain the purpose, dosage, schedule, and route of administration of any prescribed drugs, as well as side effects to report to the physician or nurse.

—Caution the patient to avoid over-the-counter medications containing ibuprofen and aspirin components.

—Discuss the need for lifelong factor replacement.

—Teach the patient and significant others venipuncture and intravenous administration of factor products. Allow time for return demonstration and practice.

—Teach the patient and caregiver to keep blood factor concentrate and infusion equipment available at all times, even on vacation.

—Discuss the storage of fluids and the proper disposal of equipment.

—Review adverse reactions, such as bloodborne infection and factor inhibitor development.

—Discuss common side effects of factor and blood product infusion and management of possible symptoms.

> Flushing, headache, or tingling with factor replacement may be decreased by slowing infusion.
>
> Urticaria with cryoprecipitate or plasma may be relieved with diphenhydramine. Persons who have frequent reactions should receive antihistamine 4 minutes before factor infusion.
>
> Fever and chills resulting from plasma infusion may be decreased with acetaminophen.

—Review symptoms of anaphylaxis: rapid or difficult breathing, wheezing, hoarseness, stridor, and chest tightness.

—Teach the patient or caregiver to administer epinephrine and then to contact the physician immediately.

• *Activity*

—Encourage the patient to discuss allowances and limitations with respect to occupation, recreation, and activities.

—Stress the need to avoid contact sports (e.g., soccer, football) or activities that may pose a risk of falls or injury.

—Discuss the benefits of regular aerobic exercise, such as swimming, walking, and cycling.

PSYCHOSOCIAL CARE

• Encourage verbalization about concerns and fears over how disease is affecting lifestyle.

• Encourage participation in planning home care.

• Provide counseling referral as indicated.

FOLLOW-UP CARE AND REFERRALS

- Stress the importance of regular follow-up visits for medical and laboratory evaluation. Make sure the patient has the necessary names and telephone numbers.
- Discuss the importance of wearing a MedicAlert bracelet and carrying an information card; assist the patient to obtain them.
- Assist the patient to identify community-based support services and resources.
- Refer the patient to the National Hemophilia Foundation.
- Obtain referrals for home care services and a medical social worker as indicated.

H

Hemorrhoid

—Hemorrhoid: varicose veins in the anal canal or anorectal area. Hemorrhoids may occur proximal (internal) or distal (external) to the anal sphincter. Continuous increased abdominal pressure leads to the development and enlargement of hemorrhoids. Persistent, high downward pressures during defecation subject hemorrhoids to congestion, bleeding, prolapse, and thrombosis.

CAUSES/CONTRIBUTING FACTORS

- Pregnancy
- Prolonged sitting or standing
- Straining during defecation
- Cirrhosis with portal hypertension

SIGNS/SYMPTOMS

- Rectal itching
- Rectal bleeding
- Rectal or anal discomfort
- Constipation

COMPLICATIONS

- Hemorrhage
- Infection
- Strangulation and ulceration of hemorrhoid

DIAGNOSTIC TESTS

- Describe each procedure, its purpose, and the normal feelings or sensations that are likely, as well as any preprocedural and postprocedural care.
  —Rectal examination
  —Proctoscopy or sigmoidoscopy: to confirm the diagnosis and rule out carcinoma or inflammatory disease

TREATMENT
Medical

- Therapy
  —Heat application
  —Sitz baths
- Drugs
  —Stool softeners
  —Topical anesthetics
  —Steroid preparations

Surgical

- Sclerotherapy: injection of sclerosing agent between and around hemorrhoid to cause tissue shrinkage
- Rubber band ligation (internal hemorrhoids): to cause tissue necrosis and sloughing of hemorrhoids
- Cryosurgery: freezing of hemorrhoids
- Laser removal
- Hemorrhoidectomy

HOME CARE

- Give both the patient and the caregiver *verbal* and *written* instructions. Provide them with the name and telephone number of a physician or nurse to call if questions arise.
- *General information*
  —Review any explanation about treatment and specific follow-up care.
  —Explain and discuss the development of hemorrhoids, causes or contributing factors, care, treatment, and potential for recurrence.
- *Warning signs*
  —Review the signs and symptoms that should be reported to a physician or nurse.
      Frequent, unrelieved urge to defecate
      Constipation or lack of bowel movement

- *Special instructions*
  —Discuss measures to prevent the development or enlargement of hemorrhoids.

  Eat a diet high in fiber to promote regular bowel movements and soft stools.

  Drink plenty of fluids, up to 2 to 3 liters/day, unless contraindicated.

  Use stool softeners and bulk laxatives to prevent constipation.

  Perform daily mild exercise to enhance peristalsis and promote elimination.

  Defecate promptly after the urge so that pressure in the rectum will be prevented.

  Avoid prolonged sitting (including on the toilet), squatting, or standing.

  Avoid straining during defecation, which could increase discomfort and pressure on the affected area.

  —Advise the patient to sit on thick foam pillows or pads and to avoid air or rubber doughnuts because they spread the buttocks apart.

  —Discuss the procedure for using sitz baths after bowel movements to relieve discomfort and for cleansing.

  Use warm sitz baths for brief periods to avoid hypotension secondary to vasodilation of pelvic blood vessels.

  Discontinue sitz bath when feeling dizzy or faint.

  —Stress the importance of perianal cleanliness at all times. Explain to the patient that proper hygiene helps prevent infection.

  —Instruct the patient to wipe gently after a bowel movement. Encourage the use of moist perineal wipes.

  —Discuss and demonstrate the use of cold compresses to reduce congestion and edema when hemorrhoids are inflamed.

  —Provide and demonstrate the use of warm compresses to promote circulation.

  —Advise the patient to abstain from anal intercourse until healing is complete.

- *Medications*
  —Explain the purpose, dosage, schedule, and route of administration of any prescribed drugs, as well as side effects to report to the physician or nurse.

  —Advise the patient to use topical anesthetics, astringents, and prescribed antiinflammatory preparations.

FOLLOW-UP CARE

- Stress the importance of regular follow-up visits for medical and laboratory evaluation. Make sure the patient has the necessary names and telephone numbers.

Hemorrhoidectomy

—**Hemorrhoidectomy: surgical excision of hemorrhoids that do not respond to other therapies.**

PREPROCEDURAL TEACHING

- Review the physician's explanation of the procedure and the reason for it; encourage the patient to ask questions and to discuss any fears or anxieties. Explain the need for informed consent.

Review of Preprocedural Care

- Explain that the procedure may be performed on an outpatient basis.

Review of Postprocedural Care

- Discuss postoperative care, including pain management, rectal packing, and bowel elimination.
- Inform the patient that early ambulation will be encouraged to promote peristalsis.
- Explain that a postoperative bowel movement will be encouraged to prevent complications such as anal strictures. Tell the patient that the first postoperative bowel movement will be stimulated by a stool softener. Warn the patient that the movement will be painful and may cause dizziness.

SIDE EFFECTS/COMPLICATIONS

- Hemorrhage
- Infection
- Anal strictures or stenosis

🏠 HOME CARE

- Give both the patient and the caregiver *verbal* and *written* instructions. Provide them with the name and telephone number of a physician or nurse to call if questions arise.
- *General information*
  —Review any explanation about the procedure and specific follow-up care.
  —Explain and discuss the development of hemorrhoids, causes or contributing factors, care, treatment, and potential for recurrence.
- *Warning signs*
  —Review the signs and symptoms that should be reported to a physician or nurse.

    Infection: fever, purulent drainage, redness, swelling, warmth, tenderness

    Increased rectal bleeding (more than two saturated pads in 8 hours)

    Frequent, unrelieved urge to defecate

    Urinary retention

    Constipation or lack of bowel movement

- *Special instructions*
  —Discuss and demonstrate rectal packing or perianal dressing: procedure, frequency, and signs to report.
  —Assist the patient in obtaining appropriate supplies, such as dressings and perineal pads to protect clothing from post-operative oozing.
  —Advise the patient to sit on thick foam pillows or pads and to avoid air or rubber doughnuts because they spread the buttocks apart.
  —Stress the importance of perianal cleanliness at all times. Explain to the patient that proper hygiene helps prevent infection. Instruct the patient to wipe gently after a bowel movement. Encourage the use of moist perineal wipes.
  —Advise the patient to abstain from anal intercourse until healing is complete.
  —Warn the patient to anticipate some bleeding 8 to 12 days postoperatively when sutures begin to dissolve.

FOLLOW-UP CARE AND REFERRALS

- Stress the importance of regular follow-up visits. Make sure the patient has the necessary names and telephone numbers.

- Assist the patient to obtain referrals for home care services and supplies.

Hepatitis, Viral
(Hepatitis A, B, C, D, and E)

—Hepatitis, viral: inflammation of the liver caused by hepatitis viruses. Viral hepatitis may lead to liver damage, necrosis, and failure.

CAUSES/CONTRIBUTING FACTORS/RISK FACTORS

- Hepatitis A (fecal-oral)
    - —Ingestion of food, water, or shellfish contaminated with hepatitis A virus
    - —Direct fecal-oral transmission
    - —Travel to underdeveloped countries
    - —Poor sanitation
- Hepatitis B (serum)
    - —Exposure to blood, secretions, or body fluids contaminated with hepatitis B virus via direct or indirect contact with infective source
    - —History of intravenous drug use
    - —History of accidental exposure to contaminated needles or blood, body fluids, or secretions
    - —History of blood transfusion
    - —History of multiple sexual partners or homosexual contact
    - —History of household contact with an infected person
    - —Perinatal transmission
- Hepatitis C (serum)
    - —Contact with blood or serum (same as hepatitis B)
    - —Often transmitted by chronic carriers
- Hepatitis D (serum)
    - —Can cause infection only if person already has hepatitis B
    - —Blood infectious throughout hepatitis B infection

- Hepatitis E (fecal-oral)
  —Fecal-oral, food-borne; water-borne (same as hepatitis A)
  —Most frequent in persons living or traveling in parts of Asia, Africa, or countries where sanitation conditions are poor

SIGNS/SYMPTOMS

- Anorexia
- Malaise
- Tenderness and pain in the right upper quadrant
- Jaundice
- Clay-colored stools
- Dark urine
- Nausea and vomiting
- Diarrhea
- Headache
- Scleral icterus
- Fever (hepatitis A, E)
- Pruritus (hepatitis B, C, D)
- Urticaria (hepatitis B, C, D)
- Muscles or joint aches (hepatitis B, C, D)

COMPLICATIONS

- Fulminant hepatitis
- Chronic hepatitis infection
- Hepatic coma

DIAGNOSTIC TESTS

- Describe each procedure, its purpose, and the normal feelings or sensations that are likely, as well as any preprocedural and postprocedural care.
  —Serum antigen or antibody tests: to detect the antigen or antibodies and to indicate the course of the disease and immune status
  —Serum enzymes and serum bilirubin: to indicate liver dysfunction
  —Complete blood count: to detect the presence of infection
  —Prothrombin time: to assess clotting function
  —Stool specimen analysis: to detect the presence of hepatitis A or E in stool
  —Urinalysis: to reveal elevation of urobilinogen in the presence of infection
  —Liver biopsy: for pathologic examination of liver tissue

TREATMENT
Medical

- Therapy
  —Bed rest with a gradual return to normal activities as symptoms subside
  —Dietary therapy
  —Small, frequent, low-fat, high-carbohydrate feedings
  —Parenteral or enteral feedings if oral intake is not tolerated
  —Prohibition of alcoholic beverages
  —Vitamin supplements
- Drugs
  —Antiinfective agents
  —Hepatitis A: immune globulin
  —Hepatitis B and D: hepatitis B vaccine
  —H$_2$ blockers
  —Antihistamines
  —Vitamin K
  —Corticosteroids
  —Recombinant interferon
  —Antiemetics: avoid prochlorperazine (Compazine) because of excessive sedation

HOME CARE

- Give both the patient and the caregiver *verbal* and *written* instructions. Provide them with the name and telephone number of a physician or nurse to call if questions arise.
- *General information*
  —Explain and discuss hepatitis, transmission, causes and contributing factors, care, treatment, and prevention.
  —Explain that the symptomatic infected patient and the carrier patient are infectious.
- *Warning signs*
  —Review the signs and symptoms that should be reported to a physician or nurse
    Altered level of consciousness: lethargy, somnolence, stupor, coma
    Confusion and personality changes
    Asterixis
    Easy bruising; prolonged bleeding; blood in the vomitus, urine, or stool
    Edema in the extremities or abdomen
    Unexplained weight gain

- *Special instructions*
  —Discuss the infectious nature of hepatitis A, B, C, D, and E.
  —Review necessary precautions for hepatitis A and E.
    Tell the patient to wash hands thoroughly after toileting.
    Instruct the family or caregiver to wear gloves if contact with feces is possible and to boil articles (e.g., linens, clothing) soiled by feces.
    Instruct the patient not to prepare food for others during the symptomatic phase of the disease.
    Instruct the patient not to share items, such as eating utensils, toothbrushes, or toys.
    Refer close family members and friends for injection of gamma globulin.
    Refer the patient for immunization with hepatitis A virus vaccine.
  —Review necessary precautions for hepatitis B, C, and D.
    Teach the patient and caregiver to exercise blood and body fluid precautions until the patient is free of hepatitis B surface antigen (HBsAg).
    Advise the patient not to share razors, toothbrushes, or needles.
    Tell the patient to use an electric razor and soft-bristled toothbrush to help prevent bleeding.
    Advise the patient to handle cuts and lacerations cautiously.
    Offer hepatitis B vaccine to the patient's close personal contacts. Advise the patient to avoid sexual activity during the acute stage of illness and ideally until HBsAg tests are negative or until the partner has received hepatitis B vaccine.
    Explain to the patient that blood donation is no longer possible.
    Stress the importance of informing other physicians, dentists, and health care workers of the hepatitis diagnosis.
    Encourage caregivers to provide a separate bed and bathroom for the patient if possible.
  —Discuss skin care.
    Advise the patient to avoid using alkaline soaps and to use mild soaps.

Advise the patient to keep the skin moist with emollient lotions.

Encourage the patient not to scratch, but to apply pressure to the affected area.

Encourage the patient to keep nails trimmed and smooth and to use knuckles to relieve itching.

Suggest cool water showers or cool compresses for pruritus.

Encourage the patient to wear loose, soft clothing, such as cotton.

—Explain that jaundice will disappear as the disease resolves.

—Suggest wearing bright red or blue clothing to offset the jaundice.

- *Medications*
  —Explain the purpose, dosage, schedule, and route of administration of any prescribed drugs, as well as side effects to report to the physician or nurse.
  —Tell the patient to avoid using over-the-counter medications, especially aspirin or drugs containing aspirin.

- *Activity*
  —Encourage the patient to discuss allowances and limitations with respect to occupation, recreation, or activities.
  —Tell the patient to alternate planned rest periods with activities during the symptomatic phase.
  —Provide diversional activities and socialization to promote social interaction during therapeutic isolation.

- *Diet*
  —Advise the patient to avoid alcohol intake for up to 1 year after the attack.
  —Encourage small, frequent meals of low-fat, high-carbohydrate foods.
  —Encourage intake of fluids (fruit juices and carbonated beverages) up to 2 liters/day, unless contraindicated.
  —Instruct the patient to monitor and record daily weights and to report any sudden or steady decrease.

PSYCHOSOCIAL CARE

- Encourage the caregiver to verbalize feelings and concerns about precautions and adaptations for the disease process.
- Encourage the patient to verbalize concerns about body image related to jaundice.

FOLLOW-UP CARE

- Stress the importance of regular follow-up visits and liver function tests. Make sure the patient has the necessary names and telephone numbers.
- For a patient with hepatitis B, instruct the patient to return for follow-up serologic tests in 1 or 2 months to determine if HBsAG is present.
- Assist the patient to obtain a MedicAlert bracelet and information card listing the diagnosis, medications, and treatment.

REFERRALS

- Refer the patient to drug and alcohol treatment programs, if appropriate.

Herniorrhaphy
(Hernia)

—Herniorrhaphy: surgical repair of an incarcerated or strangulated hernia.

—Hernia: a protrusion of an organ, usually the intestine, through an abnormal opening in the abdominal wall. A hernia may occur as a result of a congenital opening, abdominal wall weakness, increased abdominal pressure, or trauma. Hernias may occur at any age, in both males and females. Most hernias occur in the groin. Some examples of hernia are indirect inguinal, direct inguinal, femoral, and umbilical. A hernia may be reducible (returned to proper position spontaneously or by manual manipulation), incarcerated (trapped by the narrow neck of the opening), or strangulated (becomes gangrenous).

INDICATIONS

- Incarcerated hernia
- Strangulated hernia

PREPROCEDURAL TEACHING

- See also Abdominal Surgery (p. 6).
- Review the physician's explanation of the procedure and the reason for it; encourage the patient to ask questions and to discuss any fears or anxieties. Explain the need for informed consent.

Review of Preprocedural Care

- Explain that an elective procedure may be performed on an outpatient basis; strangulated or incarcerated repairs require a hospital stay.

Review of Postprocedural Care

- Discuss anticipated postoperative care, including pain management and incisions.
- Discuss and demonstrate splinting the incision during coughing or sneezing.
- Discuss the purpose of and demonstrate the use of the incentive spirometer.
- Encourage early ambulation.
- Explain that analgesics will be given for pain management.

SIDE EFFECTS/COMPLICATIONS

- Infection
- Hemorrhage
- Impaired blood supply to the vas deferens

HOME CARE

- Give both the patient and the caregiver *verbal* and *written* instructions. Provide them with the name and telephone number of a physician or nurse to call if questions arise.
- *General information*
  —Review any explanation about the procedure and specific follow-up care.
  —Explain and discuss the development of hernias, causes or contributing factors, care and treatment, and prevention.
- *Wound/incision care*
  —Discuss and demonstrate proper wound management and dressing changes: procedures, frequency, and signs to report.
- *Warning signs*
  —Review the signs and symptoms that should be reported to a physician or nurse.

Infection: fever, pain, edema, erythema, warmth, purulent drainage, foul odor from the incision
Abdominal distention, nausea, vomiting
Hernia recurrence: firm, tender, globular, irreducible swelling in the groin

- *Special instructions*
  —Apply and demonstrate to the male patient scrotal support or ice packs to decrease scrotal edema and discomfort.
  —Assist the patient in obtaining appropriate supplies, such as sterile dressings.
- *Medications*
  —Explain the purpose, dosage, schedule, and route of administration of any prescribed drugs, as well as side effects to report to a physician or nurse.
  Analgesics
  Stool softeners
  Laxatives
- *Activity*
  —Encourage the patient to discuss allowances and limitations with respect to occupation, recreation, or activities.
  —Instruct the patient to avoid coughing, straining, stretching, constipation, heavy lifting (>10 pounds), strenuous exercise, and sports for 6 weeks.
  —Demonstrate splinting incision manually or with a pillow during coughing, sneezing, or hiccups.
  —Stress the importance of activity restrictions and splinting the incision for up to 6 weeks after surgery.
  —Demonstrate proper body mechanics for moving and lifting.
  —Advise returning to work in 2 weeks for desk workers and 6 weeks for heavy laborers.
  —Advise that sexual activity should be avoided for several weeks to avoid strain on the incision and discomfort to the scrotum, if edematous.
- *Diet*
  —Advise the patient to plan a high-fiber diet to help prevent constipation; provide the patient with a list of high-fiber foods.
  —Advise the patient to drink plenty of fluids, up to 2 to 3 liters/day, unless contraindicated.
  —Stress the importance of weight loss if the patient is obese.

PSYCHOSOCIAL CARE

- Encourage the verbalization of fears and concerns about altered sexual function secondary to impaired blood supply to the vas deferens.

FOLLOW-UP CARE

- Stress the importance of regular follow-up visits. Make sure the patient has the necessary names and telephone numbers.
- Stress the importance of smoking cessation to eliminate the smoker's cough as a contributing factor to hernia development.

REFERRALS

- Provide information and refer the patient to community resources for weight loss and smoking cessation, if indicated.

Hip Replacement

—Hip replacement: total hip replacement (arthroplasty) is removal of the hip joint (including femoral and acetabular sides) and its replacement with a prosthesis. Total hip replacement is performed when the joint has been severely affected by conditions that result in significant pain and dysfunction. Partial hip replacement involves replacement of only the femoral head with a prosthesis.

INDICATIONS

- Total hip replacement
  - —Osteoarthritis
  - —Rheumatoid arthritis
  - —Ankylosing spondylitis (Marie-Strümpell disease)
  - —Legg-Calvé-Perthes disease
  - —Benign and malignant bone tumors
  - —Severe hip trauma
- Partial hip replacement
  - —Avascular necrosis of the head of the femur, caused by systemic steroid therapy, sickle cell anemia, and alcohol abuse
  - —Fractures of the femoral head

COMPLICATIONS

- Infection
- Neurovascular dysfunction
- Disabling pain
- Deep vein thrombosis
- Loosening of implant
- Dislocation of the prosthesis
- Atelectasis
- Pneumonia
- Hemorrhage

PREPROCEDURAL TEACHING

- Review the physician's explanation of the procedure and the reason for it; encourage the patient to ask questions and to discuss any fears or anxieties.

Review of Preprocedural Care

- Explain that the patient will be admitted on the day of surgery or the night before and will remain in the hospital for 3 to 5 days.
- Explain that IV antibiotics may be started before surgery and will be continued during surgery and for at least 3 to 5 days after surgery.
- Review routine preoperative procedures.
  —Blood and urologic studies, type and crossmatch, chest x-ray, electrocardiogram
  —NPO from midnight the night before
  —Bowel preparation with enema the night before
  —Shower and shampoo the night before
  —Skin preparation: cleansing with bactericidal soap and shave at operative site
- Explain that the hip will be x-rayed and measured to determine the size of the prosthesis.

Review of Postprocedural Care

- Discuss the importance of exercises and teach the patient to perform them.
  —Coughing and deep breathing
  —Foot exercises (dorsiflexion and plantar flexion)
  —Gluteal and abdominal contractions and quadriceps setting
  —Range of motion of unaffected extremities

- Provide instruction on the use of ambulatory aids: crutches, cane, walker.
- Tell the patient that the diet will be NPO for the first 24 hours and then progress to a regular diet as tolerated.
- Explain that a drainage tube will be inserted to remove excess blood and fluid around the wound.
- Tell the patient that antiembolic stockings will be applied.
- Inform the patient that bed rest will be maintained for 24 to 48 hours and then the patient can get up with an ambulatory aid as prescribed by the physician.
- Discuss the importance of postoperative body position and measures to keep the hip from bending beyond 90 degrees and dislocating the prosthesis.
  —Use of continuous passive motion device
  —Use of knee immobilizer to prevent knee-hip flexion
  —Use of an abduction pillow to keep the legs apart and prevent them from turning inward (internal rotation)
- Explain that physical therapy will be started to strengthen muscles around the new hip, regain the hip's range of motion, and permit walking.

HOME CARE

- Give both the patient and the caregiver *verbal* and *written* instructions. Provide them with the name and telephone number of a physician or nurse to call if questions arise.
- *General information*
  —Review any explanation about the procedure and specific follow-up care.
- *Wound/incision care*
  —Discuss and demonstrate proper care of the incision.
- *Warning signs*
  —Review the signs and symptoms that should be reported to a physician or nurse.
      Infection: fever; chills; redness; swelling; drainage from incision; deep, dull aching pain in operative area
      Deep venous thrombosis: pain or soreness in calf, redness, swelling along vein lines
      Neurovascular impairment: loss of sensation or movement of affected foot and leg, coolness, pallor, numbness, tingling in affected extremity

- *Special instructions*
  —Advise the patient to obtain self-help devices to limit hip bending: raised toilet seat, bath bench, long-handled grippers. Refer the patient to a medical supply store for purchase or rental.
  —Explain that the patient should avoid putting excess weight on the hip and should use a walker, then crutches, and then a cane until completely recovered.
  —Stress the importance of participating in physical therapy to regain muscle strength and ensure adequate upper extremity strength for ambulating with a walker, crutches, or cane.
- *Medications*
  —Explain the purpose, dosage, schedule, and route of administration of any prescribed drugs, as well as side effects to report to a physician or nurse.
- *Activity*
  —Encourage the patient to discuss allowances and limitations with respect to occupation, recreation, or activities. For example, tennis and skiing are not recommended but golf and swimming may be permitted.
  —Discuss restrictions and activities to avoid loosening or displacing the prosthesis.
    Avoid crossing the legs or ankles while standing, sitting, or lying.
    Sit with the feet 6 inches apart.
    When sitting, keep the knees below the hips; sit on a pillow to keep the hips higher.
    Avoid bending over at the waist. Use a long-handled shoehorn and sock aid to assist in putting on shoes and socks.
    Do not drive for approximately 3 months or until approved by physician.
  —Discuss safety precautions to be taken at home.
    Use handrails on stairs.
    Wear low-heeled shoes.
    Be sure floors are free of objects that could cause falls, such as throw rugs, electrical cords, and clutter. Avoid wet or waxed floors.
- *Diet*
  —Encourage a diet high in protein, fiber, and vitamins to promote healing and prevent constipation.

FOLLOW-UP CARE

- Stress the importance of regular follow-up visits with the physician and physical therapist until recovery is complete. Make sure the patient has the necessary names and telephone numbers.

REFERRALS

- Assess the need for and provide referrals for home health care services, a skilled nursing facility, and a medical social worker as indicated.

Hodgkin's Disease
(Hodgkin's Lymphoma)

—Hodgkin's disease: a malignant disorder characterized by painless, progressive enlargement of the lymph node, lymphoid tissue, and spleen. Hodgkin's lymphoma is distinguished from malignant lymphomas by the presence of Reed-Sternberg cells, which proliferate and invade normal lymph tissue throughout the body. Hodgkin's disease occurs more frequently in young adults (15 to 38 years) and in men. If diagnosed in stage I or II, the disease is potentially curable.

RISK FACTORS

- Male, white
- History of infectious mononucleosis or immunodeficiency syndrome

STAGING

- Stage I: single lymph node region
- Stage II: two or more nodes limited to one side of the diaphragm
- Stage III: disease on both sides of the diaphragm, but limited to the lymph nodes and spleen
- Stage IV: involvement of the bones, bone marrow, lung parenchyma, pleura, liver, skin, gastrointestinal tract, central nervous system, etc.

All stages are classified as A or B to describe the absence (A) or presence (B) of systemic symptoms.

SIGNS/SYMPTOMS

- Painless, swollen lymph nodes (lymphadenopathy): usually cervical or supraclavicular (early sign)
- Fever, night sweats, weight loss, lethargy, malaise, anorexia, jaundice
- Edema or pain distal to swollen lymph nodes
- Splenomegaly
- Hepatomegaly

COMPLICATIONS

- Cervical node enlargement: venous occlusion, neck edema, airway obstruction
- Mediastinal node enlargement: dyspnea, cough
- Inguinal node enlargement: dysuria, frequency, painful urination, low back pain
- Infection
- Fractures
- Superior vena cava syndrome

DIAGNOSTIC TESTS

- Describe each procedure, its purpose, and the normal feelings or sensations that are likely, as well as any preprocedural and postprocedural care.
  - —Staging procedure
    - Lymph node biopsy: to detect presence of Reed-Sternberg cells
    - Chest x-ray: to detect mediastinal or hilar lymphadenopathy
    - Bone marrow biopsy
    - Computed tomography scans: liver, spleen, and bone
    - Laparotomy
    - Lymphangiography
  - —Laboratory tests
    - Test for normocytic normochromic anemia
    - White blood cell count with differential
    - Alkaline phosphatase: increase indicates bone involvement

TREATMENT
Medical

- Therapy
  —Chemotherapy in combination with radiation therapy for stages III and IV
  —Radiation therapy (stages I to III)
- Drugs
  —Interferon, monoclonal antibodies: research on effectiveness being conducted

Surgical

- Laparotomy
- Splenectomy
- Autologous bone marrow transplantation: research on effectiveness being conducted

HOME CARE

- Give both the patient and the caregiver *verbal* and *written* instructions. Provide them with the name and telephone number of a physician or nurse to call if questions arise.
- *General information*
  —Explain and discuss Hodgkin's disease/lymphoma, its causes, and contributing factors.
  —Discuss staging of the disease and the impact that various stages may have on daily living.
- *Warning signs*
  —Review the signs and symptoms that should be reported to a physician or nurse.
      Persistent fever
      Weight loss
      Enlarged lymph nodes
      Malaise
      Decreased exercise tolerance
      Infection: cough, foul-smelling sputum, pain and burning with urination, frequency, urgency, hematuria, redness, swelling at wound site, drainage (foul smelling, containing pus, discolored)
- *Special instructions*
  —Discuss the importance of avoiding large crowds and persons suspected to have an active infection because chemotherapy decreases resistance to infection.

—Stress the importance of avoiding trauma, which can cause bruising and bleeding. Thrombocytopenia commonly results from chemotherapy.

—Discuss skin care measures to decrease itching.

- *Medications*
  —Explain the purpose, dosage, schedule, and route of administration of any prescribed drugs, as well as side effects to report to the physician or nurse.
  —Explain the importance of following the chemotherapy regimen and reporting the side effects of therapy to the physician or nurse: sores in mouth or on tongue, anorexia, nausea, vomiting, malaise.

- *Activity*
  —Encourage the patient to discuss allowances and limitations with respect to occupation, recreation, or activities.
  —Discuss the need for planned rest periods. Stress the importance of avoiding overexertion. Teach stress reduction techniques.

- *Diet*
  —Stress the importance of a balanced diet to maintain nutrition.
  —Encourage small, frequent meals and oral fluids.
  —Discuss methods to maintain hydration, nutrition during periods of stomatitis, nausea, vomiting, anorexia associated with therapy: sip fluids all day, drink nectar juices, avoid spicy, hot, and citrus foods.

PSYCHOSOCIAL CARE

- Encourage verbalization and questions regarding disease and treatment options and prognosis.
- Encourage use of support services and counseling as needed.

FOLLOW-UP CARE

- Stress the importance of regular follow-up visits. Make sure the patient has the necessary names and telephone numbers.
- Emphasize the importance of planning radiation therapy and chemotherapy sessions and keeping appointments.

REFERRALS

- Refer the patient to the American Cancer Society, the Lymphoma Research Foundation, and local support groups as indicated.

Hyperparathyroidism

—Hyperparathyroidism: overactivity of one or more of the parathyroid glands. Excessive secretion of parathyroid hormone causes an increase of calcium that cannot be controlled by renal excretion or uptake in soft tissue or bones. Hyperparathyroidism is common in postmenopausal women and is classified as a primary or secondary disorder.

CAUSES/CONTRIBUTING FACTORS

- Primary hyperparathyroidism
  —Parathyroid adenoma
  —Cell hyperplasia
- Secondary hyperparathyroidism
  —Rickets
  —Chronic renal failure
  —Osteomalacia
  —Excessive intake of drugs: thiazide diuretics, calcium supplements

SIGNS/SYMPTOMS

- Polyuria, polydipsia, kidney stones
- Abdominal pain, constipation, nausea, anorexia
- Fractures of ribs, spine
- Joint or back pain
- Depression, paranoia, mood swings
- Muscular weakness and atrophy

COMPLICATIONS

- Cardiac arrhythmias, cardiac failure
- Gastric ulcers
- Skeletal problems
  —Pathologic fractures
- Renal disorder
  —Kidney stones
  —Urinary tract infection
  —Renal failure
- Pancreatitis
- Stupor/coma

DIAGNOSTIC TESTS

- Describe each procedure, its purpose, and the normal feelings or sensations that are likely, as well as any preprocedural and postprocedural care.
  - —Laboratory tests
    - Total serum calcium: greater than 11 mg/dl
    - Ionized calcium: increased
    - Parathyroid hormone: increased
    - Intact parathyroid hormone

TREATMENT
Medical

- Therapy
  - —Hydration: 2 to 3 liters/day
  - —Low-calcium diet
- Drugs
  - —Loop diuretics: to lower serum calcium levels
  - —Phosphates, calcitonin, mithramycin: to inhibit bone reabsorption

Surgical

- Parathyroidectomy

HOME CARE

- Give both the patient and the caregiver *verbal* and *written* instructions. Provide them with the name and telephone number of a physician or nurse to call if questions arise.
- *General information*
  - —Explain hyperparathyroid disease, including specific causes, contributing factors, and recurrence of symptoms of hypercalcemia.
- *Warning signs*
  - —Review the signs and symptoms that should be reported to a physician or nurse.
    - Gastric problems: nausea, vomiting, abdominal pain
    - Musculoskeletal problems: tetany, bone tenderness, pain
    - Renal problems: decreased urine output, hematuria, dysuria, flank pain, kidney stones
- *Special instructions*
  - —Advise the patient on the use of assistive devices (walker, cane) for ambulation as necessary.

—Discuss pain management as indicated.

   Teach the patient to rate pain on a scale and to describe pain so as to better monitor pain and analgesic effectiveness.

   Encourage the patient to take pain medication on schedule rather than as needed.

   Assist the patient in developing a plan for using alternative pain-relieving methods rather than relying on pain medication.

- *Medications*
  —Explain the purpose, dosage, schedule, and route of administration of any prescribed drugs, as well as side effects to report to the physician or nurse.
  —Explain the need to avoid over-the-counter drugs that contain calcium, such as antacids.
  —Advise the patient to avoid using enemas or laxatives.
- *Activity*
  —Encourage the patient to discuss allowances and limitations with respect to occupation, recreation, or activities.
  —Discuss the importance of proper body alignment and mechanics and the need to increase activity gradually according to personal tolerance. If the patient has had pathologic fractures, advise the caretaker to assist with transferring from bed to chair and ambulation.
  —Discuss safety measures to prevent accidents and injuries.
  —Tell the patient to splint the ribs while coughing and turning to decrease pain and prevent further injury (pathologic fracture).
  —Instruct the patient to monitor urine output and strain urine for kidney stones as indicated (see Urolithiasis, p. 630).
- *Diet*
  —Explain the importance of maintaining adequate fluid intake (3000 ml/day) to reduce serum calcium unless contraindicated.
  —Provide instruction on a low-calcium, low–vitamin D, high-fiber diet.

FOLLOW-UP CARE

- Stress the importance of regular follow-up visits. Make sure the patient has the necessary names and telephone numbers.

Hypertension

—Hypertension: blood pressure higher than 140/90 mm Hg (based on two or more readings at two or more visits). Blood pressure is the force that the heart muscle exerts as it pumps against the blood vessels. Optimal blood pressure is 120/80; normal blood pressure is 130/85 mm Hg. Borderline blood pressure is 130 to 139/85 to 89 mm Hg. Primary or essential hypertension is the most common form of hypertension, accounting for 90% of all cases. The cause is unknown, but certain risk factors are known to contribute to its presence. Secondary hypertension is high blood pressure related to some underlying disease such as renal disease, endocrine disease, or central nervous system disorders.

RISK FACTORS

- Family history
- Age group: persons older than age 50
- African-Americans have a higher incidence
- Obesity
- Stress
- Tobacco use: cigarettes, chewing tobacco
- Diet high in salt and saturated fats

SIGNS/SYMPTOMS

- Dizziness
- Fatigue
- Vertigo
- Palpitations
- Throbbing headache
- Nosebleed

COMPLICATIONS

- Malignant hypertension
- Stroke
- Myocardial infarction
- Kidney failure
- Heart failure
- Retinopathy

DIAGNOSTIC TESTS

- Describe each procedure, its purpose, and the normal feelings or sensations that are likely, as well as any preprocedural and postprocedural care.
  —Serial blood pressure measurements
  —Physical examination
  —Laboratory tests
  —Blood tests: potassium, blood urea nitrogen, and creatinine to assess kidney function
  —Urine tests: to assess kidney function for hypertension
  —Electrocardiogram
  —Chest x-ray
  —Intravenous pyelography: to detect kidney disease

TREATMENT
Medical

- Therapy
  —Low–saturated fat, low-salt diet; low-calorie diet for weight reduction
- Lifestyle modifications
  —Regular exercise
  —No smoking/tobacco use
  —Diet
  —Weight reduction
- Drugs
  —Diuretics
  —Beta blockers
  —Calcium channel blockers
  —Angiotensin-converting enzyme inhibitors
  —Angiotensin II receptor blockers
  —Antihypertensive agents such as alpha blockers

HOME CARE

- Give both the patient and the caregiver *verbal* and *written* instructions. Provide them with the name and telephone number of a physician or nurse to call if questions arise.
- *General information*
  —Explain the disease process, contributing factors, and complications. Assist the patient to identify individual risk factors.

—Explain what blood pressure is, its components, systolic and diastolic pressure, and interpretation of a blood pressure reading. Provide blood pressure values to achieve.

- *Warning signs*
  —Review the signs and symptoms that should be reported to a physician or nurse.
  > Headache (morning occipital)
  > Dizziness
  > Fatigue
  > Epistaxis (bloody nose)
  > Palpitations

- *Special instructions*
  —Explain that the goal of treating hypertension is one of lifestyle modification that includes diet, exercise, stress management, blood pressure self-monitoring, and regular medical follow-up.
  —Teach the patient how and when to take blood pressure measurements using home monitoring equipment if available. Instruct the patient to take blood pressure at the same time each day, to keep a record of blood pressure readings, noting any changes in diet or activities that might contribute to changes in pressure, and to report elevated blood pressure to the physician or nurse. Provide time for a return demonstration.
  —Discuss the importance of avoiding all tobacco products. Explain that nicotine increases the heart rate and constricts blood vessels, which can cause blood pressure to rise.
  —Discuss the need to prevent obesity. Explain that a 10- or 20-pound weight reduction may reduce blood pressure if the patient is overweight.

- *Medications*
  —Explain the purpose, dosage, schedule, and route of administration of any prescribed drugs, as well as side effects to report to the physician or nurse.
  —Emphasize the importance of taking medications on time and reporting side effects.
  —Instruct the patient not to stop taking medications if side effects occur without notifying the physician or even if blood pressure normalizes.

- *Activity*
  —Encourage the patient to discuss allowances and limitations with respect to occupation, recreation, or activities. Explain that isometric exercise, walking, jogging, swimming, bicycling, and aerobic exercise are permissible but weight lifting or any sport requiring muscle contractions should be avoided because they increase the work of the heart and raise blood pressure.
  —Discuss the benefits of regular exercise: eases the work of the heart, reduces stress, strengthens the heart muscle, helps to reduce or control weight, and reduces cholesterol levels. Explain that after aerobic exercise systolic pressure can be reduced 25% and that over time a regular aerobic exercise program can permanently lower at-rest diastolic pressure.
  —Caution the patient to rise slowly from a sitting position or to get out of bed slowly to prevent dizziness.
- *Diet*
  —Explain that salt causes fluid retention, which increases the pressure in the blood vessels. Tell the patient to avoid foods high in sodium (e.g., fast foods, canned goods), to read food labels for sodium content, and not to add salt to food while cooking or at the table.
  —Discuss the need to reduce or avoid foods high in saturated fats, such as butter, cream, foods high in animal fat (red meat, bacon, organ meats).
  —Refer the patient to the dietitian to assist in diet planning.
  —Explain the need to limit alcohol intake because alcohol raises blood pressure.

PSYCHOSOCIAL CARE

- Discuss how stress contributes to hypertension. Assist the patient to identify stress-producing factors. Discuss methods of stress management: relaxation techniques, guided imagery, biofeedback.
- Inform male patients that certain drugs may cause sexual dysfunction and to report such problems.

FOLLOW-UP CARE

- Stress the importance of regular follow-up visits. Make sure the patient has the necessary names and telephone numbers.

REFERRALS

- Provide the patient with a list of hospital- or community-based support services for behavior modification.
- Provide referral to home care services as indicated.
- Give the patient literature on managing hypertension. Refer the patient to the American Heart Association for further information.

H

Hyperthyroidism
(Graves' Disease)

—Hyperthyroidism: a clinical syndrome that causes tissues to be exposed to overproduction of thyroid hormones. The excessive production of thyroid hormones produces a state of hypermetabolism that is responsible for the symptoms. There are several varieties of hyperthyroidism, ranging in seriousness from mild to severe. Graves' disease (toxic diffuse goiter), the most common form, is more frequently seen in women than men during the third and fourth decades. The exact cause of Graves' disease is unknown, but it is believed to be an autoimmune disorder resulting from thyroid-stimulating immunoglobulins. Thyrotoxic crisis, or thyroid storm, is an acute manifestation of hyperthyroidism that is life threatening. Precipitating factors include stressful events such as surgery, trauma, and infection.

SIGNS/SYMPTOMS

- Lid retraction and lag
- Proptosis
- Conjunctival irritation; lacrimation
- Characteristic bright-eyed, frightened, or startled look
- Increased systolic blood pressure, widening pulse pressure
- Increased body temperature and sweating
- Tachycardia
- Palpitations
- Weight loss

- Increased appetite
- Diarrhea
- Generalized muscle wasting and weakness
- Hyperactive deep tendon reflexes
- Tremors
- Restlessness, irritability
- Decreased concentration, memory
- Insomnia
- Labile emotions and manic behavior

COMPLICATIONS

- Thyroid storm
  —Extreme restlessness
  —Confusion, delirium, disorientation
  —Stupor, coma
  —Marked tachycardia
  —Vomiting
- Dysrhythmias
- Pulmonary edema
- Shock

DIAGNOSTIC TESTS

- Describe each procedure, its purpose, and the normal feelings or sensations that are likely, as well as any preprocedural and postprocedural care.
  —Laboratory tests
    Serum thyroxine (T_4) and triiodothyronine (T_3) and serum-free T_4 and T_3: all increased
    Thyroid radioiodine uptake and scan: uptake increased in most patients with hyperthyroidism
    Thyroid-stimulating hormone: suppressed and does not respond to thyrotropin-releasing hormone
    Thyroid-stimulating immunoglobulins: present in Graves' disease

TREATMENT
Medical

- Drugs
  —Thioamides: to inhibit thyroid hormone synthesis
    Propylthiouracil
    Methimazole (Tapazole)
    Oral cholecystographic agents (Ipodate)

—Beta-adrenergic blockers: to control symptoms of hyper-thyroidism
—Iodides: to promote short-term inhibition of thyroid hormone synthesis
   Potassium or sodium iodide (SSKI, Lugol's solution)
—Radioactive iodine (^{131}I-NaI or ^{125}I-NaI): to destroy thyroid tissue
—Glucocorticoids: to inhibit thyroid hormone secretion

Surgical

• Thyroidectomy

Graves' Disease Ophthalmopathy
Medical

• Therapy
   —Irradiation of the orbit
   —0.5% Methylcellulose eyedrops for eye irritation and pain
• Drugs
   —Corticosteroids

Surgical

• Orbital decompression
• Correction of muscle imbalance

Graves' Disease Dermopathy
Medical

• Drugs
   —0.2% Fluocinolone or other corticosteroid cream for palliative treatment of extensive bulbous or ulcerated lesions

HOME CARE

• Give both the patient and the caregiver *verbal* and *written* instructions. Provide them with the name and telephone number of a physician or nurse to call if questions arise.
• Prepare the patient for thyroidectomy as ordered (see p. 613).
• *General information*
   —Explain hyperthyroidism and the effects of excessive thyroid hormones on body tissues. Review cause or contributing factors and prescribed treatments.
   —Explain thyroid storm, discussing precipitating factors, symptoms, and measures to take if a crisis is suspected.

- *Warning signs*
  —Review the signs and recurrent symptoms of hyperthyroidism (see p. 371) that should be reported to a physician or nurse. Explain that many symptoms (e.g., nervousness) will decrease if treatment is followed.
- *Special instructions*
  —Discuss measures to manage ophthalmopathy or exophthalmos.
    Tell the patient to protect eyes from bright lights, corneal ulcerations, and infections and to wear sunglasses or eye patches.
    Advise the patient to apply cool compresses to the eyes if irritated.
    Suggest that the patient apply lubricants as ordered to protect the cornea.
    Tell the patient to notify the physician or nurse of increased visual disturbances.
- *Medications*
  —Explain the purpose, dosage, schedule, and route of administration of any prescribed drugs, as well as side effects to report to the physician or nurse.
    Propylthiouracil: take medications with meals to avoid gastrointestinal distress
    Radioactive ^{131}I: review signs and symptoms of hypothyroidism; discuss the need to avoid contact with pregnant women, infants, and children for 1 week after treatment
  —Stress the importance of not using over-the-counter medications without checking with the physician or nurse.
  —Tell the patient to check all medication labels to see whether iodine is included.
- *Activity*
  —Encourage the patient to discuss allowances and limitations with respect to occupation, recreation, or activities.
  —Discuss with the patient the importance of planned rest and avoidance of excessive exercise.
  —Discuss measures to improve sleep patterns: avoid stimulants (diet, activities) before sleep, do not sleep during normal waking hours, develop regular sleep patterns.
- *Diet*
  —Discuss with the patient the need for a high-calorie, high-protein, high-carbohydrate diet until the patient's weight is stable.

PSYCHOSOCIAL CARE

- Explain that emotional outbursts are part of the disease process. Maintain a nonstimulating environment by controlling extraneous noise.

FOLLOW-UP CARE

- Stress the importance of regular follow-up visits. Make sure the patient has the necessary names and telephone numbers.
- Instruct the patient to inform all health care providers about the medical condition.
- Discuss the need to wear a MedicAlert bracelet.
- Inform a woman patient to notify the physician if menstrual irregularities occur or pregnancy is suspected. Advise pregnancy planning and provide contraceptive information.

H

Hypertrophic Cardiomyopathy

—Hypertrophic cardiomyopathy: a heart muscle disorder resulting in impaired pumping of the heart. Other terms include idiopathic hypertrophic subaortic stenosis, asymmetric septal hypertrophy, and hypertrophic obstructive cardiomyopathy. A primary disease of the heart muscle, hypertrophic cardiomyopathy is characterized by thickening of the interventricular septum, hypertrophy of the left ventricle, and small ventricular cavities. The increase in muscle tissue can also affect the mitral valve. In hypertrophic cardiomyopathy, output may be low, normal, or high. Low heart output may lead to fatal heart failure.

CAUSES

- Autosomal dominant trait resulting in abnormal heart structure
- Abnormal myocardial calcium kinetics

SIGNS/SYMPTOMS

- Dyspnea
- Orthopnea
- Chest pain

- Palpitations
- Syncope
- Lightheadedness/dizziness

COMPLICATIONS

- Left ventricular failure
- Sudden death
- Arrhythmias: atrial and ventricular
- Endocarditis

DIAGNOSTIC TESTS

- Inform the patient that several diagnostic procedures may be done to aid in diagnosis of the condition. Describe each procedure, its purpose, and the normal feelings or sensations that are likely, as well as any preprocedural and postprocedural care.
    —Chest x-ray: to determine heart size and detect signs of pulmonary congestion
    —Electrocardiogram: to detect ventricular dysrhythmias and heart enlargement
    —Echocardiogram: to detect thickening of the septum, abnormal motion of the aortic and mitral valves, and ventricular outflow
    —Holter monitor to detect dysrhythmias
    —Radionuclide studies (thallium and technetium): to detect heart muscle thickening and the amount of blood the left ventricle may hold
    —Cardiac catheterization and angiography: to detect abnormal ventricular pressures and mitral insufficiency
    —Biopsy: to determine the structure of the heart muscle

TREATMENT
Medical

- Therapy
    —Cardioversion for atrial fibrillation
- Drugs
    —Beta blockers: to reduce the work of the heart by reducing the amount of adrenaline that reaches the heart muscle; to slow the heart rate and relax the heart muscle
    —Digitalis: indicated only in the presence of atrial fibrillation to strengthen and regulate the heart rhythm

—Calcium channel blockers: to relax the arteries and thus reduce the amount of force the heart needs to pump against these arteries

—Anticoagulants in the presence of atrial fibrillation

Surgical

- Ventricular myotomy: resection of the hypertrophic septum with mitral valve replacement

▦ HOME CARE

- Give both the patient and the caregiver *verbal* and *written* instructions. Provide them with the name and telephone number of a physician or nurse to call if questions arise.
- *General information*
  —Describe the nature of hypertrophic cardiomyopathy, explaining the limitation of the disease on lifestyle and the prognosis.
  —Discuss with the patient the possibility of screening family members.
- *Warning signs*
  —Review the signs and recurrent symptoms that should be reported to a physician or nurse.
    Dyspnea
    Unusual fatigue
    Angina
- *Special instructions*
  —Explain the need to record daily weight to detect fluid retention. Tell the patient to report a sudden weight gain of 2 to 3 pounds in 1 day or 5 pounds in 1 week.
- *Medications*
  —Explain the purpose, dosage, schedule, and route of administration of any prescribed drugs, as well as side effects to report to the physician or nurse.
  —Caution the patient not to discontinue the use of beta blockers without notifying the physician. Abrupt discontinuation of a beta blocker may result in heart attack or sudden death.
  —Instruct the patient that prophylactic antibiotics will be needed before dental and surgical procedures to reduce the risk of endocarditis.

- *Activity*
  —Stress the importance of avoiding isometric exercises and strenuous activities (e.g., competitive sports such as football and soccer, jogging, and weight lifting). Advise the patient to rest when tired and after heavy tasks.
  —Encourage discussion and questions regarding occupation, recreation, and activities.
- *Diet*
  —Discuss with the patient the need for a low-salt diet.
  —Stress the importance of avoiding alcohol.

FOLLOW-UP CARE AND REFERRALS

- Stress the importance of regular follow-up visits. Make sure the patient has the necessary names and telephone numbers.
- Encourage the caregiver to learn cardiopulmonary resuscitation because of the risk of sudden cardiac death. Assist with referral to hospital or community resources.

Hypoparathyroidism

—Hypoparathyroidism: a deficiency of parathyroid hormone. Parathyroid hormone is necessary to maintain normal levels of serum calcium. A rare condition, hypoparathyroid disease may occur as the result of removal of or damage to the parathyroid glands (e.g., radiation or treatment with iodine-131).

SIGNS/SYMPTOMS

- Personality disturbances: anxiety, depression, irritability
- Paresthesias, tetany, hyperreflexia
- Nausea, vomiting, diarrhea, abdominal pain
- Dry scaly skin, brittle nails, thin patchy hair

COMPLICATIONS

- Cardiac arrhythmias
- Seizures
- Cardiac arrest

DIAGNOSTIC TESTS

- Describe each procedure, its purpose, and the normal feelings or sensations that are likely, as well as any preprocedural and postprocedural care.
  —Serum tests
      Calcium: decreased
      Parathyroid hormone: decreased or absent
      Bicarbonate: decreased
      Phosphate: increased
  —Urine tests
      Calcium: decreased
      Phosphate: decreased

TREATMENT
Medical

- Therapy
  —Dietary calcium supplement
- Drugs
  —Vitamins
  —Calcium replacement
  —Phosphate binders

HOME CARE

- Give both the patient and the caregiver *verbal* and *written* instructions. Provide them with the name and telephone number of a physician or nurse to call if questions arise.
- *General information*
  —Explain and discuss hypoparathyroidism, its specific causes, and contributing factors.
- *Warning signs*
  —Review the signs that should be reported to a physician or nurse.
      Hypocalcemia: tingling, emotional irritability, muscle stiffness, fatigue, palpitations, nausea and vomiting, abdominal pain
      Acute hypoparathyroidism: tetany (painful muscle spasms), irritability, tingling of fingers and around mouth
      Seizure activity: tremors, loss of consciousness, involuntary muscular contractions

- *Special instructions*
  —Discuss the actions to take for seizure activity.
    Stay with the person.
    Avoid restraining or interrupting the behavior.
    Protect the head and clear surrounding areas.
    After the seizure, turn the head to the side to avoid aspiration.
    Record the activity, including the length of the seizure.
    Call the physician immediately.
- *Medications*
  —Explain the purpose, dosage, schedule, and route of administration of any prescribed drugs, as well as side effects to report to the physician or nurse.
  —Stress the importance of the continued need for calcium and vitamin D supplements and the reasons for the treatment.
  —Instruct the patient to take calcium replacement medications on time to enhance the dietary intake of calcium.
- *Activity*
  —Discuss the need to exercise to tolerance, to alternate exercise with periods of rest, and to report increasing muscle weakness and fatigue.
  —Encourage the patient to discuss allowances and limitations with respect to occupation, recreation, and activities.
  —Discuss the potential for falls resulting from difficulty maintaining balance during the acute period. Inform the patient of the need for a safe home environment, and aid the patient in obtaining assistive devices or help in moving about as indicated.
- *Diet*
  —Encourage a high-calcium, high–vitamin D, low-phosphorus diet.
  —Discuss with the patient the need to maintain fluid balance, especially when nausea, vomiting, and diarrhea are present.

PSYCHOSOCIAL CARE

- Discuss with the patient and caregiver the need to decrease stressors.
- Discuss with the caregivers the symptoms of changes in mood or thought process that may require medical interventions.

FOLLOW-UP CARE

- Stress the importance of regular follow-up visits. Make sure the patient has the necessary names and telephone numbers.

Hypothyroidism
(Myxedema)

H

—Hypothyroidism: the clinical sydrome caused by a deficiency in thyroid hormones. Hypothyroidism occurs most often in women between the ages of 30 and 60 years. Myxedema coma is a severe form of hypothyroidism that is often fatal. Precipitating factors include withdrawal of thyroid medication, severe stress, or infection. Chronic autoimmune thyroiditis (idiopathic hypothyroidism, Hashimoto's disease), the most common form of hypothyroidism, is generally believed to be an autoimmune disorder. Transient autoimmune thyroiditis is a pregnancy-related form that occurs 3 to 6 months postpartum. Hypothyroidism may also follow radioiodine therapy, external neck radiation therapy, or postoperative thyroidectomy.

SIGNS/SYMPTOMS

- Decreased body temperature
- Dry, rough, scaly skin
- Puffy face, hands, and feet; periorbital edema
- Decreased blood pressure
- Bradycardia
- Decreased exercise tolerance
- Weight gain, constipation
- Anorexia
- Abdominal distention, myxedema ileus
- Nonspecific fatigue, weakness
- Delayed deep tendon reflexes
- Muscle aches and joint stiffness
- Intolerance to cold
- Slowed, slurred, monotonous speech

- Somnolence, lethargy
- Impaired memory, inattentiveness, slow cognition
- Loss of initiative
- Paranoia, depression, agitation
- Decreased libido

COMPLICATIONS

- Myxedema coma
  —Hypothermia
  —Depressed respirations
  —Stupor advancing to coma
  —Cardiovascular collapse
  —Metabolic imbalances
- Ischemic heart disease: angina, myocardial infarction
- Heart failure
- Dysrhythmias
- Intestinal obstruction
- Anemia

DIAGNOSTIC TESTS

- Describe each procedure, its purpose, and the normal feelings or sensations that are likely, as well as any preprocedural and postprocedural care.
  —Serum T_4 and T_3 and serum-free T_4 and T_3: decreased
  —Serum thyroid-stimulating hormone levels: increased
  —Radioiodide uptake test: below normal uptake

TREATMENT
Medical

- Therapy
  —Intravenous albumin and fluids
- Drugs
  —Synthetic thyroid hormones
    Levothyroxine sodium (Cytolen, Levoid, Levothroid, Synthroid sodium)
    Liothyronine sodium (Cytomel, Cytomine)
    Lotrix (Euthroid, Thyrolar)
  —Diagnostic agents
    Thyroid-stimulating hormone (Thytropar)
    Protirelin (thyrotropin-releasing hormone) (Relefact TRH, Thypinone)

🏠 **HOME CARE**

- Give both the patient and the caregiver *verbal* and *written* instructions. Provide them with the name and telephone number of a physician or nurse to call if questions arise.
- *General information*
  —Explain hypothyroidism, including the effects of deficient thyroid hormones on body tissues and personality. Review causes and contributing factors, and tell the patient that the symptoms will subside with treatment.
  —Explain myxedema coma, the precipitating factors, and emergency measures to take if they are suspected.
- *Warning signs*
  —Review the signs and symptoms that should be reported to a physician or nurse.

  > Hypothyroidism: puffy, masklike face; periorbital edema
  > Myxedema coma: decreased exercise tolerance, lightheadedness, slowing pulse, difficulty breathing, decreasing temperature
  > Pulmonary infection: temperature above normal for patient; cold or flu symptoms
  > Urinary infection: burning, urgency, and frequent urination
- *Special instructions*
  —Explain the importance of avoiding infections.
- *Medications*
  —Explain the purpose, dosage, schedule, and route of administration of any prescribed drugs, as well as side effects to report to the physician or nurse.
  —Stress the importance of not discontinuing thyroid medication because the medication is essential for life and treatment is lifelong.
- *Activity*
  —Encourage the patient to discuss allowances and limitations with respect to occupation, recreation, and activities.
  —Discuss the importance of getting adequate periods of rest and of alternating periods of exercise with rest.
  —Advise avoiding extremely cold temperature until the condition is stabilized.
- *Diet*
  —Discuss with the patient the need for a high-fiber, low-calorie diet and adequate fluid intake to prevent constipation and promote weight loss.

H

PSYCHOSOCIAL CARE

- Discuss personality changes, explaining that slowness and lethargy will recede once treatment is started. Refer the patient to counseling as indicated.

FOLLOW-UP CARE AND REFERRALS

- Stress the importance of regular follow-up visits. Make sure the patient has the necessary names and telephone numbers.
- Advise the patient to inform all physicians (e.g., gynecologist, urologist) of the disease process.
- Discuss the need to wear a MedicAlert bracelet.

Hysterectomy, Radical

—Hysterectomy, radical: surgical removal of the ovaries, tubes, uterus with the cervix, and parametrial tissue, along with lymph node dissection. The ovarian tissue is often preserved in premenopausal patients. Because of the extensiveness of the procedure, an abdominal approach is required.

INDICATIONS

- Chronic endometriosis
- Malignant neoplastic disease
- Leiomyomas

PREPROCEDURAL TEACHING

- See Abdominal Surgery (p. 6) for general preoperative and postoperative instructions.
- Review the physician's explanation of the procedure and the reason for it; encourage the patient to ask questions and to discuss any fears or anxieties. Discuss the need for informed consent.

Review of Postprocedural Care

- Explain that after surgery the patient will be maintained in a supine or low Fowler's position to prevent pelvic congestion.
- Discuss perineal care: sitz baths, heat lamps, ice packs.

- Inform the patient that an indwelling urinary catheter or suprapubic tube is required to avoid urinary retention.
- Explain that a nasogastric tube or rectal tube may be inserted to prevent abdominal distention.
- Explain that abdominal cramping with a moderate amount of drainage is expected and that the patient will have a perineal pad in place.

SIDE EFFECTS/COMPLICATIONS

- Wound infection, dehiscence
- Hemorrhage
- Urinary retention
- Urinary tract infection
- Paralytic ileus
- Pneumonia
- Thrombophlebitis
- Constipation
- Pulmonary embolus
- Ureteral fistula, ureteral ligation

HOME CARE

- Give both the patient and the caregiver *verbal* and *written* instructions. Provide them with the name and telephone number of a physician or nurse to call if questions arise.
- *General information*
  —Reinforce the physician's information about hysterectomy and correct any misconceptions. Common misconceptions about hysterectomy are that afterward a woman grows fat and flabby, develops facial hair, becomes wrinkled, old, and masculine, loses her mind, or becomes depressed and nervous. Normal concerns that should be discussed include fear of death, disfigurement, cancer, and loss of femininity and childbearing ability; pain; and changes in sexuality. Encourage the patient to verbalize her concerns with significant others.
- *Wound/incision care*
  —Instruct the patient to care for the incision with general cleanliness and daily bathing.
- *Warning signs*
  —Review the signs and symptoms that should be reported to a physician or nurse.

Elevated temperature (>100° F [37.8° C])
Incisional swelling
Redness
Purulent drainage
Foul odor
Vaginal bleeding (more than slightly bloody drainage)
Abdominal pain
Change in bowel habits
Difficulty in urinating

- *Special instructions*
  —Tell the patient to avoid constipation by taking mild laxatives and stool softeners as necessary. Demonstrate care of the suprapubic catheter (see Urinary Catheter, p. 736) if the patient is discharged with one in place. Teach clean, intermittent self-catheterization as indicated.
  —Explain that no intercourse, tampons, douching, or tub baths are allowed for 4 to 6 weeks or until permitted by the physician.
  —Explain that menstruation will no longer occur.
- *Medications*
  —Explain the purpose, dosage, schedule, and route of administration of any prescribed drugs, as well as side effects to report to a physician or nurse.
    Estrogen replacement therapy if ordered
    Analgesic
- *Activity*
  —Advise the patient of the importance of exercise and activity to tolerance.
  —Tell the patient to avoid fatigue and plan regular rest periods.
  —Explain that jarring activities, driving, and heavy lifting (>10 pounds) should be avoided for 4 to 6 weeks or as indicated by a physician.
  —Advise the patient to avoid activities that increase pelvic congestion (e.g., dancing, horseback riding, sitting for long periods) until allowed to resume them by a physician.

PSYCHOSOCIAL CARE

- Explore the patient's fears and anxieties regarding changes in body image and sexuality: loss of uterus, fertility, femininity, or sexual functioning. Inform the patient that counseling for a sexually active woman and her partner is available and that she should discuss options with her physician or nurse.

FOLLOW-UP CARE AND REFERRALS

- Stress the importance of regular follow-up gynecologic appointments. Make sure the patient has the necessary names and telephone numbers.
- Provide referrals to support services, such as the Hysterectomy Educational Resources and Services Foundation (HERS).

Implantable Cardioverter Defibrillator

—Implantable cardioverter defibrillator: a self-contained device that monitors heart activity and treats ventricular tachycardia and ventricular fibrillation. The implantable cardioverter defibrillator delivers electrical countershocks or rapid pacing in the presence of ventricular tachycardia or fibrillation via electrodes that are surgically implanted into the heart.

INDICATIONS

- Patients who have survived sudden cardiac death not associated with acute myocardial infarction
- Uncontrollable dysrhythmias
- History of multiple cardiac arrests
- Sustained ventricular tachycardia uncontrolled with antidysrhythmia medications

PREPROCEDURAL TEACHING

- Review the physician's explanation of the procedure and the reason for it; encourage the patient to ask questions and to discuss any fears or anxieties. Discuss the need for informed consent.

Review of Preprocedural Care

- Review the implantation procedure, the type of device, and the recommended surgical approach: thoracotomy, sternotomy, subxiphoid, subcostal, or transvenous.
- Instruct the patient about the need to have nothing by mouth (NPO) after midnight before the procedure.

- Review preprocedural tests: electrocardiogram, electrophysiologic study, and laboratory work, including blood type and crossmatch.
- Explain skin preparation of the chest and abdomen.

Review of Postprocedural Care

- Discuss the use of the electrocardiogram and hemodynamic monitoring after the procedure.
- Discuss fear and anxiety about the device, discharges, possible malfunction, and underlying condition.

SIDE EFFECTS/COMPLICATIONS

- Pneumothorax (collapsed lung)
- Bleeding
- Lead dislodgment
- Infection
- Atelectasis
- Pericarditis
- Malfunction of device

HOME CARE

- Give both the patient and the caregiver *verbal* and *written* instructions. Provide them with the name and telephone number of a physician or nurse to call if questions arise. Use visual aids to assist in instruction.
- *General information*
  —Review any explanation about the procedure and device and any specific follow-up care.
- *Warning signs*
  —Review the signs and symptoms that should be reported to a physician or nurse.
   Infection (incision): redness, swelling, fluid, or purulent drainage, skin irritation, tenderness, warmth, fever
   More than one shock felt in 24 hours
   Symptoms associated with rhythm disturbances: dizziness, palpitations, loss of consciousness
- *Special instructions*
  —Review the procedure to follow when the device discharges inappropriately.
   Note symptoms and call the physician.

If multiple discharges are given or the patient loses consciousness, call the physician, call the emergency number (911), or bring the patient to the emergency room.

—Describe the sensations and feelings when the device delivers a countershock: a blow, thump, or "kick in the chest" that may last 1 second. Explain that the patient may be unconscious before receiving the shock.

—Explain that someone touching the patient will not feel the shock or will feel only a tingle.

—Instruct the patient not to wear tight, restrictive clothing, such as belts and girdles.

—Stress the importance of avoiding the following:

Strong magnets and magnetic fields, such as radio or television transmitting towers

Spark plugs or running motor, such as a lawn mower or car

Handheld airport metal detectors

Rough physical contact or dangerous sports

Large stereo speakers

Television that is in operation with the back off

Direct contact over alternators, such as in a running car engine

Diathermy, magnetic resonance imaging, or electrocautery

—Instruct the patient that contact with well-grounded home appliances, such as microwave ovens and hair dryers, is not harmful.

• *Activity*

—Encourage the patient to discuss allowances and limitations with respect to occupation, recreation, or activities. Tell the patient to discuss occupational concerns with the physician.

—Tell the patient that driving is not permitted for 6 months after surgery because of the potential loss of consciousness associated with dysrhythmias. The patient must be free of discharges for 6 months before driving is permitted.

—Inform the patient that working at heights, swimming alone, or being involved in activities in which the patient or others could be injured if the patient loses consciousness should be avoided.

—Instruct the patient to avoid heavy lifting (>10 pounds) for the first 6 weeks.

—Tell the patient that sexual activity may be resumed as the patient tolerates.

—Advise the patient to report any plans to travel alone or move.

—Encourage the patient to engage in activities of daily living and exercises as tolerated.

—Teach the pateint to check pulses during exercise. Inform the patient of the cutoff rate before discharge and tell the patient not to exceed that rate.

—Explain that the life of the battery depends on the model used and the number of shocks delivered.

PSYCHOSOCIAL CARE

• Encourage the patient and caregiver to verbalize fears and concerns about device function, possible malfunction, and the underlying condition.

FOLLOW-UP CARE

• Stress the importance of regular follow-up visits to assess battery life and device function. Make sure the patient has the necessary names and telephone numbers.

• Encourage the patient to obtain a MedicAlert bracelet and identification card listing the diagnosis and the device.

• Encourage the caregiver to learn cardiopulmonary resuscitation (CPR). Provide a list of community CPR instruction sites. Instruct the patient in cough CPR.

REFERRALS

• Refer the patient and caregiver to support groups for persons with implantable defibrillators.

• Refer the patient to community monitored exercise programs.

Iron Deficiency Anemia

—Iron deficiency anemia: an inadequate absorption or excessive loss of iron. Anemia is a common hematopoietic disorder, defined as a reduced red blood cell volume or a reduced concentration of hemoglobin. The general effects of anemia result from a deficiency of the oxygen-carrying mechanism, although some effects are related to varied pathogenetic factors.

CONTRIBUTING FACTORS/RISK FACTORS

- Decreased dietary intake
- Blood loss (gastrointestinal bleeding)
- Chronic diarrhea
- Menstrual abnormalities
- Pregnancy
- Chronic disease (e.g., rheumatoid arthritis)

SIGNS/SYMPTOMS

- Brittle hair and nails
- Pallor
- Sore mouth or tongue
- Fatigue
- Decreased ability to concentrate
- Cold sensitivity
- Menstrual irregularities
- Loss of libido
- Tachycardia
- Palpitations
- Tachypnea
- Exertional dyspnea
- Nail beds: spoon-shaped, pale
- Vertigo
- Nonfood cravings (e.g., clay, ashes)

COMPLICATIONS

- Hemochromatosis (iron overdose)
- Infection

DIAGNOSTIC TESTS

- Describe each procedure, its purpose, and the normal feelings or sensations that are likely, as well as any preprocedural and postprocedural care.
  —Blood count
  —Peripheral blood smear
  —Total iron-binding capacity
  —Reticulocyte count
  —Bone marrow aspiration

TREATMENT
Medical

- Therapy
  —Increased dietary intake of iron
  —Iron replacement (ferrous sulfate, ferrous gluconate)
  —Treatment of the cause

🏠 HOME CARE

- Give both the patient and the caregiver *verbal* and *written* instructions. Provide them with the name and telephone number of a physician or nurse to call if questions arise.
- *General information*
  —Explain and discuss with the patient iron deficiency anemia, its causes, and contributing factors.
- *Warning signs*
  —Review the signs and symptoms that should be reported to a physician or nurse.
    Dyspnea
    Dizziness
    Palpitations
    Chest pain
    Headache
    Abnormalities in menstrual cycle
    Iron overdose: diarrhea, fever, stomach pain, nausea and vomiting
- *Special instructions*
  —Inform the patient that stools will appear dark or black as the result of iron replacement therapy. Discuss the importance of monitoring for blood loss in the stool when patients have gastrointestinal bleeding tendencies. Teach the proper use of guaiac tests.
- *Medications*
  —Explain the purpose, dosage, schedule, and route of administration of any prescribed drugs, as well as side effects to report to the physician or nurse.
  —Explain the need to avoid taking over-the-counter vitamins that may contain iron. Tell the patient to read labels and check with the physician.
  —Advise the patient to take oral iron with meals to maximize absorption. Advise the patient not to take iron with milk or an antacid, which could decrease absorption. Review the

need to increase vitamin C intake, which can increase iron absorption.

—Tell the patient to take liquid iron through a straw and to rinse the mouth afterward to minimize tooth staining.

• *Activity*

—Encourage the patient to discuss allowances and limitations with respect to occupation, recreation, or activities.

—Discuss the need to space activities to allow for frequent rest periods.

• *Diet*

—Emphasize the importance of a well-balanced diet, especially iron intake, which is found in foods such as red meat, green vegetables, and raisins.

—Discuss the benefits of eating six small meals spread throughout the day rather than trying to get all nutrition in three meals.

—Discuss the need to increase liquids and fiber in the diet to prevent constipation, which is common with iron supplements.

FOLLOW-UP CARE

• Stress the importance of regular medical and laboratory follow-up visits. Make sure the patient has the necessary names and telephone numbers.

Laminectomy
(Spinal Fusion, Diskectomy)

—Laminectomy: removal of a flat, bony portion of the vertebrae referred to as the lamina to access the intervertebral space for removal of protruding fragments of the ruptured disk or to remove the entire disk (diskectomy). The incision may be performed anteriorly or posteriorly in the cervical, thoracic, or lumbar region. Laminectomy is performed to relieve nerve root or spinal cord compression only after conservative treatment no longer alleviates pain.

—Spinal fusion: procedure done in conjunction with laminectomy, performed to stabilize the vertebrae. The procedure involves placing bone chips, obtained from the iliac crest or a bone bank, over the unstable portion of the spine. Wires, rods, screws, or plates are also used.

INDICATIONS

- Ruptured disk (herniated disk)
- Trauma
- Displaced fracture
- Incomplete vertebral dislocation from rheumatoid arthritis or osteoporosis

PREPROCEDURAL TEACHING

- Review the physician's explanation of the procedure and the reason for it; encourage the patient to ask questions and to discuss any fears or anxieties. Explain the need to obtain informed consent for surgery and anesthesia.

Review of Preprocedural Care

- Explain that the incision will be between 1 and 3 inches long.
- Explain that the hospital stay is usually 3 to 5 days.
- Inform the patient of the need to have nothing by mouth (NPO) from midnight the night before.
- Discuss routine blood and urine tests to detect signs of electrolyte imbalance or infection.
- Discuss the chest x-ray and electrocardiogram to evaluate signs of chronic disease.
- Inform the patient about skin preparation: cleansing the night before with bacterial soap and shaving the skin over the incisional area.
- Tell the patient that bowel preparation with an enema may be ordered the night before surgery.

Review of Postprocedural Care

- Explain that the patient will be NPO until the morning after surgery and then will be given clear fluids, advancing to a regular diet.
- Advise the patient that complete bed rest will be maintained until the evening of surgery, with turning from side to side every 2 hours. Explain that the patient will be allowed up at the

bedside the evening of surgery and up to three times daily thereafter.

- Tell the patient that frequent checks of neurovascular status, peripheral pulses, and vital signs will be performed.
- Inform the patient that the first dressing change will be done after 24 hours.
- Discuss the need to deep breathe and cough every 2 hours.
- Inform the patient of the possibility of urinary retention. Tell a male patient that he may stand to void.
- For a patient with cervical laminectomy, explain that a neck brace and a nasogastric drainage tube may be used. Explain that the drainage tube will be removed in 1 to 2 days.
- Advise the patient that incisional pain will be mild to moderate and may radiate to the shoulders and occipital area (if cervical) or to the hips and buttocks (if lumbar). Tell the patient that nerve pain may not be relieved immediately after surgery.

SIDE EFFECTS/COMPLICATIONS

- Continued nerve compression pain
- Hoarseness (cervical)
- Bleeding, hemorrhage
- Spinal cord neurovascular damage
- Wound infection
- Urinary infection, retention
- Effects of anesthesia

HOME CARE

- Give both the patient and the caregiver *verbal* and *written* instructions. Provide them with the name and telephone number of a physician or nurse to call if questions arise.
- *General information*
  —Review any explanation about the procedure.
- *Special instructions*
  —Instruct the patient in the use of antiembolism hose to prevent thrombus formation.
  —Teach techniques for ankle circling and calf pumping to increase venous circulation in legs.
  —Instruct the patient in the use of braces or corsets if prescribed. Braces are applied while in bed for the fusion procedure; braces or corsets are worn approximately 3 months to keep the operative site immobile.

—For a patient with cervical laminectomy, explain the need to wear a neck brace as directed.

—Instruct the patient in the use of assistive devices to help reduce stress on the back: reachers, elevated toilet seats, tub railings.

- *Wound/incision care*

—Instruct the patient to keep the incision site clean and dry until sutures and staples are removed, which usually takes place within 10 days after discharge.

—Instruct the patient who has had a fusion to check the donor site (usually the iliac crest) and what extra padding is needed.

- *Warning signs*

—Review the signs and symptoms that should be reported to a physician or nurse.

Wound infection: fever, chills, redness, swelling, drainage of the incisional area

Neurovascular impairment: increase or appearance of numbness (explain that some numbness as a sign of former nerve pressure may remain), tingling of extremities, coolness, pallor of extremities, increased pain

Changes in bowel or bladder function

Faintness, dizziness, headache, neck stiffness, photophobia

Calf pain, tenderness, warmth

- *Activity*

—Inform the patient that showering is usually not permitted until sutures or staples are out or until advised by the physician.

—Provide instruction on good body mechanics.

Use logrolling when getting in and out of bed to prevent back strain and twisting.

Avoid sudden turning or twisting.

Sit in straight-backed chairs; avoid soft chairs.

—Tell the patient to avoid lifting and driving for 3 to 6 weeks or longer as prescribed by a physician.

—Advise the patient to use a firm mattress (or plywood between the box spring and mattress).

—Instruct the patient to resume activities gradually. Suggest beginning by walking around the house, progressing to longer walks outdoors. Advise the patient to wear shoes with good foot and ankle support.

—Encourage discussion with the physician as to any limitations on exercise, resumption of work, and recreational activities.

—Discuss the importance of continuing with back exercises (see box on p. 97) as ordered and prescribed to increase muscle strength.
- *Diet*
  —Advise the patient that a regular diet high in protein and vitamins will aid wound healing, unless such a diet is contraindicated.
  —Explain the importance of avoiding weight gain. Refer the patient to a dietitian for diet management.

FOLLOW-UP CARE AND REFERRALS
- Stress the importance of regular follow-up visits. Make sure the patient has the necessary names and telephone numbers.
- Provide referral for home health care services to assist with activities of daily living as indicated.

Laryngeal Cancer

—Laryngeal cancer: cancer of the larynx (voice box). Laryngeal cancer occurs most commonly (60%) in the glottis (true vocal cords). Carcinoma of the supraglottic larynx (epiglottis, false cord) has a lower incidence. Ninety percent of cases of laryngeal cancer occur in men, with the highest incidence between 60 and 70 years. The death rate from laryngeal cancer is higher among blacks than whites. Squamous cell cancer of the glottic larynx is the classic smoker's cancer and generally occurs after decades of cigarette smoking. Cancer in situ may exist alone or in association with invasive disease. Malignancies of the supraglottis are usually in an advanced stage when diagnosed. Malignancy rarely develops in the subglottic larynx.

RISK FACTORS
- Cigarette smoking
- Alcohol abuse

SIGNS/SYMPTOMS

- Persistent hoarseness and other vocal complaints
- Aspiration on swallowing
- Dysphagia
- Foreign body sensation
- Unilateral sore throat
- Earache
- Neck mass (supraglottic)
- Dyspnea

DIAGNOSTIC TESTS

- Describe each procedure, its purpose, and the normal feelings or sensations that are likely, as well as any preprocedural and postprocedural care.
    —Indirect mirror examination: to see the lesion on the larynx
    —Direct laryngoscopy and biopsy: to see the lesion on the larynx and detect the presence of malignant cells
    —Anterior laryngeal tomography: to detect subglottic extension of tumor
    —Pulmonary function studies: to assess preoperative respiratory status
    —Chest x-ray: to detect other pulmonary disease such as lung cancer

TREATMENT
Medical

- Therapy
    —Radiation therapy: external beam
    —Chemotherapy
        Cisplatin
        5-Fluorouracil (5-FU)
        Adjuvant chemotherapy with methotrexate and 5-FU

Surgical

- Endoscopic laser excision: for small tumors
- Partial laryngectomy: removal of half or more of larynx
    —Supraglottic laryngectomy
    —Epiglottidectomy
    —Cordectomy
    —Anterior commissure resection

—Vertical hemilaryngectomy
—Frontolateral and extended frontolateral partial laryngectomy
—Near-total laryngectomy

- Total laryngectomy: removal of larynx; voice permanently lost; tracheostomy performed
- Total laryngectomy with radical neck dissection: removal of larynx and surrounding lymph nodes, tissue, muscle, and blood vessels
- Reconstruction: skin flap

HOME CARE

- Give both the patient and the caregiver *verbal* and *written* instructions. Provide them with the name and telephone number of a physician or nurse to call if questions arise. Use visual aids and permit time for return demonstration before discharge.
- For a patient who will undergo laryngectomy, see p. 400. Discuss the extent of the planned surgery and clarify any misconceptions.
- For radiation therapy, see p. 721; for chemotherapy, see p. 667.
- *General information*
  —Review the physician's explanation of the disease and the type of prescribed treatment: radiation therapy or surgery. Explain that treatment depends on the stage and site of the tumor.

PSYCHOSOCIAL CARE

- Encourage verbalization of feelings and questions regarding disease and treatment options.

FOLLOW-UP CARE

- Stress the importance of regular follow-up visits. Make sure the patient has the necessary names and telephone numbers.

REFERRALS

- If a patient is to undergo laryngectomy, arrange a meeting with a laryngectomy survivor before surgery and with a support group to help the patient deal with changes of body image.

Laryngectomy

—Laryngectomy: surgical removal of the larynx with or without neck resection to treat malignancies.

TYPES OF LARYNGECTOMY

- Partial laryngectomy: removal of half or more of the larynx
  - —Supraglottic laryngectomy: hyoid bone, epiglottis, and false cords removed; negative effect on swallowing
  - —Epiglottidectomy, cordectomy, anterior commissure resection
  - —Vertical hemilaryngectomy: removal of one true cord, one false cord, arytenoid cartilage, one half thyroid cartilage; patient has hoarse but usable voice
  - —Frontolateral and extended frontolateral partial laryngectomy
  - —Partial laryngectomy laryngofissure: one vocal cord removed; patient has hoarse but usable voice
- Total laryngectomy: removal of larynx, hyoid bone, epiglottis, false and true cords, cricoid cartilage, two or three rings of trachea; patient has loss of voice as a result of tracheolaryngectomy; swallowing is normal; procedure may be done with radical neck dissection

PREPROCEDURAL TEACHING

- Review the physician's explanation of the procedure and the reason for it; encourage the patient to ask questions and to discuss any fears or anxieties. Discuss the need for informed consent for surgery and anesthesia.

Review of Preprocedural Care

- Inform the patient that the skin will be cleansed with bactericidal soap or antiseptic solutions to remove bacteria.
- Discuss preprocedural tests: complete blood count and urinalysis to check for infection and bleeding.
- Tell the patient that NPO status must be maintained from midnight of the night before surgery.
- Provide preparatory instruction in suctioning (oral and tracheal) and wound care.
- Teach the patient to do own tube feedings.
- Review the use of a magic slate or paper and pencil, flash cards, or a communication board.

- Prepare the patient for permanent loss of speech if total laryngectomy is to be performed.
- Have a speech therapist visit the patient to discuss and plan for alternative means of speech.
- Discuss issues and fears related to the surgery and body image changes.

Review of Postprocedural Care

- Explain that the patient will be in the high Fowler's position to lessen edema, increase coughing and deep breathing, ease suctioning, and provide comfort.
- Explain that the patient will be given mechanical ventilation via a tracheostomy tube and that suctioning will be done frequently to maintain a clear airway for breathing.
- Discuss the importance of frequent deep breathing and coughing.
- Demonstrate the use of intermittent positive-pressure breathing devices and ultrasonic nebulization treatments.
- Explain the presence of pressure dressings and neck drainage tubes. Discuss the use of a nasogastric tube to assist with feedings (bolus or continuous drip based on patient tolerance).
- Explain that swallowing and speech rehabilitation will begin soon after surgery, with the need based on the type and extent of surgery.

SIDE EFFECTS/COMPLICATIONS

- Hemorrhage
- Airway obstruction
- Infection
- Thoracic duct leakage
- Nerve injury

HOME CARE

- Give both the patient and the caregiver *verbal* and *written* instructions. Provide them with the name and telephone number of a physician or nurse to call if questions arise. Use visual aids to assist in instruction.
- *General information*
    —Review any explanation about the procedure and any specific follow-up care.

- *Wound/incision care*
  —Instruct the patient and caregiver to inspect the incision site daily and to change the dressing using sterile supplies as demonstrated by the nurse.
- *Warning signs*
  —Review the signs and symptoms that should be reported to a physician or nurse.
    Infection of the stoma or incision: redness, drainage, pain, warm to touch, fever
    Dyspnea without exertion
    Difficulty swallowing
- *Special instructions*
  —Teach the patient to avoid voice strain and to whisper or use alternative methods of communication when the voice needs rest. If the voice is gone (total laryngectomy), have the patient work with a speech therapist to develop an alternative method of communicating.
- *Medications*
  —Provide pain management, encouraging the patient to use mild analgesics when possible (see Pain Management, p. 708).
- *Activity*
  —Remind the patient to plan frequent rest periods to avoid shortness of breath.
  —Assist the patient to begin self-care as soon as possible, including tracheostomy care (see p. 727) and taking food and fluids by mouth.
- *Diet*
  —Plan a diet with the patient and caregivers that will avoid the possibility of choking or aspirating. For example, the patient may initially receive tube feedings and progress to soft foods and liquids as the swallowing reflex returns.

PSYCHOSOCIAL CARE

- Encourage questions and verbalization of fear and anxieties regarding body image changes, including possible loss of the voice.

FOLLOW-UP CARE

- Stress the importance of regular follow-up visits. Make sure the patient has the necessary names and telephone numbers.

REFERRALS

- Assist the patient to obtain referral services, supplies, and information about support groups from the Lost Cord Club/ International Association of Laryngectomees, sponsored by the American Cancer Society.
- Arrange a reconstructive surgery consultation as needed.

Leukemia

—Leukemia: malignant proliferation of abnormal immature white blood cells. These abnormal cells, which accumulate in the bone marrow, infiltrate body tissues and blood vessels and eventually cause malfunction by encroachment, hemorrhage, or infection. Acute leukemia, the most common type, affects children under 5 years of age and older adults. There are two forms: acute lymphocytic leukemia (ALL), which involves the lymphocytes and lymphoid organs, and acute myelocytic leukemia (AML), which affects adults older than 65 years and involves the hematopoietic cells (granulocytes, erythrocytes, and platelets). In chronic leukemia the white blood cells produced are more mature and accumulate much more slowly. Chronic leukemia occurs in adults after age 20 and is classified as chronic lymphocytic leukemia (CLL) and chronic myelocytic (granulocytic) leukemia (CML).

CAUSES/RISK FACTORS

- Idiopathic
- Chromosomal abnormality
- Overexposure to radiation, chemicals, drugs, or viruses

SIGNS/SYMPTOMS

- Low-grade fever
- Pallor
- Chills
- Fatigue and weakness
- Gingivitis
- Easy bruising
- Nosebleeds

- Prolonged menstruation
- Acute indicators (crisis)
  —High fever
  —Diffuse petechiae
  —Bruising
  —Nosebleeds
  —Anorexia
  —Nausea and vomiting
  —Headaches
  —Visual disturbances
  —Weakness
  —Lethargy
  —Seizures

COMPLICATIONS

- Hemorrhage
- Stroke, seizures
- Myocardial infarction
- Infection
- Organ failure (renal, liver)

DIAGNOSTIC TESTS

- Describe each procedure, its purpose, and the normal feelings or sensations that are likely, as well as any preprocedural and postprocedural care.
  —White blood cell components elevated
      T cell (ALL)
      Blasts
      Lymphocytes (ALL)
      Auer rods (AML)
      Phi bodies (AML)
  —Reticulocytopenia
      Normochromic (AML)
      Normocytic
  —Anemia
  —Thrombocytopenia
  —Prothrombin time and partial thromboplastin time: increased
  —Serum copper: elevated
  —Zinc: decreased
  —Hypergammaglobulinemia (AML)
  —Urine uric acid: elevated
  —Bone marrow aspiration: proliferation of blast cells

TREATMENT
Medical

- Therapy
  —Radiation therapy
  >CLL: local irradiation of spleen, lymph nodes, and painful bony lesions
  >CML: whole brain irradiation or leukapheresis
  —Blood and blood product transfusion
  —Fluid therapy
  —Chemotherapy
  >ALL: vincristine sulfate, prednisone, and daunorubicin with or without L-asparaginase and methotrexate
  >AML: daunorubicin hydrochloride, cytarabine, and thioguanine
  >CLL: chlorambucil or cyclophosphamide and prednisone to produce remission
  >CML: busulfan and hydroxyurea (during stable chronic phase); daunorubicin, cytarabine, vincristine, prednisone, and thioguanine (during acute phase)
  —Analgesics
  —Bone marrow transplantation: ALL, CML

Surgical

- CML: splenectomy if destroying platelets

⊞⊡ HOME CARE

- Give both the patient and the caregiver *verbal* and *written* instructions. Provide them with the name and telephone number of a physician or nurse to call if questions arise.
- *General information*
  —Explain the particular leukemic disorder, possible causes, and precipitating factors.
  —Discuss disease progression and the possibility of exacerbations as well as remissions.
- *Warning signs*
  —Review the signs and symptoms that should be reported to a physician or nurse.
  >Acute crisis: high fever, easy bruising, bleeding, lethargy, headaches, visual blurring
  >Infection: high fever, cough, chills
  >Bleeding: oozing of blood from gums and mucous membranes, ears, nose; bruising; petechiae

- *Special instructions*
  —Discuss measures for preventing infections.
  > Avoid persons who are suspected of having infection.
  > Avoid large crowds.
  > Change air and furnace filters on a regular basis.
  > Maintain good personal hygiene.
  > Maintain good oral hygiene (brushing and flossing regularly; when mouth sores are present, use oral rinses and avoid brushing and flossing).

  —Discuss measures to take for bleeding.
  > Apply direct pressure and ice to the area.
  > Seek medical attention if unable to control the bleeding.

- *Medications*
  —Explain the purpose, dosage, schedule, and route of administration of any prescribed drugs, as well as side effects to report to the physician or nurse.
  —Discuss the side effects of particular chemotherapeutic agents and procedures for managing these symptoms (see Chemotherapy, p. 667).

- *Activity*
  —Encourage the patient to discuss allowances and limitations with respect to occupation, recreation, or activities.
  —Discuss the need to maintain activities as tolerated to prevent depression and physical debilitation.
  —Discuss bleeding precautions: use an electric razor and soft-bristled toothbrush; avoid activities that increase the risk of trauma or injury, such as contact sports and working with sharp tools and instruments.
  —Encourage pacing of activities and the use of assistance to avoid overexertion.

- *Diet*
  —Explain the need for nutritious foods and liquids to 2500 ml/day.
  —Encourage the patient to continue normal eating patterns to enhance appetite.
  —Discuss alternative resources for delivery of meals to the home as appropriate (e.g., Meals on Wheels).
  —Teach the patient methods of maintaining nutritional intake during times of anorexia, nausea, vomiting, stomatitis, and other symptoms.

PSYCHOSOCIAL CARE

- Encourage the verbalization of feelings and fears regarding the diagnosis and treatment options.
- Discuss the need to maintain open communications with family, friends, the physician, and the nurse, to discuss needs and how they can be met.

FOLLOW-UP CARE

- Stress the importance of regular follow-up visits. Make sure the patient has the necessary names and telephone numbers.
- Discuss the importance of informing all medical and dental personnel of bleeding tendencies before any procedures (e.g., dental cleanings, injections).
- Instruct the patient to wear a MedicAlert bracelet and carry an identification card with a list of medications at all times.

REFERRALS

- Provide referrals for home care and social services.
- Encourage the use of formal cancer support and educational services: American Cancer Society, local cancer support groups, and the Leukemia Society of America.

Liver Biopsy

—Liver biopsy: percutaneous introduction of a needle into the liver to obtain tissue for pathologic examination and diagnosis of liver diseases.

INDICATIONS

- Abnormal liver function
- Cirrhosis
- Hepatitis
- Hepatomegaly or hepatosplenomegaly of unexplained origin
- Suspected malignancy of the liver
- Suspected systemic or infiltrative disease, such as sarcoidosis
- Routine evaluation for rejection in a transplanted liver

PREPROCEDURAL TEACHING

- Review the physician's explanation of the procedure and the reason for it; encourage the patient to ask questions and to discuss any fears or anxieties. Discuss the need for informed consent.

Review of Preprocedural Care

- Review preprocedural laboratory tests: type and crossmatch, prothrombin time, hemoglobin, hematocrit, and platelet count.
- Inform the patient of the need to be NPO for 4 to 8 hours before the biopsy.
- Explain that the patient will be asked to void before the biopsy.
- Discuss instructions for the patient during the biopsy.
  —Instruct the patient to lie still during the biopsy. Local anesthetic will be administered.
  —Instruct and coach the patient to hold his or her breath at the end of expiration to maximally elevate the liver.
  —Stress the importance of sustaining expiration because failure to do so may result in puncture of the lung.

Review of Postprocedural Care

- Explain that vital signs will be monitored, breath sounds will be auscultated for 6 to 8 hours, and the patient will be observed for complications.
- Inform the patient that sedatives and analgesics will be administered as ordered.
- Tell the patient that it will be necessary to lie on the right side for the first 6 hours to keep pressure on the site and remain on bed rest for 8 to 12 hours after the biopsy to minimize the risk of hemorrhage.
- Discuss the resumption of a normal diet.

SIDE EFFECTS/COMPLICATIONS

- Hemorrhage
- Pneumothorax
- Peritonitis

HOME CARE

- Give both the patient and the caregiver *verbal* and *written* instructions. Provide them with the name and telephone number of a physician or nurse to call if questions arise.

- *General information*
  —Review any explanation about the procedure and any specific follow-up care.
- *Warning signs*
  —Review the signs and symptoms that should be reported to a physician or nurse.
  - Severe abdominal pain
  - Abdominal distention and rigidity
  - Rebound tenderness
  - Nausea and vomiting
  - Pallor
  - Respiratory distress
  - Fever
  - Tachycardia
- *Medications*
  —Provide pain management, encouraging the patient to use mild analgesics when possible (see Pain Management, p. 708).
  —Advise the patient to avoid taking nonsteroidal antiinflammatory drugs (NSAIDs) and hepatotoxic medications.
  —Provide a list of NSAIDs and hepatotoxic medications to avoid.
- *Activity*
  —Instruct the patient to avoid strenuous activity or heavy lifting for the first day or as instructed.
- *Diet*
  —Advise the family or caregiver to provide assistance with eating as needed for 24 hours.
  —Explain that a regular diet can be resumed as prescribed by the physician for the underlying disease.

FOLLOW-UP CARE

- Stress the importance of regular follow-up visits. Make sure the patient has the necessary names and telephone numbers.

Lung Cancer
(Bronchogenic)

—Lung cancer: cancer of the lung, the leading cause of cancer-related deaths for both men and women. Approximately 80% of lung tumors are linked to cigarette smoking. Contributing factors include exposure to carcinogenic substances and industrial air pollutants, genetic predisposition, and vitamin A deficiency. Types of lung cancer include non–small cell lung cancer, which is usually treated surgically and includes squamous cell (epidermoid), adenocarcinoma, and large cell undifferentiated, and small cell lung cancer, or oat cell cancer, which is aggressive but highly sensitive to chemotherapy and radiation therapy.

SIGNS/SYMPTOMS

- Chronic cough
- Change in volume or odor of sputum
- Shortness of breath
- Dull chest pain
- Upper respiratory infection
- Fatigue
- Chest tightness
- Aching joints
- Later signs
  - —Blood in sputum
  - —Clubbing of fingers
  - —Weight loss
  - —Pleural effusion
  - —Edema of neck and face
  - —Paralysis of diaphragm
  - —Hoarseness
  - —Shoulder and arm pain or numbness

COMPLICATIONS

- Superior vena cava syndrome
- Paraneoplastic syndromes: hypercalcemia, dermatomyositis, clubbed fingers, Cushing's syndrome, anemia, disseminated intravascular coagulation

DIAGNOSTIC TESTS

- Describe each procedure, its purpose, and the normal feelings or sensations that are likely, as well as any preprocedural and postprocedural care.
    - —Bronchoscopy, mediastinoscopy, thoracentesis, and sputum cytology: to detect the presence of tumor and malignant cells
    - —Chest x-ray: to determine the size and location of the tumor
    - —Computed tomography scan and magnetic resonance imaging: to determine precise size and density and invasion or compression of blood vessels
    - —Tissue biopsy (scalene, supraclavicular node, bone marrow): to detect the presence of malignant cells
    - —Pulmonary function tests: to determine the impact of the tumor on vital capacity
    - —Computed tomography, ultrasound scan, magnetic resonance imaging: to detect evidence of metastatic disease

TREATMENT
Medical

- Therapy
    - —Radiation therapy
        - External beam
        - Interstitial/endobronchial bradytherapy with iridium-192
    - —Endobronchial laser therapy (photodynamic therapy)
    - —Sclerosis: treatment of pleural effusion
    - —Chemotherapy
        - For advanced non–small cell lung cancer (NSCLC)
        - ○ VdP (vindesine, cisplatin)
        - ○ VbP (vinblastine, cisplatin)
        - ○ CAMP (cyclophosphamide, doxorubicin, methotrexate, procarbazine)
        - ○ MVbP (mitomycin, vinblastine, cisplatin)
        - ○ PtVP-16 (etoposide [VP-16], cisplatin)
        - ○ CAP (cyclophosphamide, doxorubicin, cisplatin)
        - ○ CBP (cyclophosphamide, bleomycin, cisplatin)
        - ○ FOMi (5-fluorouracil, vincristine, mitomycin C)
        - ○ Vinorelbine as a single agent or in combination with paclitaxel (Taxol)
        - For small cell lung cancer
        - ○ CAV (cyclophosphamide, doxorubicin, vincristine)
        - ○ CEA (cyclophosphamide, etoposide, doxorubicin)

○ CEV (cyclophosphamide, etoposide, vincristine)
○ EVAC (etoposide, vincristine, doxorubicin, cyclophosphamide)

Hansen's (cyclophosphamide, lomustine, vincristine, methotrexate)

Hansen's VP (cyclophosphamide, lomustine, vincristine,
etoposide)

VP-16+P (etoposide, cisplatin)

—Biologic response modifiers
—Monoclonal antibody KC4 for NSCLC

Surgical

• Indications
—Choice of treatment for patients with NSCLC
—Removal of limited primary or secondary tumor, and lymph
node resection
—Extended resection for widespread disease

• Procedures
—Thoracotomy: surgical incision of chest wall, collection of
biopsy specimen; limited pulmonary resection (segmental,
wedge)
—Lobectomy: removal of lobe of lung and regional node
dissection
—Pneumonectomy: surgical removal of an entire lung
—Extended resection: en bloc removal of portions of the chest
wall, vertebral body, left atrium, and diaphragm

🏠 HOME CARE

• Give both the patient and the caregiver *verbal* and *written*
instructions. Provide them with the name and telephone number
of a physician or nurse to call if questions arise.
• For surgery, see Thoracentesis, p. 608.
• For radiation therapy, see p. 721.
• For chemotherapy, see p. 667.
• *General information*
—Review the physician's explanation of the type of cancer and
prescribed treatment. Use illustrations to identify the tumor's
location.
—Evaluate respiratory function: need for O_2 therapy at home.
—Encourage questions and verbalization of feelings and
concerns about the disease prognosis and changes in lifestyle.

—Explain and outline prescribed treatment protocols, length of therapies, and expected outcomes and results.

—Stress the importance of not smoking or using tobacco products. Provide referral to smoking cessation programs as indicated.

—Evaluate diet and daily oral intake.

- *Warning signs*
  —Review the signs and symptoms that should be reported to a physician or nurse.

  Shoulder or arm pain

  Difficulty with memory

  Fatigue

  Weight loss

  Increased coughing or hemoptysis

- *Medications*
  —Explain the purpose, dosage, schedule, and route of administration of any prescribed drugs, as well as side effects to report to the physician or nurse.

- *Activity*
  —Discuss any limitations and restrictions necessary.
  —Discuss the importance of exercising to tolerance each day; alternate activities and periods of rest.

- *Diet*
  —Instruct the patient to eat a diet high in protein and calories.

PSYCHOSOCIAL CARE

- Encourage verbalization of feelings and fears regarding disease progression and treatment options.

FOLLOW-UP CARE

- Stress the importance of regular follow-up visits. Make sure the patient has the necessary names and telephone numbers.

REFERRALS

- Assist the patient to obtain referral services, such as the American Cancer Society and the American Lung Association, that can provide information, support groups, and equipment.

Lupus Erythematosus, Systemic

—Lupus erythematosus: systemic lupus erythematosus (SLE) is a chronic, autoimmune inflammatory disease of the connective tissues that produces biochemical and structural changes in skin, joints, and muscles. There is no characteristic clinical pattern. SLE usually involves multiple organs and is characterized by periods of exacerbation and remission. Women are 9 times more likely to have SLE than men and 15 times more likely in the childbearing years. SLE is most prevalent in Asians and African-Americans. Discoid lupus erythematosus (DLE) affects only the skin.

RISK FACTORS

- Stress
- Streptococcal or viral infections
- Exposure to sunlight or ultraviolet light
- Immunization
- Pregnancy
- Abnormal estrogen metabolism

SIGNS/SYMPTOMS

- Cutaneous lesions: raised, red, scaling rash on sun-exposed skin areas
- Facial erythema (butterfly rash)
- Fever
- Arthritis
- Mouth sores
- Light sensitivity
- Serositis (inflamed serous membranes)
- Anorexia
- Weight loss
- Malaise
- Fatigue
- Abdominal pain
- Irregular menstruation or amenorrhea

COMPLICATIONS

- Stroke
- Cardiac arrest

- Renal failure
- Seizures
- Gangrene (fingers, toes)

DIAGNOSTIC TESTS

- Describe each procedure, its purpose, and the normal feelings or sensations that are likely, as well as any preprocedural and postprocedural care.
  —Chest x-ray: pleurisy or lupus pneumonitis
  —Electrocardiogram: conduction defect, pericarditis
  —Electroencephalogram, brain scan, magnetic resonance imaging: to detect central nervous system involvement
  —Renal biopsy: positive for renal disease
  —Laboratory findings
      Serum complement (C3 and C4): decreased
      Complete blood count with differential: decreased red blood cells, white blood cells, and platelets
      Erythrocyte sedimentation rate: increased
      Electrophoresis: hypergammaglobulinemia
      Urine studies: positive for red blood cells, white blood cells, urine casts and sediment, and protein loss
      Lupus-specific blood tests
      ○ Antinuclear antibodies (anti-DNA, anti-Smith): positive
      ○ Anti–deoxyribonucleic acid: positive
      ○ Lupus erythematosus cell test: positive

TREATMENT
Medical

- Drugs
  —Mild disease
      Nonsteroidal antiinflammatory drugs: aspirin for arthritis
      Corticosteroids: for skin lesions
      Antimalarials
  —Acute exacerbations
      Corticosteroids (prednisone)
      Cytotoxic agents (azathioprine, cyclophosphamide, methotrexate): to delay or prevent renal deterioration
      Antihypertensive drugs
      Antiinfectives: for secondary infections
      Warfarin: to prevent clotting caused by antiphospholipid antibodies

HOME CARE

- Give both the patient and the caregiver *verbal* and *written* instructions. Provide them with the name and telephone number of a physician or nurse to call if questions arise.
- *General information*
  —Explain the disease process, causes, and precipitating factors. Stress the importance of avoiding factors that can trigger exacerbation.
  —Stress that preventive measures can reduce flareups: exercise, diet, support groups.
- *Warning signs*
  —Review the signs and symptoms that should be reported to a physician or nurse.
    Fever
    Cough
    Rash
    Increase in chest, abdominal, muscle, or joint pain
- *Special instructions*
  —Explain that a woman with SLE can have a successful pregnancy, but pregnancies must be planned. Provide information and referrals for information about appropriate contraception.
  —Advise the patient to report any menstrual abnormalities.
  —Teach the patient to monitor for organ involvement.
    Renal: weight gain, hypertension
    Neurologic: personality changes, depression, drooping of eyelids, double vision
    Hematologic: bleeding (urine, stool, sputum)
    Skin: hair loss, petechiae, sores, pallor, bruising
    Immunologic: infection (fever, cough)
  —Teach skin care.
    Use only nonallergenic skin and hair care products.
    Avoid sun exposure; wear protective clothing (hats, long-sleeved shirts and blouses, pants) and use factor-15 sunscreen.
    Avoid hair dyes.
    Avoid fluorescent or ultraviolet lights.
  —Caution the patient to avoid infections by staying away from large crowds and persons known to have active infections.
  —Discuss the need for meticulous oral care to prevent infection.

- *Medications*
  —Explain the purpose, dosage, schedule, and route of administration of any prescribed drugs, as well as side effects to report to the physician or nurse.

  Corticosteroids (see Steroid Therapy, p. 590).

  Warfarin (see Anticoagulation Therapy, p. 648).

  —Advise the patient to avoid penicillin, sulfa, phenytoin, and oral contraceptives.
  —Warn against trying "miracle" drugs for arthritis without consulting the physician.
- *Activity*
  —Encourage the patient to discuss allowances and limitations with respect to occupation, recreation, or activities.
  —Encourage regular exercise to maintain range of motion and prevent contractures. Teach the patient to use heat packs to relieve joint pain and stiffness.
  —Stress the importance of avoiding physical exertion; discuss the need for planning regular rest periods and pacing activities.
  —Encourage the use of assistive devices such as splints, walker, or cane, as indicated.
- *Diet*
  —Encourage a balanced diet with foods high in protein, vitamins, and iron to help maintain nutrition and prevent anemia.
  —Encourage small, frequent meals.

PSYCHOSOCIAL CARE

- Encourage verbalization of fears and concerns about the disease.
- Stress the importance of avoiding emotional stress; discuss stress reduction methods: imagery, meditation, relaxation.

FOLLOW-UP CARE

- Stress the importance of regular follow-up visits. Make sure the patient has the necessary names and telephone numbers.
- Discuss the importance of wearing a MedicAlert bracelet and carrying an identification card at all times.

REFERRALS

- Refer the patient to the Lupus Foundation of America and the Arthritis Foundation as indicated.

- Provide referrals for a medical social worker as indicated.
- Encourage cessation and/or avoidance of negative behaviors such as smoking or alcohol use. Provide cessation referrals as indicated.

Lyme Disease

—Lyme disease: an acute inflammatory disease transmitted by a tick-borne spirochete via an animal vector (such as a deer). First described in 1975 in Lyme, Connecticut, the disease has been reported primarily in New York, New Jersey, and Connecticut but has also been reported in other states and sporadically in other countries. It can occur in all age groups. Flulike symptoms appear in recurrent episodes, lasting about 1 week and occurring at intervals from 1 to several weeks over a 2- to 3-year period. Other symptoms such as joint manifestations mimic diseases like arthritis. Lyme disease is also known as Lyme arthritis.

SIGNS/SYMPTOMS

- Early stage
    - —Spreading red, circular (target lesion) rash appearing at site of tick bites (axillae, thighs, groin)
    - —Flulike symptoms
        Headache
        Stiff neck
        Aches, pain
        Joint tenderness and swelling
        Fever, chills
        Nausea, vomiting
- Later stage
    - —Palpitations, mild shortness of breath
    - —Memory loss, confusion
    - —Limb weakness, sensory loss
    - —Bell's palsy

—Arthritic symptoms
  Joint swelling
  Redness
  Limited movement

COMPLICATIONS

- Arthritis
- Meningitis
- Encephalitis
- Cerebellar ataxia
- Cranial or peripheral neuropathies
- Cardiac: heart block, myocarditis, pericarditis, congestive heart failure

DIAGNOSTIC TESTS

- Describe each procedure, its purpose, and the normal feelings or sensations that are likely, as well as any preprocedural and postprocedural care.
  —Serologic tests
    Enzyme-linked immunosorbent assay (ELISA): positive
    Indirect immunofluorescence assay: elevated
    Erythrocyte sedimentation rate: sometimes elevated
    Rheumatoid factor: negative
    Culture of specimen of blood into animal tissue: positive for spirochete
    Microscopic examination of skin specimen: positive for spirochete

TREATMENT
Medical

- Therapy (depends on symptoms and stage of illness)
  —Bed rest: to allow inflamed tissues to be rested and recover strength, especially with cardiac and neurologic involvement
  —Physical therapy: for muscle weakness, paralysis, arthritis
- Drugs
  —Antibiotics: oral in early stage, intravenous in later stage
  —Analgesics, antipyretics: for pain and fever

HOME CARE

- Give both the patient and the caregiver *verbal* and *written* instructions. Provide them with the name and telephone number of a physician or nurse to call if questions arise.

- *General information*
  —Explain the disease process and causes. Assist the patient to identify the possible site of the tick bite.
- *Warning signs*
  —Review the signs and symptoms of recurrence and complication that should be reported to a physician or nurse.
  > Muscle weakness
  > Altered mental functioning
  > Excessive drowsiness
  > Flulike symptoms
- *Special instructions*
  —Reinforce ways to prevent recurrence.
  > Avoid tick-infested areas.
  > Wear shirt tucked into pants and long pants tucked into boots when going into a wooded area.
  > Apply insect repellent before going into the woods.
  > Check body surfaces and clothing every 3 to 4 hours for ticks after being in the woods or infested areas.
  > Remove tick immediately with tweezers or forceps, using a firm steady traction. Notify the physician or nurse of a tick bite.
  > Detick dogs regularly to minimize tick population near residence.
- *Medications*
  —Explain the purpose, dosage, schedule, and route of administration of any prescribed drugs, as well as side effects to report to the physician or nurse.
  —Explain that antibiotic treatment will continue up to 20 days if symptoms persist.
  —Stress the importance of continuing medications as prescribed.
- *Activity*
  —Explain the need to avoid fatigue, to plan regular rest periods, and to maintain bed rest as ordered.
  —Instruct the patient in range-of-motion exercises to unaffected joints to maintain strength, but advise the patient to avoid overexertion.

FOLLOW-UP CARE

- Stress the importance of regular follow-up visits until recovery is complete.

Lymphoma, Malignant
(Non-Hodgkin's Lymphoma)

—Lymphoma, malignant: neoplasms of the lymphoid tissues, which are classified by degree and differentiation of cellular content. Non-Hodgkin's lymphoma is characterized by spread to adjacent nodes and is likely to involve other organs. Non-Hodgkin's lymphoma is often widespread before detection. It affects adults 50 years of age and older and is more common than Hodgkin's lymphoma. The cause is largely unknown.

RISK FACTORS
- Male, white, Jewish ancestry
- History of autoimmune disorders and congenital disorders
- Immunosuppressant therapy (e.g., transplant patients)

STAGING
- Stage I: single lymph node region
- Stage II: two or more node regions limited to one side of the diaphragm
- Stage III: disease on both sides of the diaphragm but limited to the lymph nodes or spleen
- Stage IV: involvement of the bones, bone marrow, lung parenchyma, pleura, liver, skin, gastrointestinal tract, central nervous system, etc.

All stages are subclassified as A or B to describe the absence (A) or presence (B) of systemic symptoms.

SIGNS/SYMPTOMS
- Painless, swollen lymph nodes (lymphadenopathy): swelling and size fluctuate (early sign)
- Enlarged tonsils and adenoids
- Fever
- Night sweats
- Weight loss
- Lethargy

- Malaise
- Anorexia
- Edema or pain distal to swollen lymph nodes

COMPLICATIONS

- Cervical node enlargement: venous occlusion, neck edema, airway obstruction
- Mediastinal node enlargement: dyspnea, cough
- Inguinal node enlargement: dysuria, frequency, painful urination, low back pain
- Infections
- Fractures

DIAGNOSTIC TESTS

- Describe each procedure, its purpose, and the normal feelings or sensations that are likely, as well as any preprocedural and postprocedural care.
  - —Staging procedures
    - Lymph node biopsy
    - Chest x-ray
    - Bone marrow biopsy
    - Liver and spleen biopsy, scans
    - Laparoscopy: to view peritoneal organs
    - Computed tomography scans: bone, liver, spleen, abdomen
    - Lymphangiography: to evaluate nodal involvement in abdomen and pelvis
  - —Laboratory tests
    - Normocytic, normochromic anemia
    - White blood cells with differential
    - Erythrocyte sedimentation rate
    - Hypercalcemia
    - Alkaline phosphatase: increased (indicates bone involvement)
    - Copper: elevated
    - Lactate dehydrogenase: elevated
    - Antiglobulin (Coombs') test: positive
    - Hypoalbuminemia or hypergammaglobulinemia
    - Monoclonal immunoglobulin spikes

TREATMENT
Medical

* Therapy
  —Radiation therapy for stages I and II
  —Autologous bone marrow transplant: research being conducted to determine effectiveness
* Drugs
  —Chemotherapy in combination with radiation therapy for stages III and IV
  —Intrathecal chemotherapy if central nervous system involvement is present
  —Interferon, monoclonal antibodies: research being conducted as to effectiveness

Surgical

* Laparotomy
* Splenectomy

HOME CARE

* Give both the patient and the caregiver *verbal* and *written* instructions. Provide them with the name and telephone number of a physician or nurse to call if questions arise.
* *General information*
  —Discuss non-Hodgkin's lymphoma, its possible causes, and contributing factors.
  —Discuss staging of the disease and the impact that various stages may have on daily living.
  —Discuss prescribed treatment (see Chemotherapy, p. 667, and Radiation Therapy, p. 721).
* *Warning signs*
  —Review the signs and symptoms of problems that should be reported to a physician or nurse.
    Persistent fever
    Weight loss
    Enlarged lymph nodes
    Malaise
    Decreased exercise tolerance
    Infection (urinary tract, upper respiratory tract): cough, foul-smelling sputum, pain and burning with urination, frequency, urgency, hematuria, redness

- *Special instructions*
  —Discuss the importance of avoiding injury and trauma, which can cause bruising and bleeding.
  —Discuss the importance of avoiding large crowds and persons suspected of having an active infection.
  —Discuss the signs and symptoms of complications related to non-Hodgkin's lymphoma.
- *Medications*
  —Explain the purpose, dosage, schedule, and route of administration of any prescribed drugs, as well as side effects to report to the physician or nurse.
  —Explain the importance of following the chemotherapy regimen and of reporting the side effects of therapy (e.g., sores in the mouth and on the tongue, anorexia, nausea, vomiting, malaise) to the physician or nurse.
- *Activity*
  —Encourage the patient to discuss allowances and limitations with respect to occupation, recreation, and activities.
  —Discuss the need for planned rest periods. Stress the importance of avoiding overexertion.
  —Teach stress reduction techniques.
- *Diet*
  —Stress the importance of a balanced, high-calorie, high-protein diet to maintain nutrition.
  —Encourage small, frequent meals.
  —Discuss methods to maintain hydration and nutrition during periods of stomatitis, nausea, vomiting, and anorexia associated with therapy (sip fluids all day; drink nectar juices; avoid spicy, hot, and citrus-type foods).

PSYCHOSOCIAL CARE

- Encourage verbalization of feelings and fears regarding disease progression and treatment options.

FOLLOW-UP CARE

- Stress the importance of regular follow-up visits for medical and laboratory evaluation. Make sure the patient has the necessary names and telephone numbers.
- Discuss the need to plan radiation therapy and chemotherapy sessions and to keep appointments.

REFERRALS

- Refer the patient to the American Cancer Society and local support groups as indicated and to the Lymphoma Research Foundation.

Mitral Stenosis

—Mitral stenosis: narrowing of the mitral valve because of calcification, fibrosis, or fusion of the leaflets.

CAUSES/CONTRIBUTING FACTORS/RISK FACTORS

- Rheumatic fever
- Female gender
- Endocarditis
- Systemic lupus erythematosus
- Rheumatoid arthritis

SIGNS/SYMPTOMS

- Shortness of breath with activity
- Orthopnea, paroxysmal nocturnal dyspnea
- Weakness
- Fatigue
- Palpitations
- Chest pain
- Right ventricular failure (see Heart Failure, p. 333)
- Pulmonary edema
- Hemoptysis

COMPLICATIONS

- Atrial fibrillation
- Systemic embolism
- Bronchitis
- Pulmonary embolism
- Endocarditis
- Pulmonary hypertension

M

DIAGNOSTIC TESTS

- Describe each procedure, its purpose, and the normal feelings or sensations that are likely, as well as any preprocedural and postprocedural care.
    - —Cardiac catheterization: to measure pulmonary and intracardiac pressures; to assess severity of the stenosis
    - —Chest x-ray: to show enlargement of the heart or pulmonary edema
    - —Echocardiography: to establish diagnosis and severity of the stenosis; to detect abnormal leaflet motion and enlargement of the left atrium
    - —Electrocardiogram: to detect right ventricular hypertrophy or dysrhythmias

TREATMENT
Medical

- Drugs
    - —Antibiotics
    - —Diuretics
    - —Digoxin
    - —Beta blockers
    - —Calcium channel blockers
    - —Oral anticoagulants

Surgical

- Mitral commissurotomy
- Percutaneous mitral valve balloon valvuloplasty
- Mitral valvotomy
- Mitral valve replacement

HOME CARE

- Give both the patient and the caregiver *verbal* and *written* instructions. Provide them with the name and telephone number of a physician or nurse to call if questions arise. Use heart models or diagrams to assist in instruction.
- *General information*
    - —Discuss the disease process, contributing factors, the cause of obstruction, and the signs and symptoms of disease progression. Explain that treatment is guided by disease progression. Show the patient the location of the affected valve and explain its role in the arterial circulation.

—Instruct the patient for balloon angioplasty or surgery as recommended (see Valve Repair/Replacement, p. 635).

- *Warning signs*
  —Review the signs and symptoms that should be reported to a physician or nurse.
    Palpitations
    Chest pain
    Shortness of breath
    Dyspnea on exertion
    Swelling of ankles and feet
    Signs of emboli: syncope (faintness, muscle weakness, paresthesia, confusion)

- *Special instructions*
  —Explain the risk of endocarditis, discussing the causes and means of prevention. Tell the patient to alert the dentist or any other medical personnel (urologist, gynecologist) of valve disease.
  —Explain the importance of good oral hygiene and regular dental care. Explain the need for antibiotic prophylaxis before dental care and other invasive procedures (dilation and curettage, cystoscopy) for prevention.
  —Provide female patients with instruction regarding contraception and risk of pregnancy. Emphasize the importance of pregnancy planning. Tell the patient to avoid the use of estrogen-based contraceptives or intrauterine devices.

- *Medications*
  —Explain the purpose, dosage, schedule, and route of administration of any prescribed drugs, as well as side effects to report to the physician or nurse.
  —Provide specific instructions for a patient discharged with a prescription for anticoagulants (see p. 648).

- *Activity*
  —Stress the importance of avoiding strenuous activity (e.g., heavy lifting, pushing a car or changing a tire, engaging in competitive sports).
  —Encourage the patient to discuss allowances and limitations with respect to occupation, recreation, and activities.
  —Explain the need for moderate activity such as walking for conditioning.
  —Encourage frequent rest periods and avoidance of fatigue.

- *Diet*
  —Discuss the need to restrict salt intake to 3000 mg/day. Explain that further sodium restrictions may be necessary in the presence of heart failure.

FOLLOW-UP CARE AND REFERRALS

- Stress the importance of regular follow-up visits for medical and laboratory evaluation. Make sure the patient has the necessary names and telephone numbers.
- Stress the importance of not smoking or using tobacco products. Provide information on and referral to smoking cessation programs as necessary.

Mitral Valve Insufficiency or Regurgitation

—Mitral valve insufficiency or regurgitation: incomplete closure of valve that results when rigidity, calcification, and fusion of the valve leaflets with the chordae tendineae cause the leaflets to shorten and retract.

CAUSES/CONTRIBUTING FACTORS/RISK FACTORS

- Myocardial infarction
- Coronary artery disease
- Papillary muscle dysfunction
- Cardiomyopathy
- Inflammatory heart disorders
- Rheumatic fever
- Mitral valve prolapse
- Ruptured chordae tendineae or papillary muscle
- Mitral annular calcification
- Endocarditis
- Congenital heart disease

SIGNS/SYMPTOMS

- Pulmonary edema
- Fatigue

- Angina
- Palpitations
- Shortness of breath
- Anxiety

COMPLICATIONS

- Heart failure
- Pulmonary hypertension
- Endocarditis
- Systemic emboli
- Pulmonary edema
- Atrial fibrillation

DIAGNOSTIC TESTS

- Describe each procedure, its purpose, and the normal feelings or sensations that are likely, as well as any preprocedural and postprocedural care.
    —Cardiac catheterization: to determine severity of insufficiency; to measure pulmonary and intracardiac pressures
    —Echocardiography: to visualize the valves and determine the severity of the insufficiency
    —Electrocardiogram: to detect evidence of past infarction and left ventricular hypertrophy; dysrhythmias
    —Chest x-ray: to identify heart enlargement

TREATMENT
Medical

- Drugs
    —Antibiotics
    —Digitalis
    —Oral anticoagulants
    —Vasodilators
    —Diuretics

Surgical

- Commissurotomy
- Valvuloplasty
- Valvotomy
- Mitral valve replacement

🏠 HOME CARE

- Give both the patient and the caregiver *verbal* and *written* instructions. Provide them with the name and telephone number of a physician or nurse to call if questions arise.
- Use heart models or diagrams to assist in instruction.
- Instruct and prepare the patient for valve replacement as recommended (see p. 635).
- *General information*
  —Discuss the disease process and underlying and contributing factors. Show the patient the location of the affected valve.
- *Warning signs*
  —Review the signs and symptoms of disease progression that should be reported to a physician or nurse.
    Exertional dyspnea
    Orthopnea
    Paroxysmal nocturnal dyspnea
    Fatigue
    Palpitations
    Chest pain
- *Special instructions*
  —Explain the risk of endocarditis, discussing the causes and means of prevention. Tell the patient to alert the dentist or any other medical personnel (urologist, gynecologist) of valve disease.
  —Explain the importance of good oral hygiene and regular dental care. Explain the need for antibiotic prophylaxis before dental care and other invasive procedures (dilation and curettage, cystoscopy) for prevention.
  —Provide female patients with instruction regarding contraception and risk of pregnancy. Emphasize the importance of pregnancy planning.
  —Stress the importance of not smoking or using tobacco products.
- *Medications*
  —Explain the purpose, dosage, schedule, and route of administration of any prescribed drugs, as well as side effects to report to the physician or nurse.
- *Activity*
  —Stress the importance of avoiding strenuous activity.
  —Encourage the patient to discuss allowances and limitations with respect to occupation, recreation, and activities.

—Explain the need for moderate activity.

—Encourage frequent rest periods and avoidance of fatigue.

- *Diet*

  —Discuss the need to restrict salt intake. Explain that further sodium restrictions may be necessary in the presence of heart failure.

FOLLOW-UP CARE AND REFERRALS

- Stress the importance of regular follow-up visits. Make sure the patient has the necessary names and telephone numbers.
- Provide information on and referral to smoking cessation programs as necessary.

Mitral Valve Prolapse

—Mitral valve prolapse: a usually benign condition diagnosed in healthy people. One of the two mitral leaflets is displaced (prolapses) into the atrium during heart systole. In the majority of cases this does not impair valve closure. In rare cases mitral regurgitation results. An estimated 2% to 3% of the population has mitral valve prolapse. Most people are asymptomatic, although some report mild symptoms. The condition occurs in men and women 20 to 40 years of age but is more common in women.

CAUSES

- A primary connective tissue abnormality
- A normal or abnormal variation

SIGNS/SYMPTOMS

- Primarily asymptomatic
- Fatigue
- Palpitations
- Shortness of breath
- Panic attacks
- Anxiety
- Migraine (headache)
- Chest pain

COMPLICATIONS

- Arrhythmias
- Mitral regurgitation
- Endocarditis
- Rupture of chordae tendineae
- Transient ischemic attack or stroke
- Rarely sudden death

DIAGNOSTIC TESTS

- Describe each procedure, its purpose, and the normal feelings or sensations that are likely, as well as any preprocedural and postprocedural care.
    —Echocardiogram: to show how the heart structures move and how large the heart chambers are; to reveal the presence of valve deformities
    —Electrocardiogram: to record how well the heart's electrical system is working; to detect cardiac rhythm abnormalities and to identify cardiac hypertrophy
    —Holter monitor or ambulatory electrocardiogram: to record the heart's activities as the patient follows a normal routine; correlates symptoms with actual cardiac events and the patient's activities
    —Treadmill electrocardiogram recording during exercise: to identify the heart's response to exercise; to diagnose the cause of chest pain and identify cardiac arrhythmias
    —Tilt table test: to check blood pressure and heart rate in an upright and prone position; to identify neurogenic cause of syncope

TREATMENT
Medical

- Drugs
    —Beta blockers: to slow heart rate and prevent headache
    —Calcium channel blockers: to reduce workload of the heart

 HOME CARE

- Give both the patient and the caregiver *verbal* and *written* instructions. Provide them with the name and telephone number of a physician or nurse to call if questions arise.
- Use visual aids or heart models to help the patient understand the location of the mitral valve and its role in the heart function.

- *Warning signs*
  —Review the signs and symptoms associated with this condition and the need to report any change in the condition to a physician or nurse.
- *Special instructions*
  —Describe the condition and explain that in the majority of cases the diagnosis is based on a "clicking" sound heard during a routine examination. Tell the patient that the clicking sound alone in an otherwise asymptomatic person is usually benign and requires no treatment. Provide reassurance that the patient can expect to live a perfectly normal life.
  —Instruct an asymptomatic patient that the disease is not life threatening and that symptoms are usually treated with beta blockers.
  —Provide specific instruction for a patient with mitral regurgitation (see p. 428).
  —Assist the patient to identify precipitating factors of palpitations, anxiety, or panic attacks.
  —Suggest ways of reducing stress levels and practicing relaxation techniques to prevent the occurrence of symptoms.
- *Activity*
  —Inform the patient that full activity is permitted with no restrictions if the patient feels well and does not have significant mitral regurgitation.
- *Diet*
  —Explain that a regular diet can be followed but that patients with palpitations and anxiety should avoid caffeine beverages, alcohol, stimulants, and use of tobacco products.

FOLLOW-UP CARE AND REFERRALS

- Explain to the patient the importance of notifying the dentist, urologist, and gynecologist of mitral valve prolapse only if prescribed by a physician. Generally, asymptomatic patients with simple prolapse are exempt from this notification, but emphasize that the patient should check with the physician for specific instructions. Make sure that the patient has the necessary phone numbers.

Multiple Sclerosis
(Disseminated Sclerosis)

—**Multiple sclerosis: a chronic, progressive neurologic disease characterized by scattered demyelination of nerve fibers in the brain and spinal cord. Multiple sclerosis affects women slightly less often than men, with onset of symptoms commonly occurring between 20 and 40 years of age. The symptoms, severity, duration, and prognosis of multiple sclerosis vary. Remission and exacerbation of symptoms occur with multiple sclerosis. The exact cause is unknown.**

CAUSES/CONTRIBUTING FACTORS/RISK FACTORS

- Autoimmune processes
- Viral infection
- Allergic reactions to infections
- Familial tendencies
- Cool, temperate climates

SIGNS/SYMPTOMS

- Sensory impairment: numbness, tingling, anesthesia, paresthesia, pain
- Loss of joint sensation and proprioception
- Loss of sense of position
- Motor impairment: paresis, paralysis, dragging of foot, spasticity
- Fatigue, especially after a hot bath or shower
- Facial palsy
- Poor coordination: staggering gait, tremors, spasticity of extremities, ataxia (lack of muscle coordination)
- Dizziness
- Visual disturbances: diplopia, blurred vision, optic neuritis (pain with eye movement), decreased visual field, nystagmus, visual clouding
- Slurred speech
- Muscular spasms
- Difficulty chewing and swallowing
- Mental changes: mood swings, depression, euphoria, irritability, inattention, apathy, poor judgment

- Fecal or urinary incontinence or retention
- Impotence

COMPLICATIONS

- Respiratory failure
- Pneumonia
- Neurologic deficits: paralysis
- Urinary tract infections
- Sexual dysfunction
- Contractures

DIAGNOSTIC TESTS

- Describe each procedure, its purpose, and the normal feelings or sensations that are likely, as well as any preprocedural and postprocedural care.
  —Cerebrospinal fluid sampling: to evaluate levels of protein, oligoclonal bands of immunoglobulin G, gamma globulin, and lymphocytes in the cerebrospinal fluid
  —Magnetic resonance imaging: to reveal the presence of plaques and demyelination; the test of choice when multiple sclerosis is suspected
  —Computed tomography scan: to reveal the presence of plaques and demyelination
  —Positron emission tomography: to detect areas of altered cerebral glucose metabolism
  —Evoked potential studies: to evaluate the integrity of certain nerve pathways
  —Electroencephalogram: to assess for abnormal slowing of brain activity

M

TREATMENT
Medical

- Therapy
  —Physical therapy
  —Occupational therapy
  —Rehabilitation
  —Bowel and bladder retraining
  —Speech therapy
  —Nutritional counseling
  —Counseling, including sexual counseling
  —Bed rest during acute exacerbation
  —Assistive devices: braces, walkers, wheelchairs, splints

—Plasmapheresis: to remove antimyelin antibodies; provides short-term improvement only

- Drugs
  —Antiinflammatory agents
  —Pituitary hormones
  —Corticosteroids
  —Muscle relaxants
  —Smooth muscle relaxants or stimulants
  —Beta-adrenergic blockers
  —Antianxiety and antidepression agents
  —Immunosuppressive agents
  —Interferon beta

Surgical

- Peripheral nerve block with rhizotomy or contralateral thalamotomy

HOME CARE

- Give both the patient and the caregiver *verbal* and *written* instructions. Provide the name and telephone number of a physician or nurse to call if questions arise. Use visual aids in instruction.
- *General information*
  —Explain and discuss the development of multiple sclerosis, causes or contributing factors, care, and treatment.
  —Discuss factors that exacerate the symptoms of multiple sclerosis, and emphasize the importance of avoiding them.
    Overexertion
    Extreme hot and cold temperatures, such as with bath water or weather
    Fever
    Emotional stress
    High humidity
    Pregnancy
    Infections
- *Warning signs*
  —Review the signs and symptoms that should be reported to a physician or nurse.
    Disease progression: memory deficits, confusion, disorientation, scanning speech (slow speech with pauses between syllables)

Urinary tract infection: urinary frequency, urgency, retention, or incontinence; suprapubic distention; pain or burning with urination; malodorous urine; cloudy or bloody urine; fever; chills; flank pain

Flu or cold symptoms: fever, chills, fatigue

- *Special instructions*
—Advise the patient to regulate bath water temperature because of the loss of sense of temperature.
—Stress the importance of avoiding persons with upper respiratory infections.
—Assist the patient in obtaining appropriate devices, such as assistive aids for ambulation and self-care. Assist the patient to identify and correct hazards in the home: remove small scatter rugs, arrange furniture to provide a clear pathway, provide rails for support, provide a ramp for wheelchairs.
—Refer the patient to a bladder retraining program. Teach intermittent self-catheterization and Credé maneuver.
—Suggest incontinence pads or garment protectors for incontinence. Advise the patient to establish regular bowel routines.
—Advise the patient to avoid constipation.
—Stress the importance of pregnancy planning for female patients and the need to consult their physician prior to becoming pregnant.

- *Medications*
—Explain the purpose, dosage, schedule, and route of administration of any prescribed drugs, as well as side effects to report to a physician or nurse.

For corticosteroids and adrenocorticotropic hormones: perform and record daily weights; take medication with food, milk, or buffering agents; avoid aspirin or caffeine while taking these medications; do not discontinue medication abruptly; assist the patient to plan a diet high in potassium and low in sodium; provide a list of specific foods that are high in potassium and low in sodium; report anorexia, nausea, muscle weakness (signs and symptoms of potassium deficiency), abrupt weight gain, and black, tarry stools to the physician or nurse.

For baclofen or dantrolene (muscle relaxants): take medications with food, milk, or buffering agents; avoid activities that require alertness; for patients with diabetes mellitus, monitor blood glucose levels and adjust insulin dosage as needed; advise the family to provide assistance and support for ambulation initially after the patient takes medication; advise the patient to avoid exposure to the sun and to use sunscreens when exposure is unavoidable; report fever, jaundice, dark urine, clay-colored stools, and pruritus (signs and symptoms of hepatitis) and severe diarrhea to the physician or nurse.

For cholinergic and anticholinergic agents: suggest sugarless gum or hard candy to relieve mouth dryness; advise slow position changes to prevent dizziness and fainting.

—Stress the importance of not taking over-the-counter medications without consulting the physician.

* *Activity*

—Encourage the patient to discuss allowances and limitations with respect to occupation, recreation, or activities.

—Encourage the patient to resume activities of daily living, work, chores, and recreational activites as tolerated and to take regular rest breaks.

—Stress the importance of avoiding fatigue and overwork.

—Provide diversional activities with planned rest periods.

—Advise the family or caregiver to assist with activities of daily living but to allow independence as much as possible.

—Teach the family or caregiver to support the patient when ambulating.

—Teach the patient to walk with a wide base.

—Instruct the patient to perform stretching exercises and range-of-motion exercises to reduce muscle spasms and tightness.

—Demonstrate range-of-motion exercises to the family or caregiver and instruct them to assist the patient with exercises.

—Instruct the patient and caregiver on proper skin care and positioning if the patient is confined to a bed or wheelchair.

—Advise the patient that sleeping in a prone position may help decrease spasms in hips and knees.

—Discuss the need to avoid factors that may exacerbate symptoms: excessive exertion, infection, fever, exposure to cold, and emotional stress.

- *Diet*
  —Assist the patient to plan a high-fiber diet or a soft, semisolid diet as ordered.
  —Encourage the patient to drink plenty of fluids, up to 3 liters/day, unless contraindicated.

PSYCHOSOCIAL CARE

- Encourage the patient to maintain socialization with significant others.
- Encourage the patient to verbalize anxiety and concerns related to disease, disability, body image changes, and feelings of powerlessness, grief, and loss.
- Encourage the caregiver to verbalize concerns related to disease, disability, and effect on lifestyle.

FOLLOW-UP CARE

- Stress the importance of regular follow-up visits with the physician and physical, occupational, and rehabilitation therapists. Make sure that the patient has the necessary phone numbers.
- Assist the patient to obtain a MedicAlert bracelet and identification card listing diagnosis, medications, and treatment.

REFERRALS

- Refer the patient to a social worker for further support and counseling.
- Refer the patient for psychotherapy.
  —Male: for sexual dysfunction, primarily impotence, caused by multiple sclerosis
  —Female: for birth control and reproductive counseling, since pregnancy may exacerbate symptoms
- Refer to home health or custodial care services, if indicated.
- Assist the patient and caregiver to obtain referral to community resources, local support groups, and the National Multiple Sclerosis Society, 733 3rd Ave., Sixth Floor, New York, NY 10017, (212) 986-3240, (800) 344-4867.

Muscular Dystrophy

—Muscular dystrophy: a hereditary, degenerative neuromuscular disease characterized by chronic, progressive wasting and weakness of the voluntary muscles. In muscular dystrophy, defective muscle cells leak proteins and other molecules. Muscle fibers undergo degenerative changes and are replaced by connective and fatty tissues, which make muscles appear hypertrophic or pseudohypertrophic (varying in size). The different types of muscular dystrophy vary in the age at onset, rate of symptom progression, and clinical manifestations. The types include Duchenne (pseudohypertrophic); limb-girdle; facioscapulohumeral; myotonic; and Becker. Muscular dystrophy occurs more commonly in males than females and affects both children and young adults.

SIGNS/SYMPTOMS
- Hypertrophied muscles
- Progressive, bilateral weakness of voluntary muscles
- Difficulty walking, running, or climbing stairs
- Waddling gait
- Difficulty raising from supine position
- Lordosis
- Weakness of facial, neck, oropharyngeal, shoulder, or pelvic girdle muscles
- Mental retardation

COMPLICATIONS
- Neuromuscular deficits
- Cardiac failure
- Respiratory failure
- Infections: pneumonia, urinary tract

DIAGNOSTIC TESTS
- Describe each procedure, its purpose, and the normal feelings or sensations that are likely, as well as any preprocedural and postprocedural care.
    - Serum creatine kinase: to detect marked elevation
    - Electromyography: to detect myopathic changes

—Muscle biopsy: to detect degenerative and myopathic changes

—Electrocardiogram: to detect changes in cardiac musculature as disease progresses

TREATMENT
Medical

* Therapy
  —Physical therapy
  —Assistive devices, such as ambulation aids
  —Muscle stretching and resistive exercises

🏠 HOME CARE

* Give both the patient and the caregiver *verbal* and *written* instructions. Provide them with the name and telephone number of a physician or nurse to call if questions arise. Use visual aids in instruction.
* *General information*
  —Explain and discuss the progression of muscular dystrophy, causes, management of progressive disabilities, and steps to take to prevent them. Explain that there is no cure for muscular dystrophy; interventions are supportive.
* *Warning signs*
  —Review the signs and symptoms that should be reported to a physician or nurse.
      Difficulty chewing or swallowing
      Cardiac or respiratory distress
* *Special instructions*
  —Assist the patient in obtaining appropriate devices, such as aids for ambulation and self-care activities.
  —Assist the patient to identify adaptations in the home environment, such as bed trapezes, handrails, raised toilet seats, and widened doorways and ramps for wheelchairs.
  —Instruct the patient and family on proper skin care and positioning, if the patient is confined to a bed or wheelchair.
  —Provide instruction in pain management techniques to deal with chronic pain: visualization, guided imagery, meditation, relaxation, and biofeedback.
* *Medications*
  —Explain the purpose, dosage, schedule, and route of administration of any prescribed drugs, as well as side effects to report to a physician or nurse.

M

- *Activity*
  —Encourage the patient to discuss allowances and limitations with respect to occupation, recreation, or activities.
  —Stress the importance of performing stretching and resistive exercises to preserve range of motion, prevent or minimize contractures, decrease atrophy, and promote mobility.
  —Instruct the patient to avoid moving a joint beyond the point of resistance.
  —Instruct the patient to avoid applying force; movements should be gentle and slow.
  —Instruct the patient to stop exercises when feeling pain.
  —Teach the patient to avoid factors that increase spasticity: fatigue, tightening of muscles, maintaining a position too long, cold temperatures.
  —Explain that physical inactivity may contribute to weight gain.
- *Diet*
  —Assist the patient to plan a balanced diet with fruits, vegetables, milk, poultry, and fish.
  —Advise smaller, frequent meals.

PSYCHOSOCIAL CARE

- Assist the patient to establish realistic goals and identify alternative methods for communication and mobility when physical disabilities increase.
- Encourage the patient to verbalize anxiety and concerns related to disease, disability, loss of mobility, body image changes, and feelings of grief.
- Encourage the caregiver to avoid overprotectiveness.
- Encourage decision making and promote independence in the patient.
- Encourage the caregiver to verbalize concerns related to disease, disability, and effect on lifestyle.

FOLLOW-UP CARE

- Stress the importance of regular follow-up visits with the physician and physical, occupational, and rehabilitation therapists. Make sure that the patient has the necessary phone numbers.
- Assist the patient to obtain a MedicAlert bracelet and identification card listing diagnosis, medications, and treatment.

REFERRALS

- Refer the patient to a social worker for further support and counseling, if appropriate.
- Assist the patient and caregiver to obtain referral to community resources, local support groups, home health care, custodial care services, and the Muscular Dystrophy Association (see Appendix F).
- Refer the patient and caregiver to genetic counseling so that familial carriers of the gene can be identified and affected infants can be identified in utero via amniocentesis.

Myasthenia Gravis

—**Myasthenia gravis: an autoimmune neuromuscular disease that produces sporadic but progressive weakness exacerbated by exercise and improved by rest and anticholinergic drugs. Myasthenia gravis is a chronic disorder that follows an unpredictable course of recurring exacerbation and remission. No cure is known. Myasthenia gravis occurs as a result of loss of the acetylcholine receptors at the postsynaptic neuromuscular junction. Although it may occur at any age, between 20 and 40 years women are more commonly affected and after 50 years men are more commonly affected.**

M

SIGNS/SYMPTOMS

- Eye muscles
  - —Ocular palsy
  - —Ptosis (unilateral or bilateral)
  - —Diplopia
- Facial muscles
  - —Masklike expression and mobility (weakness) of face
  - —Weak voice that may fade to a whisper
  - —Dysphagia
  - —Choking
  - —Aspiration, impaired swallowing
  - —Drooling
  - —Nasal speech

- Neck muscles
  —Head bobbing up and down
- Respiratory muscles
  —Shallow respirations
  —Breathlessness
  —Respiratory weakness
- Other muscles
  —Stress incontinence
  —Anal sphincter weakness
  —Sexual impairment
  —Muscle weakness
- *Myasthenic crisis:* rapid or significant worsening of ocular, bulbar, and generalized weakness; urgent threat is to the respiratory system; may require mechanical ventilatory support
  —Respiratory distress
  —Tachycardia
  —Tachypnea
  —Generalized muscular weakness
  —Extreme fatigue
  —Anxiety
  —Restlessness
  —Irritability
  —Facial weakness
  —Dysphagia
  —Inability to chew
  —Elevated temperature
  —Ptosis
  —Speech impairment
  —Hypertension
- *Cholinergic crisis:* secondary to overmedication in relation to muscular requirement; may mimic myasthenic crisis; *only* cholinergic crisis will produce excessive drooling and twitching or cramping of muscles
  —Respiratory distress
  —Vertigo
  —Blurred vision
  —Sweating
  —Lacrimation
  —Salivation
  —Anorexia
  —Dysarthria
  —Dysphasia

—Abdominal cramps, diarrhea
—Nausea and vomiting
—Muscular spasms or cramps
—Generalized muscle weakness
—Dyspnea and wheezing
—Bradycardia
—Hypotension

COMPLICATIONS

- Myasthenic crisis and cholinergic crisis
- Aspiration of secretions, choking
- Pneumonia
- Respiratory failure

DIAGNOSTIC TESTS

- Describe each procedure, its purpose, and the normal feelings or sensations that are likely, as well as any preprocedural and postprocedural care.
  —Edrophonium (Tensilon) test: injection produces a sudden improvement in muscle function; also used to differentiate a myasthenic crisis from a cholinergic crisis (worsens if crisis is cholinergic)
  —Electromyography: to differentiate nerve disorders
  —Nerve conduction studies: to measure the speed at which electrical impulses travel along a nerve
  —Chest x-ray or computed tomography scan: to identify a thymoma
  —Cerebrospinal fluid protein levels: elevated as disease progresses
  —Serum: acetylcholine receptor antibody (anti-AChR) may be elevated

TREATMENT

- Appropriate health care is usually on an outpatient basis, with the inpatient setting used for myasthenic or cholinergic crisis. Medical management of myasthenia gravis is difficult and best handled by a specialist in that field. It is important to be alert for myasthenic crisis and cholinergic crisis, which may often be quite difficult to differentiate, and which can be made dramatically worse by overmedication.
- Establish an accurate neurologic and repiratory baseline: tidal volume, vital capacity, and inspiratory force.

Medical

- Therapy
    —Plasmapheresis: done before thymectomy, during a respiratory crisis, or as an adjunct treatment to reduce drug dosages
- Drugs
    —Cholinergic agents: pyridostigmine (Mestinon)
    —Corticosteroids

Surgical

- Thymectomy

HOME CARE

- Give both the patient and the caregiver *verbal* and *written* instructions. Provide them with the name and telephone number of a physician or nurse to call if questions arise.
- *General information*
    —Discuss and describe the disease process and factors that can exacerbate symptoms: infection, stress, and surgery.
- *Warning signs*
    —Review the signs and symptoms of impending myasthenic or cholinergic crisis (see above; primarily increased muscle weakness, respiratory distress, difficulty talking and chewing) that should be reported to a physician or nurse.
- *Special instructions*
    —Assure the patient that an experienced myasthenia gravis patient is often the best judge of his or her treatment requirements.
    —Advise and assist the patient in obtaining necessary supportive equipment and devices as the disease advances (e.g., suctioning equipment, adaptive devices).
    —Advise the patient to use an eye patch over the affected eye or a frosted lens to improve vision if diplopia persists.
    —Instruct the patient with ptosis to apply artificial tears to keep the corneas moist and free of abrasions.
- *Medications*
    —Explain the purpose, dosage, schedule, and route of administration of any prescribed drugs, as well as side effects to report to a physician or nurse.
    —Teach the patient to recognize adverse effects of cholinergic drugs: headache, weakness, sweating, abdominal cramps, nausea, vomiting, excessive salivation, and bronchospasm.

—Teach the patient to recognize adverse effects of corticoste-roids: decreased or blurred vision; increased thirst; frequent urination; rectal bleeding, burning, and itching; restlessness; depression.

- *Activity*
  —Advise the patient to plan daily activities to coincide with energy peaks, which usually occur in the morning or after a nap.
  —Stress the importance of rest periods throughout the day.
  —Advise the patient to avoid strenuous exercise, stress, infection, needless exposure to the sun or cold weather, and exposure to people with infections (e.g., upper respiratory infections).
  —Explain that periodic remissions, exacerbations, and day-to-day fluctuations are common.

- *Diet*
  —Discuss swallowing precautions. Teach the patient that as swallowing becomes more difficult, soft, semisolid foods (applesauce, mashed potatoes) instead of liquids will lessen the risk of choking and eating warm (not hot) foods can ease swallowing. Instruct the patient to eat slowly, cut food into small pieces, and chew thoroughly.
  —Advise the patient to avoid alcohol because it increases weakness.

PSYCHOSOCIAL CARE

- Stress the importance of psychologic support. Encourage the patient to verbalize concerns, fears, and feelings about the disease process.

FOLLOW-UP CARE

- Stress the importance of regular follow-up visits. Make sure that the patient has the necessary phone numbers.
- Assist the patient to obtain a MedicAlert bracelet and identification card listing diagnosis, medications, and treatment.

REFERRALS

- Provide information for home health, social services, and physical therapy referrals as indicated.
- Encourage contact with a national support group and provide the following address for the patient to obtain printed materials

and other forms of family support information: Myasthenia Gravis Foundation, 123 W. Madison Ave., Suite 800, Chicago, IL 60602, (312) 853-0522. The Muscular Dystrophy Association is the umbrella organization for myasthenia gravis research and can provide materials and clinical services. Their address is: Muscular Dystrophy Association, 3300 E. Sunrise Drive, Tucson, AZ 85718-3208, (800) 572-1717.

Myelogram

—**Myelogram: study in which contrast material is injected through a lumbar or cisternal puncture to visualize the spinal canal and nerve roots. Myelography aids in the diagnosis of spinal stenosis or obstruction within the spinal canal caused by a ruptured or herniated nucleus pulposus. The entire canal from lumbar to cervical area can be examined. The *myelogram* is a roentgenographic procedure in which a needle is inserted into a disk space below the spinal cord and 2 to 15 ml of spinal fluid is removed. A contrast solution or air is injected and distributed to the various tissues and structures to be examined, and x-rays are taken frequently. Flow of the solution depends on the tilt of the table and patient position. With the needle in place, the patient is placed in the prone position on a tilt table with the head down. A foot support and shoulder brace or harness keeps the patient from sliding. Fluoroscopy shows flow of the contrast solution. The procedure takes 45 minutes and requires that the patient be positioned on the stomach on a tilt table to permit flow of the dye. In a *computed tomography myelogram* a water-soluble contrast material is instilled into the subarachnoid space. Films are taken at the time of contrast injection and followed by computed tomography scan of the appropriate regions. This procedure is particularly useful in cervical spondylosis in which magnetic resonance imaging may not demonstrate detail of an osteophyte or herniated disk.**

INDICATIONS

- Severe back pain
- Localized signs and symptoms of spinal cord injury or disease

PREPROCEDURAL TEACHING

- Review the physician's explanation of the procedure and the reason for it; encourage the patient to ask questions and to discuss any fears or anxieties. Explain the need for informed consent.

Review of Preprocedural Care

- Identify any possible allergies, particularly to iodine.
- Verify the list of current medications; tell the patient to stop anticoagulants at the appropriate time as determined by the physician.
- Review laboratory tests: complete blood count, prothrombin time/international normalized ratio (INR) if the patient has previously received anticoagulation therapy.
- Explain the need to avoid phenothiazines, tricyclic antidepressants, central nervous system stimulants, and amphetamines, which could decrease the seizure threshold.
- Inform the patient of the need to have no food or fluids for 4 hours before the procedure.
- Discuss the type of contrast material that will be used, and explain that a patient receiving water-soluble contrast material should be well hydrated.
- Inform the patient that baseline vital signs and neurologic assessment will be performed.
- Explain that the patient will be tilted into an up-and-down position on a table so that the dye can properly fill the spinal canal and provide adequate visualization of the desired area.
- Instruct the patient to empty the bladder and bowel before the procedure.
- Explain the importance of lying still during the procedure.

Review of Postprocedural Care

- Explain that after the procedure the patient will be closely monitored for 24 hours or until discharge for signs of meningeal irritation or seizure activity.
- Tell the patient that vital signs and neurologic status will be checked every 30 minutes for 2 hours, every 60 minutes for the next 2 hours, and every 4 hours for the next 24 hours.

M

- Discuss the need for proper positioning after the procedure.
  —If air myelography is done, the patient is positioned with the head lower than the trunk to prevent air from gravitating to the cerebral space and causing headaches. This position should be maintained for 48 hours to allow absorption of the air. Then the head is elevated.
  —If water-soluble contrast material is used, the patient is positioned upright at a 30- to 45-degree angle for 12 hours; then bed rest upright or flat is maintained for 12 hours.
  —If oil-based contrast material is used, the patient is kept flat for 8 to 12 hours.
- Explain that there will be pain at the puncture site.

SIDE EFFECTS/COMPLICATIONS

- Headache
- Herniation of the brain
- Meningitis
- Seizures
- Allergic reaction to iodinated dye: mild flushing, itching, urticaria, life-threatening anaphylaxis

HOME CARE

- Give both the patient and the caregiver *verbal* and *written* instructions. Provide them with the name and telephone number of a physician or nurse to call if questions arise.
- *General information*
  —Review the physician's explanation of the procedure and any initial findings.
- *Warning signs*
  —Review the signs and symptoms that should be reported to a physician or nurse.
    Meningeal irritation: fever, stiff neck, occipital headache, photophobia
    Nausea and vomiting
    Severe headache
    Change in level of consciousness
    Seizure activity
- *Special instructions*
  —Advise the patient to lower the bed to the flat position to relieve a headache; inform the patient that mild analgesics may be ordered for persistent pain.

—Advise the patient not to take phenothiazines for nausea and vomiting; these agents can increase symptoms of toxicity.

—Explain the need to increase fluid intake to enhance excretion of the dye and to replace cerebrospinal fluid, if not contraindicated.

Myocarditis

—**Myocarditis: an inflammatory process of the myocardium affecting portions or all of the heart muscle. It may be acute or chronic and affects persons of any age. Recovery is usually complete, but the disease may cause myofibril disarray and myocyte necrosis, leading to ventricular failure. Myocarditis may be uncomplicated and self-limiting.**

CAUSES

- Viral infections
- Bacterial infections
- Rheumatic fever
- Postcardiotomy syndrome
- Radiation therapy
- Chemical poisons, such as alcohol
- Environmental toxins including lead, arsenic, and carbon monoxide
- Parasitic infections
- Collagen vascular disease

SIGNS/SYMPTOMS

- Fatigue
- Myalgias
- Dyspnea
- Palpitations
- Fever
- Chest pain

COMPLICATIONS

- Dilated cardiomyopathy
- Arrhythmias

- Thromboembolism
- Congestive heart failure

DIAGNOSTIC TESTS

- Describe each procedure, its purpose, and the normal feelings or sensations that are likely, as well as any preprocedural and postprocedural care.
  —Blood tests
      Cardiac enzymes and troponin I
      Elevated antibody titers
      Elevated cardiac isoenzymes
      White blood cells
      Erythrocyte sedimentation rate
  —Cultures: throat, stool
  —Electrocardiogram
  —Echocardiography
  —Endomyocardial biopsy
  —Chest x-ray

TREATMENT
Medical

- Therapy
  —Treatment of underlying infection
  —Bed rest: to decrease myocardial oxygen demand
- Drugs
  —Digoxin
  —Vasodilators
  —Angiotensin-converting enzyme inhibitors
  —Antibiotics
  —Anticoagulants

HOME CARE

- Give both the patient and the caregiver *verbal* and *written* instructions. Provide them with the name and telephone number of a physician or nurse to call if questions arise.
- *General information*
  —Review the disease process, explaining the cause and prescribed treatment. Explain that medical treatment is aimed at treating the underlying cause and preventing and treating complications.

- *Warning signs*
  - —Review the signs and symptoms that should be reported to a physician or nurse.
    - Chest pain that persists and is unrelated to exertion
    - Shortness of breath at rest, on exertion, or at night
    - Swelling of feet or ankles
    - Palpitations
- *Medications*
  - —Explain the purpose, dosage, schedule, and route of administration of any prescribed drugs, as well as side effects to report to a physician or nurse.
  - —Review the symptoms of digitalis toxicity if the patient is discharged with a prescription for digitalis.
- *Activity*
  - —Instruct the patient to restrict activities and to resume normal activities slowly or as directed to reduce work of the heart and promote healing.
  - —Tell the patient to take regular rest periods during the day.
  - —Stress the importance of avoiding physical exertion and competitive sports.
  - —Advise the patient not to exercise or do demanding physical activities when a cold, flu, or other infection is present.
- *Diet*
  - —Instruct the patient to follow a low-salt diet, especially if the patient has signs of heart failure (see Heart Failure, p. 333).
  - —Instruct the patient to avoid alcohol.

FOLLOW-UP CARE AND REFERRALS

- Stress the importance of regular follow-up visits. Make sure that the patient has the necessary phone numbers.

Nephrectomy

—**Nephrectomy: surgical removal of part or all of a kidney. *Radical nephrectomy,* usually done for a malignant tumor, is removal of the entire kidney, surrounding tissue and fat, adrenal gland, part of the ureter, and the lymph nodes.**

INDICATIONS

- Malignant tumor
- Polycystic kidney disease
- Donation of a kidney
- Trauma
- Large stones
- Hydronephrosis
- Congenital deformity
- Chronic pyelonephritis
- Vascular disease or narrowed renal arteries

PREPROCEDURAL TEACHING

- Review the physician's explanation of the procedure and the reason for it; encourage the patient to ask questions and to discuss any fears or anxieties. Explain the need for informed consent for surgery, anesthesia, and blood transfusion.

Review of Preprocedural Care

- Explain that hospital admission may be on the day of surgery.
- Review the preoperative tests that may be performed.
  —Chest x-ray and electrocardiogram
  —Blood tests: complete blood count, electrolytes, coagulation studies, tissue compatibility tests
  —Urine studies: urinalysis, culture and sensitivity, creatinine clearance
  —Intravenous pyelography
  —Urogram
  —Renal angiography (see box on p. 455)
- Inform the patient that a cleansing enema (e.g., Fleet) will be performed the night before the procedure.
- Discuss the need for a shower and shampoo with bactericidal soap (Safeguard, Dial, Hibiclens) the night before or morning of the procedure.
- Explain that the skin over the abdomen and flank may be shaved before surgery.
- Explain the need for nothing by mouth (NPO) status from midnight of the night before.
- Review the possibility of renal angiography (see box on p. 455) before surgery to decrease bleeding during and after surgery.

RENAL ANGIOGRAPHY

Renal angiography evaluates the status of both kidneys. Under local anesthesia a small catheter is inserted through a needle in the groin and is threaded up to the renal artery under fluoroscopy. Contrast medium is injected while x-ray pictures are obtained. The patient may feel a flushing sensation, a "funny taste" in the mouth, or nausea when the contrast medium is injected, but the symptoms pass quickly. After removal of the catheter, a pressure dressing is applied and a sandbag is placed. The patient must lie still for several hours before being allowed to leave. Further instructions include no heavy lifting (>10 pounds) and no strenuous exercise for several days. The test is performed on an outpatient basis.

Review of Postprocedural Care

- See posteroperative care under Abdominal Surgery, p. 6.
- Tell the patient that the hospital stay after surgery will be 3 to 5 days.
- Stress the importance of turning, coughing, and deep breathing.
- Discuss the purpose of the incentive spirometer and demonstrate its use.
- Explain the purpose of wearing thigh-high elastic compression stockings and alternating pressure stockings while in bed.
- Emphasize the importance of getting out of bed (usually the second day) and moving about.
- Explain that drainage tubes may be needed after surgery and describe the various possibilities: chest tube, nasogastric tube, urinary drainage tube from bladder, nephrostomy tube from kidney through flank, Penrose drain from incisional area.
- Explain the need for frequent dressings soon after the procedure.
- Inform the patient that the urine will be blood colored (bright red) but will become normal appearing in several days.
- Discuss the need for pain relief medication and antibiotics.

SIDE EFFECTS/COMPLICATIONS

- Hemorrhage and shock
- Infection
- Atelectasis
- Pneumonia

HOME CARE

- Give both the patient and the caregiver *verbal* and *written* instructions. Provide them with the name and telephone number of a physician or nurse to call if questions arise.
- *General information*
  —Review the purpose and explain the type of procedure performed: partial or total nephrectomy.
  —If the nephrectomy is total, prepare the patient for dialysis (see p. 674).
- *Wound/incision care*
  —Instruct the patient on caring for the incision and changing the dressing.
    Wash hands.
    Inspect the incision for signs of infection.
    Cleanse the area with Betadine.
    If there is no evidence of drainage, leave the site open to the air. Otherwise, cover the incision with sterile gauze squares held in place with tape.
    If Steri-Strips were used, do not remove them; allow them to drop off.
  —Teach the patient how to care for the nephrostomy tube, if present.
- *Special instructions*
  —Inform the patient that showering and bathing may be resumed as recommended by the physician.
  —Explain how to measure urine output as indicated.
- *Warning signs*
  —Review the signs and symptoms that should be reported to a physician or nurse.
    Infection: incision red, warm to touch, painful, with increased or purulent drainage
    Urinary tract infection: fever, chills, hematuria, flank pain, sudden increase in urinary output
- *Activity*
  —Discuss the need to exercise to tolerance and to plan frequent rest periods. Explain that fatigue is common.

—Encourage the patient to discuss allowances and limitations with respect to occupation, recreation, and activities.

—Tell the patient to avoid heavy lifting (>10 pounds) for at least 6 weeks.

—Advise the patient to avoid contact sports (e.g., wrestling, football) that could endanger the remaining kidney.

- *Diet*

—Inform the patient that a regular diet can be followed unless there are restrictions related to the underlying reason for the nephrectomy.

—Encourage the patient to drink 8 to 10 glasses of fluids per day unless restrictions of the underlying disease apply.

FOLLOW-UP CARE

- Stress the importance of regular follow-up visits. Make sure the patient has the necessary names and telephone numbers.

Neurogenic Bladder

—Neurogenic bladder: dysfunctional bladder caused by interruption of normal bladder innervation as a result of lesions or injuries. Types of neurogenic bladder dysfunction include reduced bladder capacity, no control of urination, and decreased perception of bladder fullness.

CONTRIBUTING FACTORS

- Spinal cord injury or tumor
- Stroke
- Brain tumor
- Parkinson's disease
- Multiple sclerosis
- Alzheimer's disease
- Aging
- Diabetes mellitus and resultant peripheral innervation
- Chronic alcoholism
- Systemic lupus erythematosus

- Heavy metal toxicity (e.g., mercury)
- Vascular disease
- Herpes zoster

SIGNS/SYMPTOMS
- Urinary frequency, dribbling
- Voiding in small amounts
- Overflow incontinence
- Reduced bladder capacity
- Loss of reflex to urinate
- Loss of sensation of bladder fullness
- Inability to empty the bladder completely (residual urine)

COMPLICATIONS
- Urinary tract infection
- Dysreflexia (associated with spinal cord injuries)
- Urinary tract stones
- Total incontinence
- Septic shock

DIAGNOSTIC TESTS
- Describe each procedure, its purpose, and the normal feelings or sensations that are likely, as well as any preprocedural and postprocedural care (see Urinary Incontinence, p. 749).

TREATMENT
Medical
- Therapy
  —Hydration: to prevent infection and stone formation
  —Bladder training: Credé's method, Kegel exercises
  —Urinary catheterization: intermittent or continuous
  —Reflex triggering techniques: timed voiding
- Drugs
  —For underlying cause

Surgical
- Implantation of artificial urinary sphincter
- Implantation of neuroprosthetics (bladder pacemaker)
- Continent vesicostomy: surgical closure of the urethra at the bladder junction and an artificial opening made to the outside; a special valve is in place to allow the client to self-catheterize (see Urinary Diversion, p. 740)

☷☷ HOME CARE

- Give both the patient and the caregiver *verbal* and *written* instructions. Provide them with the name and telephone number of a physician or nurse to call if questions arise.
- *General information*
  —Explain the factors contributing to the disorder.
- *Warning signs*
  —Review the signs, symptoms, and problems that should be reported to a physician or nurse.

  > Urinary tract infection: fever, chills, flank pain
  > Kidney stones: acute colicky pain in the flank or lower abdomen
  > Problems with the indwelling catheter (see Urinary Catheter, p. 736)
  > Mechanical malfunction

  —Review the signs and symptoms of autonomic dysreflexia, explaining that it may be life threatening if not corrected and that it is usually caused by a distended bladder, fecal impaction, a full rectum, or sexual stimulation.

  > Headache
  > Decrease (<60) or increase (>100) in heart rate
  > High blood pressure (>140/90 mm Hg)
  > Blurred vision
  > "Gooseflesh" and pallor below the level of the spinal injury
  > Cold sweat of the head and neck
  > Metallic taste in the mouth
  > Nasal congestion
  > Paresthesia (numbness, tingling, prickling, increased sensitivity)

- *Special instructions*
  —Discuss and demonstrate bladder training programs (see Urinary Incontinence, p. 749).
  —Advise the patient on how and where to obtain supplies.
  —Explain how to avoid autonomic dysreflexia by setting up a schedule for emptying the bladder (or rectum) and maintaining free flow of urine through the tubing.
  —Explain how to recognize the signs of bladder distention by visually inspecting the bladder area, feeling the bladder, and tapping the bladder area. The bladder area will be swollen

N

and feel like a full balloon. Tapping it with the fingertips will produce a kettle drum sound and may cause dribbling.

—Demonstrate Credé's method to assist in emptying of the bladder. Tell the patient to place the outside part of the hand against the abdomen right below the umbilicus and bear down as if having a bowel movement until urination starts. The patient may have to do this several times before urination begins. When urination starts, the motion should be continued every 30 seconds until urine flow stops.

—Review the techique for intermittent or indwelling catheterization (see Urinary Catheter, p. 736).

—Explain the option of an external condom catheter for men (see Urinary Incontinence, p. 749).

—Review the instructions for the care of implanted mechanical devices and explain the signs and symptoms of malfunction or infection.

Wound infection or erosion at the bulb site: redness, tenderness, warmth, purulent drainage

Problems with the artificial sphincter: urinary tract infection, urinary retention or incontinence, pain, swelling, fever, blood in urine

Pacemaker malfunction: bladder does not empty

- *Medications*
  —Explain the purpose, dosage, schedule, and route of administration of any prescribed drugs, as well as side effects to report to a physician or nurse.
- *Activity*
  —Encourage the patient to verbalize concerns about changes in lifestyle imposed by the disorder. Encourage questions about allowances and limitations with respect to occupation, recreation, and sports.
- *Diet*
  —Explain that a regular diet or one prescribed by the physician for the underlying disease should be followed.
  —Advise the patient to reduce calcium intake and increase fluids to prevent the formation of renal calculi.

FOLLOW-UP CARE

- Stress the importance of regular follow-up visits. Make sure that the patient has the necessary phone numbers.

• Assist the patient to obtain a MedicAlert bracelet and identification card listing diagnosis, medications, and treatment.

REFERRALS

• Provide information on home health referrals as indicated.
• Assist the patient to obtain psychologic support.

Orchiectomy

—Orchiectomy: surgical removal of one (unilateral) or both (bilateral) testes.

INDICATIONS

• Prostate cancer
• Testicular cancer
• Trauma

PREPROCEDURAL TEACHING

• Review the physician's explanation of the procedure and the reason for it. Discuss the need for informed consent for surgery and anesthesia. Encourage the patient to ask questions and to discuss fears or anxieties about loss of sexual function and manhood.
• Explain that fertility may be affected and provide the patient with information on sperm banking.

Review of Preprocedural Care

• Explain that the patient is usually admitted on the day of surgery and stays overnight after the procedure.
• Review preprocedural diagnostic tests.
  —Alpha-fetoprotein (AFP) and human chorionic gonadotropin (HCG) for tumor markers
  —Pregnancy test for certain types and stages of tumors
  —Intravenous pyelogram and urogram
  —Radionuclide imaging
  —Lymphangiogram: injection of contrast dye into the lymph vessels to determine blockage

- Inform the patient that he will be asked to shower and shampoo with bactericidal soap (Safeguard, Dial, Hibiclens) the night before or morning of the procedure.
- Explain the need for nothing by mouth (NPO) status from the night before the procedure.
- Discuss the possibility that the pubic hair will be shaved.

Review of Postprocedural Care

- Explain that analgesics and antiemetics will be administered as needed.
- Stress the importance of turning, coughing and deep breathing, and getting out of bed and moving about.
- Demonstrate use of the incentive spirometer.
- Explain that a scrotal support will be used to relieve pain and scrotal swelling; the scrotum will be elevated on a towel roll and an ice pack may be applied. Tell the patient that the pain usually lasts 24 to 48 hours.
- Advise the patient to avoid sitting for long periods, since this increases scrotal swelling.

SIDE EFFECTS/COMPLICATIONS

- Persistent pain
- Swelling
- Hemorrhage
- Wound infection
- Infertility

HOME CARE

- Give both the patient and the caregiver *verbal* and *written* instructions. Provide them with the name and telephone number of a physician or nurse to call if questions arise.
- Prepare the patient for chemotherapy (see p. 667) or radiation therapy (see p. 721), if ordered.
- *General information*
  —Review the procedure that was performed: unilateral (diseased testis removed, scrotum left intact) or bilateral orchiectomy. Discuss the underlying reason for the procedure (see Testicular Cancer, p. 604, or Prostate Cancer, p. 520).
  —For unilateral orchiectomy, explain that the scrotum is left intact so reconstructive surgery (placement of a gel-filled

testicular implant) can be done later, that sexual function resumes once the incision is healed, that monthly testicular self-examination of the remaining testis is important, and that one healthy testis can compensate for loss of function of the other so male characteristics are not affected.

—For bilateral orchiectomy, explain that the procedure is usually done for testicular cancer, that it renders the male sterile and will cause impotence if the nerves or vasculature is damaged, and that synthetic hormones may be given to replace male hormones. Provide information on impotence (see Erectile Dysfunction, p. 278).

- *Wound/incision care*
  —Demonstrate care of the surgical wound and dressing changes as needed. Explain that the dressing can be placed over the incision and held by the scrotal support.
- *Warning signs*
  —Review the signs and symptoms that should be reported to a physician or nurse.
  Difficulty urinating or inability to urinate
  Severe or persistent pain
  Wound infection: redness, warmth, tenderness, purulent drainage, fever, chills
  Nausea and vomiting
  Appearance of a mass in the opposite testicle, inguinal area, or neck
- *Medications*
  —Explain the purpose, dosage, schedule, and route of administration of any prescribed drugs, as well as side effects to report to a physician or nurse.
- *Activity*
  —Encourage the patient to discuss allowances and limitations with respect to occupation, recreation, and activities.
  —Instruct the patient to plan frequent rest periods, gradually increasing activity as tolerated. Tell him that normal activity can usually resume within 1 week.
  —Advise the patient to avoid stair climbing and sitting for long (more than 2-hour) periods.
  —Suggest that the patient avoid lifting more than 10 pounds, working or exercising strenuously, or playing contact sports for the period of time specified by the physician.

* *Diet*
    —Inform the patient that he may follow a regular diet unless the physician has prescribed a special one.

PSYCHOSOCIAL CARE

* Encourage the patient to verbalize his feelings about perceived or actual changes in body image, sense of loss of manhood, fear of losing sexual function, and feminization.

FOLLOW-UP CARE

* Stress the importance of regular follow-up visits. Make sure the patient has the necessary names and telephone numbers.

REFERRALS

* Provide information about reproduction and fertility as needed, and refer the patient to medical or community-based counseling.

Osteomalacia

—Osteomalacia: a metabolic disease characterized by loss of mineralization of bones, resulting in softening, brittleness, and deformity. Similar to rickets in children, osteomalacia occurs when vitamin D deficiency leads to reduced absorption of phosphorus and calcium. Weight-bearing bones such as those in the spine, pelvis, and lower extremities are mostly affected and are prone to fractures. The elderly and women are at highest risk.

CONTRIBUTING FACTORS

* Inadequate dietary intake of vitamin D
* Calcium deficiency
* Lack of sun exposure
* Defective metabolism of vitamin D
* Intestinal malabsorption of vitamin D
    —Liver disease

—Hypoparathyroidism
—Small intestinal disease
- Chronic renal failure
- Chronic anticonvulsant therapy

SIGNS/SYMPTOMS

- Abnormal bowing and bending of long bones and vertebral column
- Bone pain and limb tenderness
- Muscle weakness and cramps
- Decreased joint range of motion
- Generalized weakness, malaise, fatigue

COMPLICATIONS

- Degenerative joint disease
- Bone deformities
- Bone fractures

DIAGNOSTIC TESTS

- Describe each procedure, its purpose, and the normal feelings or sensations that are likely, as well as any preprocedural and postprocedural care.
    —Blood tests: serum calcium, serum alkaline phosphatase, vitamin D, sedimentation rate
    —X-rays: to identify calcification of bones, fractures
    —Bone biopsy: to show excessive uncalcified bone

TREATMENT
Medical

- Therapy
    —Adjunctive therapy
    —Diet therapy: high calcium, high phosphorus
    —Physical therapy
- Drugs
    —Vitamin D replacement
    —Calcium supplements
    —Analgesics

Surgical

- Fracture repair as indicated

🏠 HOME CARE

- Give both the patient and the caregiver *verbal* and *written* instructions. Provide them with the name and telephone number of a physician or nurse to call if questions arise.
- *General information*
  —Discuss the disorder, explaining the role that vitamin D plays in calcium and phosphorus absorption, which is required for bone calcification.
  —Review the sources of vitamin D: diet, vitamin supplements, exposure to ultraviolet light. Explain that sunlight is a good source of vitamin D formation.
  —Discuss avoiding the use of aluminum-containing antacids because aluminum prevents absorption of phosphate.
- *Warning signs*
  —Review the signs and symptoms that should be reported to a physician or nurse.
    Increase in or sudden appearance of bone or joint pain
- *Special instructions*
  —Discuss ways to prevent injury through maintenance of a safe environment: side rails; nonskid surfaces; clean, dry floors; adequate lighting.
- *Medications*
  —Explain the purpose, dosage, schedule, and route of administration of any prescribed drugs, as well as side effects to report to the physician or nurse.
  —Advise the patient to watch for and report any signs of vitamin D toxicity: headache, nausea, diarrhea, renal calculi.
- *Activity*
  —Encourage the patient to discuss allowances and limitations with respect to occupation, recreation, and activities.
  —Advise the patient on the use of ambulatory assistance devices such as a cane or crutches to lessen strain and load on weak bones and joints. Assist the patient to obtain the equipment.
  —Encourage and instruct the patient in range-of-motion and muscle-strengthening exercises to help maintain muscle strength and joint mobility.
  —Discuss the exercise regimen for retaining calcium in bones: isometric and resistive.
  —Advise the patient to be careful when doing activities that could lead to strain, severe stress, and fractures (e.g., rising from a chair, deep bending, exercising).

—Discuss the need to avoid activities that can cause injury (e.g., bowling and horseback riding, which can cause vertebral decompression).
- *Diet*
  —Discuss the importance of increasing dietary calcium and vitamin D through foods such as dairy products, egg yolks, tuna, liver oil, and salmon. Refer the patient to a dietitian for assistance with meal planning.

FOLLOW-UP CARE AND REFERRALS

- Stress the importance of regular follow-up visits. Make sure the patient has the necessary names and telephone numbers.
- Provide referrals to home health care, a skilled nursing facility, or a medical social worker as indicated.

Osteomyelitis

—Osteomyelitis: an acute or chronic infection of the bone caused by a bacterial, fungal, or viral organism. The most commonly involved organisms are *Staphylococcus aureus, Escherichia coli, Klebsiella,* and *Pseudomonas*. Chronic osteomyelitis is a bone infection that persists for years, flaring up intermittently after minor trauma to the area or when systemic resistance is low. Primary osteomyelitis is a direct invasion of bone as a result of compound fractures, penetrating wounds, bone marrow aspiration, or surgery. Secondary osteomyelitis (acute hematogenic osteomyelitis) is an infection of the bone via the patient's blood or adjacent soft tissues; it may be related, for example, to pressure sores, intravenous drug abuse, joints involved with septic arthritis, or radiation therapy.

CONTRIBUTING FACTORS/RISK FACTORS

- Undernourishment
- Old age
- Diabetes mellitus
- Tuberculosis
- Chronic obstructive pulmonary disease

- Sickle cell disease
- Malignancies
- Peripheral vascular disease
- IV drug abuse
- Penetrating trauma

SIGNS/SYMPTOMS

- Acute osteomyelitis
  —Abrupt onset of localized pain
  —Fever, chills, sweats
  —Redness, heat, swelling, infected bone
  —Malaise
  —Headache
  —Nausea
  —Limited motion
  —Restlessness
  —Irritability
- Chronic osteomyelitis
  —Persistent purulent drainage from old pocket

COMPLICATIONS

- Chronic osteomyelitis
- Amputation
- Abscess formation
- Pathologic fracture
- Joint contractures
- Limb shortening

DIAGNOSTIC TESTS

- Describe each procedure, its purpose, and the normal feelings or sensations that are likely, as well as any preprocedural and postprocedural care.
  —Blood tests
      White blood cell count: elevated
      Erythrocyte sedimentation rate: elevated
      Blood cultures: to identify causative organism
  —Bone biopsy: to obtain material for culture and sensitivity studies
  —Bone scan: to show the area of inflammation or avascularization
  —X-rays: to reveal destructive process

—Computed tomography: to detect bone changes and spread of infection to surrounding tissues

—Magnetic resonance imaging: to determine extent of acute or chronic infection

TREATMENT
Medical

- Therapy
  —Bed rest
  —Frequent dressing changes
  —Compresses: warm, moist, or alternate warm and cold
  —Hyperbaric oxygen chamber
  —Splints, casts, slings to immobilize weakened bones
- Drugs
  —Intravenous antibiotics: therapy prescribed for 4 to 6 weeks
  —Topical antibiotics
  —Analgesics, antipyretics

Surgical

- Surgical decompression of infected bone: holes are drilled into the bone to localize sites of exudate; the overlying infected bone is removed; the cavity is loosely packed for drainage purposes and to keep wound open
- External fixation devices: to stabilize bones and prevent fractures
- Saucerization (sequestrectomy): removal of necrotic bone and scar tissue to provide a healthy surface for regeneration of bone
- Bone grafting
- Microsurgical free muscle transfer: to cover the wound and eliminate dead space
- Amputation of limb: for life-threatening or persistent infections

HOME CARE

- Give both the patient and the caregiver *verbal* and *written* instructions. Provide them with the name and telephone number of a physician or nurse to call if questions arise.
- *General information*
  —Discuss the disease process, causes and contributing factors, and the potential for chronic infection. Stress the importance of continuing the prescribed antibiotic therapy.

- *Wound/incision care*
  —Explain and demonstrate wound care using aseptic technique for dressing changes. Discuss proper disposal of contaminated dressings and removal of soiled linens. Stress the importance of maintaining wound isolation.
- *Warning signs*
  —Review the signs and symptoms of infection that should be reported to a physician or nurse.
    Fever
    Chills
    Increased pain
    Malaise
    Recurring drainage from wound
  —Review the signs of neurovascular impairment that need to be reported promptly:
    Diminished sensation
    Numbness
    Tingling
    Pain
    Coolness
- *Special instructions*
  —Review care of a casted extremity if indicated (see p. 656).
  —Review care of the external fixator device if indicated (see p. 284).
  —Teach the patient how to use and care for the Hickman catheter or other intravenous access device for home antibiotic therapy (see p. 659). Provide referrals for home care.
- *Medications*
  —Explain the purpose, dosage, schedule, and route of administration of any prescribed drugs, as well as side effects to report to the physician or nurse.
  —Explain that antibiotic therapy may continue for 3 to 6 months.
  —Advise the patient to watch for and report any side effects of antibiotics: nausea, vomiting, diarrhea, abdominal pain.
- *Activity*
  —Explain the need for rest to conserve energy and promote healing.
  —Teach the patient range-of-motion exercises and encourage their use to maintain muscle strength and joint mobility.
  —Explain the importance of immobilizing the affected part to decrease the spread of purulent material.

—Instruct the patient in the use of ambulatory aids (crutches, cane, splint, wheelchair, or walker, as indicated) when he or she is allowed out of bed. Assist the patient to obtain the equipment.

* *Diet*
—Encourage the patient to follow a nutritionally sound diet high in protein and vitamins C and D to enhance and promote healing.
—Advise the patient to consume at least 2 to 3 liters of fluids per day (unless contraindicated) to prevent urinary calculi and other complications of immobility.

FOLLOW-UP CARE AND REFERRALS

* Stress the importance of regular follow-up visits. Make sure the patient has the necessary names and telephone numbers.
* Provide referral for home health care to assist with activities of daily living as indicated.

Osteoporosis

—Osteoporosis: an overall reduction in bone mass or density that occurs because bone resorption (breaking down of bone for other body uses) is greater than bone formation. Osteoporosis causes bone to become brittle and susceptible to fractures. Bones store calcium for other body functions; the body takes the calcium out for use through resorption. With age the process of resorption normally occurs faster than bone formation, calcium absorption becomes impaired, and vitamin D formation decreases from lack of estrogen. These changes result in a gradual decrease in bone mass or density.

RISK FACTORS

* Women
—After menopause because of decreased estrogen production and inactivity
—Petite, white, or Asian because of small amount of bone mass
—Nulliparity

- Others
  - —In young people after severe injury because of prolonged inactivity or immobility
  - —History of rheumatoid arthritis, liver disease, certain cancers, overactive thyroid, diabetes mellitus, malabsorption syndrome, chronic obstructive pulmonary disease (COPD)
  - —Sedentary lifestyle, lack of exercise and weight-bearing activities
  - —Smoking or alcohol abuse: interferes with calcium absorption
  - —Long-term use of drugs (e.g., corticosteroids, antacids, heparin, phenytoin, isoniazid): suppresses the activity of bone-building cells
  - —High caffeine intake: decreases absorption of calcium
  - —Family history
  - —Inadequate calcium intake

SIGNS/SYMPTOMS

- Dull, aching, constant pain in bones
- Muscle spasms
- Fractures
  - —Dorsal and lumbar vertebral bodies
  - —Neck and intertrochanteric regions of femur (hip fracture)
  - —Distal radius
  - —Vertebral compression fractures leading to:
    - Loss of height
    - Kyphosis (back hump)
    - Back discomfort
    - Constipation
- Decreased strength in muscles and joints

COMPLICATIONS

- Fractures of vertebrae, hip, wrist
- Respiratory compromise caused by severe kyphosis
- Immobility
- Deformity

DIAGNOSTIC TESTS

- Describe each procedure, its purpose, and the normal feelings or sensations that are likely, as well as any preprocedural and postprocedural care.

—Blood tests
   Serum alkaline phosphatase: decreased
   Serum hydroxyproline: increased
—X-ray examination: to document osteoporotic fractures, spinal curvature
—Radiogrammetry, photodensitometry, single- and dual-photon absorptiometry: to measure skeletal density and detect loss of bone mass
—Computed tomography: to measure vertebral (spinal) bone density; to detect herniated or fractured vertebral disks

TREATMENT
Medical

- Therapy
   —Application of back corset or neck support to prevent stress fractures
   —Heat and massage for muscle spasm
   —Moderate weight-bearing exercises to hold calcium in bone
   —Passive exercises if unable to do active exercises
   —High-calcium, high-protein diet
   —Nutritional supplements: calcium carbonate and vitamin D
- Drugs
   —Estrogen replacement therapy for postmenopausal women
   —Analgesics
   —Antiresorptive agents to prevent further loss of bone mass
   —Calcitonin

Surgical

- Repair of fractures (e.g., hip, wrist)
- Laminectomy to relieve pressure on the spinal nerves or cord if vertebrae are involved (fractures, ruptured disk)

HOME CARE

- Give both the patient and the caregiver *verbal* and *written* instructions. Provide them with the name and telephone number of a physician or nurse to call if questions arise.
- *General information*
   —Explain and discuss the disease process and the causes and contributing factors.
   —Instruct all patients at risk early in their lives about preventive measures because of the prolonged time involved in development of this disease.

- *Warning signs*
  —Review the signs and symptoms of pathologic fractures that should be reported to a physician or nurse.
    Deformity
    Pain
    Edema
    Ecchymosis
    Limb shortening
    False motion, decreased range of motion
    Loss of bladder or bowel control
    Paralysis
- *Special instructions*
  —Discuss the importance of establishing home safety measures to prevent falls and injuries: placing a handrail in the bathtub, installing nightlights, and avoiding the use of throw rugs.
  —Advise the patient to use ambulatory assist devices such as a cane or walker as indicated to relieve stress on the back and joints; this will help the patient maintain balance and reduce the risk of falling.
  —Remind the patient of the need for sunlight (15 minutes/day) to allow activation of vitamin D.
- *Medications*
  —Explain the purpose, dosage, schedule, and route of administration of any prescribed drugs, as well as side effects to report to the physician or nurse.
  —Discuss the use of calcium supplements. Explain that calcium should be taken 2 hours before or after other medications because it can reduce absorption of other drugs. Inform the patient that increased calcium can result in kidney stone formation. This can be prevented by increasing daily fluid intake and not taking calcium supplements with iron, since iron absorption would be impaired.
- *Activity*
  —Explain the importance of weight-bearing exercises to increase bone mass. Encourage activities such as walking, tennis, and dancing to activate bone formation, improve circulation, and enhance calcium absorption.
  —Advise the patient to be careful when doing any activity (e.g., getting up from a chair or bending deeply), since falling or straining can cause severe stress and lead to fractures.

- *Diet*
    —Encourage the patient to eat foods high in calcium, including cheese, milk, dark green leafy vegetables, eggs, peanuts, sesame seeds, and oysters.
    —Instruct the patient in planning menus that provide a sufficient daily intake of foods high in or fortified with calcium and vitamin D, such as eggs, halibut, herring, dairy products, liver, salmon, and sardines.
    —Tell the patient to limit intake of alcohol and caffeine.
    —Remind the patient to drink plenty of fluids (2 to 3 liters of water per day) to reduce the risk of renal calculi.

FOLLOW-UP CARE

- Stress the importance of regular follow-up visits. Make sure the patient has the necessary names and telephone numbers.

Ovarian Cancer

—Ovarian cancer: a rapidly growing tumor that is seldom diagnosed in the early stages because of the lack of signs or symptoms. More than 60% of women with ovarian cancer have advanced disease at the time of diagnosis. The most common type of ovarian cancer is serous cystadenocarcinoma; other types are mucinous, endometrioid, or clear cell. Most ovarian cancer arises in the epithelium. Between 5% and 10% of tumors have their primary source in another body organ, usually the breast. Dissemination occurs through implantation of cells into the surface of the pelvic peritoneum, sigmoid colon, cecum, or terminal ileum and omentum, as well as via submesothelial lymphatics.

RISK FACTORS

- Uninterrupted ovulation
- Age older than 50 (postmenopausal)
- Nulliparity, celibacy, infertility
- Long history of menstrual irregularity

- Higher socioeconomic status
- High-fat diet
- Exposure to industrial chemicals such as asbestos and talc

Other risk factors being studied are age at menopause, history of rubella and mumps, family history of ovarian cancer, family size, and ovarian malfunctions.

SIGNS/SYMPTOMS

- Ascites, abdominal or pelvic pain or fullness
- Weight loss
- Gastrointestinal complaints: dyspnea, indigestion
- Urinary complaints: frequency, urgency
- Menstrual irregularities: abnormal uterine bleeding

DIAGNOSTIC TESTS

- Describe each procedure, its purpose, and the normal feelings or sensations that are likely, as well as any preprocedural and postprocedural care.
  —Pelvic examination with bimanual manipulation: to palpate the ovaries for size and shape
  —Laparoscopy with biopsy: to detect ovarian abnormality and the presence of malignant cells
  —Lymphangiography: to detect the involvement of retroperitoneal nodes
  —Cancer antigen 125 (CA-125): tumor marker elevated in the presence of ovarian cancer

TREATMENT
Medical

- Therapy
  —Radiation therapy
    Intracavity
    External beam
  —Single-agent chemotherapy
    Chlorambucil
    Melphalan
    Doxorubicin
    Cyclophosphamide
    5-Fluorouracil
    Methotrexate
    Vinblastine

Bleomycin
Cisplatin
Nitrogen mustard
Thiotepa
Tetracycline
Paclitaxel (Taxol)
—Combination chemotherapy (including cisplatin)

Surgical

- Simple salpingo-oophorectomy
- Total abdominal hysterectomy with bilateral salpingo-oophorectomy and partial or complete omentectomy

🏠 HOME CARE

- Give both the patient and the caregiver *verbal* and *written* instructions. Provide them with the name and telephone number of a physician or nurse to call if questions arise. Use visual aids in instruction.
- *General information*
  —Review the physician's explanation of the disease process. Explain that prescribed treatment will be based on the stage of cancer and age of the patient.
  —Provide information about the prescribed treatment: hysterectomy (see p. 384), chemotherapy (see p. 667), or radiation therapy (see p. 721).
- *Warning signs*
  —Review the signs and symptoms that should be reported to a physician or nurse.
    Infection: redness, drainage, fever, pain
    Bleeding
    Urinary obstruction: distention, decreased output
    Bowel obstruction: distention, abdominal discomfort, flatulence, nausea, loss of appetite
    Pleural effusion: shortness of breath, fever
- *Special instructions*
  —Teach the patient methods of managing abdominal discomfort and other gastrointestinal complaints: medications; heat; small, frequent meals.
  —Discuss pain management techniques: relaxation, imagery, biofeedback.

- *Medications*
  - —Explain the purpose, dosage, schedule, and route of administration of any prescribed drugs, as well as side effects to report to the physician or nurse.
- *Activity*
  - —Encourage the patient to exercise as tolerated. Explain that walking is especially helpful in relieving abdominal discomfort.
- *Diet*
  - —Stress the importance of adequate intake of fluids and food and obtaining sufficient calories. Suggest dietary supplements as needed.

PSYCHOSOCIAL CARE

- Encourage verbalization of fears and feelings regarding disease progression and treatment options.
- Encourage the patient and family to seek psychosocial counseling.

FOLLOW-UP CARE

- Stress the importance of follow-up medical and gynecologic examinations as ordered. Make sure the patient has the necessary names and telephone numbers.
- Advise other women in the family including young daughters to begin annual gynecologic examinations at onset of sexual activity or age 18.

REFERRALS

- Assist the patient to obtain referrals for home health care and social services. Refer to support groups as needed.

Paget's Disease
(Osteitis Deformans)

—Paget's disease: a chronic inflammatory disease that results in thickening, softening, and eventual bowing of bones. Paget's disease is characterized by an initial phase of excessive bone resorption (breaking down of bone for other body uses), followed by excessive abnormal bone formation. The diseased bone is structurally weak and fragile, causing painful deformities, and is prone to fractures. Paget's disease usually affects the femur, tibia, lower spine, pelvis, and skull. It occurs worldwide but is extremely rare in Asia, the Middle East, Africa, and Scandinavia. In the United States it affects 3% of people older than 40 years of age (mostly men). The cause of the disease is unknown.

SIGNS/SYMPTOMS

- Bone pain: mild to severe, aggravated by weight bearing or pressure, worse at night
- Increased warmth over involved sites
- Backache
- Skeletal deformities: kyphosis, barrel-shaped chest, bowing of the tibia or femur
- Easily bendable bones
- Pathologic fractures
- Cranial nerve compression: visual deficits, hearing loss, headaches, dysphagia
- Skull enlarged, soft, thick

COMPLICATIONS

- Pathologic fractures
- Renal calculi
- Heart failure
- Hearing loss
- Visual changes
- Sarcoma

DIAGNOSTIC TESTS

- Describe each procedure, its purpose, and the normal feelings or sensations that are likely, as well as any preprocedural and postprocedural care.
  - —Standard x-rays: to document typical lesions of the disease, pathologic fractures, deformed bone structure
  - —Blood tests: to detect elevated alkaline phosphatase, indicating new bone growth
  - —Bone biopsy: to confirm the diagnosis
  - —Bone scans: to identify active bone lesions

—Magnetic resonance imaging: to detect areas of bone breakdown and bone growth

TREATMENT
Medical
- Therapy
  —Orthotics (e.g., external splints, casts): to maintain reduction and help straighten bone
- Drugs
  —Hormones: to retard bone formation
  —Calcitonin
  —Etidronate
  —Cytotoxic antibiotic (mithramycin): to produce remission of symptoms
  —Analgesics: to control pain
  —Nonsteroidal antiinflammatory drugs: to control pain

Surgical
- Repair of pathologic fractures by closed or open reduction

🏠 HOME CARE
- Give both the patient and the caregiver *verbal* and *written* instructions. Provide them with the name and telephone number of a physician or nurse to call if questions arise.
- *General information*
  —Explain the disease process and prescribed treatment.
- *Warning signs*
  —Review the signs and symptoms that should be reported to a physician or nurse.
  > Cranial and spinal involvement: decreased hearing, headache, paresthesia (numbness, tingling), paralysis, visual defects (pupil inequality), changes in speech patterns, difficulty in swallowing
  > Kidney stones: dysuria, hematuria
  —Discuss the high risk of pathologic fracture, and explain that signs or symptoms should be reported immediately to a physician.
  > Sudden increase in pain
  > Hearing or sensing a bone crack
  > Experiencing the inability to bear weight or use bone normally

- *Special instructions*
  —Teach the patient to self-inject calcitonin. Permit time for practice, and stress the need to rotate injection sites.
- *Medications*
  —Explain the purpose, dosage, schedule, and route of administration of any prescribed drugs, as well as side effects to report to the physician or nurse.
  —Tell the patient to avoid over-the-counter products such as antacids and vitamins without checking with a physician.
  —Instruct the patient taking etidronate to schedule medication doses 2 hours before or after meals. Advise not taking the medication with milk or foods high in calcium, since they impair absorption.
- *Activity*
  —Encourage the patient to maintain activity levels as tolerated. Encourage range-of-motion exercises of the unaffected joints to maintain joint mobility.
  —Advise the patient to avoid excessive activity but also to avoid immobility.
  —Instruct the patient in the use of ambulatory assist devices and aids (crutches, cane, walker).
  —Discuss home safety measures to prevent falls: removal of throw rugs, electrical cords, and other obstacles.
  —Advise the patient to move cautiously, avoiding sudden jerking movements, to lessen the probability of fracture.
- *Diet*
  —Instruct the patient to increase intake of foods containing vitamin D (milk, certain seafoods), calcium dairy products, and dark green vegetables.
  —Encourage fluid intake of 6 to 8 glasses/day to minimize renal calculus formation.

FOLLOW-UP CARE

- Stress the importance of follow-up visits. Make sure the patient has the necessary names and telephone numbers.

Pancreatic Cancer

—**Pancreatic cancer: a highly malignant tumor that is insidious in onset and, because there are no early signs, is frequently diagnosed late in the course. Pancreatic tumors are usually adenocarcinomas arising in the head of the pancreas.**

RISK FACTORS (KNOWN AND SUSPECTED)

- Medical history of diabetes or pancreatitis
- Cigarette smoking
- Dietary fat
- Alcoholism
- Organic chemicals such as coke, coal gas, beta-naphthylamine, and benzidine

SIGNS/SYMPTOMS

- Weight loss, often gradual and progressive
- Pain: midepigastric, steady, dull, usually worse at night, more common in the left upper quadrant when the tumor is in the body or tail of the pancreas; lower abdominal pain in a small number of patients
- Back pain: aggravated by lying flat and relieved by sitting up and bending forward or lying curled in a fetal position
- Jaundice with itching of arms, legs, and abdomen: worse in evening and at night
- Weight loss
- Constipation, bloating, flatulence
- Depression

COMPLICATIONS

- Thrombophlebitis
- Diabetes mellitus
- Bleeding tendencies
- Ascites

DIAGNOSTIC TESTS

- Describe each procedure, its purpose, and the normal feelings or sensations that are likely, as well as any preprocedural and postprocedural care.

—Computed tomography, ultrasound: to determine the size and location of the lesion
—Fine-needle aspiration biopsy: to identify the type of tumor
—Endoscopic retrograde cholangiopancreatography: to determine more precisely the size and location of the tumor
—Angiography: to determine vascular involvement of the tumor
—Laparoscopy: to detect metastatic abdominal lesions
—Cancer antigen 19-9, carcinoembryonic antigen: nonspecific tumor markers elevated in the presence of pancreatic cancer

TREATMENT
Medical

- Therapy
  —Radiation therapy
      High-dose external beam
      Interstitial seed of iodine-125 or iridium-192
      Brachytherapy
      Intraoperative radiation therapy
- Drugs
  —5-Fluorouracil alone or with radiation therapy
  —Nitrosoureas, mitomycin C, doxorubicin
  —Gemcitabine as single agent

Surgical

- Pancreatoduodenectomy (Whipple procedure)
- Total pancreatectomy
- Palliation: anastomosis of jejunum to distended common bile duct to relieve jaundice and itching

 HOME CARE

- Give both the patient and the caregiver *verbal* and *written* instructions. Provide them with the name and telephone number of a physician or nurse to call if questions arise.
- *General information*
  —Review the physician's explanation of the disease process and prescribed treatment.
- *Warning signs*
  —Review the signs and symptoms that should be reported to a physician or nurse.
      Weight loss, dehydration

Anorexia, constipation, bloating, flatulence, or other signs and symptoms of gastrointestinal distress

Pain uncontrolled by prescribed medication

- *Special instructions*
  —Teach the patient to use frequent baths, lotions, and ointments to soothe skin and lessen itching.
  —Discuss pain management early in treatment.
  —Teach the patient alternative methods of pain management to supplement or enhance pain medications (see Pain Management, p. 708).
- *Medications*
  —Explain the purpose, dosage, schedule, and route of administration of any prescribed drugs, as well as side effects to report to the physician or nurse.
  —Teach the self-administration of insulin if diabetes develops (see Diabetes Mellitus, p. 233).
  —Encourage the patient to use pain medications regularly to maintain an acceptable level of comfort.
- *Diet*
  —Stress the importance of adequate intake of fluids and food. Encourage small, frequent meals and the use of nutritional supplements.

PSYCHOSOCIAL CARE

- Encourage expressions of fear and feelings about death. Assist the patient and family to seek counseling.
- Encourage independence as much as possible.

FOLLOW-UP CARE

- Stress the importance of follow-up visits. Make sure the patient has the necessary names and telephone numbers.

REFERRALS

- Assist the patient to obtain referral for home care, social services, and hospice care.

Pancreatitis

—Pancreatitis: inflammation of the pancreas. Acute pancreatitis has a sudden onset, usually following a large meal or large intake of alcohol. The acute form is a type of autodigestion of the pancreas by its own enzymes, progressing to a necrotic form. Chronic pancreatitis is progressive functional damage to the pancreas.

CONTRIBUTING FACTORS
- Excessive use of alcohol
- Gallbladder disease
- Cancer
- Physical trauma to abdomen
- Duodenal ulcer
- Mumps
- Drug toxicity: oral contraceptives, glucocorticoids, sulfonamides, chlorothiazides, azathioprine

SIGNS/SYMPTOMS
- Acute
  —Constant, severe epigastric pain
  —Pain radiating to back or left shoulder, somewhat relieved by sitting
  —Nausea and vomiting
  —Extreme malaise
  —Decreased urine output
  —Jaundice with gallbladder involvement
  —Fever, chills
  —Rapid pulse, low blood pressure, shallow respirations
  —Discoloration of the flank or abdomen
  —Agitation, confusion related to electrolyte imbalance
  —Diminished or absent bowel sounds
- Chronic
  —Constant, dull epigastric pain
  —Sharp pain with radiation to the back
  —Pain relieved by sitting forward
  —Pain increased by eating or lying flat
  —Greasy, foul-smelling stools

—Weight loss
—Nausea and vomiting
—Malnutrition
—Fat-soluble vitamin deficiencies
—Symptoms of diabetes mellitus

COMPLICATIONS

- Acute
  —Acute respiratory distress syndrome
  —Electrolyte imbalance, cardiac dysrhythmias
  —Circulatory or renal failure
  —Shock, hemorrhage
  —Disseminated intravascular coagulation
- Both acute and chronic
  —Jaundice
  —Paralytic ileus
  —Hyperglycemia
  —Infection and abscesses
  —Pancreatic pseudocyst
  —Pancreatic rupture
  —Wound infection
  —Surgical fistulas

DIAGNOSTIC TESTS

- Describe each procedure, its purpose, and the normal feelings or sensations that are likely, as well as any preprocedural and postprocedural care.
  —Stool for fat analysis
  —X-ray of abdomen
  —Ultrasound of abdomen
  —Computed tomography of abdomen
  —Upper gastrointestinal series
  —Cholangiography
  —Acute
     Urine studies: urinalysis, amylase
     Blood studies: complete blood count, blood urea nitrogen, glucose, calcium, albumin
     Pancreatic enzymes, amylase, lipase
  —Chronic
     Urinalysis

Blood studies: complete blood count, glucose, alkaline phosphatase, amylase, bilirubin

Endoscopic retrograde cholangiopancreatography

TREATMENT
Medical

- Therapy
  —Acute pancreatitis
  - Intravenous hydration and electrolyte replacement
  - Nothing by mouth (NPO) and nasogastric tube
  - Bed rest
  - Peritoneal lavage
  - Nutritional support (total or partial parenteral nutrition, jejunostomy feeding)
- Drugs
  —Acute pancreatitis
  - Analgesics
  - Antacids
  - Antibiotics
  - Anticholinergics
  - Histamine (H$_2$) blocker
  - Antiemetics
  —Chronic pancreatitis
  - Analgesics, digestants (pancreatic enzyme supplements)
  - Antacids
  - Histamine (H$_2$) blocker
  - Insulin or oral hypoglycemic agents

Surgical

- Acute pancreatitis
  —Surgical drainage of pseudocysts
  —Surgical drainage of pancreatic abscesses
  —Surgery for gallbladder duct obstruction
- Chronic pancreatitis
  —Secondary treatment for pain complications (cysts, abscesses)
  —Surgery involving the pancreas or small intestine
  —Islet cell (or insulin) preservation
  —Autotransplantation of islet cell preparations
  —Autotransplantation of pancreas segments
  —Closed-loop insulin infusion system

HOME CARE

- Give both the patient and the caregiver *verbal* and *written* instructions. Provide them with the name and telephone number of a physician or nurse to call if questions arise.
- *General information*
  —Explain the disease process, underlying cause, and contributing factors. Stress the importance of initiating measures to prevent further attacks.
  —Describe prescribed treatment. Explain that surgery is generally not indicated for pancreatic pseudocysts in abscess form.
- *Warning signs*
  —Review the signs and symptoms that should be reported to a physician or nurse.
    Severe epigastric pain relieved by sitting
    Nausea and vomiting
    Greasy, foul-smelling or clay-colored stools
    Weight loss
    Dark urine
    Pseudocyst: epigastric pain radiating to the back
    Fever
- *Special instructions*
  —Discuss skin care, including the use of nonalcoholic lotions or creams to treat itchy, dry skin.
  —Discuss nonmedication measures for coping with pain, such as relaxation techniques and guided imagery.
  —Encourage activity and mobilization as prescribed.
- *Medications*
  —Explain the purpose, dosage, schedule, and route of administration of any prescribed drugs, as well as side effects to report to the physician or nurse.
  —Teach the patient how and when to take prescribed enzyme therapy. Instruct the patient to take enzymes with meals or snacks, and not to take pancreatin with hot foods or drinks.
  —Teach the self-administration of insulin if diabetes develops (see Diabetes Mellitus, p. 233).
- *Diet*
  —Inform the patient that a high-carbohydrate, high-protein, low-fat diet or one prescribed by the physician should be followed.

—Stress the importance of avoiding alcohol, caffeinated beverages (coffee, tea, soda), and spicy or irritating, gas-producing foods.

—Advise the patient to eat small, frequent meals to alleviate bloating, nausea, and cramps.

FOLLOW-UP CARE

• Stress the importance of follow-up visits. Make sure the patient has the necessary names and telephone numbers.

REFERRALS

• Obtain counseling and refer the patient to a community-based alcohol treatment program as needed.

Parkinson's Disease
(Paralysis Agitans)

—Parkinson's disease: a syndrome characterized by progressive muscle rigidity, bradykinesia (slowing of the ability to initiate voluntary movements), and involuntary tremors. Parkinson's disease often develops after age 60, and deterioration progresses for an average of 10 years, with death usually resulting from aspiration pneumonia or some other infection. Parkinson's disease involves degeneration of dopamine-producing cells in the brain, which leads to degeneration of neurons in the basal ganglia. Once cell loss reaches 80%, symptoms appear. There is no definable cause.

CONTRIBUTING FACTORS

• Drug exposure (e.g., neuroleptic drugs or reserpine)
• Carbon monoxide poisoning
• Manganese poisoning
• Tumors or infarcts involving the midbrain

SIGNS/SYMPTOMS

- Initial symptoms
  —Muscle fatigue/weakness
  —Resting tremble (usually in one hand)
  —Slowness or awkwardness of affected limb
  —Some loss of facial expression
  —Deliberate quality of speech
  —Tendency to posture arm flexed at elbow
  —May progress to other side of body after 1 to 2 years
- Autonomic dysfunction
  —Skin: oily perspiration, seborrhea
  —Intermittent, profuse diaphoresis
  —Gastric retention
  —Urgency or hesitation in urination
  —Urinary retention
  —Orthostatic hypotension
  —Dysphasia
- Equilibrium
  —Festination (leaning of trunk farther with each step)
  —Propulsion (forward stepping with leaning of trunk)
  —Retropulsion (backward stepping with leaning of trunk)
  —Lateropulsion (sidewise stepping with leaning of trunk)
- Face
  —Masklike facies (blank facial expression)
  —Decreased eye blinking
- Hands
  —Fingers extended with metacarpophalangeal joints flexed approximately 30 degrees
  —Handwriting
  —Letters becoming progressively smaller (micrographia)
  —Tremulous writing
- Nutrition
  —Impaired deglutition
  —Drooling, excessive salivation
  —Weight loss
  —Failure of cricopharyngeal muscles to relax; choking
  —Constipation
- Posture and rigidity
  —Shuffling gait without arm swing
  —Akinesia (most evident in spinal musculature)
  —Stooped body posture
  —Impaired mobility; self-care deficits

- Speech
  - —Involuntary repetition of sentences
  - —Decreased amplitude
  - —Monotone: voice becomes soft, whisperlike, and muffled
- Tremors
  - —Lips, jaw, tongue, facial muscles, axial muscles, limb muscles
  - —Fingers: pill-rolling movement
  - —Head: to-and-fro tremor
  - —Usually resting tremors (most apparent when affected area is at rest): paralysis agitans
  - —Exaggerated by stress and anxiety
- Gradual dementia
  - —Initial
    - Forgetfulness
    - Minor confusional episodes
    - Depression
  - —Later
    - Irritability, nervousness
    - Mood swings
    - Paranoia and visual hallucinations
    - Frank delirium
    - Social isolation

P

COMPLICATIONS

- Aspiration pneumonia
- Injury: fall
- Social isolation
- Urinary tract infection
- Constipation

DIAGNOSTIC TESTS

- Describe each procedure, its purpose, and the normal feelings or sensations that are likely, as well as any preprocedural and postprocedural care.
  - —Serum examination: mild microcytic anemia
  - —Chest x-ray: slight scoliosis
  - —Computed tomography, skull x-ray: normal results, or computed tomography may show cerebral atrophy when there is history of chronic dementia

—Electroencephalogram: normal results or slowing and disorganization

—Cineradiographic study of swallowing: abnormal pattern

—Gastrointestinal studies: hypomotility; delayed emptying of stomach, varying degrees of large bowel distention (frank megacolon in patients with severe constipation)

TREATMENT
Medical

- Therapy
  —Treatment is done on an outpatient basis except for complications or elective surgery. The patient's physical limitations may require many adjustments in the home for activities of daily living.
- Drugs
  —Dopamine agonists
  —Monoamine oxidase (MAO) B inhibitors
  —Dopamine replacement
  —Anticholinergic drugs
  —Antidepressants
  —Antihistamines
  —Vitamin E in a high dose; 2000 IU daily may be suggested to prevent dementia

Surgical

- Stereotactic thalamotomy: to control tremors by producing a small lesion in the ventrolateral nucleus of the thalamus
- Pallidotomy: performed when rigidity, hypokinesia, and tremor are present
- Deep brain stimulation

HOME CARE

- Give both the patient and the caregiver *verbal* and *written* instructions. Provide them with the name and telephone number of a physician or nurse to call if questions arise.
- *General information*
  —Discuss the causes, symptoms, and treatment modalities for Parkinson's disease and explain procedures as they occur.
  —Explain to the patient that emotional stress, infection, overwork, and exposure to cold can exacerbate symptoms.

- *Medications*
  —Explain the purpose, dosage, schedule, and route of administration of any prescribed drugs, as well as side effects to report to the physician or nurse.
  —Stress the importance of taking medications on schedule; assist the patient to schedule taking medication to achieve the peak effect at times the patient needs mobility most.
  —Instruct the patient to chew gum or eat hard candy to ease dry mouth that may occur.
  —Explain that the patient must take medications with food to reduce gastric irritation and nausea.
- Activity
  —Encourage the patient to discuss allowances and limitations with respect to occupation, recreation, and activities but stress the potential risk of injury (e.g., falls) as disease progresses.
  —Discuss the need to evaluate the home environment for potential dangers: loose rugs, stairs.
  —Urge the patient to maintain activity to whatever degree is possible.
  —Advise the patient to use a cane as necessary for walking.
  —Instruct the patient in safety measures to prevent injury.
  —Explain the need for speech therapy.
  —Stress the importance of frequent skin care and oral hygiene.
  —Explain that following a daily exercise program can slow progression of the disease.
  —Advise the patient about the importance of diversional activities.
  —Emphasize the need for independence; tell caregivers to avoid overprotection and to permit the patient to perform self-care, including feeding, dressing, and walking.
  —Stress the importance of room temperature control.
- *Diet*
  —Encourage the patient to follow a high-residue, high-bulk, high-roughage diet to promote gastrointestinal motility.
  —Maintain a weight chart.
  —Advise the use of natural laxatives such as prune juice to maintain regular bowel evacuation.
  —Instruct the patient to limit protein intake to minimize blocking of L-dopa.

—Encourage a fluid intake of 2000 ml/day, unless contraindicated, to maintain voiding.

—Suggest acidifying the urine by drinking orange or cranberry juice to minimize the potential for infection.

—Inform the patient of the need for a high-calorie, soft diet, and instruct the patient to take small bites and eat slowly.

—Discuss strategies to help with meals: cut food for the patient; place all utensils within easy reach; use a blender for thicker foods; use braces or splints to help with tremor; use a straw and bib to help with drooling.

PSYCHOSOCIAL CARE

• Explain to the family the need to encourage social participation.

• Explain that although physically disabled, the patient is intellectually normal.

• Stress the importance of verbalization about loss of self-esteem, sexuality, and body functions.

• Advise the patient of the importance of expressing feelings.

FOLLOW-UP CARE

• Stress the importance of continued outpatient care: physician visits, physical therapy, and home nursing care. Make sure the patient has the necessary names and telephone numbers.

REFERRALS

• Assist with referrals for home care services including speech, occupational, and physical therapy as indicated.

• Ensure that the patient has the following addresses and phone numbers to obtain printed information: Parkinson's Disease Foundation, 710 W. 168th St., New York, NY 10032, phone (800) 457-6676; or National Parkinson's Foundation, phone (800) 327-4545.

Percutaneous Transluminal Coronary Angioplasty (PTCA), Intracoronary Stenting

—Percutaneous transluminal coronary angioplasty: nonsurgical, invasive procedure in which a balloon-tipped catheter is introduced, usually through an artery in the groin. Under fluoroscopy, the catheter is moved to specific areas of the coronary arteries of the heart that are narrowed by atherosclerotic plaque. The balloon is inflated to flatten the plaque and allow more blood and oxygen to reach the tissues.

—Intracoronary stenting: sometimes a tiny mesh wire tube is implanted and left in the coronary artery to prevent reocclusion.

INDICATIONS

- Occluded or nearly occluded coronary arteries

PREPROCEDURAL TEACHING

- Review the physician's explanation of the procedure and the reason for it; encourage the patient to ask questions and to discuss any fears or anxieties.

Review of Preprocedural Care

- See Cardiac Catheterization (p. 154).
- Obtain informed consent.

Review of Postprocedural Care

- Explain that the introductory catheter sheath may remain in place after the procedure and if so, the patient will spend 10 to 36 hours in the coronary care unit (CCU) for continuous monitoring.
- Stress the importance of flat bed rest. Explain that the head may be raised 15 degrees for meals only and only while the sheath is in place.
- Inform the patient that the physician may use a plug such as an Angio-Seal that occludes the vessel and there will be no sheath.

- Emphasize the need to keep the catheterized leg straight. Tell the patient that a light restraint may be applied as a reminder.
- Explain that frequent checks of vital signs, the groin, leg pulses, color, and temperature will be done.
- Inform the patient that a urine catheter or condom catheter may be in place overnight.
- Explain that intravenous hydration will continue overnight.
- Discuss removal of the sheath. Explain that it will occur 6 to 12 hours after the procedure; that pressure will be applied to the groin for 20 to 30 minutes manually or by a special C clamp or a FemoStop until there is no evidence of bleeding, with a 5-pound sandbag for 6 to 8 hours afterward; that flat bed rest will be maintained for 6 to 8 hours afterward, with bed rest overnight; and that vital signs, including pedal pulses and groin check, will be monitored frequently.
- Explain that the patient is usually moved out of the CCU after the sheath is removed and the condition is stabilized.
- Inform the patient that he or she will probably be allowed out of bed the next morning and may walk around. If heparin is being administered intravenously, the patient may get out of bed, take a few steps, and sit in the chair. The urine catheter is removed.

COMPLICATIONS

- Failure to dilate coronary arteries
- Bleeding (groin) or hematoma
- Rupture or dissection of coronary artery(ies)
- Heart attack
- Cardiac arrest
- Clot formation (leg or coronary arteries)
- Renal hypersensitivity to contrast dye (decreased urine) or acute renal failure
- Abrupt reclosure of the coronary artery
- Infection

HOME CARE

- Give both the patient and the caregiver *verbal* and *written* instructions. Provide them with the name and telephone number of a physician or nurse to call if questions arise.
- *General information*
  —Review the explanation of the procedure and findings.

- *Warning signs*
  —Review the signs and symptoms that should be reported to a physician or nurse.
    Infection: redness, swelling, warm to touch, purulent drainage
    Active bleeding of the groin or an enlarging hematoma of the area: discoloration, firmness, tenderness
    Numbness, tingling, coolness, or cyanosis of the affected extremity
    Angina unrelieved or shortness of breath
    Irregular pulse, lightheadedness, dizziness
    Constipation
- *Special instructions*
  —Explain that a Band-Aid over the puncture site may be changed and may not be needed after a day or two.
  —Inform the patient that if bleeding does occur at the groin site, pressure should be applied immediately, the patient should lie flat, and the physician should be called at once.
- *Medications*
  —Explain the purpose, dosage, schedule, and route of administration of any prescribed drugs, as well as side effects to report to a physician or nurse.
  —Explain that if a stent is in place, antiplatelet therapy such as ticlopidine (Ticlid) or clopidogrel (Plavix) will be taken for 4 to 6 weeks.
- *Activity*
  —Encourage the patient to discuss allowances and limitations with respect to occupation, recreation, or activities.
  —Discuss the need to avoid heavy lifting (>10 pounds), heavy exercise, straining with bowel movements, and sexual relations for about a week after the procedure or as advised by the physician.
  —Tell the patient that showering or bathing is permitted but that very hot water should not be used.
- *Diet*
  —Emphasize the need to limit or avoid alcohol as advised by the physician.

FOLLOW-UP CARE

- Stress the importance of regular follow-up visits. Make sure the patient has the necessary names and telephone numbers.

Pericardiocentesis

—Pericardiocentesis: withdrawal of blood or fluid from the pericardial sac via percutaneous needle puncture.

INDICATIONS

- Relief of cardiac compression and withdrawal of pericardial fluid for analysis secondary to pericarditis or pericardial effusion

PREPROCEDURAL TEACHING

- Review the physician's explanation of the procedure and the reason for it; encourage the patient to ask questions and to discuss any fears or anxieties. Explain the need for informed consent.

Review of Preprocedural Care

- Instruct the patient not to eat or drink for 4 to 6 hours before the procedure.
- Explain that the procedure will be performed under local anesthesia and sedation will be given.
- Inform the patient that the skin will be cleansed from the left costal margin to the xiphoid process.
- Explain that the patient will be positioned with the head of the bed elevated 20 to 30 degrees.
- Tell the patient that laboratory tests and a 12-lead electrocardiogram will be completed before the procedure.
- Explain that vital signs will be monitored throughout the procedure, including pulsus paradoxus and pulse pressure.
- Inform the patient that emergency treatment and medications will be readily available.
- Explain that oxygen will be administered by mask or cannula.

Review of Postprocedural Care

- Inform the patient that signs and symptoms of complications or recurrence of cardiac tamponade or effusion will be monitored.
- Explain that bed rest will be ordered.

- Tell the patient that heart sounds and blood pressure will be monitored.
- Inform the patient that the catheter may be left in place for several hours to allow gravity drainage of fluid.

SIDE EFFECTS/COMPLICATIONS

- Puncture of coronary artery, ventricle, or lung
- Dysrhythmias, including ventricular fibrillation
- Laceration of the lung
- Pneumothorax
- Air embolism
- Cardiac tamponade
- Myocardial injury

 HOME CARE

- Give both the patient and the caregiver *verbal* and *written* instructions. Provide them with the name and telephone number of a physician or nurse to call if questions arise.
- *General information*
    —Review any explanation of the procedure and specific follow-up care.
- *Warning signs*
    —Review the signs and symptoms that should be reported to a physician or nurse.
    Dyspnea
    Palpitations
    Chest pain
    Lightheadedness
    Fever

FOLLOW-UP CARE

- Stress the importance of regular follow-up visits for care of the specific disease process. Make sure the patient has the necessary names and telephone numbers.

P

Pericarditis

—Pericarditis: inflammatory process of the outer lining of the heart, which leads to the formation of a serous fluid and fibrous adhesion. The thickening and scarring of the lining can restrict the movement of the heart muscles and may lead to pericardial effusion. The condition may be acute or chronic.

CAUSES/CONTRIBUTING FACTORS/RISK FACTORS

- Infection: bacterial, viral, fungal
- Myocardial infarction
- Trauma from surgery
- Tuberculosis
- Tumors
- Drugs
- Radiation
- Autoimmune diseases
- Blunt chest trauma
- Idiopathic factors

SIGNS/SYMPTOMS

- Sudden sharp chest pain radiating to the shoulder, back, and arm
- Pain that worsens when lying down or coughing or with inspiration and is relieved by leaning forward
- Fever and chills
- Nausea
- Shortness of breath
- Anxiety
- Fatigue

COMPLICATIONS

- Pericardial effusion
- Cardiac tamponade
- Chronic constriction of myocardium

DIAGNOSTIC TESTS

- Describe each procedure, its purpose, and the normal feelings or sensations that are likely, as well as any preprocedural and postprocedural care.

—Blood tests: white blood cell count, fungal serology, blood urea nitrogen, erythrocyte sedimentation rate, cardiac enzymes
—12-Lead electrocardiogram: to identify diffuse ST elevation
—Chest x-ray: to detect enlarged cardiac silhouette
—Echocardiogram: to detect accumulation of fluid around the heart

TREATMENT
Medical

- Therapy
  —Pericardiocentesis: needle aspiration of excess fluid from pericardial sac
- Drugs
  —Nonsteroidal antiinflammatory drugs
  —Steroids
  —Analgesics
  —Antibiotics

Surgical

- Pericardial window: open pericardial drainage
- Pericardiectomy: surgical removal of visceral and parietal pericardium

HOME CARE

- Give both the patient and the caregiver *verbal* and *written* instructions. Provide them with the name and telephone number of a physician or nurse to call if questions arise.
- *General information*
  —Discuss the development of pericarditis, causes and contributing factors, care, and treatment.
- *Warning signs*
  —Review the signs and symptoms that should be reported to a physician or nurse.
    Recurrence of symptoms
    Chest pain
    Fever
    Signs and symptoms of cold and flu
- *Special instructions*
  —Instruct the patient to avoid people with colds or flu and to get medical attention at once if an infection, cold, or flu is suspected.

—Advise the patient that sitting up and leaning forward on a table may ease chest discomfort.

—Inform the patient that a feeling of wellness does not necessarily mean that inflammation is completely resolved.

- *Medications*
  —Explain the purpose, dosage, schedule, and route of administration of any prescribed drugs, as well as side effects to report to the physician or nurse.
  —Stress the importance of not stopping medications without notifying the physician.
- *Activity*
  —Explain the need to increase activity gradually, avoid activities that require large amounts of energy, and take frequent rest periods during the day.
- *Diet*
  —Advise the patient to follow the prescribed diet.

FOLLOW-UP CARE AND REFERRALS

- Stress the importance of follow-up visits. Make sure the patient has the necessary names and telephone numbers.

Pernicious Anemia
(Hyperchromic Macrocytic Anemia)

—Pernicious anemia: an anemia caused by decreased absorption of vitamin B_{12}. Deficiency of an intrinsic factor essential for absorption of vitamin B_{12} causes production of red blood cells with increasingly fragile cell membranes, which leads to widespread destruction of the cells and results in low hemoglobin levels. Deficiency of vitamin B_{12} causes gastric, intestinal, and neurologic abnormalities.

CAUSES/CONTRIBUTING FACTORS/RISK FACTORS

- Primary
  —Genetic predisposition

—Immunologically related diseases (thyroiditis, myxedema, Graves' disease)
- Secondary
  —Surgical removal of a portion of the stomach, limiting the amount of productive mucosa

SIGNS/SYMPTOMS

- Classic trilogy of signs: weakness; beefy red, sore tongue; numbness and tingling in the extremities
- Gastrointestinal
  —Nausea and vomiting
  —Anorexia
  —Weight loss
  —Flatulence
  —Diarrhea
  —Constipation
  —Pallor
  —Jaundice
- Neurologic
  —Lack of coordination
  —Impaired fine finger movement
  —Lightheadedness
  —Headache
  —Altered vision (blurred, double vision)
  —Ringing in the ears
  —Irritability
  —Depression
  —Poor memory
  —Impaired judgment
  —Paresthesias of hands and feet

COMPLICATIONS

- Paralysis
- Psychotic behavior: paranoia, hallucinations, delusions
- Loss of bowel and bladder control
- Fatal if left untreated
- Cardiomegaly, congestive heart failure
- Gastritis
- Infections: pulmonary, urinary
- Peptic ulcer disease (4 to 5 times greater in this population)

DIAGNOSTIC TESTS

- Describe each procedure, its purpose, and the normal feelings or sensations that are likely, as well as any preprocedural and postprocedural care.
  —Schilling test: definitive for diagnosis of pernicious anemia
  —Bone marrow biopsy: increased megaloblasts
  —Gastric analysis: elevated pH, no free hydrochloric acid
  —Therapeutic trial with parenteral vitamin B_{12}: increased reticulocyte count in 4 to 5 days after injection
  —Laboratory tests
     Red blood cells: <3 million
     Mean corpuscular volume, mean corpuscular hemoglobin concentration: elevated
     White blood cell count, mean corpuscular hemoglobin: decreased
     Bilirubin: unconjugated forms elevated
     Serum vitamin B_{12}: decreased
     Serum folate: decreased
     Hemoglobin: decreased

TREATMENT
Medical

- Therapy
  —Blood transfusions
  —Diet high in vitamin B_{12}
- Drugs
  —B_{12} replacement therapy
  —Folic acid (Folvite)
  —Iron replacement
  —Ferrous sulfate (Feosol); ferrous gluconate (Fergon)
  —Digestants: hydrochloric acid
  —Antifungal, analgesic mouth rinse

HOME CARE

- Give both the patient and the caregiver *verbal* and *written* instructions. Provide them with the name and telephone number of a physician or nurse to call if questions arise.
- *General information*
  —Explain and discuss pernicious anemia, its causes, and contributing factors.
  —Review symptoms of the disease. Explain that most symptoms will recede with treatment.

- *Warning signs*
  —Review the signs and symptoms that should be reported to a physician or nurse.
     Pulmonary infection: fever, cough, production of sputum
     Urinary tract infection: frequency, urgency, burning with urination, foul-smelling urine
     Neurologic disturbances: increasing weakness, lack of coordination, irritability, confusion
- *Special instructions*
  —Explain that the weakened condition may predispose the patient to infection. Stress the importance of avoiding large crowds and individuals who have or are suspected of having infections.
  —Discuss oral care if the mucous membranes and tongue are red, swollen, and painful.
     Rinse the mouth every 2 hours while awake with dilute mouthwash or normal saline.
     Use a soft-bristled toothbrush or sponge cleaners as indicated. Use water-soluble jelly on the lips.
     Medicate with topical analgesics as ordered for severe discomfort.
  —Discuss safety measures.
     Advise a patient who has sensory deficits to avoid exposure of the extremities to extreme heat and cold.
     Encourage the use of assistive devices for ambulation (walker, cane) as indicated.
     Encourage the use of nonslip, well-fitting shoes.
     Instruct the patient to remove hazards such as loose rugs and furniture that blocks walkways.
- *Medications*
  —Explain the purpose, dosage, schedule, and route of administration of any prescribed drugs, as well as side effects to report to the physician or nurse.
  —Explain the importance of taking vitamin B_{12} on a lifelong basis.
  —Instruct the patient to avoid taking over-the-counter medications without first consulting the physician or nurse.
  —Teach the patient or caregiver the proper injection technique for administering vitamin B_{12}, or arrange for monthly clinic visits for injection.
  —For injections administered by the patient or caregiver, provide information about obtaining vitamin B_{12}, needles,

syringes, and alcohol sponges. Teach the proper method for disposing of needles and syringes.

- *Activity*
  —Encourage the patient to discuss allowances and limitations with respect to occupation, recreation, and activities.
  —Encourage the patient to pace activities, allow for frequent rest periods, and avoid overexertion.
  —Encourage the patient to participate in regular exercise as tolerated to prevent complications from motor deficits.
- *Diet*
  —Encourage a diet that is high in vitamin B_{12} (eggs, fish, meat, milk).
  —Encourage the patient to take 2500 ml of fluid daily (unless contraindicated) and to avoid hot liquids.
  —Teach the patient to eat small, frequent meals and between-meal snacks to enhance appetite.
  —Discuss the need to avoid foods that may irritate the gastrointestinal tract (spicy, flatus-forming, and caffeine).
  —Encourage the patient to weigh daily at the same time of day and in the same clothing and to record and report steady or rapid weight losses to the physician.

FOLLOW-UP CARE

- Stress the importance of follow-up medical and laboratory evaluations. Make sure the patient has the necessary names and telephone numbers.

Pheochromocytoma
(Chromaffin Tumor)

—Pheochromocytoma: a chromaffin cell tumor of the sympathetic nervous system that produces excessive amounts of epinephrine and norepinephrine. Pheochromocytoma is characterized by paroxysmal or sustained hypertension, increased metabolism, and hyperglycemia and occurs most commonly in women between the ages of 30 and 40. Although this disorder is potentially fatal, the prognosis is generally good with treatment. Most tumors are benign.

CAUSES/PRECIPITATING FACTORS

- Adrenal chromaffin cell tumor in adrenal medulla or sympathetic ganglia
- Extraadrenal chromaffin cell tumor in abdomen, thorax, urinary bladder, or neck
- Inherited as an autosomal dominant trait
- Postural drainage
- Exercise
- Laughing
- Smoking
- Urination
- Change in body or environmental temperature
- Vasovagal stimulus
- Anything that puts pressure on the tumor (e.g., pregnancy)

SIGNS/SYMPTOMS

- Persistent or paroxysmal hypertension
- Headache
- Palpitations
- Visual blurring
- Nausea and vomiting
- Weight loss
- Severe diaphoresis
- Feelings of impending doom
- Precordial or abdominal pain
- Tachypnea
- Pallor or flushing
- Tremors

COMPLICATIONS

- Cerebrovascular accident
- Retinopathy
- Heart disease
- Dysrhythmia
- Kidney failure

DIAGNOSTIC TESTS

- Describe each procedure, its purpose, and the normal feelings or sensations that are likely, as well as any preprocedural and postprocedural care.
    —Computed tomography or magnetic resonance imaging: to identify adrenal gland lesions
    —Computed tomography, x-ray, or abdominal aortography: to identify extraadrenal lesions
    —Laboratory tests
        Total plasma catecholamine: 10 to 50 times higher than normal
        24-Hour urinalysis: increased secretion of catecholamines and metabolites

TREATMENT
Medical

- Drugs
    —Alpha-adrenergic blocking agents
        Phentolamine (Regitine)
        Phenoxybenzamine (Dibenzyline)
    —Beta-adrenergic blocking agents
        Propranolol (Inderal)
    —Tyrosine inhibitors
        Alpha-methylparatyrosine
    —Glucocorticoids, mineralocorticoids: for surgical patients
    —Analgesics: for headache, postsurgical pain

Surgical

- Removal of pheochromocytoma

🏠 HOME CARE

- Give both the patient and the caregiver *verbal* and *written* instructions. Provide them with the name and telephone number of a physician or nurse to call if questions arise.
- *General information*
    —Discuss pheochromotytoma and its causes and precipitating factors. Explain that surgery is the preferred treatment.
    —Provide the patient with information about adrenalectomy if performed (see p. 16).
- *Warning signs*
    —Review the signs and symptoms of an acute attack that should be reported to a physician or nurse.

Headache

Nausea

Dizziness

Palpitations

Dyspnea

Diaphoresis

- *Special instructions*
  - —Demonstrate to the patient and caregiver how to measure and record blood pressure at home. Permit time for practice. Advise the patient on where to obtain equipment.
  - —Instruct the patient to weigh daily at the same time, on the same scale, and wearing the same clothing.
  - —Review precipitating events and discuss how to avoid them.
  - —Teach stress reduction techniques: meditation, breathing exercises, imagery.
  - —Instruct surgical patients to monitor for infection (respiratory or urinary tract): fever; cough; foul-smelling sputum; burning, frequency, or urgency with urination; foul-smelling urine.
  - —Instruct the patient to inspect the surgical site daily for signs of infection: drainage, separation of suture line, redness, swelling.
- *Medications*
  - —Explain the purpose, dosage, schedule, and route of administration of any prescribed drugs, as well as side effects to report to the physician or nurse.
  - —Instruct the patient to avoid taking over-the-counter medications without first consulting the physician or nurse.
- *Activity*
  - —Encourage the patient to discuss allowances and limitations with respect to occupation, recreation, and activities.
- *Diet*
  - —Advise the patient to avoid tyramine-containing foods (e.g., aged cheese, wine).
  - —Encourage the patient to eat small, frequent meals.

FOLLOW-UP CARE

- Stress the importance of follow-up medical and laboratory evaluations. Make sure the patient has the necessary names and telephone numbers.
- Discuss the need to wear a MedicAlert bracelet and carry an identification card at all times.

Photodynamic Therapy
(Laser Therapy)

—Photodynamic therapy: treatment involving injecting a patient with an intravenous photosensitizing agent such as dihematoporphyrin ether (DHE), waiting 48 to 72 hours for the drug to concentrate in malignant cells, and then exposing the cancerous area to laser light delivered through a scope such as a cystoscope or bronchoscope.

INDICATIONS
- Possible cure for early stages of skin and bladder cancers
- Palliation of advanced lung, esophageal, and pelvic cancers
- Alleviation of symptoms caused by obstructive primary or secondary cancer
- Tumor debulking with relief of bleeding, infection, pain, and symptoms of obstruction

PREPROCEDURAL TEACHING
- Review the physician's explanation of the procedure and the reason for it; encourage the patient to ask questions and to discuss any fears or anxieties.

Review of Preprocedural Care
- Assure the patient that the procedure is painless.

Review of Postprocedural Care
- Teach the patient to stay out of sunlight for up to 6 weeks after treatment because of tissue photosensitivity.
- If the procedure is used to treat bladder cancer, inform the patient that severe urinary frequency and urgency may be experienced and bladder capacity decreased; that bladder capacity usually returns to normal within 3 months; and that oral analgesics, antispasmodics, and prophylactic antibiotics may be prescribed.

Pleural Effusion

—Pleural effusion: accumulation of fluid (blood, pus, chyle, serous fluid) in the pleural space between visceral and parietal pleura (lining of the lung). Types of effusion include exudate, which is an often dark yellow or amber fluid resulting from a disease of the pleural surface or an obstruction in the lymphatic system, and transudate, which is fluid produced when the flow of protein-free fluid is disturbed.

CAUSES/CONTRIBUTING FACTORS

- Exudate
  - —Neoplastic diseases
  - —Viral infections
  - —Tuberculosis
  - —Empyema pneumonia
  - —Chest trauma
  - —Pancreatitis
  - —Rheumatic fever
  - —Collagen-vascular disease
  - —Uremia
  - —Pulmonary embolism
  - —Subphrenic abscess
- Transudate
  - —Peritoneal dialysis
  - —Pericarditis
  - —Cirrhosis
  - —Congestive heart failure
  - —Myxedema
  - —Sarcoidosis
  - —Hypoproteinemia
  - —Nephrotic syndrome
  - —Atelectasis

SIGNS/SYMPTOMS

- Shortness of breath
- Respiratory difficulty
- Localized chest pain
- Asymmetric chest expansion

- Elevated temperature
- Fatigue
- Cough

COMPLICATIONS

- Pneumothorax
- Atelectasis
- Empyema
- Reaccumulation of pleural fluid after thoracentesis
- Cardiopulmonary compromise

DIAGNOSTIC TESTS

- Describe each procedure, its purpose, and the normal feelings or sensations that are likely, as well as any preprocedural and postprocedural care.
  —Chest x-ray
  —Thoracentesis
  —Pleural biopsy

TREATMENT
Medical

- Therapy
  —Bed rest
  —Chest tube insertion
  —Thoracentesis
- Drugs
  —Antibiotics
  —Antipyretics
  —Pain management medications
  —Sclerosing pleurodesis: nitrogen mustard instillation or tetracycline via chest tube

⊞:: HOME CARE

- Give both the patient and the caregiver *verbal* and *written* instructions. Provide them with the name and telephone number of a physician or nurse to call if questions arise.
- *General information*
  —Explain the underlying cause and contributing factors.
- *Warning signs*
  —Review the signs and symptoms that should be reported to a physician or nurse.
    Difficulty in breathing

Chest pain
Elevated temperature
Persistent cough
Symptoms of cold or flu

- *Special instructions*
  —Discuss measures to prevent respiratory infections: avoiding persons with infections, especially upper respiratory infections; obtaining influenza vaccinations as ordered.
  —Instruct and demonstrate coughing and deep breathing to maintain lung aeration, and encourage the patient to perform them.
  —Demonstrate the use of the incentive spirometer.
- *Medications*
  —Explain the purpose, dosage, schedule, and route of administration of any prescribed drugs, as well as side effects to report to the physician or nurse.
  —Instruct the patient to avoid taking over-the-counter medications without first consulting the physician or nurse.
- *Activity*
  —Advise the patient of the importance of exercising to tolerance, avoiding fatigue, and planning rest periods.

FOLLOW-UP CARE

- Stress the importance of follow-up visits. Make sure the patient has the necessary names and telephone numbers.
- Emphasize the importance of not smoking and of avoiding secondhand smoke.

Pneumonia and Pneumonitis

—Pneumonia: an inflammatory process of the respiratory bronchioles and alveolar spaces caused by infection. Bacterial pneumonia is usually caused by *Streptococcus, Staphylococcus,* or *Haemophilus.* The infection can start from an upper respiratory infection such as "strep" throat or from inhaling fluid or other foreign substances into the lungs. Viral pneumonia is commonly caused by influenza A. It is transmitted by respiratory droplets. *Mycoplasma* pneumonia, which is most common in school-age children and young adults, spreads among family members. Transmission is believed to be by infected respiratory secretions. Aspiration pneumonia syndrome occurs as a result of aspiration when the patient is in an altered state of consciousness (e.g., seizure, use of drugs or alcohol, anesthesia, acute infection, or shock).

—**Pneumonitis: noninfectious bronchial and alveolar inflammation.**

SIGNS/SYMPTOMS
- Chills and fever (102° to 106° F [38.8° to 41.1° C])
- Difficult and painful respirations
- Pleuritic pain
- Shortness of breath and grunting
- Tachypnea
- Diaphoresis
- Loss of appetite or upset stomach
- Generalized fatigue that is worse than you would expect from a cold
- Cough that produces greenish yellow sputum progressing to pink or rusty
- Restlessness
- Cyanosis
- Disorientation or confusion and low-grade fever in elderly
- Anxiety

COMPLICATIONS
- Atelectasis
- Empyema
- Acute respiratory distress syndrome
- Superinfection pericarditis
- Lung abscess
- Septic shock
- Bacteremia

DIAGNOSTIC TESTS
- Describe each procedure, its purpose, and the normal feelings or sensations that are likely, as well as any preprocedural and postprocedural care.

—Chest x-ray: to evaluate the pulmonary system; to detect patchy or diffuse infiltrates
—Sputum examination for Gram stain and culture and sensitivity tests: to identify microorganisms present so that appropriate antiinfective agents can be prescribed
—White blood cell count: increased (>11,000/µl) in the presence of bacterial pneumonia; normal or low in viral or *Mycoplasma* pneumonia
—Blood culture and sensitivity: to determine the presence of bacteremia and aid in identification of the causative organism
—Serologic studies: to diagnose viral pneumonia; relative rise in antibody titer suggests viral infection
—Arterial blood gases
—Bronchoscopy

TREATMENT
Medical

- Therapy
  —Rest
  —Suctioning
  —Fluid management
  —Parenteral therapy
  —Oxygen therapy
  —Chest physiotherapy
  —Artificial airway or mechanical ventilation support
- Drugs
  —Antipyretics
  —Antibiotics
  —Bronchodilators
  —Mucolytics

HOME CARE

- Give both the patient and the caregiver *verbal* and *written* instructions. Provide them with the name and telephone number of a physician or nurse to call if questions arise.
- *General information*
  —Explain the underlying cause and contributing factors.
- *Warning signs*
  —Review the signs and symptoms that should be reported to a physician or nurse.

Elevated temperature
Diaphoresis
Difficulty in breathing
Persistent cough
Cold or flu

- *Special instructions*
  —Explain the importance of avoiding transmission of disease: turn head away when coughing, cover mouth with tissue, use tissue only once, dispose of tissue in waste container, and wash hands after handling soiled tissues and before and after using the bathroom.
  —Explain the need to avoid recurrence of disease: avoid persons with infections, especially upper respiratory infections.
  —Administer the influenza vaccine as ordered.
  —Demonstrate and explain the importance of postural drainage and deep breathing exercises. Tell the patient to continue deep breathing exercises four times a day for 6 to 8 weeks.
  —Explain the need to use a vaporizer or humidifier at home. Advise the patient on obtaining the equipment from a drugstore or pharmacy.
  —Instruct the patient on methods of clearing secretions, such as coughing, positioning, splinting chest wall, or suctioning.
  —Instruct the patient on adaptive breathing techniques to decrease the work of breathing.
  —Encourage the patient to avoid smoking.
- *Medications*
  —Explain the purpose, dosage, schedule, and route of administration of any prescribed drugs, as well as side effects to report to the physician or nurse.
      Antibiotics
      Antipyretics
      Analgesics: for chest pain
      Cough suppressants: for nonproductive cough
  —Instruct the patient to avoid taking over-the-counter medications without first consulting the physician or nurse.
- *Activity*
  —Explain the importance of a gradual convalescence.
  —Explain the need to limit exercise and activity to tolerance, to avoid fatigue, and to plan two or three rest periods during the day.
  —Explain the need for 7 to 8 hours of sleep every night.

- *Diet*
  —Explain the importance of maintaining a diet as tolerated.
  —Advise the patient to drink at least 6 to 8 glasses of fluids (up to 300 ml) daily unless contraindicated.

FOLLOW-UP CARE AND REFERRALS

- Stress the importance of follow-up visits. Make sure the patient has the necessary names and telephone numbers.
- Provide referrals to smoking cessation programs in the community.

Polycystic Kidney Disease

—**Polycystic kidney disease: hereditary kidney disease characterized by multiple fluid-filled cysts that enlarge and eventually compress and replace the functioning kidney tissue. In the adult form the onset is insidious, symptoms appear between 30 and 50 years of age, and the disease progresses slowly to renal failure.**

SIGNS/SYMPTOMS

- Early
  —Hypertension
  —Increased urine output
  —Urinary tract infection
- Late
  —Abdominal pain and distention
  —Lumbar pain
  —Widening abdominal girth
  —Palpable kidneys
  —Hematuria
  —Proteinuria
  —Decreased urine output

COMPLICATIONS

- Ruptured cysts causing infection and bleeding
- Severe hypertension

P

- Abscesses
- Ureteral obstruction from clots
- Renal failure

DIAGNOSTIC TESTS

- Describe each procedure, its purpose, and the normal feelings or sensations that are likely, as well as any preprocedural and postprocedural care.
    - —Blood studies: electrolytes, protein, blood urea nitrogen, creatinine
    - —Urine studies: urinalysis, culture and sensitivity, 24-hour urine for creatinine clearance
    - —X-ray of kidney, ureter, bladder (KUB)
    - —Intravenous pyelogram, urogram
    - —Renal computed tomography

TREATMENT
Medical

- Therapy
    - —Bed rest if bleeding
    - —Dietary restrictions on sodium, potassium, protein
    - —Dialysis for end-stage renal disease
- Drugs
    - —Antihypertensives
    - —Diuretics
    - —Antibiotics

Surgical

- Intervention if cysts break and cause abscesses or bleeding (see Abdominal Surgery, p. 6)
- Nephrectomy
- Kidney transplant

▦ HOME CARE

- Give both the patient and the caregiver *verbal* and *written* instructions. Provide them with the name and telephone number of a physician or nurse to call if questions arise.
- *General information*
    - —Explain the disease process and outcome.

- *Warning signs*
  —Review the signs and symptoms that should be reported to a physician or nurse.

    Sudden change in urine: color, blood, decreased amount, odor

    Sudden onset of flank pain

    Fever, chills

    Urinary tract infection: fever; chills; painful urination; low back or flank pain; cloudy, foul-smelling urine (ammonia or fishy smell); blood in urine

- *Special instructions*
  —Instruct the patient in prevention of urinary tract infections: increased fluid intake (amount will depend on stage of disease), regular emptying of bladder, good perineal area care after urination and defecation, and thorough handwashing before and after toileting.
  —Instruct the patient to take, monitor, and record blood pressure and provide parameters to report.
  —Instruct the patient to weigh daily at the same time, using the same scale, and wearing the same clothing.

- *Medications*
  —Explain the purpose, dosage, schedule, and route of administration of any prescribed drugs, as well as side effects to report to the physician or nurse.

- *Activity*
  —Advise the patient to identify and avoid activities that may precipitate pain.
  —Encourage the patient to discuss allowances and limitations with respect to occupation, recreation, and activities.
  —Tell the patient to exercise to tolerance but to avoid contact sports (e.g., football, soccer, basketball).
  —As the disease advances, encourage the patient to take frequent rest periods and avoid fatigue.

- *Diet*
  —Explain that the diet depends on the stage of the disease and includes restrictions on sodium, potassium, and protein. Fluids are encouraged at first and then restricted if kidney function decreases.

PSYCHOSOCIAL CARE

- Encourage verbalization of fears and concerns regarding disease progression.
- Provide support and encourage family counseling.

FOLLOW-UP CARE AND REFERRALS

- Stress the importance of follow-up visits. Make sure the patient has the necessary names and telephone numbers.
- Discuss the need for genetic counseling because this is an autosomal dominant disease. Provide referrals as indicated.

Prostate Cancer

—Prostate cancer: cancer of the prostate gland, the most common site of cancer in men. Prostate cancer is rare in men younger than 50 years of age. The incidence and mortality are increasing, especially among African-Americans. Most prostate cancers are adenocarcinomas, which grow slowly, spread via the lymphatics through the pelvic region and into the pelvic bones, and spread via the blood to the lungs, liver, kidneys, and bones (vertebrae, pelvis, femur, and ribs). The rest are ductal (transitional cell and squamous cell carcinoma, endometrioid cancer, or sarcoma). Acinar dysplasia/prostatic intraepithelial neoplasia is a premalignant lesion.

CAUSES/CONTRIBUTING FACTORS

- Influence of endogenous hormones, especially dihydrotestosterone
- Genetic influences
- Dietary fat
- Exposure to certain viruses, pathogens, or industrial chemicals
- Urbanization

SIGNS/SYMPTOMS

- Early
  —Weak urinary stream
  —Frequency

—Dysuria
—Difficulty starting and stopping urination
- Pain in lower back, pelvis, or upper thighs
- Bilateral obstruction with renal insufficiency
- Late
  —Hematuria
  —Bone pain, urinary frequency, decreased stream, dribbling

DIAGNOSTIC TESTS

- Describe each procedure, its purpose, and the normal feelings or sensations that are likely, as well as any preprocedural and postprocedural care.
  —Digital rectal examination: to palpate the prostate gland and detect abnormalities
  —Needle biopsy via perineal or transrectal route: to detect malignant cells
  —Transrectal ultrasonography: to determine the presence and characteristics of the lesion
  —Computed tomography and magnetic resonance imaging: to determine the size and extent of the lesion
  —Lymphangiography: to determine the extent of paraaortic and pelvic node involvement
  —Prostate-specific antigen (PSA): tumor marker that is elevated in the presence of prostate cancer

TREATMENT
Medical

- Therapy
  —Radiation therapy
    External beam
    Interstitial implant
    General preprocedural and postprocedural care (see Radiation Therapy, p. 721)
- Drugs
  —Single-agent chemotherapy
    Cyclophosphamide
    5-Fluorouracil
    Doxorubicin
    Methotrexate
    Cisplatin
    Mitomycin C
    Dacarbazine

—Hormone therapy
  Diethylstilbestrol
  Conjugated estrogens (Premarin)
  Estradiol
  Diethylstilbestrol (Stilphostrol)
  Estramustine phosphate
—Medical adrenalectomy
  Aminoglutethimide
  Ketoconazole
  Spironolactone
  Glucocorticoids
—Antiandrogens
  Cyproterone acetate
  Flutamide
  Megestrol acetate
—Gonadotropin-releasing hormone agonists
  Leuprolide
  Goserelin (Zoladex)
  Buserelin

Surgical

- Transurethral resection
- Radical prostatectomy
- Bilateral orchiectomy
- General preprocedural and postprocedural care (see Prostatectomy, p. 523)

🏠 HOME CARE

- Give both the patient and the caregiver *verbal* and *written* instructions. Provide them with the name and telephone number of a physician or nurse to call if questions arise.
- *General information*
  —Review the physician's explanation of the disease, possible causes or contributing factors, type and stage of tumor, and prescribed treatment.
  —Discuss actual and potential sexual dysfunction associated with the prescribed therapy. Encourage questions. (See Erectile Dysfunction, p. 278.)
- *Warning signs*
  —Review the signs and symptoms that should be reported to a physician or nurse.
    Decreased output

Edema
Hypertension
Weight gain
- *Special instructions*
  —Discuss methods of pain management (see Pain Management, p. 708).
- *Medications*
  —Explain the purpose, dosage, schedule, and route of administration of any prescribed drugs, as well as side effects to report to the physician or nurse.
- *Activity*
  —Stress the importance of adequate fluid intake, exercise, and rest.

PSYCHOSOCIAL CARE

- Encourage the verbalization of feelings regarding body image, self-esteem, and actual or perceived loss of sexual function.
- Provide education about erectile dysfunction as indicated (see p. 278).

FOLLOW-UP CARE

- Stress the importance of follow-up visits, including an annual digital rectal examination and PSA if the prostate was not removed. Make sure the patient has the necessary names and telephone numbers.

REFERRALS

- Assist the patient to obtain referral services, access to support groups, and sexual counseling services.

Prostatectomy

—**Prostatectomy: removal of part or all of the prostate gland to relieve obstruction of urinary flow.** *Transurethral resection of the prostate* **(TURP) is removal of part of the hypertrophied prostate by means of a cystoscope or rectoscope inserted through the urethra. A spinal or light general anesthetic is** used, and the hospital day is 3 or more days. *Laser ablation prostatectomy* is the passage of a laser scope through the urethra to ablate part of the prostate. The patient is under general or spinal anesthesia. The surgery is performed on the day of admission and the patient usually stays overnight. *Open prostatectomy* is surgical removal of part of the prostate through an incision in the lower abdomen or perineum because of an enlarged prostate or complications such as recurrent bladder stones, bladder diverticula, immobile hip joints, or localized cancer. *Radical prostatectomy* is removal of the entire prostate, including the covering capsule and ducts within, through a surgical incision in the lower abdomen. Removal is based on diagnosis of cancer, including the capsule.

INDICATIONS

- Benign prostatic hypertrophy
- Prostate cancer

PREPROCEDURAL TEACHING

- Review the physician's explanation of the procedure and the reason for it; encourage the patient to ask questions and to discuss any fears or anxieties. Explain the need for informed consent for surgery, anesthesia, and blood transfusions.
- Encourage the patient to discuss sperm banking if treatment will affect fertility.

Review of Preprocedural Care

- Inform the patient that routine blood and urine studies, a chest x-ray, and an electrocardiogram will be performed.
- Explain that bowel preparation with an enema will be needed the night before.
- Instruct the patient to shower and shampoo with bactericidal soap (e.g., Dial, Safeguard, Hibiclens) the night before.
- Discuss the need for NPO status from midnight the night before.
- Mention the possibility that the pubic hair will be shaved before the operation.
- Explain that some procedures can affect sexual function.
    - —TURP or open prostatectomy: semen may go into the bladder rather than out during ejaculation (retrograde ejaculation); does not cause impotence; affects fertility

  —Radical prostatectomy: depends on extent of surgery and whether nerves are spared; may or may not affect ejaculatory function

  —Laser ablation prostatectomy: ejaculatory function often preserved, although diminished in volume

- Provide information on erectile dysfunction as indicated (see p. 278).

Review of Postprocedural Care

- For general postoperative care, see Abdominal Surgery (p. 6).
- Explain that the urine will be blood colored (bright red), then turn a darker tea color, and then lighten within about 1 week. Tell the patient that the urine may become pink-tinged with excessive walking or sitting.
- Explain that stress incontinence or dribbling after urinary catheter removal may occur and that pelvic (Kegel) exercises may improve the condition.
- Explain the possibility of frequent dressing changes with the flat Penrose drain.
- Tell the patient that sitting for long periods (more than 2 hours) may stimulate bleeding during the first week.
- Discuss care after TURP.
  —Explain that the patient will be remain in the hospital for 3 or more days.
  —Inform the patient that drainage tubes will be in place after surgery: a three-way urinary catheter in the urethra for continuous bladder irrigation.
  —Tell the patient that traction of the urinary catheter will be in place for a time after surgery.
  —Discuss the use of elastic stockings or alternating pressure stockings while the patient is in bed.
  —Stress the importance of deep breathing and coughing.
- Discuss care after laser ablation prostatectomy.
  —Tell the patient that surgery will be on the day of admission and an overnight stay will be required.
  —Explain that a urinary catheter usually stays in place about 5 days.
- Discuss care after open and radical prostatectomy.
  —Tell the patient that surgery will be performed on the day of admission and a 3- to 5-day stay will be needed.
  —Explain the drainage tubes that may be used: urinary catheter for 7 to 10 days or more; suprapubic catheter; flat Penrose

P

drainage tube under the tissue near the incision; Jackson-Pratt (self-suction) drain near the incision.

COMPLICATIONS

- TUR syndrome (TURP)
- Shock
- Blood clots in legs or elsewhere
- Stress incontinence
- Dribbling
- Retrograde ejaculation
- Impotence
- Pain
- Infection: fever, chills, redness, tenderness at incision site
- Paralytic ileus
- Constipation

HOME CARE

- Give both the patient and the caregiver *verbal* and *written* instructions. Provide them with the name and telephone number of a physician or nurse to call if questions arise.
- *General information*
  —Explain the type of procedure and the reason for it. Discuss the drainage catheters and tubes that will be left in place.
- *Warning signs*
  —Review the signs and symptoms that should be reported to a physician or nurse.
  > Obstructed urinary catheter: feeling of fullness in bladder, feeling of need to urinate, spasms of bladder, leakage of urine around catheter, decreased or no urine in bag for 4 hours
  > Infection: fever, chills, redness, swelling, purulent drainage from the operative area
  > Urinary tract infection (see Urolithiasis, p. 630)
  > Epididymitis, especially after TURP (see Epididymitis, p. 276)
  > Persistent pain in operative area
  > Gross blood or clots from catheter
  > Constipation
- *Special instructions*
  —Advise the patient on how and where to obtain supplies.
  —Explain and demonstrate care of the urinary catheter (see Urinary Catheter, p. 736).

—Instruct the patient to avoid sexual activity until permitted by the physician (different with each procedure). Remind the patient that retrograde ejaculation may occur after TURP.

—Teach Kegel exercises to tighten the perineum and encourage return of sphincter control after removal of the urethral catheter (see Urinary Incontinence, p. 749).

—Tell the patient to shower daily. Suggest the use of sitz baths to ease perineal discomfort.

—Discuss the need to avoid use of rectal suppositories or enemas unless ordered by the physician.

- *Medications*
  —Explain the purpose, dosage, schedule, and route of administration of any prescribed drugs, as well as side effects to report to a physician or nurse.
  —Advise the patient to avoid using over-the-counter medications without discussing them with the physician.
- *Activity*
  —Encourage the patient to discuss allowances and limitations with respect to occupation, recreation, or activities.
  —Instruct the patient to allow for frequent rest periods, gradually increasing activity as allowed and tolerated.
  —Advise the patient to avoid long car rides (more than 2 hours) or rides over bumpy roads.
- *Diet*
  —Inform the patient that a regular diet or one prescribed by the physician for the underlying condition should be followed.
  —Caution the patient to avoid alcohol for 1 month.
  —Advise avoiding caffeine (coffee, tea, cola) as directed.
  —Encourage a high-fiber diet to prevent constipation and facilitate bowel movements. Explain that straining can cause bleeding.
  —Encourage intake of water or juices (cranberry, prune, plum), 6 to 10 glasses/day, to induce frequent urination.

PSYCHOSOCIAL CARE

- Assist the patient, family, and caregiver to obtain emotional support.
- Encourage verbalization of feelings, fears, and perceived or actual changes in body image and sexual function.

FOLLOW-UP CARE

- Stress the importance of regular follow-up visits. Make sure the patient has the necessary names and telephone numbers.

REFERRALS

- Assist the patient to obtain home health care if needed.
- Provide a list of local support groups.

Pulmonary Embolism

—Pulmonary embolism: an obstruction of a pulmonary blood vessel by an embolus. An embolus is a clot made up of blood, fat, air, or amniotic fluid. The emboli cause decreased perfusion of the lung, resulting in decreased oxygenation (hypoxemia). Damage to the lung depends on the number of clots and the extent of obstruction to pulmonary circulation. The most common source of pulmonary embolism is venous thrombosis of the leg, thigh, or pelvis.

CONTRIBUTING FACTORS

- Venostasis (e.g., prolonged bed rest, obesity, advanced age, pregnancy, postpartum period)
- Fractures, injury of pelvis, trauma
- Increased blood coagulability (e.g., use of oral contraceptives high in estrogen [>100 μg per pill])
- Systemic disease: chronic lung disease, congestive heart failure, atrial fibrillation, thromboembolism, thrombophlebitis or vascular surgery, diabetes mellitus, major surgery, myocardial infarction

SIGNS/SYMPTOMS

- Shortness of breath
- Complaints of pain when breathing
- Restlessness
- Apprehension
- Diaphoresis
- Cyanosis, pallor

- Tachypnea
- Tachycardia
- Bloody sputum (rare)
- Cough
- Decreased blood pressure
- Elevated temperature

COMPLICATIONS

- Extended or recurrent pulmonary embolism
- Pulmonary infarction
- Atelectasis
- Pulmonary hypertension
- Right ventricular failure
- Decreased cardiac output
- Shock
- Cardiopulmonary arrest

DIAGNOSTIC TESTS

- Describe each procedure, its purpose, and the normal feelings or sensations that are likely, as well as any preprocedural and postprocedural care.
    —Chest x-ray: to evaluate the pulmonary and cardiac systems
    —Lung (ventilation/perfusion) scan: to identify defects in blood perfusion of the lung
    —Pulmonary angiogram: definitive study for pulmonary embolism
    —Electrocardiogram: to differentiate between pulmonary embolism and myocardial infarction
    —Arterial blood gases: to determine acid-base balance and need for oxygen
    —Serum assays: elevated lactate dehydrogenase, bilirubin, fibrin split products, and fibrin degradation

TREATMENT
Medical

- Therapy
    —Bed rest
    —Oxygen therapy
    —Antiembolism stockings
- Drugs
    —Anticoagulants: heparin, warfarin (Coumadin)

—Thrombolytics: streptokinase, urokinase; to speed the process of clot lysis

Surgical

• Insertion of umbrella filter for multiple emboli

HOME CARE

• Give both the patient and the caregiver *verbal* and *written* instructions. Provide them with the name and telephone number of a physician or nurse to call if questions arise.
• *General information*
   —Explain the disorder, underlying causes, and contributing factors.
   —Provide information on prevention for patients at risk for pulmonary embolism.
   —Stress the importance of not smoking or using tobacco products. Explain to the patient that nicotine causes constriction and damage to intimal cells.
• *Warning signs*
   —Review the signs and symptoms that should be reported to a physician or nurse.
      Sudden, sharp chest pain
      Bloody sputum
      Elevated temperature
      Tachypnea
      Shortness of breath
• *Medications*
   —Explain the purpose, dosage, schedule, and route of administration of anticoagulants, as well as side effects to report to the physician or nurse (see Anticoagulation Therapy, p. 648).
   —Tell the patient to avoid medications that enhance the response to warfarin (Coumadin), such as aspirin, nonsteroidal antiinflammatory drugs (ibuprofen), cimetidine, trimethaphan. Drugs that decrease the response to warfarin (Coumadin) include antacids, diuretics, oral contraceptives, and barbiturates.
   —Explain the need to check for bleeding in urine, stools, and sputum if the patient is sent home with a prescription for anticoagulants.

- *Activity*
  —Discuss the importance of exercising to tolerance with planned rest periods. Tell the patient to perform regular exercise such as walking.
  —Teach strategies to prevent venous pooling: avoid sitting or standing for long periods, elevate legs while sitting, and avoid crossing the legs. Demonstrate proper application of antiembolic stockings if ordered.

FOLLOW-UP CARE AND REFERRALS

- Stress the importance of medical and laboratory follow-up visits. Make sure the patient has the necessary names and telephone numbers.
- Provide information and referral to smoking cessation programs as indicated. Provide literature prepared by the American Heart Association.
- Explain the importance of laboratory testing for anticoagulant therapy.
- Tell the patient to inform all health care providers of the anticoagulant therapy.

Pulmonary Hypertension

—Pulmonary hypertension: increased pulmonary artery pressure resulting from progressive disease of the pulmonary vessels or lung tissue. Pulmonary hypertension occurs as a primary disease or secondary to existing cardiac or pulmonary disease. In primary pulmonary hypertension the small pulmonary arteries become narrow as a result of thickening of the intimal lining of the lung. Primary hypertension affects primarily women between 20 and 40 years of age.

CAUSES/CONTRIBUTING FACTORS

- Primary pulmonary hypertension
  —Unknown
- Secondary pulmonary hypertension
  —Congenital heart disease that causes left-to-right shunting

—Acquired heart disease that results in left ventricular failure (e.g., rheumatic valvular heart disease)
—Chronic hypoxia related to chronic obstructive pulmonary disease
—Pulmonary embolus
—Pulmonary stenosis

SIGNS/SYMPTOMS

- Increasing dyspnea on exertion and at rest
- Tachypnea
- Chest pain
- Dizziness
- Syncope
- Apprehension, fear
- Excessive fatigue
- Cyanosis (secondary hypertension)

COMPLICATIONS

- Right-sided heart failure
- Sudden death

DIAGNOSTIC TESTS

- Describe each procedure, its purpose, and the normal feelings or sensations that are likely, as well as any preprocedural and postprocedural care.
    —Chest x-ray: to detect enlargement of the pulmonary artery and right atrium and ventricle
    —Electrocardiogram: to detect arrhythmias
    —Echocardiogram: to evaluate the structure and function of the heart
    —Arterial blood gases: to determine acid-base balance and the need for oxygen
    —Cardiac catheterization: invasive procedure to visualize the heart and major blood vessels

TREATMENT
Medical

- Therapy
    —Oxygen therapy
    —Hemodynamic monitoring
    —Isovolumetric phlebotomy (secondary hypertension)

- Drugs
  —Primary hypertension: vasodilators such as prostacyclin, diuretics, calcium channel blockers, anticoagulation agents

Surgical

- Lung transplantation

HOME CARE

- Give both the patient and the caregiver *verbal* and *written* instructions. Provide them with the name and telephone number of a physician or nurse to call if questions arise.
- *General information*
  —Explain the disorder, underlying causes, and contributing factors.
- *Warning signs*
  —Review the signs and symptoms that should be reported to a physician or nurse.

  Decreased activity tolerance

  Changes in skin color or consistency of sputum

  Increased cough

  Swelling of legs, ankles, or abdomen

  Erythrocytosis: headache, muscle aches, blurred vision, increased fatigue, hemoptysis, epistaxis
- *Special instructions*
  —For patients with secondary hypertension, explain that a compensatory polycythemia (erythrocytosis) occurs as a result of shunting (arteriovenous mixing) and that a hematocrit greater than 45% may be within normal limits for the patient. Provide individual hematocrit parameters.
  —Provide the patient with information regarding oxygen therapy (see p. 700) if ordered and assist the patient to obtain equipment from medical supply houses.
  —Demonstrate and provide information on adaptive breathing techniques.
  —Explain the value of relaxation techniques, such as music therapy, deep breathing, meditation, and biofeedback.
  —Stress the importance of not smoking or using tobacco products. Explain that smoking increases the workload of the heart by causing vasoconstriction.
  —For female patients explain that pregnancy is contraindicated, and advise the patient not to use estrogen-based oral contraceptives.

- *Medications*
    - —Explain the purpose, dosage, schedule, and route of administration of any prescribed drugs, as well as side effects to report to the physician or nurse.
    - —Demonstrate preparation and administration of IV prostacyclin and care for the IV catheter.
    - —Tell the patient to avoid taking aspirin or iron; advise checking labels of all over-the-counter medications.
- *Activity*
    - —Discuss the importance of exercising to tolerance, avoiding fatigue, and planning rest periods. Confer with the physician about the type of exercise.
    - —Tell the patient to avoid activities involving sudden strenuous movement, push-pull exercise, or heavy lifting.
    - —Advise the patient to avoid exertion on hot, humid, or smoggy days.
    - —Explain that activities involving isotonic exercises (walking, bicycling, swimming) are permissible as long as the patient is aware of actions to take during episodes of fatigue or dyspnea (e.g., stop the activity and take a rest).
    - —Teach energy-saving procedures: sitting while shaving, combing hair, dressing, cooking, and taking a shower.
    - —Stress the importance of avoiding dehydration by drinking fluids on hot days and avoiding strenuous activity.
    - —Advise the patient to avoid extreme hot or cold temperatures.

PSYCHOSOCIAL CARE

- Encourage verbalization of fears and concern over lifestyle changes imposed by the disease.
- Provide emotional support and referral for counseling as indicated.

FOLLOW-UP CARE AND REFERRALS

- Stress the importance of follow-up visits. Make sure the patient has the necessary names and telephone numbers.
- Provide information on and referral for smoking cessation programs and pulmonary rehabilitation programs for exercise guidelines as indicated.

Pyelonephritis

—Pyelonephritis: inflammatory disease process from acute and chronic effects caused by bacterial infection of the lower urinary tract. The incidence is greater in females because they have a shorter urethra and lack the antibacterial secretions of the prostate that men have.

CONTRIBUTING FACTORS

- Lower urinary tract infection
- Urologic procedures involving a catheter or instrument
- Urethral obstruction caused by stone, clots, stricture, or tumor
- Congenital weakness of the bladder and ureter junction (allows reflux of urine)
- Neurogenic bladder
- Glomerulonephritis
- Polycystic kidney disease
- Diabetes mellitus
- Analgesic abuse (e.g., Tylenol)
- Benign prostatic hypertrophy
- History of unexplained fevers or bed-wetting
- Pregnancy

SIGNS/SYMPTOMS

- Urinary frequency, urgency, burning
- Decreased urine output
- Cloudy, foul-smelling urine (ammonia like or fishy)
- Blood in urine
- Flank pain and tenderness
- High fever
- Shaking chills
- Malaise, fatigue, weakness
- Loss of appetite
- Nausea and vomiting

COMPLICATIONS

- Generalized bacterial infection (septic shock)
- Scarring of the kidney tissue
- Kidney abscess

- Kidney stones
- Necrosis of kidney tissue

DIAGNOSTIC TESTS

- Describe each procedure, its purpose, and the normal feelings or sensations that are likely, as well as any preprocedural and postprocedural care.
  —Urinalysis, culture and sensitivity
  —X-ray of kidneys, ureter, bladder (KUB)
  —Intravenous pyelogram and urogram
  —Blood culture and sensitivity for persistently high temperature

TREATMENT
Medical

- Therapy
  —Hydration intravenously or orally to achieve urine output of at least 2000 ml/day
- Drugs
  —Antibiotics
  —Antipyretics
  —Analgesics

Surgical

- Intervention only if obstruction present (see Urolithiasis, p. 630, and Nephrectomy, p. 453).

🏠 HOME CARE

- Give both the patient and the caregiver *verbal* and *written* instructions. Provide them with the name and telephone number of a physician or nurse to call if questions arise.
- *General information*
  —Explain the disease process, underlying causes, and contributing factors.
- *Warning signs*
  —Review the signs and symptoms that should be reported to a physician or nurse.
      Recurrence of symptoms, elevated temperature
- *Special instructions*
  —Discuss methods of preventing recurrent urinary tract infection: empty the bladder regularly (every 3 to 4 hours and

once during the night); avoid prolonged bladder distention; wash hands before and after toileting.

—For a female patient, advise her to keep the perineal area clean and dry, wipe from front to back after toileting, avoid the use of feminine hygiene sprays, urinate before and after sexual intercourse to prevent (re)infection, report vaginal discharge and follow through with treatment, wear cotton underpants and avoid nylon underpants, and wear loose, nonrestrictive clothing.

—Teach the patient the method of obtaining midstream urine samples for culture and sensitivity.

—Teach the self-monitoring urine test for bacteria.

- *Medications*

—Explain the purpose, dosage, schedule, and route of administration of any prescribed drugs, as well as side effects to report to the physician or nurse.

—Stress the importance of completing the antibiotic course even if feeling better.

- *Activity*

—Encourage the patient to discuss allowances and limitations with respect to occupation, recreation, and activities.

- *Diet*

—Tell the patient to follow a regular diet or the one prescribed by the physician.

—Stress the importance of drinking 10 to 15 glasses of clear fluids (water or cranberry, plum, or prune juice) per day.

—Tell the patient to avoid caffeinated beverages (coffee, tea, cola) and alcohol, especially during a urinary tract infection episode.

FOLLOW-UP CARE

- Stress the importance of follow-up medical and laboratory evaluations. Make sure the patient has the necessary names and telephone numbers.

Renal Failure

—Renal failure: inability to meet normal demands of kidney function. Acute renal failure is the sudden and rapid deterioration of kidney function resulting from obstruction, decreased blood flow, or renal disease. Acute renal failure is usually reversible but has high morbidity and mortality if not treated. Chronic renal failure is the slow, progressive loss of kidney function, leading to end-stage renal disease. It is an irreversible process, requiring dialysis or kidney transplantation.

CAUSES/CONTRIBUTING FACTORS

- Acute renal failure
  —Nephrotoxic exposure: drugs, chemicals, metals, contrast dyes
  —Infection
  —Shock: hemorrhagic, septic, cardiogenic, hypovolemic
  —Trauma: burns
- Chronic renal failure
  —Renal thrombus, stenosis, obstructions (calculi)
  —Chronic renal failure
  —Diabetes mellitus
  —Glomerulonephritis
  —Chronic pyelonephritis
  —Polycystic kidneys
  —Small kidneys
  —Tuberculosis
  —Tumors
  —Recent surgery (cardiac or vascular)
  —Several organ failure
  —Advanced age

SIGNS/SYMPTOMS

- Acute renal failure
  —Decrease (<400 ml/24 hr) or absence of urine output
  —Lethargy, confusion, irritability, headache
  —Nausea, vomiting, constipation, diarrhea
  —Shortness of breath on exertion or when flat

- Chronic renal failure
  —General malaise and fatigue, sleepiness, apathy, confusion
  —Loss of appetite, metallic taste, nausea, vomiting
  —Skin: itching; dry, discolored skin; easy bruising; sallow color; thin, brittle nails and hair
  —Decreased urine output, anuria
  —Peripheral neuropathy: burning, pain of soles of feet or "restless legs"
  —Cardiovascular: anemia, hypertension, shortness of breath, peripheral edema
  —Amenorrhea in women, impotence in men

COMPLICATIONS

- Acute renal failure
  —Pericarditis
  —Fluid and electrolyte imbalance
  —Infection and sepsis
  —Chronic renal failure
- Chronic renal failure
  —Cardiovascular: dysrhythmias, pericarditis, congestive heart failure, accelerated atherosclerosis
  —Pulmonary edema
  —Musculoskeletal: calcium deposits in blood vessels or joints, bone disease and disturbed vitamin D metabolism
  —Peripheral neuropathy
  —Metabolic encephalopathy
  —Peptic ulcer disease
  —Fluid-electrolyte imbalance

DIAGNOSTIC TESTS

- Describe each procedure, its purpose, and the normal feelings or sensations that are likely, as well as any preprocedural and postprocedural care.
  —Blood tests: blood urea nitrogen, creatinine, electrolytes, uric acid
  —Urine tests: urinalysis, osmolality, electrolytes, creatinine clearance, uric acid
  —X-ray of kidneys, ureter, bladder (KUB)
  —Renal computed tomography (CT) scan
  —Intravenous urogram
  —Renal biopsy
  —Renal ultrasound

TREATMENT
Medical

- Therapy
  —Treatment of underlying cause
  —Fluid and electrolyte management
  —Dialysis
  —Nutritional support: diet high in calories; low in protein, potassium, sodium, and phosphate
- Drugs
  —Alkalinizing agents
  —Potassium-removing resins
  —Diuretics
  —Phosphate binders
  —H_2 receptor antagonists
  —Antihypertensives

Surgical

- Single or bilateral nephrectomy
- Kidney transplant

⊞ HOME CARE

- Give both the patient and the caregiver *verbal* and *written* instructions. Provide them with the name and telephone number of a physician or nurse to call if questions arise.
- *General information*
  —Explain the underlying cause or contributing factors of the condition. Explain the type of renal failure and disease process.
  —Explain and prepare the patient for dialysis as ordered (see p. 674).
- *Warning signs*
  —Review the signs and symptoms that should be reported to a physician or nurse.
    Urine output decreased (<1 cup/8 hr) or absent
    Elevated blood pressure (>140/90 mm Hg)
    Rapid weight gain (>2 pounds in 24 hours)
    Swelling (edema) of feet, ankles, abdomen
    Excessive muscle weakness
    Palpitations or irregular pulse
    Shortness of breath on exertion or flat

General malaise and fatigue, increased sleepiness, drowsiness

Loss of appetite, loss of weight

Burning feet or "restless legs," paresthesias

Muscle cramps (especially legs), twitching

Excessive bruising or easy bruising

- *Special instructions*
  —Discuss skin care and grooming: keep nails short and clean; bathe daily but avoid long hot baths or showers; avoid vigorous towel rubbing; use lanolin, nonalcohol, superfatted soaps and emollient lotions for itchy skin; use mild shampoo with conditioners; avoid scratching the skin to prevent skin breaks and infection.
  —Instruct the patient in oral hygiene: brush the teeth using a soft-bristled toothbrush; use mouthwash after each meal for breath control; eat hard or sour candy for breath control and dry mouth.
  —Discuss the need for perineal care after toileting.
  —Instruct the patient in and demonstrate techniques for taking and recording blood pressure, temperature, and pulse (rest 5 minutes before taking). Provide a timetable and parameters to report. Allow time for practice using home blood pressure equipment.
  —Explain the need to weigh daily at the same time and wearing the same clothes, after urination, and before eating. Instruct the patient to keep a log of weight and to report weight gains of >2 pounds in 24 hours.
  —Discuss ways of avoiding infections including handwashing techniques and avoiding persons with upper respiratory infections.
- *Medications*
  —Explain the purpose, dosage, schedule, and route of administration of any prescribed drugs, as well as side effects to report to the physician or nurse.
  —Remind the patient that certain drugs must be taken with meals.
  —Advise patients taking diuretics to take them in the morning to avoid having to get up in the night.
- *Activity*
  —Discuss the need to pace activities as tolerated.
  —Instruct the patient in the use of ambulatory aids as needed (walker, cane, wheelchair).

—Discuss energy-conserving techniques and the use of home assist devices such as a shower chair or bath bars as needed.
—Tell the patient to schedule rest periods between activities.
—Encourage the patient to discuss allowances and limitations with respect to occupation, recreation, and activities.

• *Diet*
—Review the prescribed diet with the patient.
—Discuss the need to restrict sodium, potassium, phosphate, and protein. Explain that salt intake can be reduced by not eating "fast" or convenience-type foods, avoiding use of table salt, not cooking with salt, reading all labels, and rinsing canned vegetables before cooking and eating.
—Advise the patient to eat foods high in calories.
—Encourage a diet high in fiber to prevent constipation.
—Instruct a patient who is nauseated to take antiemetics half an hour before eating and to eat smaller, more frequent meals.
—Review prescribed fluid restrictions. Explain that levels are usually based on the previous day's urine output plus 500 to 800 ml over intake. Encourage the patient to spread fluid intake over the day, particularly during mealtimes and when active. Suggest using ice chips to control thirst.
—Arrange for the patient and family to meet with a dietitian before discharge.

PSYCHOSOCIAL CARE

• Encourage the patient and caregiver to verbalize fears and feelings about the disease process.
• Encourage independence and participation in planning care. Refer the patient to counseling to help the patient and caregiver cope with the disease and its outcomes.

FOLLOW-UP CARE

• Stress the importance of follow-up medical and laboratory evaluations. Make sure the patient has the necessary names and telephone numbers.
• Encourage and assist the patient to obtain a MedicAlert bracelet and identification card.

REFERRALS

• Provide referrals for home health care, social services, and community resources.

Renal Transplant

—**Renal transplant: implantation of a kidney from a living relative or a cadaver donor into a recipient to restore renal function. Implantation of the donor organ is preceded by nephrectomy of the diseased kidney.**

INDICATIONS

- End-stage renal disease

PREPROCEDURAL TEACHING

- Review the physician's explanation of the procedure and the reason for it; encourage the patient to ask questions and to discuss any fears or anxieties. Explain the need for informed consent for surgery, anesthesia, and blood transfusions.

Review of Preprocedural Care

- Explain that when a suitable donor is found, the patient will be called in for the transplantation.
- Review the comprehensive workup and evaluation for a patient awaiting transplant.
  —Blood studies for blood typing and tissue typing for compatibility, as well as electrolytes, creatinine, and blood urea nitrogen
  —Cystometrogram to evaluate bladder capacity and urination reflex
  —Voiding cystourethrography to evaluate bladder filling and emptying
  —Urine studies of creatinine and blood urea nitrogen
  —Transplant coordinator workup
  —Social worker and psychiatry workup
- Discuss the preoperative procedures once the donor is identified.
  —Hemodialysis (depending on time of last run)
  —Urinalysis to evaluate for infection
  —Blood studies for electrolytes, creatinine, blood urea nitrogen
  —Electrocardiogram, chest x-ray
- Explain that the patient will have nothing by mouth (NPO) from the time of notification (if a cadaver kidney) or from the night before (if donor is a living relative).

- Discuss the need for a small cleansing enema.
- Inform the patient of the need to shower with bactericidal soap (e.g., Hibiclens, Safeguard, Dial).
- Discuss the probability that the abdomen and pubic area will be shaved.
- Review the regimen of oral immunosuppressants.
- Inform the patient that the surgery lasts 3 to 4 hours or more and the patient will be under general anesthesia.

Review of Postprocedural Care

- For general postprocedural care, see Abdominal Surgery (p. 6).
- Explain that the patient is usually in the intensive care unit for the night after the surgery.
- Explain that the patient may be returned to surgery for removal of the transplanted kidney if hyperacute rejection occurs.
- Describe the drainage tubes that may be used: urethral catheter for 2 to 3 days or more (urine will be blood tinged for several days), Jackson-Pratt bulb (self-suction) drain near the incision line.
- Inform the patient that analgesics will be available for pain. Stress the importance of explaining the type and severity of pain.
- Explain that dialysis may be needed until the kidney starts working (2 to 30 or more days with cadaver kidney). A kidney from a living related donor usually starts working immediately.

COMPLICATIONS

- Rejection of transplanted kidney
- Wound infection
- Urinary tract infection
- Pulmonary problems
- Hemorrhage, shock
- Paralytic ileus
- Renal artery stenosis, thrombosis, or aneurysm
- Side effects of immunosuppressants
- Gastrointestinal bleeding
- Diabetes
- Glaucoma
- Cushing's syndrome

HOME CARE

- Give both the patient and the caregiver *verbal* and *written* instructions. Provide them with the name and telephone number of a physician or nurse to call if questions arise.
- *General information*
  —Review renal transplantation, reinforcing the importance of lifelong immunosuppressant treatment.
  —Review the signs of rejection, explaining that it may occur at any time, even years later.
- *Wound/incision care*
  —Demonstrate wound care and dressing change (see Nephrectomy, p. 453). Assist the patient to obtain necessary supplies.
- *Warning signs*
  —Review the signs and symptoms that should be reported to a physician or nurse.
    Infection: redness, tenderness, pain, swelling, warm to touch, purulent drainage
    Rejection: decreased or absent urine output; large amounts of dilute urine; hematuria; flulike symptoms (elevated temperature [>100° F], malaise, nausea, vomiting, diarrhea); reddening, swelling, and tenderness of the transplant area; sudden weight gain (>3 pounds/day); increased blood pressure; increased pulse (>100)
    Urinary tract infection
    Sudden onset of acute pain in operative area
    Inability to take medications
- *Special instructions*
  —Stress the importance of avoiding exposure to crowds and persons with known or suspected infections for at least 3 months after surgery.
  —Explain the importance of recording daily weight (weighing at the same time, with the same clothing, after urination, and before eating). Instruct the patient to report a gain of 2 or more pounds a day or 4 or more pounds a week.
  —Explain and demonstrate how to measure and record intake and output for the first 3 weeks.
  —Explain the importance of taking and recording temperature, pulse, and blood pressure (same arm, same time, 5-minute rest period before measurement) twice daily. Help the patient obtain equipment for home use.

R

—Inform the patient that strong or direct sunlight should be avoided because immunosuppressants increase susceptibility to skin cancer (especially lymphoma). They also decrease susceptibility to cancer of the cervix, vulva, and perineum and Kaposi's sarcoma.

- *Medications*
  —Explain the purpose, dosage, schedule, and route of administration of any prescribed drugs, as well as side effects to report to a physician or nurse.
  —Provide detailed instructions on immunosuppressant therapy and side effects.
  —Tell the patient to avoid over-the-counter medications unless approved by the physician.
  —Stress the importance of not missing doses of medications.
- *Activity*
  —Encourage the patient to discuss allowances and limitations with respect to occupation, recreation, or activities.
  —Tell the patient to begin exercise slowly and increase the level gradually, taking frequent rest breaks.
  —Advise the patient to avoid heavy lifting (>10 pounds) and contact sports such as football, soccer, and basketball.
  —Discuss the need to avoid driving for 2 weeks.
  —Instruct the patient to avoid positions that place pressure on the transplant site (lap seat belt on long car trip).
  —Explain the need to refrain from sexual activity for at least 6 weeks or until advised by the physician. Advise women that they should avoid pregnancy until it is approved by a physician. Provide contraceptive information.
- *Diet*
  —Tell the patient to follow a regular diet or one prescribed by the physician.
  —Advise the patient of the tendency to overeat because steroids stimulate the appetite.
  —Explain the need for a low-potassium diet if the patient is taking cyclosporine.
  —Tell the patient not to drink alcohol until allowed by the physician.

PSYCHOSOCIAL CARE

- Encourage expression of concern and fears about transplant and need for life-long immunosuppression.
- Encourage use of counseling services as indicated.

FOLLOW-UP CARE

- Stress the importance of life-long follow-up medical and laboratory visits. Make sure the patient has the necessary names and telephone numbers. Remind the patient to take the log of medications, weight, and vital signs to each medical appointment.
- Explain the importance of notifying the physician of dentist appointments, having eye examinations every 6 months for glaucoma and cataracts, and having annual pelvic examinations (for females).
- Encourage and assist the patient to obtain a MedicAlert bracelet and identification card listing the diagnosis, medication, and other information.

REFERRALS

- Assist the patient, family, or caregiver to obtain emotional support and family planning counseling as needed.
- Provide referrals for home care or community-based support services as indicated.

Replacement of Knee or Shoulder

—**Total knee replacement: replacement of the knee joint with a prosthesis to provide stability and motion. The femoral condylar cartilage and the tibial condylar surfaces are replaced with the prosthesis.**

—**Total shoulder replacement: placement of a prosthesis into the humeral shaft after removal of the head of the humerus.**

INDICATIONS

- Degenerative disease: rheumatoid arthritis, osteoarthritis

PREPROCEDURAL TEACHING

- Review the physician's explanation of the procedure and the reason for it; encourage the patient to ask questions and to discuss any fears or anxieties. Explain the need for informed consent for surgery and anesthesia.

Review of Preprocedural Care

- Review properative studies: x-rays, serologic and urologic studies to show the presence of infection, anemia, and electrolyte status.
- Explain that the patient will be NPO from midnight of the night before.
- Inform the patient of the need to shower with bactericidal soap (e.g., Hibiclens, Safeguard, Dial).
- Discuss the probability that the operative site will be shaved.
- Explain that ice may be applied before surgery to lessen edema (knee replacement).

Review of Postprocedural Care

- Explain that the patient will be in the hospital for 4 to 5 days.
- Inform the patient that bed rest will be required for 24 to 48 hours. After knee replacement, the operative leg will be elevated on a pillow.
- Discuss the drainage tubes (Hemovac) that may be used, and explain that wound drainage will be moderate, decreasing in amount.
- Tell the patient that a regular diet will be resumed in 2 to 3 days.
- Discuss the frequency of checks for vital signs, peripheral pulse, and neurovascular status.
- Explain that after shoulder replacement a sling and swathe may be used for joint immobilization or a shoulder spica or airplane splint may be used with the arm elevated on a pillow.
- Review postoperative exercises: range of motion for unaffected joints; isometric exercises; quadriceps setting, gluteal contractions, and flexion-extension exercises (for knee replacement); exercises of fingers, wrist, and elbow (for shoulder replacement).
- Introduce the use of the continuous passive motion (CPM) device (after knee replacement). Explain that the operative extremity is positioned in a sling in the device and the leg is moved through preset limits of range of motion.
- Review activity levels. After knee replacement, ambulation without weight bearing is permitted in 3 to 5 days and weight bearing in 10 to 14 days. After shoulder replacement, ambulation as tolerated with a shoulder immobilizer is permitted after 48 hours.

COMPLICATIONS

- Hemorrhage/hematoma formation
- Infection
- Thrombophlebitis
- Fat embolus
- Compartment syndrome (after knee replacement)
- Intraoperative fracture
- Atelectasis
- Pneumonia
- Nerve weakness
- Displacement of prosthesis
- Limb length inequality

HOME CARE

- Give both the patient and the caregiver *verbal* and *written* instructions. Provide them with the name and telephone number of a physician or nurse to call if questions arise.
- *General information*
  —Review the type of procedure performed and any specific limitations.
- *Warning signs*
  —Review the signs and symptoms that should be reported to a physician or nurse.
    - Increased pain in knee or shoulder area
    - Redness, swelling, redness in calf of one leg
    - Fever
    - Shortness of breath or chest pain
    - Decreased ability to move shoulder, arm, or knee
- *Special instructions*
  —Instruct the patient in the proper use of ambulatory aids: walker, crutches, and cane (for knee replacement).
- *Medications*
  —Explain the purpose, dosage, schedule, and route of administration of any prescribed drugs, as well as side effects to report to a physician or nurse.
    - Antibiotics
    - Analgesics
    - Anticoagulants
  —Stress the importance of having prothrombin time checked and observing for bleeding if the patient is taking anticoagulants (see p. 648).

- *Activity*
  —Advise the patient that full movement takes 3 to 6 months to return after joint replacement surgery. Review strengthening and range-of-motion exercises to help strengthen muscles and regain joint mobility and flexibility.

FOLLOW-UP CARE AND REFERRALS

- Stress the importance of regular follow-up visits with the physician and physical therapist until recovery is complete. Make sure the patient has the necessary names and telephone numbers.
- Provide referrals for home care services or a skilled nursing facility as indicated.

Restrictive Cardiomyopathy

—Restrictive cardiomyopathy: cardiomyopathy is a heart muscle disorder resulting in impaired function of the heart's pumping action. A less common form, restrictive cardiomyopathy, occurs when the heart loses its elasticity and cannot fill completely and contract effectively. This occurs when fibroelastic tissue infiltrates the heart, resulting in a thick and stiff heart.

CAUSES

- Endomyocardial fibroelastosis
- Infiltrative and storage disorder (sarcoidosis, amyloidosis)
- Scleroderma
- Radiation

SIGNS/SYMPTOMS

- Exercise intolerance
- Fatigue
- Dyspnea
- Orthopnea
- Chest pain
- Peripheral edema
- Abdominal discomfort, liver tenderness

COMPLICATIONS

- Heart failure
- Sudden death
- Arrhythmias
- Systemic emboli
- Heart failure

DIAGNOSTIC TESTS

- Inform the patient that several diagnostic procedures may be done to aid in the diagnosis of this condition. Describe each procedure, its purpose, and the normal feelings or sensations that are likely, as well as any preprocedural and postprocedural care.
    - —Chest x-ray: to show the enlarged heart and increased pressure in the pulmonary arteries
    - —Electrocardiogram: to determine the extent and location of muscle involvement and show low voltage and conduction disturbance
    - —Echocardiogram: to detect thickness of the heart muscle or fluid in the pericardial sac and the ability or inability of the heart muscle to move
    - —Radionuclide studies: to show infiltration of the heart muscle and detect its pumping ability
    - —Cardiac catheterization: to identify a decrease in heart muscle, elevated pressures during the filling of the heart, and the cause of the restriction
    - —Endomyocardial biopsy: to determine the cause

TREATMENT
Medical

- Drugs
    - —Digitalis: to strengthen and regulate the heart
    - —Diuretics: to aid the kidney in eliminating salt and fluid
    - —Oral vasodilators: to reduce the amount of blood coming into the heart and thus reduce the heart's workload; to relax the muscles against which the heart pumps
    - —Anticoagulants: to prevent clots from forming
    - —Heart transplantation: for patients with refractory symptoms

HOME CARE

- For home care see Heart Failure (p. 333).

Retinal Detachment

—Retinal detachment: partial or complete separation of the sensory layers of retina (the inner lining of the eyeball) from the posterior retinal lining, creating a subretinal space that fills with fluid. The retina is an extension of the central nervous system that receives images and transmits them to the brain. Retinal detachment is usually unilateral and spontaneous. It occurs more often in males. A retinal tear is a jagged break in the retina. A retinal hole is a break in the retina that allows liquid vitreous to seep between retinal layers; the condition is associated with trauma and aging.

CONTRIBUTING FACTORS

- Myopia
- Cataract surgery
- Eye trauma
- Degenerative changes caused by aging
- Systemic diseases
  —Severe hypertension
  —Chronic glomerulonephritis
  —Diabetes
  —Retinal vein occlusion
  —Retinal tumors, inflammation

SIGNS/SYMPTOMS

- Floating spots
- Recurrent flashes of light
- Blurred or sooty vision
- Unilateral vision loss: gradual and painless

COMPLICATIONS

- Vision impairment
- Blindness

DIAGNOSTIC TESTS

- Describe each procedure, its purpose, and the normal feelings or sensations that are likely, as well as any preprocedural and postprocedural care.

—Ophthalmoscopy: to show retinal pallor; hanging retina; crescent-shaped, red-orange tear(s); bulging retina

TREATMENT
Surgical

- Retinal tears and holes
  —Photocoagulation: to burn and eventually seal localized tears or breaks; used frequently in torn areas that are small or with retinal holes to prevent further detachment
  —Cryothermy: placement of a frozen metal probe on the conjunctiva near the tear, causing scleral inflammation, which leads to scar tissue formation and reattachment
  —Diathermy: application of a heated probe to the scleral surface over the site of the retinal break, causing burning that leads to an inflammatory response and eventual scarring and healing
- Retinal detachment
  —Scleral buckling: placement of a band similar to a piece of belt around the sclera at the site of detachment, drawing the sclera closer to the retina to facilitate attachment

PREPROCEDURAL TEACHING

- Review the physician's explanation of the procedure and the reason for it; encourage the patient to ask questions and to discuss any fears or anxieties.
- Explain that retinal detachment rarely heals spontaneously and that surgical correction is necessary to seal the retina.

Review of Preprocedural Care

- Inform the patient that complete bed rest is necessary to restrict eye movements.
- Explain that sedation is used and bilateral eye patches are applied to restrict eye movement and that the head will be positioned to promote reattachment.
- Tell the patient that mydriatics and cycloplegics are given to dilate the pupil and decrease movement of intraocular structures.
- Explain the need to cleanse the face with bactericidal soap and the possibility that the eyelashes will be cut off to minimize the chance of infection.

Review of Postprocedural Care

- Explain the importance of avoiding activities that increase intraocular pressure: straining, coughing, sneezing, bending, vomiting.
- Tell the patient that to minimize excessive eye movement, the patient will need to avoid shaving, brushing teeth, washing the face, and combing the hair.
- Explain that moderate pain can be expected in the first 24 to 48 hours but can be relieved with prescribed analgesics. Instruct the patient to report the presence of *sudden severe pain,* which can signal occurrence of hyphema.
- Advise the patient that eye patches will be worn for several days after eye surgery to prevent eye movement.
- Discuss the need for the patient to be placed in a specific position for several days according to the location of the detachment (e.g., may be prone) and type of surgical procedure; bed rest is maintained if there is macular involvement.
- Explain that the eyelid may be swollen after surgery and that ice packs will be applied.

🏠 HOME CARE

- Give both the patient and the caregiver *verbal* and *written* instructions. Provide them with the name and telephone number of a physician or nurse to call if questions arise.
- *General information*
    - —Explain the underlying cause or contributing factors of the condition. Discuss the purpose and type of procedure performed.
- *Warning signs*
    - —Review the signs, symptoms, and complications that should be reported to a physician or nurse.
        - Sudden loss of vision
        - Severe pain in eyeball
        - Heavy shower of floaters
        - Flashing lights
        - Purulent drainage
        - Persistent redness
        - Swelling
        - Fever
        - Postsurgical complications: hyphema, retinal re-detachment, infection, thrombophlebitis

- *Special instructions*
  —Remind the patient to lie in the recommended position following the scleral buckling procedure.
  —Advise the patient to apply cold compresses to the eye to reduce swelling and ease discomfort.
  —Explain the importance of wearing dark glasses to minimize photophobia and pain when eyedrops (mydriatics) are used.
  —Instruct the patient to wear an eye shield at night for protection (for 2 to 4 weeks).
  —Discuss lid hygiene: remove any drainage with a cotton ball moistened with tap water; gently sweep the cotton ball from the inner to outer aspect of the lid, using a new cotton ball with each sweeping motion.
  —Explain that floaters may appear after surgery and can disappear in weeks or last for years.
  —Explain the importance of avoiding rubbing, touching, and bumping of the operative eye.
- *Medications*
  —Explain the purpose, dosage, schedule, and route of administration of any prescribed drugs, as well as side effects to report to the physician or nurse.
  —Tell the patient to avoid using over-the-counter eyedrops or ointments without checking with the physician.
  —Teach the patient the procedure for administering eyedrops and emphasize the importance of washing the hands thoroughly before administration.
- *Activity*
  —Explain the importance of avoiding activities that can increase intraocular pressure: constipation (straining); sneezing; jarring head movements; heavy exercise; heavy lifting; bending; driving. Tell the patient to avoid sexual activity for 4 to 6 weeks or as prescribed by a physician.
  —Inform the patient that watching television is permitted but reading should generally be avoided for the first week or as directed by the physician.
  —Discuss the need to remove hazards at home to avoid injury (e.g., remove loose rugs).

FOLLOW-UP CARE

- Stress the importance of follow-up visits until recovery is complete. Make sure the patient has the necessary names and telephone numbers.

Rheumatic Fever

—Rheumatic fever: a systemic inflammatory disease that develops following a group A streptococcal infection of the upper respiratory tract (e.g., tonsillitis, nasopharyngitis, otitis media). Rheumatic fever most commonly involves the heart, synovial joint linings, skin, and central nervous system. The mitral valve is affected in 75% to 80% of cases and the aortic valve in less than 5%. Healing may be complete, or scarring may develop because of chronic inflammation.

SIGNS/SYMPTOMS
- Fever
- Migratory joint pains (growing pains): polyarthritis
- Swelling, redness, effusion of joints
- Skin lesions: trunk, extremities
- Subcutaneous nodules: knuckles, wrists, knees
- Chorea (purposeless jerky movements)
- Carditis

COMPLICATIONS
- Heart failure
- Pericarditis
- Endocarditis
- Myocarditis
- Valvular heart disease: mitral and aortic most commonly affected
- Cardiac arrhythmias

DIAGNOSTIC TESTS
- Describe each procedure, its purpose, and the normal feelings or sensations that are likely, as well as any preprocedural and postprocedural care.
  - White blood cell count, C-reactive protein, sedimentation rate: to determine the inflammatory process
  - Streptomycin or antistreptolysin O titer: to detect streptococcal infection
  - Throat cultures
  - Electrocardiogram

—Chest x-ray
—Echocardiogram

TREATMENT
Medical

- Therapy
  —Bed rest during acute phase
- Drugs
  —Antibiotics: penicillin, erythromycin
  —Antipyretics, salicylates: aspirin
  —Nonsteroidal antiinflammatory agents
  —Steroids

HOME CARE

- Give both the patient and the caregiver *verbal* and *written* instructions. Provide them with the name and telephone number of a physician or nurse to call if questions arise.
- *General information*
  —Explain the disease process, causes, contributing factors, care, and treatment.
- *Warning signs*
  —Review the signs and symptoms that should be reported to a physician or nurse.
    Recurrent streptococcal infections: sudden sore throat, throat redness, swollen lymph glands, pain on swallowing, fever, headache, nausea
    Reaction to penicillin therapy: rash, fever, chills
- *Special instructions*
  —Review potential sources of reinfection and discuss preventive measures.
    Maintain good oral hygiene, with daily care and regular visits to the dentist.
    Change toothbrush regularly.
    Avoid persons with upper respiratory infection. Report and treat all skin boils (furuncles).
    Avoid scratching and infecting skin acne.
  —Explain the signs of cardiac complications and instruct the patient to watch for them: chest pain (pericarditis), shortness of breath, increasing fatigue, palpitations, swelling of ankles and feet (heart failure, valvular heart involvement).

—Explain the need for prophylactic antibiotic therapy before invasive procedures that predispose to bacteremia if there has been valve involvement, including dental or gum therapy, urologic and gynecologic procedures, childbirth.

- *Medications*
  —Explain the purpose, dosage, schedule, and route of administration of any prescribed drugs, as well as side effects to report to the physician or nurse.
  —Stress the importance of completing antibiotic therapy to prevent recurrence and discuss the need for lifelong prophylactic antibiotic coverage in the presence of valve involvement.
  —Discuss the hypersensitivity reaction to penicillin. Warn the patient that reaction after long-term use is possible. Instruct the patient to stop penicillin therapy and call the physician immediately if a reaction occurs.

- *Activity*
  —Explain the need for strict bed rest that may continue for up to 5 weeks during the acute phase. As activities are resumed, instruct the patient to avoid fatigue, plan regular rest periods, and avoid strenuous activities.
  —Encourage the patient to discuss allowances and limitations with respect to occupation, recreation, and activities.
  —Suggest nonstressful diversional activities during the convalescent period. For adolescents and young adults, suggest home study and tutoring programs.

FOLLOW-UP CARE

- Stress the importance of regular follow-up visits. Make sure the patient has the necessary names and telephone numbers.
- Emphasize the importance of informing the dentist and other physicians of rheumatic fever and the possible need for prophylactic antibiotic therapy if heart valves are affected.

Ruptured Disk
(Herniated or Slipped Disk, Herniated Nucleus Pulposus)

—Ruptured disk: a chronic condition occurring when all or part of the nucleus pulposus, the soft, gelatinous, cushioning center of cartilage between each two vertebrae, is pushed through the disk's weakened or torn outer ring (anulus fibrosus). This results in exertion of pressure on the spinal nerves as they exit the spinal canal, causing back pain and other signs of nerve root irritation (sciatica). Ruptured disk typically occurs in adult men younger than 45 years of age. The lumbar and lumbosacral regions are most frequently affected (95%). Cervical disks may also rupture, usually because of degenerative changes.

CAUSES/CONTRIBUTING FACTORS

- Severe trauma or strain
- Intervertebral joint degeneration caused by aging

SIGNS/SYMPTOMS

- Sciatica: severe low back pain radiating to the buttocks, legs, and feet
- Sudden pain following coughing, sneezing, bending, or lifting
- Muscle spasm and tenseness
- Loss of sensation and motor control to the extremities

COMPLICATIONS

- Paresis
- Motor weakness
- Sensory changes
- Footdrop
- Loss of bowel, bladder control

DIAGNOSTIC TESTS

- Describe each procedure, its purpose, and the normal feelings or sensations that are likely, as well as any preprocedural and postprocedural care.

—Straight leg raising test: positive when the patient complains of posterior leg (sciatic) pain versus back pain when the leg is lifted; pain is increased with foot dorsiflexion
—Back x-rays: to document decreased disk space
—Computed tomography: to show disk rupture
—Magnetic resonance imaging: to confirm disk rupture and show compression sites on the spinal nerve
—Myelogram: to show the site of rupture
—Diskogram: to show disk degeneration and rupture

TREATMENT
Medical

- Therapy
  —Skin traction with pelvic belt
  —Bed rest on firm mattress during acute rupture for 1 to 3 days
  —Williams' position in bed (head of bed elevated) and knee gatch at 45 degrees (or pillow under knee) to relax lumbosacral muscles
  —Ice massage of lumbosacral area to lessen edema
  —Back support or metal back brace
  —Ultrasound diathermy with back massage
  —Exercise regimen after acute pain and inflammation have subsided; to strengthen back and abdominal muscles
- Drugs
  —Antiinflammatory (nonsteroidal) medications
  —Analgesic and antipyretic medications
  —Muscle relaxants
  —Narcotics
  —Antianxiety agents

Surgical

—Percutaneous diskectomy: removal of the disk by insertion of a metal canal under fluoroscopy
—Microdiskectomy: removal of the affected disk by microscopic surgery through a 1-inch incision
—Arthroscopic diskectomy
—Nuclear diskectomy
—Laminectomy: excision of part of the lamina and removal of the protruding disk
—Spinal fusion: to stabilize the spine; indicated if more than one disk is involved

—Chemonucleolysis: injection of enzyme (chymopapain) directly into the disk to dissolve prolapsed tissue (done infrequently)

—Intradiskal electrothermal (IDET) therapy to shrink bulging disk

HOME CARE

- Give both the patient and the caregiver *verbal* and *written* instructions. Provide them with the name and telephone number of a physician or nurse to call if questions arise.
- *General information*
  —Discuss the disorder and contributing factors.
- *Warning signs*
  —Review the signs and symptoms that should be reported to a physician or nurse.
      Continued presence of pain
      Paresthesia (numbness, tingling sensation in extremities)
      Muscle spasms
      Changes in bowel, bladder function
- *Special instructions*
  —Explain and instruct the patient in the use and application of the back brace, support, or belt. Discuss use of the skin traction belt. Advise and assist the patient to obtain the necessary home equipment.
- *Medications*
  —Explain the purpose, dosage, schedule, and route of administration of any prescribed drugs, as well as side effects to report to the physician or nurse.
  —Discuss nonsteroidal antiinflammatory drugs (NSAIDs), and warn the patient not to take over-the-counter analgesics or muscle relaxants with NSAIDs without checking with the physician.
- *Activity*
  —Explain the need for initial complete bed rest (3 to 5 days) to decrease inflammatory responses and to reduce pressure in the spine, which relieves pressure on the irritated nerve root and decreases pain. Instruct the patient to assume the position of greatest comfort: semi-Fowler's or side lying with knees always flexed. Caution the patient not to lie on the stomach.
  —Advise the patient to use a urinal, bedpan, or bedside commode during the period of bed rest to avoid walking. Assist the patient to obtain the equipment.

R

—Teach body mechanics and principles of lifting, moving, and carrying (see p. 95) once acute pain eases.

—Demonstrate back exercises to strengthen muscles (see box on p. 97).

- *Diet*

—Explain the importance of a high fluid intake and a diet high in fiber roughage to prevent constipation during the period of bed rest.

—Discuss the need to maintain a weight appropriate for age, sex, and height. If the patient is overweight, explain that excess body weight aggravates the strain on the spine. Refer the patient to a dietitian for a weight control diet.

FOLLOW-UP CARE AND REFERRALS

- Stress the importance of regular follow-up visits to the physician and physical therapist until recovery is complete. Make sure the patient has the necessary names and telephone numbers.

Saphenous Vein Ligation and Stripping

—Saphenous vein ligation and stripping: a procedure used in the treatment of varicose veins. Such enlarged, tortuous, dilated veins usually occur in the lower extremities. As the veins dilate and venous valve function decreases, they become less functional, resulting in venous stasis and thrombus formation.

INDICATIONS

- Varicose veins

PREPROCEDURAL TEACHING

- Review the physician's explanation of the procedure and the reason for it; encourage the patient to ask questions and to discuss any fears or anxieties. Explain the need for informed consent.
- Explain that hospital admission may be on the day of surgery.

Review of Preprocedural Care

- Tell the patient that all hair will be removed from the surgical leg.
- Instruct the patient to take two showers with hexachlorophene within 12 hours before the procedure.
- Instruct the patient not to eat or drink after midnight before the procedure.
- Explain that all visible varicose veins that are to be stripped will be marked with dye with the patient standing.

SIDE EFFECTS/COMPLICATIONS

- Ecchymosis, bleeding
- Numbness
- Ulceration
- Infection
- Thromboembolic disease
- Scars

HOME CARE

- Give both the patient and the caregiver *verbal* and *written* instructions. Provide them with the name and telephone number of a physician or nurse to call if questions arise.
- *General information*
  —Review any explanation about the procedure and specific follow-up care.
- *Wound/incision care*
  —Discuss and demonstrate proper care of the incision.
- *Warning signs*
  —Review the signs and symptoms that should be reported to a physician or nurse.
    Fever
    Redness, warmth, pain, edema, or purulent drainage from incision sites
- *Special instructions*
  —Instruct the patient to wear support stockings. Assist the patient to obtain appropriate supplies and proper size.
  —Advise the patient to avoid wearing constrictive clothing and knee-high stockings.
- *Medications*
  —Explain the purpose, dosage, schedule, and route of administration of any prescribed drugs, as well as side effects to report to a physician or nurse.

—Encourage the patient to take pain medications.
- *Activity*
  —Advise the patient to take frequent rest periods during the day and elevate the legs above the heart while sitting for at least 6 weeks after the procedure.
  —Tell the patient to avoid prolonged periods of sitting and standing and to change positions at frequent intervals.
  —Advise the patient to not cross legs while sitting.
  —Encourage the patient to initiate a walking program.
  —Stress the importance of weight reduction, if indicated. Provide referral to community resources and weight reduction programs.

FOLLOW-UP CARE

- Stress the importance of regular follow-up visits. Make sure the patient has the necessary names and telephone numbers.

Sarcoidosis

—Sarcoidosis: a multisystem granulomatous disorder of unknown etiology, characteristically producing pulmonary infiltrates, lymphadenopathy, and skin lesions. In most cases the process is benign and self-limiting without residual effects. Sarcoidosis is most common in young adults and African-Americans between 20 and 40 years of age.

SIGNS/SYMPTOMS

- Weight loss, anorexia
- Fever, night sweats, joint pain, fatigue
- Respiratory: clubbing of fingers, dyspnea, cough
- Palpitations
- Skin nodules: over face, neck, and extremities
- Bone cysts in hands and feet
- Nasal mucosal lesions
- Hair loss
- Blurred vision, eye pain, drainage, infection

COMPLICATIONS
- Pulmonary fibrosis
- Cor pulmonale

DIAGNOSTIC TESTS
- Describe each procedure, its purpose, and the normal feelings or sensations that are likely, as well as any preprocedural and postprocedural care.
  - Kveim skin test: positive 3 to 6 weeks
  - Skin and lymph node biopsy
  - Bronchoscopy: transbronchial biopsy, open lung biopsy, bronchoalveolar lavage
  - Gallium-67 scan
  - Chest x-ray
  - Pulmonary function tests
  - Serum tests: complete blood count, creatinine protein, erythrocyte sedimentation rate, angiotensin-converting enzyme level

TREATMENT
Medical
- Therapy
  - Chest physiotherapy
  - Heat therapy and joint supports for arthritis
- Drugs
  - Systemic or topical steroids
  - Azathioprine (Imuran)
  - Optic agents: methylcellulose eyedrops
  - Antiarrhythmic agents
  - Calcium-chelating medication
  - Antiarthritic treatment: salicylates, nonsteroidal antiinflammatory drugs, corticosteroids
  - Vitamin D supplements

HOME CARE
- Give both the patient and the caregiver *verbal* and *written* instructions. Provide them with the name and telephone number of a physician or nurse to call if questions arise.
- *General information*
  - Explain and discuss sarcoidosis, its causes, and contributing factors.

S

- *Warning signs*
  - —Review the signs, symptoms, and complications that should be reported to a physician or nurse.

    Shortness of breath

    Red, watery eyes

    Dizziness

    Chest pain

    Swollen joints

    Unusual fatigue

    Fever

- *Special instructions*
  - —Teach the importance of chest physiotherapy (breathing exercises, postural drainage) as prophylaxis or treatment of chronic pulmonary disease.
  - —Stress the importance of avoiding large crowds and individuals who are known to have active infections.
  - —Instruct the patient to weigh daily to detect steady weight loss.

- *Medications*
  - —Explain the purpose, dosage, schedule, and route of administration of any prescribed drugs, as well as side effects to report to the physician or nurse.

    Topical and systemic corticosteroids (see Steroid Therapy, p. 590)
  - —Teach the patient aseptic technique for administering eyedrops to avoid contamination.

    Wash any drainage from the eye.

    Wash hands.

    Look up toward the ceiling.

    Pull down the lower lid while holding the medication tip 1 to 2 cm from the eye.

    Instill drop(s).

    Wipe any excess medication from the face.
  - —Teach the patient aseptic technique for administering ointment.

    Wash any drainage from the eye.

    Wash hands.

    Pull down the lower lid and apply a thin stream of ointment just inside the lower lid without touching the eye or surrounding area.

    Close the eyes and rotate them to distribute medication.

    Replace the cap and store as directed.

- *Activity*
  —Encourage the patient to discusss allowances and limitations with respect to occupation, recreation, and activities.
  —Discuss energy conservation and breathing exercises.
  —Encourage the patient to pace activities, allow for adequate rest periods, and avoid overexertion.
- *Diet*
  —Encourage a low-salt, low-potassium, low-calcium diet with vitamin D supplements.
  —Advise the patient to eat small, frequent meals to meet nutritional needs.

FOLLOW-UP CARE AND REFERRALS

- Stress the importance of follow-up medical and laboratory evaluations. Make sure the patient has the necessary names and telephone numbers.
- Discuss the need for routine chest x-rays and pulmonary function tests to monitor the disease process.
- Emphasize the importance of wearing a MedicAlert bracelet and carrying an identification card at all times.
- Provide referrals for resources and support services as needed.

Seizure Disorder
(Epilepsy)

S

—Seizure disorder (epilepsy): a chronic neurologic disorder characterized by repeated occurrence of any of various forms of seizures. Some seizure disorders have a familial tendency. The seizures, or convulsions, are paroxysmal episodes in which sudden discharge of abnormal electrical brain activity produces involuntary muscle contractions, resulting in disturbances in consciousness, behavior, sensation, and autonomic functioning. For half the reported cases there is no specific known cause.

CLASSIFICATION

- Partial: seizures arising from localized area of the brain, causing specific symptoms
  —Simple: consciousness not impaired
     Motor (jacksonian)
     Sensory
     Psychomotor
  —Complex: consciousness impaired
- Generalized: seizures causing generalized electrical abnormality in the brain
  —Tonic-clonic (grand mal)
  —Absence (petit mal)
  —Myoclonic
  —Clonic
  —Atonic

CAUSES

- Idiopathic (no specific cause)
- Brain tumor
- Vascular anomalies
- Trauma
- Infections: encephalitis, meningitis
- Metabolic disturbances: hypoglycemia, hypocalcemia
- Fever
- Toxins

PRECIPITATING FACTORS

- Drug withdrawal/noncompliance
- Fatigue, lack of sleep
- Flashing lights

SIGNS/SYMPTOMS

- General
  —Involuntary recurrent muscle movements
  —Jerking, patting, rubbing
  —Sudden contractions of muscle groups
  —Fluttering of eyelids
  —Facial jerking
  —Lip smacking
  —Movements confined to one area or spreading from one side to the other
  —Head and eyes deviating to the side

- Specific
  —Tonic-clonic: lasts 2 to 5 minutes
    Tonic phase: body stiffens
    Clonic phase: alternates between muscle spasm and relaxation
    Other signs
    ○ Tongue biting
    ○ Incontinence
    ○ Dyspnea, apnea
    ○ Cyanosis
    ○ After seizure: postictal sleep
  —Petit mal: lasts 5 to 30 minutes
    Change in consciousness (absence)
    Blinking, rolling of eyes, blank stare

COMPLICATIONS

- Physical injury (fracture, tongue or lip laceration)
- Aspiration
- Respiratory impairment
- Status epilepticus

DIAGNOSTIC TESTS

- Describe each procedure, its purpose, and the normal feelings or sensations that are likely, as well as any preprocedural and postprocedural care.
  —Computed tomography scan
  —Magnetic resonance imaging
  —Skull x-rays
  —Echoencephalogram
  —Cerebral angiography
  —Electroencephalogram
  —Urine screening
  —Serum chemistry/screen (hypoglycemia, increased blood urea nitrogen, alcohol)
  —History and neurologic examination

TREATMENT
Medical

- Drugs
  —Anticonvulsants
    Carbamazepine (Tegretol)
    Phenytoin (Dilantin)

Barbiturates
○ Phenobarbital (Luminal)
○ Primidone (Mysoline)
Ethosuximide (Zarontin)
Mephenytoin (Mesantoin)
Felbamate (Felbatol)
Gabapentin (Neurontin)
Lamotrigine (Lamictal)
Trimethadione (Tridione)
Valproic acid (Depakene)
Clonazepam (Klonopin)
Diazepam (Valium)
Methsuximide (Clontin)

Surgical

- Excision of epileptogenic focus
- Excision of underlying cause (e.g., brain tumor)
- Vagal nerve stimulation

HOME CARE

- Give both the patient and the caregiver *verbal* and *written* instructions. Provide them with the name and telephone number of a physician or nurse to call if questions arise.
- *General information*
  —Explain the type of seizure disorder involved, causes, and possible precipitating factors.
  —Assist the patient and family to recognize and record prodromal symptoms or auras.
- *Special instructions*
  —Explain the course of action to take during and after a grand mal seizure.
    Do not restrain the patient during a seizure; prevent or break the fall by easing the person to the floor.
    Stay with the person during the seizure.
    Protect the head by clearing the surrounding area and padding the floor.
    Note the time and type of seizure activity.
    Do not place anything in the person's mouth.
    After the seizure, turn the person to the side to prevent aspiration. Loosen tight clothing. Call the physician and report the activity.

Reassure and reorient the person.

Maintain a quiet environment.

—Explain the course of action to take during and after a petit mal seizure.

Remain with the patient. Do not startle or attempt to awaken the patient.

Be aware that there are no prodromal symptoms and that the patient will resume normal activity once the seizure passes.

—Advise a female patient that seizure activity may increase or decrease during menses or pregnancy. Stress the importance of planning all pregnancies. Discuss the risks associated with pregnancy: seizures may cause fetal death and antiepilepsy drugs are associated with birth defects. Provide birth control information and encourage questions.

—Assist the patient to identify and avoid stimuli that precipitate seizure activity (e.g., flashing lights, loud music).

- Advise the patient to lower water heater temperature to avoid scalding during a shower or bath if a seizure occurs.
- Teach stress management and progressive relaxation techniques to control excessive stress or emotional excitement that might trigger seizures.
- *Medications*
    —Explain the purpose, dosage, schedule, and route of administration of any prescribed drugs, as well as side effects to report to the physician or nurse.

    —Stress the importance of taking the prescribed medication regularly and on schedule and not discontinuing the medication without a physician's guidance. Explain that missing a dose can precipitate seizure activity many days later.

    —Explain that medications cannot be taken prn and that lack of seizure activity does not mean that the drug is unnecessary.

    —Stress that abrupt withdrawal of antiepilepsy medication can cause seizures and that discontinuing these medications is the most common cause of status epilepticus.

    —Discuss that the need for medications to prevent seizures may be lifelong.

    —Explain the importance of maintaining a therapeutic level of antiepileptic medication by checking blood regularly.

    —Discuss with the patient methods to help the patient remember to take medication, to monitor the drug supply, and to reorder medications 2 weeks before running out.

—Discuss side effects of all medications that should be reported to the physician or nurse.

Bruising, bleeding, jaundice

Nausea, vomiting

Ataxia

Diplopia

Nystagmus

Dizziness

—Instruct the patient to notify the physician or nurse of any significant weight loss or gain because the medication dosage may need to be changed.

—Stress the need to avoid alcoholic beverages and over-the-counter medications with alcohol, aspirin, or antihistamines without first consulting a physician, since these substances may affect the potency of antiepilepsy medication.

—Stress the importance of avoiding recreational/illicit drugs.

• *Activity*

—Discuss with the patient the need to evaluate activities for the potential risks and to have a buddy when participating in high-risk activities (e.g., climbing, bicycling, swimming).

—Stress the need to continue with normal work and recreation routines as much as possible; assure the patient that activity may inhibit seizure activity.

—Advise the patient to check state regulations about driving an automobile.

—Advise the patient not to operate heavy or dangerous equipment until the patient is seizure free for the time specified by the physician or nurse.

—Explain the importance of avoiding excessive visual stimulation, e.g., video games.

• *Diet*

—Stress the importance of a well-balanced diet with meals spaced throughout the day to avoid hypoglycemia. Avoid stimulants or depressants (caffeine or alcohol), since withdrawal from them may cause seizures.

PSYCHOSOCIAL CARE

• Assist the patient to gain understanding of seizure disorder. Explore and clarify any misinformation and myths associated with the disorder. Encourage questions.

- Stress the importance of verbalizing feelings of shame, humiliation, anxiety, and fears regarding the seizure disorder.
- Emphasize the need to avoid overprotection.

FOLLOW-UP CARE AND REFERRALS

- Stress the importance of regular follow-up visits to ensure adequate medical management of the disease process. Make sure the patient has the necessary names and telephone numbers.
- Discuss with the patient the need for routine blood draws to determine that therapeutic levels of antiepilepsy medications are being maintained.
- Discuss the importance of wearing a MedicAlert band and carrying an information card that describes seizures and medications at all times.
- Provide referrals to support services such as Epilepsy Foundation of America, (800) EFA-1000.

Sickle Cell Anemia

—Sickle cell anemia: a chronic hemolytic disorder that occurs as the result of a genetic mutation transmitted from parent to child. Sickle cell anemia is characterized by abnormal, crescent-shaped, rigid, and elongated red blood cells. These "sickled" cells interfere with circulation because they cannot get through the microcirculation and are destroyed in the process. Sickle cell crises occur in two forms: vasoocclusive and aplastic. In vasoocclusive crisis, the more common form, the collection of misshapen red blood cells in the smaller blood vessels (e.g., peripheral, renal) results in blockage of blood flow, tissue hypoxia, and death. In aplastic crisis, infection results in a decreased availability of functioning red blood cells because of bone marrow aplasia, iron deficiency, or splenic destruction of red blood cells. Sickle cell anemia is seen primarily in African-Americans.

CAUSES

- Genetic hereditary disorder

SIGNS/SYMPTOMS

- General
  - —Fatigue
  - —Dyspnea on exertion
  - —Delayed sexual maturity
- Crisis
  - —Severe pain: bone, abdomen, chest, joints, muscles
  - —Jaundice
  - —Pallor
  - —Joint swelling
  - —Fever (low-grade)
  - —Lethargy
  - —Leg ulcers

COMPLICATIONS

- Stroke
- Renal failure
- Respiratory failure
- Myocardial infarction
- Hemolytic anemia

DIAGNOSTIC TESTS

- Describe each procedure, its purpose, and the normal feelings or sensations that are likely, as well as any preprocedural and postprocedural care.
  - —Stained blood smear
  - —Sickle cell slide preparation of blood
  - —Sickle turbidity test (hemoglobin S [HbS])
  - —Hemoglobin electrophoresis (HbS)
  - —Red blood cell life span

TREATMENT
Medical

- Therapy
  - —Rest
  - —Oxygen
  - —Intravenous fluids and electrolytes
- Drugs
  - —Pneumococcal and flu vaccines
  - —Analgesics
  - —Antiinfectives (low-dose penicillin)
  - —Deferoxamine (chelating agent)

—Sedatives
—Iron supplements

 HOME CARE

- Give both the patient and the caregiver *verbal* and *written* instructions. Provide them with the name and telephone number of a physician or nurse to call if questions arise.
- *General information*
  —Explain and discuss sickle cell disorder, its causes, and contributing factors.
- *Warning signs*
  —Review the signs, symptoms, and complications that should be reported to a physician or nurse.
  - Jaundice
  - Dyspnea
  - Severe joint or abdominal pain
  - Headaches
  - Vertigo
  - Sleepiness with difficulty awakening
  - Persistent fever (more than 2 days)
  - Hematuria
- *Special instructions*
  —Alert the patient to avoid factors that precipitate sickle cell crisis: high altitude, drinking iced liquids, vigorous exercise, smoking.
  —Discuss the importance of avoiding persons with infections, such as upper respiratory infections. Tell the patient to seek early treatment of infection.
  —Stress the importance of seeking early treatment for crisis. Explain that hospitalization may be necessary.
  —Teach the patient to blow the nose gently, avoid coughing, and avoid straining on elimination.
  —Teach the patient to avoid trauma and extremes of temperature and to protect extremities from injury because of impaired circulation.
  —Demonstrate how to monitor oral intake, urinary output, and urine protein level.
  —Alert the patient to the need to have family members tested for HbS. Refer carriers to genetic counseling.
  —For a female patient, explain that women have a high risk for pulmonary or renal complications. Stress the importance of planning pregnancies and provide birth control information.

S

- *Medications*
  —Explain the purpose, dosage, schedule, and route of administration of any prescribed drugs, as well as side effects to report to the physician or nurse.
- *Activity*
  —Encourage the patient to discuss allowances and limitations with respect to occupation, recreation, and activities.
  —Teach range-of-motion exercises and encourage regular physical activity to prevent bone mineralization.
  —Explain the need for balance between activity and rest.
- *Diet*
  —Discuss the need for a well-balanced diet.
  —Encourage the patient to eat small, frequent meals.
  —Encourage fluid intake to prevent dehydration.

PSYCHOSOCIAL CARE

- Encourage verbalization of fears and questions about how disease may alter lifestyle and activities of daily living.
- Encourage participation in home care planning.

FOLLOW-UP CARE

- Stress the importance of follow-up medical and laboratory evaluations. Make sure the patient has the necessary names and telephone numbers.

REFERRALS

- Assist the patient to obtain psychosocial or supportive counseling as needed. Refer to hospital and community support groups as indicated.
- Refer patients planning to have children to genetic counseling.

Sigmoidoscopy

—Sigmoidoscopy: passage of a rigid or flexible scope for direct visualization of mucosa or biopsy of lesions of the sigmoid colon, rectum, and anal canal.

INDICATIONS

- Changes in bowel habits
- Rectal bleeding
- Diverticulosis
- Polyps
- Ulcerative colitis
- Crohn's disease
- Irritable bowel syndrome
- Benign tumors
- Anorectal fistulas
- Weight loss
- Anemia
- Cancer screening

PREPROCEDURAL TEACHING

- Review the physician's explanation of the procedure and the reason for it; encourage the patient to ask questions and to discuss any fears or anxieties. Discuss the need for informed consent.

Review of Preprocedural Care

- Explain that preprocedural care varies according to the suspected diagnosis.
- Inform the patient that light meals or a clear liquid diet may be ordered for 48 hours before the procedure.
- Discuss the need to have nothing by mouth (NPO) for 8 hours before the procedure.
- Explain that bowel preparation consisting of laxatives or enemas may be ordered.
- Discuss what will happen during the procedure.
  - —The patient is positioned in a knee-chest position on a tilting table or a left lateral position with the right buttock elevated.
  - —Air may be insufflated to allow better passage of the scope and better visualization.
  - —A light sedative or analgesics will be given; atropine may be given to limit gastrointestinal secretions.
- Reassure the patient that safety and privacy will be ensured.

Review of Postprocedural Care

- Explain that the patient will remain at rest in bed for 1 to 2 hours after the procedure to allow monitoring for signs and symptoms of complications.

S

- Explain that flatus will result from air inserted during the procedure and cannot be controlled, but is temporary and may be relieved with ambulation.

COMPLICATIONS

- Bowel perforation
- Vasovagal stimulation

HOME CARE

- Give both the patient and the caregiver *verbal* and *written* instructions. Provide them with the name and telephone number of a physician or nurse to call if questions arise.
- *General information*
  —Review any explanation about the procedure and specific follow-up care. Advise the patient that there may be slight rectal bleeding if biopsy specimens were taken.
- *Warning signs*
  —Review the signs and symptoms that should be reported to a physician or nurse.
    Abdominal pain and distention
    Rectal bleeding
    Fever
    Pallor and diaphoresis
- *Activity*
  —Explain that the patient should avoid vigorous activity on the day of the procedure but then may resume activities as tolerated.
- *Diet*
  —Tell the patient that a regular diet or one prescribed by the physician for the underlying disease may be followed.

FOLLOW-UP CARE

- Stress the importance of regular follow-up visits. Make sure the patient has the necessary names and telephone numbers.

Spinal Cord Injury

—Spinal cord injury (for chronic care after acute rehabilitation): physical injury that transects, lacerates, stretches, or
compresses the spinal cord, resulting in compromised blood
supply, hemorrhage, edema, or ischemia. Neurologic deficits
are caused by the interruption in neuronal function and
transmission of nerve impulses. The neurologic deficits depend
on the lesions and the level of injury. Spinal cord injuries are
classified according to type, cause, site, mechanism of injury,
stability, and degree of spinal cord function loss.

CAUSES/CONTRIBUTING FACTORS/RISK FACTORS
- Motor vehicle accidents
- Diving or other sports accidents
- Industrial accidents
- Falls
- Assaults, including gunshot wounds
- Degenerative changes or diseases of the spinal cord

SIGNS/SYMPTOMS
- Signs and symptoms depend on degree, type, and level of injury
- Loss of muscle function below the level of injury, including
  respiratory muscles
- Loss of sensation: proprioception, pain, temperature, touch, and
  pressure below the level of injury
- Loss of spinal reflexes below the level of injury
- Pain at or below the level of injury
- Loss of vasomotor tone
- Bladder and bowel dysfunction
- Priapism: abnormal prolonged or constant penile erection,
  seldom associated with sexual arousal
- Autonomic dysreflexia: bradycardia, sweating above the level
  of injury, elevated temperature, headache, nausea, nasal
  congestion, paroxysmal hypertension

COMPLICATIONS
- Contractures
- Pressure ulcers

- Urinary calculi and urinary tract infection
- Pneumonia
- Autonomic dysreflexia
- Sexual dysfunction
- Paralytic ileus
- Respiratory failure
- Sepsis
- Spinal shock
- Muscle spasms

DIAGNOSTIC TESTS

- Describe each procedure, its purpose, and the normal feelings or sensations that are likely, as well as any preprocedural and postprocedural care.
    —X-ray of spine: to detect fracture, deformity, or displacement of vertebrae
    —Computed tomography (CT) or magnetic resonance imaging (MRI): to detect changes in the spinal cord or vertebrae
    —Myelography: to show disruption of the spinal canal
    —Arterial blood gases: to assess effectiveness of respirations

TREATMENT
Medical

- Therapy
    —Stryker or Foster frame or kinetic treatment table
    —Skeletal traction
    —Cervical collar
    —Assistive devices: splints, braces, wheelchair
    —Nerve stimulation
    —Physical therapy
    —Occupational therapy
    —Neurologic rehabilitation
    —Psychologic counseling, including sexual counseling
    —Bladder and bowel retraining program
    —Nutritional counseling
    —NPO until chewing, swallowing, and gastrointestinal functioning are established
    —Feedings parenteral or enteral
    —Antiembolic stockings
    —Intermittent urinary catheterization
    —Respiratory therapy

- Drugs
  —Corticosteroids
  —Osmotic diuretics
  —Anticoagulants
  —Analgesics
  —Antacids and H_2 blockers
  —Stool softeners and laxatives
  —Antianxiety agents
  —Muscle relaxants
  —Antispasmodics
  —Antibiotics
  —Anticholinergics
  —Antihypertensives

Surgical

- Laminectomy: to relieve compression from a hematoma; to remove bone fragments or penetrating objects
- Spinal fusion: to stabilize the spine
- Cervical tongs or halo traction: to immobilize the cervical spine
- Body cast or Harrington rods: to immobilize the thoracic spine
- Tracheostomy: to provide long-term ventilatory support
- Tenotomies, myotomies, neurectomies, rhizotomy, muscle transplants: to treat spasticity

HOME CARE (FOR CHRONIC CARE AFTER LONG-TERM REHABILITATION)

- Give both the patient and the caregiver *verbal* and *written* instructions. Provide them with the name and telephone number of a physician or nurse to call if questions arise. Provide spinal cord injury instruction sheets to assist in instruction.
- *General information*
  —Explain and discuss the spinal cord injury, care, treatment, and rehabilitation needs.
- *Warning signs*
  —Review the signs, symptoms, and complications that should be reported to a physician or nurse.
    Skin breakdown or poor response to decubitus treatment
    Urinary tract infection: urinary frequency, urgency, retention, or incontinence; suprapubic distention; pain or burning with urination; malodorous urine; cloudy or bloody urine; fever; chills; flank pain

S

Renal calculi: pain that may be sharp, sudden, and intense or dull and aching in the flank area; urinary frequency; voiding in small amounts; hematuria

Upper respiratory infection: changes in respirations, color change in sputum, fever

Respiratory distress

Autonomic dysreflexia: bradycardia, sweating above level of injury, elevated temperature, headache, nausea, nasal congestion, paroxysmal hypertension

Lack of bowel movement for more than 3 days or impaction

Thrombophlebitis: erythema, warmth, edema in calves or thighs

Sudden changes in motor or sensory function

Loose or dislodged pins or vest

- *Special instructions*
  —Discuss skin care.

   If the patient is confined to bed or wheelchair, instruct the patient to use a mirror to check skin for breakdown.

   Instruct the caretaker on perineal care after elimination: wash gently with mild soap, rinse well with warm water, pat dry, and apply skin protector.

   Advise the removal of sharp objects, crumbs, and wrinkles from bed and chairs.

   Advise the patient to regulate bath water temperature and avoid application of extreme hot and cold temperatures because of loss of temperature sensation.

   Instruct the patient to change position at least every 15 to 30 minutes when in the wheelchair and at least every 2 hours when in bed. Instruct the patient to set an alarm clock to wake during the night to turn.

  —Discuss urinary elimination.

   Stress the importance of following the bladder retraining program.

   Teach the patient to observe for urinary distention every 2 to 4 hours.

   Reinforce or teach methods to stimulate the voiding reflex.

   Teach intermittent self-catheterization.

   Teach and demonstrate care of the indwelling urinary catheter.

—Discuss bowel elimination.

> Stress the importance of following the bowel retraining program.
>
> Attempt to establish the previous bowel pattern with regular, convenient times or 30 minutes after meals.
>
> Reinforce or teach methods to stimulate a bowel movement.
>
> Massage the abdomen from the right side to the left to stimulate the gastrointestinal tract.
>
> Suggest bearing down, bending forward, or applying manual abdominal pressure during defecation.
>
> Teach the patient the signs of rectal fullness: goosebumps, perspiration, rising of hair on arms and legs, and sense of fullness.
>
> Instruct the patient to sit on the bedpan, toilet, or commode at the scheduled time for bowel movement. Encourage the patient to sit erect during defecation, if possible.
>
> Tell the patient to avoid sitting on the bedpan, toilet, or commode for more than 20 minutes.
>
> Teach the patient the signs of impaction: no formed stools for more than 3 days or semiliquid stools.

—Teach the patient or caregiver about preventing and managing autonomic dysreflexia, including noxious stimuli that cause autonomic dysreflexia.

—Explain the need to use anesthetic jelly liberally for urinary catheterization and insertion of suppository or enema.

—Stress the importance of following the prescribed rehabilitation program for the specific spinal cord injury.

—Assist the patient in obtaining assistive aids for self-care, mobility, support, and physical exercises.

—Assist the patient and caregiver to identify adaptations needed in the home environment: obtaining special beds with trapeze or special mattress, widening doorways, installing ramps for wheelchairs.

—Provide alternative methods of dealing with chronic pain: visualization, guided imagery, meditation, relaxation, biofeedback.

- *Medications*
  —Explain the purpose, dosage, schedule, and route of administration of any prescribed drugs, as well as side effects to report to the physician or nurse.

—Stress the importance of not taking over-the-counter medications without consulting the physician.

- *Activity*
  —Encourage the patient to discuss allowances and limitations with respect to occupation, recreation, and activities.
  —Demonstrate range-of-motion exercises to the family or caregiver and give instructions on how to assist the patient with exercises.
  —Advise the patient that the prone position may help relieve pressure on susceptible areas and help decrease contractures and spasms in hips and knees.
  —Stress the importance of performing range-of-motion, muscle-strengthening, and stretching exercises.
  —Instruct the patient to schedule rest periods with activities and exercises.
  —Explain the need to plan activities to avoid fatigue.
  —Discuss ways to protect the legs from injury during movement and transfers.
  —Advise the patient to take warm baths and massage to help prevent spasticity.
  —Instruct the patient on the use of splints or high-top shoes that are cut off at the toes to help prevent foot contractures in patients with spasticity.
  —Advise the patient to avoid stimuli that trigger spasm: cold, anxiety, fatigue, emotional distress, infection, bowel or bladder distention, ulcers, pain, tight clothing, maintaining one position for too long. Advise the family and caregivers that touch should be firm, gentle, and steady.
- *Diet*
  —Assist the patient to plan a high-calorie, high-protein, high-fiber diet.
  —Advise the patient to avoid foods that cause an upset stomach or diarrhea.
  —Provide the patient with a list of specific gas-producing foods to avoid.
  —Encourage the patient to drink plenty of fluids, up to 2 liters/day, unless contraindicated.
  —Encourage the patient to drink cranberry juice or take vitamin C to decrease urine pH.
  —Encourage the patient to drink prune juice to help prevent constipation.

—Advise the patient to drink fluids at even intervals throughout the day.

—Instruct the patient to restrict fluid intake before bedtime.

—Advise the patient to avoid alcohol and caffeine-containing foods and beverages. Provide the patient with a list of specific caffeine-containing foods and beverages.

—Advise the patient to limit milk and dairy products to minimize the risk of renal calculi.

—Instruct the family and caregiver to assist with feedings as necessary.

PSYCHOSOCIAL CARE

- Assist the patient to establish realistic goals and implement alternative methods for communication and mobility.
- Encourage the patient to continue to express concerns related to injury, disability, loss of mobility, body image changes, and feelings of grief.
- Advise the family to avoid overprotectiveness.
- Encourage decision making and promote independence in the patient.
- Encourage the family to verbalize concerns related to injury, disability, and effects on their lifestyle.
- Offer specific suggestions of ways to achieve sexual gratification or manage common problems related to spinal cord injury and sexual activity.
- Allow the patient and partner to verbalize concerns regarding sexual activity.

FOLLOW-UP CARE

- Stress the importance of follow-up medical and laboratory evaluations. Make sure the patient has the necessary names and telephone numbers.
- Assist the patient in obtaining a MedicAlert bracelet and identification card listing diagnosis, medication, and treatment.

REFERRALS

- Refer the patient to a social worker for further support, counseling, and financial assistance, if appropriate.
- Refer the patient for sexual counseling.
  —For males: sexual dysfunction, primarily inability to ejaculate

—For females: for contraceptive and reproductive counseling because uterine contractions of labor may cause autonomic dysreflexia in women with spinal cord injuries at T8 or above
- Assist the patient to obtain referral to home health care or custodial care services.
- Refer the patient to community resources, local support groups, and vocational rehabilitation agencies.
- Assist the patient to obtain referral to spinal cord injury organizations.
  —National Spinal Cord Injury Association, (310) 588-6959
  —Information Center for Individuals with Disabilities, (617) 450-9888.
  —Christopher Reeve Paralysis Foundation, (800) 225-0292 or, in New Jersey, (973) 379-2690
  —Spinal Cord Injury Hotline, (800) 526-3456

Sprains and Strains

—Sprains and strains: muscle and ligament injuries. Sprains and strains vary in severity and tissues affected, but the treatment is often the same. A sprain is a tear, usually in a muscle but sometimes in a ligament or tendon, that may be partial or complete tearing of the fibers from their attachments. A strain is a "pull" caused by an acute or chronic overstretching or overuse; it may involve a muscle but usually affects ligaments or tendons. The tearing or stretching caused by these injuries leads to bleeding into tissues, which sets up an inflammatory reaction. Both sprains and strains are classified according to severity.

SIGNS/SYMPTOMS
- First-degree strain: excess pull or stretch
  —Mild pain
  —Edema with some bruising (bleeding into tissues)
  —Muscle spasm
  —Tenderness
  —Slight loss of function or strength

- First-degree sprain: ligament fibers partially torn
  —Mild pain
  —Slight edema
  —Local tenderness
  —No joint instability
  —Slight change in function for a short time
- Second-degree strain: tear or disruption of some muscle fibers
  —Increased pain and edema
  —Redness
  —Bleeding
  —Change in function
  —Local heat
- Second-degree sprain: incomplete tear of ligament
  —Moderate edema
  —Local pain and tenderness
  —Moderate joint instability
  —Inability to carry out usual activities
- Third-degree strain: complete disruption of muscle fibers, with possible rupture of fascia
  —Severe pain
  —Muscle spasm
  —Pronounced edema
  —Marked ecchymosis with hematoma formation
  —Marked tenderness
  —Loss of function
- Third-degree sprain: full or complete tear of ligament or tendon
  —Severe pain
  —Edema: minimal to marked
  —Joint disability
  —Loss of function

COMPLICATIONS

- Chronic joint disability
- Neurovascular dysfunction of extremity
- Posttraumatic arthritis

DIAGNOSTIC TESTS

- Describe each procedure, its purpose, and the normal feelings or sensations that are likely, as well as any preprocedural and postprocedural care.
  —Stress radiographs: to evaluate severity of injury

—Magnetic resonance imaging: to confirm the extent of ligamentous injury or disruption

—Arthrogram: to identify torn or weakened ligaments

TREATMENT
Medical

- Therapy
  —"RICE"

  Rest: let the injured area rest; how long depends on severity of injury

  Ice: apply ice packs to the affected area to decrease swelling and bruising

  Compression: elastic or Ace bandages to wrap injured area; cast or splint for severe sprains or strains; bandage should be wrapped firmly around the injury, but not so much that blood flow is restricted

  Elevation: raising the injured area above the heart to reduce swelling (foot higher than knee; hand higher than elbow)

  —Range-of-motion (ROM) and muscle-strengthening exercises started after appropriate period of immobilization (several days to 3 weeks)
- Drugs
  —Analgesics
  —Antiinflammatory agents

Surgical

- Indicated for third-degree sprains or strains
- Open reduction and repair of torn or avulsed tissues: to restore full joint function
- Ligament or tendon reattachment or removal: if severely damaged
- Arthroscopy: to rule out concurrent intraarticular pathologic conditions or trauma

🏠 HOME CARE

- Give both the patient and the caregiver *verbal* and *written* instructions. Provide them with the name and telephone number of a physician or nurse to call if questions arise.
- *General information*
  —Explain the nature and extent of injury (first, second, or third degree).

- *Warning signs*
  —Review the signs and symptoms of neurovascular impairment caused by tightness of the cast or dressing. Explain that they should be reported to a physician or nurse.
    Skin color: red, blue, purple
    Skin temperature: injured tissues are cooler than surrounding tissue; warm or hot skin
    Swelling: injured area will be swollen, but the skin around it should not be tight
    Sudden increase in pain
    Inability to bend fingers or toes of affected extremity
    Numbness and tingling in fingers or toes
    Decreased capillary refill: pink color takes longer than 4 seconds to return when pressure is applied to the fingernails or toenails of injured limb
- *Special instructions*
  —Instruct the patient in the use of required ambulatory aids (e.g., crutches, cane).
  —Teach the patient the proper method of applying Ace bandages: from distal to proximal on the limb to aid venous constriction and venous return. Advise the patient to loosen the bandage if signs of neurovascular impairment are noted.
  —Instruct the patient to apply ice packs for the first 24 to 72 hours or longer to lessen bleeding and edema, depending on injury.
- *Medications*
  —Explain the purpose, dosage, schedule, and route of administration of any prescribed drugs, as well as side effects to report to the physician or nurse.
- *Activity*
  —Depending on the severity of injury, discuss how long mobility will be impaired: 24 to 72 hours for first-degree sprains and strains; 10 days to 3 or more weeks for second- and third-degree injuries.
  —Stress the importance of maintaining rest and immobilization of the affected limb for the prescribed time. Explain that returning to activity while there is still swelling or bleeding may cause further injury and delayed healing and recovery.
  —Discuss the need to elevate the injured limb. Instruct the patient not to elevate it too high because this could reduce blood flow and thus increase swelling.

S

—Instruct the patient in progressive active range-of-motion and rehabilitative exercises as prescribed by the physician depending on severity of injury.

FOLLOW-UP CARE

• Stress the importance of follow-up medical and laboratory evaluations. Make sure the patient has the necessary names and telephone numbers.

Steroid Therapy
(Corticosteroid Therapy)

—Steroid therapy: use of corticosteroids as replacement therapy for adrenal insufficiency, for inflammation suppression, for control of allergic reactions, and for reducing the risk of graft rejection in transplantation. The length of time the patient remains on steroid therapy depends on the underlying condition for which it is prescribed; it can be lifelong or temporary. Corticosteroids are classified according to their biologic activities: glucocorticoids (carbohydrate and protein metabolism), mineralocorticoids (electrolyte and water metabolism), and androgens (anabolic and masculinizing). They are administered systemically (parenteral or oral) or topically (skin).

CAUTIONS

• Hypertension and diabetes mellitus can be exacerbated.
• Concurrent infections can be masked.
• Therapy should be used with caution in patients who are predisposed to peptic ulceration, thrombophlebitis, adrenal suppression, and mood swings.
• Gradual withdrawal of exogenous corticosteroids is necessary to prevent adrenal insufficiency.
• Women taking oral steroids are at increased risk for bone loss.

COMPLICATIONS

- Steroid-induced diabetes
- Hypertension
- Osteoporosis
- Peptic ulcer
- Thromboembolism
- Hypokalemia
- Pseudotumor cerebri
- Development of Cushing's syndrome

HOME CARE

- Give both the patient and the caregiver *verbal* and *written* instructions. Provide them with the name and telephone number of a physician or nurse to call if questions arise.
- Initiate the teaching plan as soon as it is known that the patient will be discharged with a prescription for steroid therapy.
- *General information*
  —Review the explanation of the condition that requires steroid therapy, the type of steroid therapy (systemic or topical) that is prescribed, benefits, dosage, time of administration, side effects, the importance of taking the medication at the prescribed time and not skipping a dose, and what to do if a dose is missed.
- *Warning signs*
  —Review the signs and symptoms that should be reported to a physician or nurse.
  - Euphoria (mood swings)
  - Gastrointestinal pain or bleeding
  - Bruising
  - Visual changes
  - Polydipsia, polyuria
  - Weight gain
  - Hirsutism
  - Fractures
- *Special instructions*
  —Tell the patient to refill medication prescriptions 1 to 2 weeks before the supply runs out and to store medication in a cool place, avoiding extremes of temperature.
  —Explain that normal signs of infection may be masked by steroid therapy and that the physician or nurse should be consulted at the onset of symptoms.

S

—Instruct the patient to take oral steroids with milk or antacids to decrease gastric irritation.

—Explain that the oral form of the medication comes in various dosages and that the patient must be sure to take the appropriate dose at the prescribed time.

—Discuss the need for and process of gradually withdrawing oral medication. Instruct the patient to monitor for and report the return of symptoms during withdrawal.

—Caution female patients to notify the physician or nurse if taking oral contraceptives because oral contraceptives raise serum levels of steroids.

—If the medication is administered topically, discuss the dosage and appropriate administration. Caution the patient to use the medication only as prescribed.

- *Activity*

  —Encourage the patient to discuss allowances and limitations with respect to occupation, recreation, or activities.

  —Encourage weight-bearing exercises if the patient is taking oral steroids.

- *Diet*

  —Instruct the patient to increase protein intake to combat osteoporosis.

FOLLOW-UP CARE AND REFERRALS

- Stress the importance of regular follow-up visits that include regular checks of blood pressure for patients receiving long-term therapy. Make sure the patient has the necessary names and telephone numbers.

- Discuss the possible need for bone density studies and annual eye examinations if the patient is receiving long-term oral steroid therapy.

- Provide a referral for home care blood pressure checking if indicated.

- Discuss the importance of wearing a MedicAlert bracelet and carrying an information card giving the name and dosage of the drug.

Stroke
(Cerebrovascular Accident)

—Stroke: a disruption in oxygen supply to cerebral cells, resulting in ischemia of an area of the brain and associated neurologic deficits.

CAUSES/CONTRIBUTING FACTORS/RISK FACTORS

- Ischemic stroke
  - —Thrombosis: atherosclerosis, hypertension, hematologic disorders
  - —Embolus: atrial fibrillation, extracranial clot formations, valvular heart disease
  - —Systemic hypoperfusion: circulatory failure, hypovolemia, systemic hypotension, hypoxia
- Hemorrhagic stroke
  - —Hypertension
  - —Aneurysm
  - —Vascular malformations
  - —Systemic hemorrhagic disorders

SIGNS/SYMPTOMS

- Location and size of the lesion and extent of injury determine symptoms; they may appear on the side of the body opposite the lesion or may occur bilaterally
- Altered level of consciousness: drowsiness, stupor, coma
- Behavioral changes: apathy, irritability, memory loss, disorientation
- Loss of sensation and reflexes: usually unilateral; may be temporary or permanent
- Flaccid or spastic muscle tone
- Unequal pupils
- Ptosis of eyelid
- Visual disturbances: blurring or loss of vision
- Drooping mouth
- Weakness or paralysis: unilateral or bilateral
- Communication dysfunction
  - —Aphasia: expressive or receptive language impairment

S

—Apraxia: impairment in the ability to perform purposeful acts or to manipulate objects

—Agnosia: impairment in the ability to recognize familiar objects or persons

- Dysphagia
- Bowel and bladder incontinence
- Nausea and vomiting
- Seizures
- Syncope

COMPLICATIONS

- Increased intracranial pressure
- Herniation
- Seizures
- Aspiration
- Contractures, pressure sores
- Respiratory and cardiac disturbances

DIAGNOSTIC TESTS

- Describe each procedure, its purpose, and the normal feelings or sensations that are likely, as well as any preprocedural and postprocedural care.

—Computed tomography or magnetic resonance imaging: to assess size of infarction, hematoma, shift of brain structures, cerebral circulation, cerebral edema

—Electroencephalogram: to assess lesion location and brain wave activity

—Cerebral angiography: to assess lesion size and location; to identify collateral circulation

—Transcranial Doppler ultrasonography: to assess pressure and flow in the intracranial arteries

—Positron emission tomography: to assess cerebral metabolism and circulation

—Phonoangiography or Doppler ultrasonography: to identify the presence of bruits in the carotid arteries

—Skull x-rays: to reveal intracranial calcifications

—Lumbar puncture and cerebrospinal fluid analysis: to assess for erythrocytes, proteins, and presence of infection

TREATMENT
Medical

- Therapy
  —Acute care
  > For ischemic stroke: thrombolytic therapy given within 1 to 6 hours from onset of symptoms
  > Intracranial pressure monitoring
  > Mechanical ventilation: to maintain patent airway and adequate ventilation
  > Electrocardiographic monitoring: to assess for cardiac dysrhythmias
  > Hemodynamic monitoring: to assess fluid volume status
  > Nasogastric tube: to aspirate gastric contents and free air
  > Indwelling urethral catheter: to monitor urinary output

  —Physical therapy and rehabilitation
  —Occupational therapy
  —Speech therapy
  —Bowel and bladder retraining
  —Diet: may advance to fluids, pureed, soft, or chopped foods, or tube feedings depending on the level of consciousness and ability to chew and swallow; a low-sodium, low-fat, low-cholesterol diet may be prescribed

- Drugs
  —Anticoagulants
  —Antiplatelet agents (ticlopidine, aspirin)
  —Antihypertensives
  —Diuretics
  —Corticosteroids
  —Anticonvulsants
  —Analgesics
  —Antacids
  —H$_2$ blockers
  —Stool softeners

Surgical

- Cerebral artery bypass surgery: to provide collateral cerebral circulation to the area distal to the stenosis
- Craniotomy: to evacuate intracerebral hematoma, repair ruptured aneurysm, apply arterial clips
- Carotid endarterectomy: surgical removal of plaque in the obstructed carotid artery to increase blood supply to the brain

---

SIGNS AND SYMPTOMS OF STROKE

Sudden appearance of any of the following should alert patient or family to impending stroke and be reported.
* Weakness or numbness of face, arm, or leg
* Difficulty speaking or inability to understand speech (garbled language)
* Change in vision: dimness or loss of vision
* Severe headache
* Dizziness or loss of balance

HOME CARE

* Give both the patient and the caregiver *verbal* and *written* instructions. Provide them with the name and telephone number of a physician or nurse to call if questions arise.
* *General information*
  —Explain and discuss cerebrovascular accident, causes or contributing factors, care, and treatment.
  —Review the explanation of type of stroke, degree of neurologic impairment, and discharge plans that may include a rehabilitation center or skilled nursing facility.
* *Warning signs*
  —Review the signs and symptoms that should be reported to a physician or nurse.
    Headache, vertigo, visual disturbances
    Changes in mentation and level of consciousness
    Seizure activity
    Lack of bowel movement for more than 3 days
    Respiratory distress
    Progression of sensory-motor-perception deficits
  —Alert the family to signs and symptoms of another stroke (see box above).
  —Stress the importance of getting the patient to an emergency room within 3 hours of onset of symptoms.
* *Special instructions (for patients being discharged to home)*
  —Assist the patient and caregiver in obtaining appropriate devices, such as walkers, specialty beds, and aids to safety, feeding, toileting, and grooming.

—Discuss alternative methods to deal with chronic pain: visualization, guided imagery, meditation, relaxation, bio-feedback.

—Discuss measures to provide a safe environment.

Orient the patient to the environment.

Provide good lighting.

Remove unnecessary furniture and objects, especially sharp and hazardous objects such as scissors.

Arrange furniture to provide a clear pathway.

Position the bed and personal objects within reach and in the unaffected visual field.

Protect the neglected side during activities.

Identify hazards or needed adaptations in the home, such as ramps, widening doorways to accommodate a wheelchair, rails, removal of scatter rugs, shower safety, and flat shoes.

—Encourage the patient to use vision on the affected side.

Gradually move objects, including meals, to the affected side.

Gradually move from the unaffected visual field to the patient's neglected side while communicating with the patient.

Encourage the patient to scan the affected visual field.

Initially place the patient with the unaffected side toward the most active part of the room. Gradually shift interactions and objects to the patient's neglected side.

—Encourage the patient to use the affected side in self-care.

Instruct the patient to include the affected extremities in performing activities of daily living.

Instruct the patient to attend to the affected site in grooming, care, and proper positioning.

Stimulate different sensations in the affected extremities with touch, scented lotions, or textured materials.

—Encourage the patient to use hearing on the affected side.

Move across the patient's field to the affected side while speaking and continue to speak on that side to stimulate the patient's attention to the neglected side.

—Encourage and demonstrate use of the unaffected extremity to assist the affected side in positioning and movement.

Demonstrate positioning the affected extremities using pillows or other support aids and elevating the extremities.

Provide and demonstrate use of a sling for the affected arm to support the arm and shoulder.

Instruct the patient to support affected extremities when repositioning.

Instruct the patient to limit turning to and lying on the affected side to 1 hour.

Instruct the patient to perform range-of-motion exercises of the affected extremities, using the unaffected extremities.

Instruct the patient to watch the affected leg while walking.

Instruct the family to provide restraints or belts for support and protection if body-spatial orientation is impaired.

—Instruct the patient to protect the affected side from extreme temperatures if tactile perception is impaired.

—Instruct the patient or caregiver to supervise all activities if judgment of position, distance, or spatial orientation is impaired.

—Assist and demonstrate performing activities of daily living using the unaffected side.

—Provide and instruct the patient in use of support devices in toileting, such as raised seat, commode, handrails, and undergarments that are easy to remove and replace.

—Provide and instruct the patient in use of aids in dressing and bathing, such as Velcro closures, zippers, or elastic waists.

—Instruct the patient to plan for regular rest periods to avoid fatigue.

—Encourage physical mobility.

Encourage weight-bearing and pivoting on the stronger side.

Teach the patient to transfer toward the unaffected side. Instruct the patient to position the unaffected side next to the bed or chair to which the patient is transferring.

—Encourage effective communication.

Explain the type of the patient's communication dysfunction.

Refer the patient to speech therapy.

Ensure that the patient is well rested when initiating communication exercises.

Stand within the patient's visual field. Maintain eye contact.

Reduce environmental distractions, such as television, music, or other conversations.

Speak to the patient in a normal voice. Do not shout or speak loudly.

Speak slowly in simple sentences and vocabulary that the patient understands. Repeat as necessary.

Use nonverbal gestures to supplement communication.

Limit each conversation to one clearly defined subject.

Use the same word each time a question or sentence is repeated.

Record the words to be used each time.

Ask yes-or-no questions.

Allow time for the patient to respond to questions.

Avoid finishing the patient's sentences.

Provide feedback. Correct errors and praise efforts. If the patient's verbal communication is unclear, ask the patient to repeat the statement or point to objects.

For a patient with right hemisphere damage, if the patient diverges from the subject of conversation, return the patient to the subject. Explain sounds that the patient hears by identifying the object producing the sounds.

For a patient with left hemisphere damage, provide objects for the patient to touch and name.

Provide flashcards with pictures and words the patient can point to for communication or a slate board if appropriate.

Avoid instructing the patient with concepts involving numbers or time.

Avoid using metaphors. Speak in clear, concrete terms.

—Assist the patient with elimination.

Offer an elimination opportunity every 2 hours and after fluid intake.

Monitor daily bowel movements.

Stress the importance of taking stool softeners as prescribed.

Provide incontinence pads or waterproof undergarments.

- *Medications*

—Explain the purpose, dosage, schedule, and route of administration of any prescribed drugs, as well as side effects to report to the physician or nurse.

- *Activity*
  —Encourage the patient and caregiver to discuss abilities to resume occupation, recreation, and activities.
  —Advise the caregiver to encourage independent activities as much as possible.
  —Teach the caregiver and patient to perform range-of-motion exercises.
  —Assist the patient with supportive devices such as walkers and wheelchairs.
  —Assist the patient with progression of activities and ambulation. Instruct the caregiver to stand on the affected side when ambulating with the patient.
- *Diet*
  —Assist with tube feedings as ordered.
  —Assist with oral feedings as necessary.
    Position food and utensils within reach.
    Use assistive aids for self-feeding, such as large handles on utensils or a plate guard.
  —Assist the patient and family to plan a diet to include preferred foods that are easy to swallow with increased bulk (see Appendix C).
  —Instruct the patient and family to avoid milk and foods that are thin and smooth.
  —Instruct the patient to take small portions and chew thoroughly.
  —Instruct the patient to place food on the unaffected side of the mouth.
  —Position the patient on one side with the head of the bed elevated if feeding in bed.
  —Encourage fluid intake up to 2 liters/day, unless contraindicated.

PSYCHOSOCIAL CARE

- Advise the caregiver to avoid overprotectiveness.
- Assist the caregiver to establish realistic, achievable goals.
- Praise the patient's accomplishments and progress.
- Encourage the patient and family to express concerns about adjustment to the disability: behavioral, psychosocial, and functional changes.
- Inform the patient that emotional lability and depression are common.

• Refer the patient to a social worker for further support and counseling.

FOLLOW-UP CARE

• Stress the importance of follow-up medical care with the physician, rehabilitation program, speech therapy, physical therapy, and occupational therapy. Make sure the patient and caregiver have the necessary names and telephone numbers.

REFERRALS

• Assist the patient and family to obtain referral to support groups, government and community resources, and home health support services.
• Refer the patient to physical, speech, and occupational therapy.
• Provide referral to the National Stroke Association, 8480 E. Orchard Rd., Suite 1000, Englewood, CO 80111, (303) 771-1700 or (800) 787-6537 and to the American Heart Association (AHA Stroke Connection National Center, 7272 Greenville Ave., Dallas, TX 75231, [800] AHA-USA1).

Tendinitis, Epicondylitis, and Bursitis

—Tendinitis (tenosynovitis): inflammation of the tendon-covering sheath around one or a group of tendons.

—Epicondylitis: inflammation of the tendons where they insert into condyles of bones such as the humerus and femur.

—Bursitis: inflammation of a bursa, an enclosed sac between muscles and tendons and bony prominences.

— Tendinitis and epicondylitis generally occur together, and the symptoms are similar. The cause of these conditions is repetitive motion and overuse, which lead to tears, bleeding, edema, and pain in the affected tendons. Both conditions tend to occur in younger age groups and are often caused by sports injuries. For example, lateral epicondylitis, commonly called tennis elbow, is caused by repetitive twisting and swinging movements of the elbow that accompany swinging a tennis racket. Medial epicondylitis is called golfer's elbow because it is related to repetitive swings of the elbow made by a golfer. In older age groups epicondylitis and tendinitis are related to overuse syndromes, often from repetitive motions as in office workers, clerks, writers, and meat cutters. Tendinitis also affects people with rheumatoid arthritis and diabetes and occurs in all age groups. Bursitis is usually caused by constant friction between the skin and musculoskeletal tissues around the joint. Rarely, it results from a foreign body such as calcium or infection. Since a bursa is enclosed within other tissues, the inflammation spreads to those tissues. One or more bursae can become inflamed, but the most commonly affected are bursae of the shoulder, elbow, greater trochanter lateral to the hip, and upper tibia. Bursitis is most common in athletes who perform repetitive motions.

SIGNS/SYMPTOMS
- Tenderness and pain around joint (increases with motion)
- Limitation of motion
- Heat, redness, swelling in joint
- Fever, malaise (if pathogen involved)

COMPLICATIONS
- Chronic inflammation
- Degenerative arthritis
- Avulsion tears
- Calcification in joints
- Loss of range of motion of joints
- Muscle weakness

DIAGNOSTIC TESTS
- Describe each procedure, its purpose, and the normal feelings or sensations that are likely, as well as any preprocedural and postprocedural care.
    - X-rays: may show enlarged bursa with or without calcified deposits (bursitis); calcified areas, tears in a specific tendon, or degenerative changes (tendinitis or epicondylitis)

TREATMENT
Medical

- Therapy
    - Ice applications to inflamed area
    - Moist heat after ice applications
    - Use of orthotics
        Heel pads or shoe inserts for Achilles tendinitis
        Sponge rubber knee pads (bursitis)
        Forearm band for lateral epicondylitis (tennis elbow)
        Application of splint to forearm (lateral or medial epicondylitis)
        Ace or elastic bandages if bursa is accessible to reduce edema
- Drugs
    - Corticosteroids, orally or injected into the inflamed area to relieve pain and inflammation
    - Analgesic-antipyretic agents
    - Nonsteroidal antiinflammatory drugs
    - Antibiotics

Surgical

- Excision of the bursal wall and calcified deposits
- Removal of exostosis (bone projection) around the lateral epicondyle
- Removal of the degenerated tendon sheath

HOME CARE

- Give both the patient and the caregiver *verbal* and *written* instructions. Provide them with the name and telephone number of a physician or nurse to call if questions arise.
- *General information*
    - Describe the type of injury, explaining that it is usually managed medically with rest and medication and that surgery is seldom indicated.
- *Special instructions*
    - Instruct the patient in the use of orthotics (pads, shoe inserts), an immobilizer, or a splint to ease pressure on vulnerable tissues. Advise the patient where to obtain equipment.
    - Explain how to use heat and cold applications as ordered and the importance of protecting the skin from thermal injury.

Teach the patient to cover the heat or cold container with a dry cotton cover.

• *Medications*

—Explain the purpose, dosage, schedule, and route of administration of any prescribed drugs, as well as side effects to report to the physician or nurse.

—Advise the patient not to take nonsteroidal antiinflammatory drugs on an empty stomach.

—If the patient is given a steroid injection, explain that pain may increase after injection for the first 24 hours but is followed by significant pain relief and increasing range of motion.

• *Activity*

—Emphasize the need to rest the affected part because this allows the inflamed tissues to begin healing. Explain that full healing takes 4 to 6 weeks.

—Caution the patient to avoid activities that could prevent healing of present inflammation or cause a recurrence.

Lower extremities: kneeling, running, aerobic exercises, especially high impact

Upper extremities: repetitive motion: raising arms above head, swinging a golf club or tennis racket, throwing or hitting a ball

—Instruct the patient in the importance of range-of-motion exercises to maintain function once inflammation has subsided.

FOLLOW-UP CARE

• Stress the importance of follow-up visits. Make sure the patient and caregiver have the necessary names and telephone numbers.

Testicular Cancer

—Testicular cancer: cancer of the testes, the most common cancer in men 15 to 35 years of age. Testicular cancer occurs more often in whites and in higher socioeconomic groups. The prognosis depends on cell type and stage of cancer. For stage I seminoma the cure rate is as high as 90%. Testicular cancers are most commonly seminomas or teratomas of germ cell origin. They may also be heterogeneous, nonseminomatous germ cell tumors.

CAUSES/CONTRIBUTING FACTORS

- Cryptorchidism (undescended testes)
- Atrophic testis
- In utero exposure to diethylstilbestrol (DES) or other exogenous hormones
- Familial history of testicular cancer
- History of trauma, mumps, or orchitis

SIGNS/SYMPTOMS

- Small, hard, painless lump in testicles (first sign)
- Sensation of scrotal heaviness
- Sudden fluid accumulation in scrotum
- Perineal pain or discomfort
- Episodic testicular pain
- Low back, groin, or abdominal ache, "dragging pain"
- Breast enlargement or tenderness (gynecomastia)
- Advanced signs
  —Cough
  —Dyspnea
  —Hemoptysis
  —Back pain

COMPLICATIONS

- Metastases
  —Ureteral obstruction
  —Pulmonary lesion

DIAGNOSTIC TESTS

- Describe each procedure, its purpose, and the normal feelings or sensations that are likely, as well as any preprocedural and postprocedural care.
  —Palpation and transillumination of testes: to detect lesion
  —Biopsy: to detect presence of malignant cells
  —Excretory urography: to determine placement of ureters or kidney by lesion

—Abdominal computed tomography, ultrasound, lymphangiography: to detect extratesticular involvement
—Chest x-ray, chest computed tomography, whole lung tomography: to detect presence of pulmonary metastases
—Serum alpha-fetoprotein (AFP), human chorionic gonadotropin (HCG): tumor markers elevated in presence of testicular cancer

TREATMENT
Medical

- Therapy
  —Radiation therapy
    External beam; complications: fatigue, bone marrow suppression, diarrhea, decreased sperm count
  —Chemotherapy
    For seminomas: cyclophosphamide
    For nonseminomas: PVB (cisplatin, vinblastine, bleomycin)
  —Alternative to chemotherapy for nonseminomas: surveillance program with monthly follow-up for 12 months (physical examination, tumor markers, chest x-ray)

Surgical

- Inguinal exploration and orchiectomy: removal of testis, epididymis, portion of vas deferens, portion of gonadal lymphatics and their blood supply
- Bilateral retroperitoneal lymph node dissection: removal of all perivascular tissue from area bounded superiorly by renal arteries and veins, inferiorly by common iliac arteries to the bifurcation, and laterally by ureters; usually unilateral

PREPROCEDURAL TEACHING

- Review the physician's explanation of the procedure and the reason for it; encourage the patient to ask questions and to discuss any fears or anxieties. Explain the need for informed consent.

Review of Preprocedural Care

- Inform the patient that the skin will be cleansed with bactericidal soap or antiseptic solution to remove bacteria.
- Explain that a complete blood count and urinalysis will be performed to check for infection and bleeding.

- Discuss the need for nothing by mouth (NPO) status from midnight of the night before the procedure.

Review of Postprocedural Care

- Inform the patient that an orchiectomy necessitates a high inguinal incision and a retroperitoneal lymphadenectomy usually requires a transabdominal incision.
- Discuss the need for a nasogastric tube for suctioning until bowel sounds return and a Foley catheter to facilitate urinary drainage.
- Explain that vital signs will be monitored for early signs of hemorrhage and shock.
- Tell the patient that the dressing will be checked for the amount and type of drainage.
- Discuss issues of fertility and sexual potency. Provide information about sperm banking and emotional support.

HOME CARE

- Give both the patient and the caregiver *verbal* and *written* instructions. Provide them with the name and telephone number of a physician or nurse to call if questions arise.
- *General information*
  —Review the physician's explanation of the disease process, possible causes or contributing factors, type and stage of tumor, and prescribed treatments.
- *Special instructions*
  —For nonadvanced tumors, stress the importance of performing testicular self-examination monthly to detect new or recurrent tumors. Inform the patient that the procedure is best done after a warm shower or bath when the scrotum is relaxed. Demonstrate the procedure and permit time for practice.
    Perform the examination in a standing position.
    Place the middle and index fingers below one testis with the thumb on top.
    Gently roll the testis between thumb and fingers, palpating for rubbery, spongy consistency. The testis should be smooth and free of lumps.
    Hold one testicle in each palm and observe any difference in weight.
    Report any hard painless mass (usually occurs on lateral or anterior surface).

PSYCHOSOCIAL CARE

- Explain to the patient that one healthy testis can compensate for loss of function in the other testis, so male characteristics are not adversely affected.
- Discuss actual or potential sexual dysfunction associated with the prescribed treatment.
- Encourage verbalization of feelings regarding body image, self-esteem, and sexuality.
- Provide information and supportive guidance regarding sexual functioning.

FOLLOW-UP CARE

- Stress the importance of regular follow-up visits for medical and laboratory evaluation. Make sure the patient has the necessary names and telephone numbers.
- Explain that if the patient remains free of cancer after 1 year, follow-up examinations may be performed every 2 months for the second year, then every 6 months for life. Patients who have relapses receive salvage combination chemotherapy.

Thoracentesis

—Thoracentesis: puncture of the chest wall with a large-gauge needle to remove air or fluid from the pleural space.

INDICATIONS

- Pleural effusion
- Suspected malignancy

PREPROCEDURAL TEACHING

- Review the physician's explanation of the procedure and the reason for it; encourage the patient to ask questions and to discuss any fears or anxieties. Discuss the need for informed consent.

Review of Preprocedural Care

- Inform the patient that movement or coughing during the procedure is prohibited to prevent inadvertent needle damage to the lung or pleura. Tell the patient that if coughing is unavoidable, the physician should be notified so he or she can withdraw the needle slightly to prevent puncture. Explain that a cough suppressant may be given before the procedure if the patient has a troublesome cough.

- Inform the patient that a local anesthetic will be used to minimize discomfort and that only pressure will be felt when the needle is inserted.
- Explain that the patient will be positioned on the edge of the bed with the feet supported and the head and arms resting on the overbed table; if the patient is unable to sit on the edge of the bed, he or she will lie on the unaffected side with the head of the bed elevated and the arm raised over the head.

Review of Postprocedural Care

- Explain that a bandage will be placed over the puncture site.
- Review signs and symptoms to report to the physician or nurse: bloody sputum, tachypnea, difficulty breathing, restlessness, fever.
- Inform the patient that a chest x-ray will be taken to check for pneumothorax.
- Explain that the patient will be able to resume regular activity within 1 hour if there is no sign or symptom of postthoracentesis complication.
- Teach and stress the importance of deep breathing every 2 to 4 hours and proper positioning to facilitate ventilatory effort.

COMPLICATIONS

- Hemothorax
- Pneumothorax
- Air embolism
- Subcutaneous emphysema
- Pulmonary edema
- Mediastinal shift

HOME CARE

- Give both the patient and the caregiver *verbal* and *written* instructions. Provide them with the name and telephone number of a physician or nurse to call if questions arise.
- *General information*
  —Explain the underlying cause for the procedure.

- *Warning signs*
  —Review the signs and symptoms that should be reported to a physician or nurse.
  Difficulty breathing
  Chest pain
  Vertigo
  Elevated temperature
  Diaphoresis
  Uncontrollable cough
  Bloody sputum
- *Special instructions*
  —Explain the importance of avoiding persons with upper respiratory tract infections.
- *Medications*
  —Explain the purpose, dosage, schedule, and route of administration of any prescribed drugs, as well as side effects to report to a physician or nurse.
  —Explain the need to avoid taking over-the-counter medications without checking with the physician.
- *Activity*
  —Explain that after discharge the patient can resume usual activities but should avoid heavy lifting. Advise the patient to check with the physician or nurse for any specific limitations.

FOLLOW-UP CARE

- Stress the importance of regular follow-up visits. Make sure the patient has the necessary names and telephone numbers.

Thrombolytic Therapy

—Thrombolytic therapy: intravenous or intracoronary administration of a clot-dissolving drug to lyse clots, restore coronary blood flow, and limit myocardial ischemia. Thrombolytic therapy is initiated when diagnostic evidence shows that a patient is in the process of myocardial infarction.

INDICATIONS

- Recent onset of chest pain (less than 12 hours)
- Acute myocardial infarction as evidenced on electrocardiogram

PREPROCEDURAL TEACHING

- Review the physician's explanation of the procedure, the reason for it, and associated risks; encourage the patient to ask questions and to discuss any fears or anxieties. Discuss the need for informed consent for thrombolytic therapy, cardiac catheterization, percutaneous transluminal coronary angioplasty (PTCA), and coronary artery bypass grafting (CABG).
- Inform the patient and family of the possibility of emergency treatment: PTCA or CABG.

Review of Preprocedural Care

- Explain that the procedure may last up to 3 hours.
- Review sensations to be felt during the intracoronary procedure: pressure during insertion but no discomfort with infusion.
- Explain that any uncomfortable feelings experienced as a result of thrombolytic therapy will be treated as they occur.
- Inform the patient that laboratory tests, baseline 12-lead electrocardiogram, and blood type and crossmatch will be completed before the procedure.
- Explain that at least two or three intravenous access sites will be established.
- Tell the patient that vital signs, electrocardiogram, and bleeding will be monitored during and after the procedure and that a complete neurologic assessment will be done before the procedure and repeated frequently for up to 24 hours after the infusion is completed.

Review of Postprocedural Care

- Tell the patient that bed rest will be maintained during the procedure and for 12 hours after an intracoronary infusion; there are no restrictions after intravenous infusions.
- Explain that frequent blood sampling will be performed to monitor clotting times and that signs and symptoms of successful myocardial reperfusion, coronary reocclusion, and bleeding will be monitored.
- Explain that signs of bleeding under the skin are expected and will clear with time.

SIDE EFFECTS/COMPLICATIONS

- Bleeding
- Hemorrhage: gastrointestinal, intracranial
- Myocardial infarction
- Reperfusion arrhythmias

🏠 HOME CARE

- Give both the patient and the caregiver *verbal* and *written* instructions. Provide them with the name and telephone number of a physician or nurse to call if questions arise.
- *General information*
  —Reinforce the physician's explanation regarding the outcome of therapy, extent of myocardial damage, and possible need for further interventions such as PTCA and CABG.
  —Instruct the patient about the development of coronary artery disease and the potential recurrence of coronary artery occlusion.
- *Warning signs*
  —Review the signs and symptoms that should be reported to a physician or nurse.
    Chest pain: dysrhythmias, tachycardia, lightheadedness, skin cool, clammy, and diaphoretic
    Bleeding: bruising, bleeding gums, hematuria, bloody emesis, black stools, flank pain, headache
- *Medications*
  —Explain the purpose, dosage, schedule, and route of administration of any prescribed drugs, as well as side effects to report to a physician or nurse.
- *Special instructions*
  —Advise the patient to avoid vigorous toothbrushing.
  —Discuss the need to modify coronary risk factors.

FOLLOW-UP CARE

- Stress the importance of regular follow-up visits. Make sure the patient has the necessary names and telephone numbers.
- Explain that follow-up coronary angiography may be necessary to evaluate the patency of the coronary arteries.

Thyroidectomy

—Thyroidectomy: surgical removal of part or all of the thyroid gland. Thyroidectomy is used in treatment of hyperthyroidism, respiratory obstruction from goiter, and thyroid cancer. Subtotal thyroidectomy, used to correct hyperthyroidism when drug therapy fails or radiation therapy is contraindicated, reduces secretion of thyroid hormone. It also effectively treats diffuse goiter. After surgery the remaining thyroid tissue usually supplies enough thyroid hormone for normal function. Total thyroidectomy may be performed for certain types of thyroid cancer, such as papillary, follicular, medullary, or anaplastic neoplasms. After this surgery the patient requires lifelong thyroid hormone replacement therapy.

SIDE EFFECTS/COMPLICATIONS

- Hemorrhage
- Hypocalcemia: tetany
- Hypothyroidism
- Laryngeal nerve damage
- Thyroid storm

HOME CARE

- Give both the patient and the caregiver *verbal* and *written* instructions. Provide them with the name and telephone number of a physician or nurse to call if questions arise.
- *General information*
  —Explain and discuss with the patient the thyroidectomy procedure, especially changes in thyroid function as a result of surgery.
- *Wound/incision care*
  —Teach the patient to keep the surgical site clean and dry.
  —Teach methods to conceal the surgical site without affecting healing. Suggest loosely buttoned collars, high-necked blouses, jewelry, or scarves.
  —Inform the patient that lotion may soften the healing scar and improve its appearance (if approved by the physician).

T

- *Warning signs*
  —Review the signs and symptoms that should be reported to a physician or nurse.
    General: respiratory distress, bleeding
    Wound infection: redness, warmth, swelling, persistent drainage from site, purulent exudate
    Total thyroidectomy: signs and symptoms of hypothyroidism (see p. 381).
    Parathyroid damage: signs of hypocalcemia: numbness, tingling, twitching, spasm, tetany
- *Special instructions*
  —Discuss methods of stress management.
- *Medications*
  —Explain the purpose, dosage, schedule, and route of administration of any prescribed drugs, as well as side effects to report to a physician or nurse.
  —Discuss the importance of not taking over-the-counter medications without checking with a physician or nurse.
  —If the patient has had a total thyroidectomy, explain the importance of taking thyroid replacement medication regularly.
  —If the patient has parathyroid damage, explain the need for calcium supplements.
- *Activity*
  —Encourage the patient to discuss allowances and limitations with respect to occupation, recreation, and activities.
  —Teach prescribed head and neck exercises: flexion, lateral movement, hyperextension.
  —Teach the importance of a balance between activity and rest.
- *Diet*
  —Discuss the need to maintain a well-balanced diet.

FOLLOW-UP CARE

- Stress the importance of regular follow-up visits to monitor thyroid levels: thyroid-stimulating hormone (TSH), thyroxine (T_4). Make sure the patient has the necessary names and telephone numbers.

Torn Knee Cartilage/Meniscectomy

—Meniscectomy: removal of menisci, **C**-shaped rings of cartilage covering the ends of the tibia with the knee joint. Although still indicated in certain cases, meniscectomy is done less frequently and has been largely replaced by therapeutic arthroscopy. The cartilages facilitate joint motion, while also absorbing some of the stress placed on the joint. They are subject to wear and tear because of trauma, or degeneration secondary to arthritis. Because cartilage has no intrinsic blood supply, it rarely heals without developing unsatisfactory scar tissue, necessitating surgical intervention to remove the damaged or degenerated cartilage from the knee joint. Meniscectomy is performed when torn meniscus is diagnosed; if left untreated, tears lead to further joint degeneration and chronic arthritis of the knee joint. The majority of meniscal tears are related to sports, particularly basketball, soccer, and football. Medial meniscal tears, resulting from internal rotation of the knee, are the most common; lateral meniscus tears are associated with external rotation.

SIGNS/SYMPTOMS

- Chronic (degenerative-osteoarthritic)
  —Joint stiffness, weakness
  —Joint pain, worsening with activity, relieved by rest
  —Joint swelling and fluid
  —Weak joint "giving way"
- Acute (occur after knee trauma)
  —Joint effusion (distention with fluid)
  —Limited range of motion
  —Locking of knee joint (inability to extend knee fully)
  —Joint pain

COMPLICATIONS

- Chronic knee arthritis if tear is left untreated
- Weakness, atrophy of quadriceps caused by disuse of knee joint secondary to pain
- Joint instability, degeneration
- Postsurgical infection, hemorrhage

- Scar formation leading to future tears
- Compartment syndrome
- Hematoma or thrombus formation

DIAGNOSTIC TESTS

- Describe each procedure, its purpose, and the normal feelings or sensations that are likely, as well as any preprocedural and postprocedural care.
    —McMurray's test: clicks or pops accompanied by pain when the leg is extended from a flexed position
    —Apley grinding test: grinding or crepitus elicited when the foot and lower leg are forced down on the femur from a knee flexed position
    —Arthrogram: injection of radiopaque dye and air into the joint to outline the area of injury
    —Arthrocentesis: extraction of synovial fluid to detect blood, indicating meniscal tear
    —Radiologic studies
        X-rays: to document injury
        Magnetic resonance imaging: to show specific tissues and indicate exact injury
        Diagnostic arthroscopy: to show meniscal and ligament injuries

TREATMENT
Medical

- Drugs
    —Analgesics for pain relief
    —Nonsteroidal antiinflammatory drugs to reduce the inflammatory process

Surgical

- Meniscectomy or arthroscopy: repair of the torn areas of the meniscus is usually done arthroscopically, but more extensive surgical exposure and repair may be required, depending on the severity of the injury (a traditional meniscectomy); the repair may be done as an inpatient or outpatient procedure, usually under local anesthesia

PREPROCEDURAL TEACHING

- Review the physician's explanation of the procedure and the reason for it; encourage the patient to ask questions and to discuss any fears or anxieties. Discuss the need for informed consent for surgery and anesthesia.

Review of Preprocedural Care

- Review preprocedural tests.
  —Blood tests: to show status of electrolytes in blood; to determine presence of infection
  —Urine tests: to document presence of infection
  —Chest x-ray and electrocardiogram (depending on age): to provide the baseline presence of potential problems
- Explain that a shower with bactericidal soap will be necessary the night before surgery.
- Tell the patient that the incisional area will be shaved on the morning of surgery.
- Discuss the need for NPO status from midnight the night before the procedure.
- Inform the patient that weight bearing as tolerated on the affected knee is permissible before surgery; instruct the patient in crutch walking for use after surgery.

Review of Postprocedural Care

- Explain that knee repair is usually done on an outpatient basis but that more extensive repair may require a 1- to 2-day hospital stay.
- Explain the use of a hinged knee brace or knee immobilizer.
- Discuss the need for a bandage applied to the knee and high support hose (thromboembolitic disease [TED] hose).
- Inform the patient of the importance of elevating the operative leg and applying ice bags to the operative site to relieve swelling.
- Discuss the need for and frequency of neurovascular checks, vital signs, and peripheral pulse checks.
- Tell the patient that bed rest will be maintained for 8 to 24 hours (depending on the specific procedure), that no weight bearing on the operative leg will be permitted for 24 hours, and that ambulation with crutches will be permitted as early as 6 to 8 hours postoperatively and continued for 6 weeks.
- Discuss the importance of beginning straight leg raising on the second or third postoperative day and active and passive range-of-motion exercises in the physical therapy department on the third to fifth postoperative day.

🏠 HOME CARE

- Give both the patient and the caregiver *verbal* and *written* instructions. Provide them with the name and telephone number of a physician or nurse to call if questions arise.
- *General information*
  —Review the procedure, type of injury, and contributing causes.
- *Warning signs*
  —Review the signs and symptoms of neurovascular impairment that should be reported to a physician or nurse.
     Pallor, coolness of extremity
     Numbness, tingling in toes
     Inability to use or lift leg
     Increased pain and swelling
     Decreased capillary refill of toes on affected extremity
  —Review signs of infection to report immediately.
     Fever, pain
     Swelling at incisional site
     Purulent drainage from incision
- *Special instructions*
  —Discuss methods to reduce swelling: elevation of extremity, application of ice bags to surgical site.
  —Discuss the need for continuing range-of-motion and muscle-setting exercises: (quadriceps, gluteal, and triceps) for long-term recovery.
- *Medications*
  —Explain the purpose, dosage, schedule, and route of administration of any prescribed drugs, as well as side effects to report to a physician or nurse.
- *Activity*
  —Instruct the patient in the proper use of crutches and proper stairwalking procedures.
  —Clarify the need to refrain from sports activities that could retraumatize unhealed tissues until permitted by the physician.

FOLLOW-UP CARE

- Stress the importance of regular follow-up visits. Make sure the patient has the necessary names and telephone numbers.

Tuberculosis, Pulmonary

—**Pulmonary tuberculosis:** a chronic, acute, or subacute infectious pulmonary disease in which fibrosis and cavitation are caused by the tubercle bacillus *(Mycobacterium tuberculosis)*. The bacilli are inhaled in airborne mucous droplets from the sputum of persons with active disease. Less frequently they are ingested or enter through a break in the skin. Susceptible individuals include children less than 3 years of age or adults over 65 years, the chronically ill, silicone and asbestos workers, and malnourished and immunosuppressed persons. The incidence is high for persons living in crowded, poorly ventilated, unsanitary conditions such as homeless shelters and tenements.

SIGNS/SYMPTOMS
- Persistent low-grade temperature
- Night sweats
- Anorexia, weight loss
- Fatigue, malaise
- Pleuritic chest pain or chest tightness
- Persistent cough with blood-tinged or mucopurulent sputum

COMPLICATIONS
- Atelectasis
- Hemoptysis
- Pneumothorax
- Pleural effusion
- Pericarditis, peritonitis, meningitis, lymphadenitis
- Multidrug-resistant tuberculosis
- Extrapulmonary tuberculosis

DIAGNOSTIC TESTS
- Describe each procedure, its purpose, and the normal feelings or sensations that are likely, as well as any preprocedural and postprocedural care.
  - Tuberculin skin test (e.g., purified protein derivative, Mantoux test)

—Sputum culture
—Chest x-ray
—Gastric washings
—Fiberoptic bronchoscopy
—Needle biopsy of pleura
—Acid-fast sputum smear

TREATMENT
Medical

- Therapy
  —Respiratory isolation as necessary
  —High-protein, high-carbohydrate diet
- Drugs
  —Isoniazid (INH)
  —Ethambutol
  —Rifampin
  —Streptomycin
  —Paraaminosalicylic acid
  —Pyrazinamide
  —Analgesics

Surgical

- Resection for persistent cavitary lesions
- Surgical intervention for massive hemoptysis, spontaneous pneumothorax, abscess drainage, intestinal obstruction, or ureteral stricture

HOME CARE

- Give both the patient and the caregiver *verbal* and *written* instructions. Provide them with the name and telephone number of a physician or nurse to call if questions arise.
- Include all household members in instruction.
- *General information*
  —Explain the disease process, underlying causes and contributing factors, and contagiousness and transmission.
- *Warning signs*
  —Review the signs and symptoms that should be reported to a physician or nurse.
      Bloody sputum
      Chest pain
      Difficulty in breathing

Fever

Increased cough

Night sweats

- *Special instructions*
  —Advise the patient on how and where to obtain supplies (e.g., drugstore, medical supply company).
  —Explain the importance of good hygiene and handwashing after handling secretions, masks, or soiled tissues to prevent transmission of disease. Instruct the patient to cough into a tissue, to turn head if coughing, and to avoid direct contact with sputum. Explain how to dispose of tissues. Tell the patient to wear a mask if unable to comply with directions.
  —Review home respiratory isolation procedures as necessary: sleep in a well-ventilated room, use disposable supplies and utensils, use waterproof plastic bags for disposal.
  —Explain the need to avoid crowds and persons with upper respiratory infections.
  —Discuss the importance of avoiding close contact with others until advised by the physician.
- *Medications*
  —Explain the purpose, dosage, schedule, and route of administration of any prescribed drugs, as well as side effects (e.g., hearing loss, vertigo) to report to a physician or nurse.
  —Inform the patient that antiinfective agents, most commonly isoniazid and rifampin, are given for 6 to 12 months. If the patient is taking rifampin, explain that body secretions (feces, saliva, tears) may appear red-orange.
  —Caution a female patient that medications may interfere with the effectiveness of oral contraceptives.
  —Explain the need to avoid taking over-the-counter medications without checking with a physician.
  —Emphasize the importance of not stopping medication unless the physician gives approval.
- *Activity*
  —Advise the patient to limit exercise and activity to tolerance, to avoid fatigue, and to plan frequent rest periods.
- *Diet*
  —Discuss the need for a high-protein, high-carbohydrate diet. If the patient's appetite is poor, suggest frequent small meals.
  —Instruct the patient to drink 2000 to 3000 ml or more daily unless contraindicated.

T

FOLLOW-UP CARE AND REFERRALS

- Stress the importance of regular medical and laboratory follow-up visits. Make sure the patient has the necessary names and telephone numbers.
- Discuss the need for the patient to inform the caregiver, friends, and all contacts to obtain skin testing at the local health department.
- Discuss the need for periodic reculturing of sputum during medical therapy.

Ulcer (Peptic)

—**Peptic ulcer: circumscribed ulceration of mucous membrane that develops in the lower esophagus, stomach (gastric), or duodenum (duodenal).**

CAUSES/CONTRIBUTING FACTORS

- Gastric ulcer
    - —Long-term use of medications (aspirin, indomethacin, steroids)
    - —Chemicals (tobacco, alcohol)
    - —Stress
    - —Heredity
    - —Infection
- Duodenal ulcer
    - —Heredity
    - —Chemicals
    - —Psychosocial stressors
    - —Medications
    - —Infection

SIGNS/SYMPTOMS

- Gastric ulcer
    - —Left to middle epigastric pain that may radiate to the back and occurs 60 to 90 minutes after eating
    - —Feeling of fullnesss
    - —Nausea and vomiting

- Duodenal ulcer
  —Right epigastric pain that may radiate to the back or thorax and occurs 2 to 4 hours after eating or may be unrelated to food intake
  —Heartburn
  —Feeling of fullness after eating
  —Nausea and vomiting
  —Abdominal tenderness
  —Belching
  —Mild diarrhea with black stools

COMPLICATIONS

- Electrolyte imbalance
- Hemorrhage
- Perforation
- Pyloric stenosis
- Shock

DIAGNOSTIC TESTS

- Describe each procedure, its purpose, and the normal feelings or sensations that are likely, as well as any preprocedural and postprocedural care.
  —Endoscopy with biopsy and cytology
  —Barium studies
  —Abdominal radiologic studies
  —Gastric analysis
  —Hematocrit; levels of hemoglobin, pepsinogen, gastrin
  —Stool for melena

TREATMENT
Medical

- Therapy
  —Dietary therapy
- Drugs
  —Analgesics
  —Aluminum-magnesium antacids: Delcid, Mylanta II
  —Histamine (H_2) receptor blockers: Cimetidine (Tagamet), Ranitidine (Zantac), Famotidine (Pepcid)
  —Sucralfate (Carafate)
  —Misoprostol (Cytotec)
  —Omeprazole (Prilosec)

U

Surgical

- Pyloroplasty
- Vagotomy
- Subtotal gastrectomy
- Total gastrectomy

HOME CARE

- Give both the patient and the caregiver *verbal* and *written* instructions. Provide them with the name and telephone number of a physician or nurse to call if questions arise.
- *General information*
  —Explain the disease process, underlying causes, and contributing factors. Assist the patient to identify factors that can exacerbate an attack and suggest measures to minimize or modify them.
- *Warning signs*
  —Review the signs and symptoms of perforation that should be reported to a physician or nurse.
    Extreme epigastric pain
    Hematemesis (frank blood or coffee-ground appearance)
    Tarry or bloody stools
    Sudden sharp epigastric or abdominal pain
    Pain radiating to shoulders
    Abdominal rigidity
    Fever
- *Special instructions*
  —Provide information for a patient undergoing surgical intervention (see Abdominal Surgery, p. 6).
    Demonstrate care of the incision line and dressing changes.
    Review signs and symptoms of wound infection to report to the physician or nurse: persistent redness, swelling, purulent drainage, local warmth, fever, foul odor.
- *Medications*
  —Explain the purpose, dosage, schedule, and route of administration of any prescribed drugs, as well as side effects to report to a physician or nurse.
  —Explain the need to avoid taking over-the-counter medications without checking with a physician.
  —Instruct the patient to take only prescribed antacids.
  —Discuss the reason for avoiding aspirin-containing drugs, ibuprofen, and steroids, and tell the patient to read all labels.

- *Diet*
  —Review dietary allowances and restrictions. Instruct the patient to follow a bland diet, avoiding distressing foods such as black pepper; chili powder; raw, spicy, or fatty foods; fruit juices; and caffeinated beverages.
  —Emphasize the importance of avoiding alcohol.
  —Instruct the patient to eat slowly, to take small frequent meals, and to have snacks between meals.
  —Refer the patient and caregiver to a dietitian for help in modifying meals.

PSYCHOSOCIAL CARE

- Discuss the role that emotional stress plays in precipitating attacks. Assist the patient in identifying coping skills and relaxation techniques (e.g., deep breathing, meditation, guided imagery).

FOLLOW-UP CARE AND REFERRALS

- Stress the importance of regular follow-up visits. Make sure the patient has the necessary names and telephone numbers.
- Explain the importance of not smoking and of avoiding passive smoke, since smoking stimulates gastric acid secretion. Provide information and referral to smoking and alcohol cessation programs as indicated.

Ulcerative Colitis
(Crohn's Disease, Inflammatory Bowel Disease)

—Ulcerative colitis and Crohn's disease: chronic inflammatory diseases of the bowel characterized by remissions and exacerbations. Ulcerative colitis produces congestion, edema, and ulcerations of the mucosa. The disease begins in the rectum and sigmoid colon but can extend the entire length of the colon. Ulcerative colitis occurs primarily between the ages of 15 and 20 years. The specific cause is unknown but may be an abnormal immune response. Crohn's disease, also known as regional enteritis, can involve any part of the gastrointestinal tract, but the terminal ileum is most frequently involved. The disease affects all layers of the mucous membranes; segments separated by normal bowel may be inflamed. There is a 20% to 40% familial incidence.

CAUSES/CONTRIBUTING FACTORS

- Bacterial infections
- Genetic factors
- Allergic reactions to certain foods
- Immunologic origin
- Emotional stress

SIGNS/SYMPTOMS

- Cramplike right lower quadrant abdominal pain
- Diarrhea (up to 20 stools/day or more)
- Liquid stools with tenesmus: blood, mucus, pus, fat
- Anorexia, weight loss
- Fever
- Nausea, vomiting
- Malaise, weakness

COMPLICATIONS

- Electrolyte imbalance
- Dehydration
- Malnutrition
- Anemia
- Intestinal obstruction, perforation
- Fistula
- Peritonitis
- Perianal abscess, fistula, fissure
- Hemorrhage, shock

DIAGNOSTIC TESTS

- Describe each procedure, its purpose, and the normal feelings or sensations that are likely, as well as any preprocedural and postprocedural care.
  —Stool examination
  —Sigmoidoscopy
  —Colonoscopy
  —Laboratory studies
  —Biopsy

—Barium studies
—Liver function tests
—Radionuclide imaging

TREATMENT
Medical

- Therapy
  —Fluid replacement
  —Nutritional support, total parenteral nutrition (TPN) for severe malnutrition
- Drugs
  —Corticosteroids
  —Antiinflammatory agents
  —Antidiarrheals
  —Antibiotics
  —Antiemetics
  —Immunosuppressive agents
  —Sulfasalazine

Surgical

- Total abdominal colectomy
- Mucosal proctectomy with ileoanal anastomosis
- Total proctocolectomy with permanent ileostomy

▦ HOME CARE

- Give both the patient and the caregiver *verbal* and *written* instructions. Provide them with the name and telephone number of a physician or nurse to call if questions arise.
- *General information*
  —Explain the disease process, underlying causes, and factors that can exacerbate an attack: stress, certain foods, fatigue, laxatives, antibiotics.
  —For ileostomy care, see p. 741.
- *Warning signs*
  —Review the signs and symptoms of perforation that should be reported to a physician or nurse.
    Unrelieved abdominal pain
    Bloating
    Fever, chills
    Distention
    Vomiting

U

Abdominal rigidity

Increase in diarrhea

Bloody stools

- *Special instructions*
  —Discuss the need for perianal care daily and after each bowel movement.
  —Teach perianal and perineal skin care: wash gently with soap and warm water, and apply protective skin care products (e.g., ointments, gels).
  —Advise the patient on how and where to obtain supplies (e.g., drugstore, medical supply company).
  —Instruct the patient to report unrelieved irritation, worsening of diarrhea, bleeding, or drainage.
  —Instruct the patient to maintain a record of stools, including number, time of occurrence, color, amount, consistency, odor, and presence of mucus, blood, or pus.

- *Medications*
  —Explain the purpose, dosage, schedule, and route of administration of any prescribed drugs, as well as side effects to report to a physician or nurse.
  —Explain the need to avoid taking over-the-counter medications without checking with the physician.
  —Discuss the importance of not stopping steroid therapy without consulting the physician, since abrupt discontinuation may cause adrenal crisis. Review withdrawal symptoms to report to the nurse or physician: weakness, lethargy, restlessness, anorexia, nausea, muscle tenderness.
  —Discuss pain management (see p. 708). Assist the patient to identify precipitating events, such as emotional stress or certain foods.

- *Activity*
  —Advise the patient to balance activity with rest, even during remission, because adequate rest is necessary to sustain remission.

- *Diet*
  —Discuss the importance that diet plays in controlling disease, alleviating symptoms, and preventing complications.
  —Encourage the patient and caregiver to work with the dietitian to modify home meals and review dietary allowances and restrictions.

—Encourage a diet that is bland, low in residue, roughage, and fat, but high in protein, calories, carbohydrates, and vitamins (see Appendix D).

—Advise the patient to avoid highly seasoned foods; raw fruits and vegetables; foods containing coarse cereals, bran, seeds, or nuts; milk; fatty or fried foods; and caffeine, alcohol, and carbonated beverages.

—Encourage the patient to eat small frequent meals and to eat slowly, take small bites, and chew well.

—Discuss the need to replace fluids. Teach the patient how to estimate fluid intake and output. Advise the patient to drink 8 to 10 glasses of fluid per day unless contraindicated. Instruct the patient to space the servings and to avoid fluids that are too hot or cold.

—Provide individual weight parameters (for size, sex, frame, and height). Instruct the patient to weigh daily at the same time, on the same scale, and wearing the same clothing and report any sudden or steady losses.

—Instruct the patient to rest after meals.

PSYCHOSOCIAL CARE

• Encourage the patient to verbalize feelings and concerns about the illness and imposed body and lifestyle changes.

• Discuss the role emotional stress plays in precipitating an attack.

• Assist the patient in identifying coping skills and using relaxation techniques (e.g., deep breathing, meditation, guided imagery). Encourage the patient to practice these techniques between attacks.

FOLLOW-UP CARE

• Stress the importance of regular laboratory and medical follow-up visits. Make sure the patient has the necessary names and telephone numbers.

REFERRALS

• Assist the patient to obtain referrals for home health care services, dietary management, supplies, medical social services, and psychotherapy as indicated.

• Provide phone numbers of community support resources, such as the Crohn's and Colitis Foundation of America.

Urolithiasis
(Kidney Stones, Renal Calculi)

—Urolithiasis: abnormal formation of stones in the kidney or urinary tract. Renal calculi are classified according to composition: calcium, uric acid, phosphate, oxalate, struvite. They vary in size and may be solitary or multiple. They occur most commonly in men 30 to 50 years of age.

CAUSES/CONTRIBUTING FACTORS

- Familial tendency
- Gender: females affected by some types of stone (e.g., "staghorn" struvite stones) more than males
- Diet rich in calcium, oxalates, or uric acid
- Dehydration
- Geographic location: southeastern United States
- Occupation: work in industrial area; textile (cotton) worker; work in sedentary position
- Repeated urinary infections
- Conditions causing urinary stasis: immobility (paralysis), inability to empty bladder completely, inability to urinate
- Conditions causing hypercalciuria: hyperparathyroidism, kidney dysfunction, bone cancer, multiple myeloma, breast cancer with metastasis
- Renal tubular acidosis
- Long-term use (years) of indwelling catheters
- Urinary diversion or conduit

SIGNS/SYMPTOMS

- Abrupt onset of colicky pain that usually starts in the flank and moves to the groin and lower back
- Nausea and vomiting
- Extreme restlessness
- Urine abnormality
  - Cloudy
  - Absent or scant
  - Hematuria
  - Sediment (sandlike material)

COMPLICATIONS

- Urinary tract infection
- Pyelonephritis
- Urinary obstruction
- Hydronephrosis
- Renal failure

DIAGNOSTIC TESTS

- Describe each procedure, its purpose, and the normal feelings or sensations that are likely, as well as any preprocedural and postprocedural care.
  - X-ray of kidney, ureter, bladder (KUB)
  - Computed tomography (CT) scan with contrast dye: to show stone location or obstruction
  - Intravenous pyelogram/urogram
  - Retrograde pyelogram
  - Blood studies: to determine presence of elements (e.g., calcium, phosphorus, uric acid); infection
  - Urinalysis or 24-hour samples
  - Stone studies: chemical analysis of stones
  - Ultrasound studies
  - Radionuclide studies: to determine the presence of kidney damage

TREATMENT
Medical

- Medications
  - Antispasmodics, narcotics: to relieve ureteral spasm and pain
  - Antiemetics
  - For calcium stones: sodium bicarbonate, citrate, thiazides
  - For uric acid stones: allopurinol, sodium bicarbonate, citrate
  - For oxalate stones: pyridoxine, cholestyramine
  - For cystine stones: penicillamine, tiopronin
- Chemolysis: to dissolve stones by oral medications or local irrigation
- Lithotripsy: to destroy stones by means of an external energy source; may be used with basket retrieval or flushing with irrigation fluids, depending on the size and location of stones
  - Extracorporeal shock wave lithotripsy: stones in the kidney or upper part of the ureter are fragmented by means of shock waves; fragments are then expelled into urine. This is a

U

noninvasive procedure that is done as same-day surgery or with an overnight stay.

—Cystoscopic lithotripsy: a basket catheter is placed through the urinary opening beyond the stone and then rotated downward to capture and remove stone. The procedure is done on an outpatient basis with local anesthesia, light sedation, or no sedation.

—Ureteroscopic lithotripsy or basket retrieval of stones in lower ureter: an endoscopic tube is threaded up the ureter to the stone, and a smaller instrument (fiberoptic ureteroscope) is threaded through. The procedure is done on an outpatient basis with local anesthesia, light sedation, or no sedation.

—Percutaneous nephroscopic stone lithotripsy or basket retrieval with or without irrigation of stones: a small incision is made into the flank to allow insertion of the nephroscope into the kidney that is used to break up large (>1 inch) stones with an ultrasonic probe (ultrasound waves), electrohydraulic probe (electric spark gap), or laser probe (laser beam). The nephrostomy tube may remain in place temporarily and is connected to a small external drainage bag. The procedure is done on an outpatient basis or with an overnight stay with local anesthesia.

• Therapy
  —Hydration (oral or parenteral fluids; oral hydration with 15 to 20 glasses/day is used to flush out stones <4 mm)
  —Diet: changes based on stone composition
• Urethral catheters or stents: to promote urethral dilation, permitting the stones to pass

Surgical

• Ureterolithotomy: removal of stones that cannot pass through the ureter; performed with general or spinal anesthesia

HOME CARE

• Give both the patient and the caregiver *verbal* and *written* instructions. Provide them with the name and telephone number of a physician or nurse to call if questions arise.
• *General information*
  —Explain urolithiasis and the reasons for it. Discuss the composition of the stone.

- *Warning signs*
    —Review the signs and symptoms that should be reported to a physican or nurse.

    Onset of colicky pain

    Decreased urine output

    Signs and symptoms of urinary tract infection: urgency, frequency, burning, low-grade fever

    Infection: redness, warm to touch, tenderness, drainage

    Leakage around nephrostomy tube

    —Assist the patient to identify early signs of an attack (restlessness, aching, flank pain) and advise the patient to notify the physician immediately. Instruct the patient to apply warm blankets or pads to the affected area. Explain that a warm bath or shower may help to relax muscles. Instruct the patient to have someone drive him or her to the emergency room if pain is severe.

- *Special instructions*
    —Discuss measures to prevent recurrences, including drugs, diet, fluids (see p. 634), regular emptying of bladder, and avoidance of or early treatment of urinary tract infections.

    —Instruct the patient in measuring and straining urine and identifying sand particles. Stress the importance of saving particles for analysis and notifying the physician or nurse. Advise the patient on how and where to obtain supplies.

    —Teach the patient how to measure urine specific gravity (SG) if ordered. Explain that to minimize stone formation, SG should be <1.010.

    —Explain nephrostomy tube care if the tube is in place at discharge.

    The tube must be securely taped at all times.

    Change the dressing only if instructed (the dressing may be retaped).

    Monitor urine for amount, color, and smell; report decrease in or absence of urine in the bag.

    Follow clean procedure when emptying the bag: wash hands, clean connection with alcohol, disconnect cap, wash hands again after recapping.

    Use the procedure outlined when changing bags for nighttime use (see Urinary Catheter, p. 736).

    Keep the drainage bag below the level of the kidney when up or lying down.

If the nephrostomy tube is in place, tell the patient to confirm procedures for showering and bathing with the physician.

- *Medications*
  —Explain the purpose, dosage, schedule, and route of administration of any prescribed drugs, as well as side effects to report to a physician or nurse.
- *Activity*
  —Encourage the patient to discuss allowances and limitations with respect to occupation, recreation, and activities.
- *Diet*
  —Encourage the patient to increase intake of clear fluids (water, juices) to 2500 ml/day; the maintenance level should be 8 to 10 glasses/day.
  —Explain that alcoholic beverages should be avoided.
  —Advise the patient to limit fluids sweetened with sugar or additives, which may contribute to stone formation.
  —Discuss dietary changes recommended on the basis of stone composition.

  > Calcium: decrease amounts of milk, ice cream, cheese, yogurt, sardines, canned salmon, dark green leafy vegetables
  >
  > Uric acid: decrease amounts of organ meats (kidney, liver, heart), legumes, and whole grains
  >
  > Oxalate: decrease amount of vegetables (asparagus, beets, spinach, rhubarb), fruits (plums, cranberries, raspberries), juices (cranberry, grape, grapefruit), nuts (almonds, cashews), chocolate, and caffeine

FOLLOW-UP CARE

- Stress the importance of regular follow-up visits. Make sure the patient has the necessary names and telephone numbers. Remind the patient to bring the collected stone specimens to appointments.
- Emphasize the importance of seeking medical help for stones even when traveling.

Valve Repair/Replacement

—Valve repair: surgical relief of stenosis by repairing the native valve. Procedures include commissurotomy or valvuloplasty.

—Valve replacement: surgical replacement of a diseased valve, commonly the aortic or mitral valve, with either a mechanical or a tissue valve.

INDICATIONS

- Valve stenosis
- Valve regurgitation

PREPROCEDURAL TEACHING

- See the discussion of preprocedural teaching in Coronary Artery Bypass Graft Surgery (p. 205).
- Review the physician's explanation of the scheduled surgery, the type of valve to be used, and associated risks and benefits. Answer any questions. Discuss the need for obtaining informed consent.

Review of preprocedural care

- Review procedures for blood donations from the patient or family.
- Have the patient obtain clearance from the dentist 10 to 14 days before surgery.
- Explain that hospital admission may be on the day of surgery.
- Instruct the patient not to eat or drink after midnight on the evening before surgery.
- Review laboratory studies, electrocardiography, and chest x-ray; check the patient's blood type and ensure crossmatch.
- Explain that the patient's skin will be cleansed and hair will be clipped.
- Teach the use of the incentive spirometer, and stress the importance of coughing and deep breathing.

Review of Postprocedural Care

- Discuss postoperative care, including routines in the intensive care unit, intravenous lines, catheters, chest tubes, ventilator, fluid therapy and restrictions, and pain management.
- Stress the importance of turning, coughing, deep breathing, and early ambulation.
- Discuss the purpose of the incentive spirometer and review its use.
- Address anticipated body image changes, such as the mediastinal incision scar, activity limitations, and valve care.

SIDE EFFECTS/COMPLICATIONS

- Perivalvular leaks
- Conduction defects or dysrhythmias
- Low cardiac output syndrome
- Endocarditis
- Hemolysis
- Malfunction or disintegration of the prosthesis
- Thromboembolism

HOME CARE

- Give both the patient and the caregiver *verbal* and *written* instructions. Provide them with the name and telephone number of a physician or nurse to call if questions arise.
- *General information*
  —Discuss the underlying valvular disease, causes or contributing factors, and follow-up care for the valve replacement.
- *Wound/incision care*
  —Demonstrate proper care of the incision site.
- *Warning signs*
  —Review the signs and symptoms that should be reported to a physician or nurse.
    Fever, chills, diaphoresis
    Redness, warmth, pain, swelling, purulent drainage from the incision site
    Shortness of breath, fatigue, palpitations, hemoptysis, orthopnea, exercise intolerance, syncope, dizziness, sudden weight gain
    For anticoagulation therapy: excessive bruising, bleeding from the nose, hemoptysis, hematuria, melena

- *Special instructions*
  —Valve replacement: discuss the type of valve inserted. For patients with a prosthetic valve, explain and stress the importance of lifelong anticoagulant therapy to prevent systemic emboli and obstruction of the valve.
  —Explain the risk of developing endocarditis, and discuss preventive measures (see Endocarditis, p. 262).
  —Discuss alternative methods for dealing with pain: visualization, guided imagery, meditation, relaxation, biofeedback.
- *Medications*
  —Explain the purpose, dosage, schedule, and route of administration of any prescribed drugs, as well as side effects to report to a physician or nurse.
  —Instruct the patient on anticoagulation therapy (see Anticoagulation Therapy, p. 648).
  —Stress the importance of not taking over-the-counter medications without consulting a physician.
- *Activity*
  —Encourage the patient to discuss allowances and limitations with respect to occupation, recreation, and activities.
  —Review activity limitations.
    Avoid heavy lifting (>10 pounds), pushing, pulling, the Valsalva maneuver, and isometric exercises for 6 weeks.
    Avoid driving for the first 4 to 6 weeks.
    Avoid sitting or driving for prolonged periods.
    Avoid abrupt position changes from sitting and standing.
    Increase activity gradually, as tolerated. Plan frequent rest periods to avoid fatigue.
    Avoid sexual activity for the first 6 to 8 weeks, then resume as tolerated. Use positions that are comfortable and do not strain the incision.
  —Assist the patient to identify changes or adaptations that will be needed in the home, such as dealing with stairs or housekeeping activities.
  —Discuss the importance of maintaining good oral hygiene, with daily care and regular trips to the dentist. Inform the patient of the need to wait 6 weeks after surgery before seeing a dentist.
  —Instruct patients receiving anticoagulants to use soft-bristled toothbrushes and electric razors.

—Stress the importance of prophylactic antibiotics before procedures that predispose patients to bacteremia.

—Provide information on contraception and pregnancy to female patients; stress the importance of planning all pregnancies and checking with the physician or nurse before conception.

* *Diet*

  —Assist the patient to plan a low-sodium, low-fat, low-cholesterol diet.

  —Advise the patient on the effects of vitamin K–rich foods if he or she is taking anticoagulants.

PSYCHOSOCIAL CARE

* Encourage the patient to express fears and concerns about the surgery, outcomes, limitations, and body image changes. Refer the patient to a social worker for further counseling, if indicated.

FOLLOW-UP CARE

* Stress the importance of follow-up visits for laboratory tests and medical care. Make sure the patient has the necessary names and telephone numbers.
* If the patient is taking anticoagulants, emphasize the need for adhering to the schedule for dosage and prothrombin time tests.
* Assist the patient with a prosthetic valve or taking anticoagulants to obtain a MedicAlert bracelet and identification card.
* Instruct the patient to inform any dentists and other physicians of the valve replacement before treatment, especially childbirth or dental, genitourinary, gynecologic, or skin procedures.

REFERRALS

* Stress the importance of not smoking. Provide referral to community resources for smoking cessation programs.
* Assist the patient to obtain home health care, a skilled nursing facility, or a medical social worker as indicated.
* Provide referrals for community-based cardiac exercise programs.

Venous Thrombosis

—Venous thrombosis: the development of a thrombus or thrombi in a vein as a result of venous stasis, intimal damage, or hypercoagulability or in association with inflammation. Other terms used to describe venous thrombosis include phlebitis (inflammation of a vein), phlebothrombosis (intraluminal thrombus with minimal or no inflammatory component), thromboembolism (dislodgment and migration of a thrombus), and thrombophlebitis (acute thrombus and inflammation in a deep or superficial vein).

CAUSES/CONTRIBUTING FACTORS/RISK FACTORS

- Venous trauma from intravenous solutions or direct injury
- Inflammation
- Coagulopathies associated with polycythemia, anemia, steroid use, and malignancies
- Inherited hypercoagulable states such as protein C, protein S, and antithrombin III deficiencies
- Stasis of blood associated with heart failure, shock, immobility from prolonged bed rest, structural disorders of the veins, or side effects of anesthesia
- Hemoconcentration
- Recent surgery (e.g., orthopedic)
- Use of estrogen-based oral contraceptives
- Obesity
- Varicose veins
- Childbirth
- Prolonged bed rest and immobility

SIGNS/SYMPTOMS

- Leg edema
- Pain and tenderness in calf or thigh
- Erythema
- Local warmth
- Prominent superficial veins
- Increased size compared with unaffected extremity
- Heavy feeling in the affected extremity
- Cramping

V

COMPLICATIONS
- Pulmonary embolism
- Chronic venous insufficiency
- Venous ulcers
- Cerebrovascular accident

DIAGNOSTIC TESTS
- Describe each procedure, its purpose, and the normal feelings or sensations that are likely, as well as any preprocedural and postprocedural care.
  —Doppler ultrasonography: to identify area of reduced blood flow
  —Duplex imaging: to assess veins for flow and pressure
  —Plethysmography: to assess blood flow distal to the obstruction
  —I-fibrinogen scan: to detect early formation of clots and identify areas of obstruction
  —Phlebography (venography): to visualize filling or absence of filling in veins
  —Coagulation studies

TREATMENT
Medical
- Therapy
  —Bed rest during acute phase
  —Warm, moist heat
  —Antiembolic stockings
- Drugs
  —Anticoagulants
  —Fibrinolytic agents
  —Antiplatelet agents
  —Analgesics

Surgical
- Thrombectomy: surgical excision of a thrombus

 HOME CARE
- Give both the patient and the caregiver *verbal* and *written* instructions. Provide them with the name and telephone number of a physician or nurse to call if questions arise.

- *General information*
  —Explain the development of venous thrombosis, causes and contributing factors, care and treatment, and preventive measures.
- *Warning signs*
  —Review the signs and symptoms that should be reported to a physician or nurse.

    Venous ulceration, skin breakdown, redness

    Pain, tenderness, redness, warmth to extremities

    Pulmonary embolism: chest pain, hemoptysis, dyspnea, tachypnea

    Increased size of affected extremity
- *Special instructions*
  —Teach the patient to measure and record the size of the affected extremity daily.
  —Teach the patient proper skin care.

    Use mild soap and rinse well.

    Dry gently and thoroughly.

    Avoid vigorous rubbing and massaging of the affected extremity.
  —Demonstrate the use of antiembolic stockings for ambulation and periods of prolonged sitting, if prescribed. Assist the patient to obtain stockings in the proper size. Instruct the patient to remove them every 8 hours to assess the leg and skin.
  —Instruct the patient on use of the bed cradle.
  —Demonstrate the application of warm packs to the affected extremity.
- *Medications*
  —Explain the purpose, dosage, schedule, and route of administration of any prescribed drugs, as well as side effects to report to the physician or nurse (see Anticoagulation Therapy, p. 648).
- *Activity*
  —Teach the patient methods to prevent thrombus formation.

    Avoid restrictive clothing, such as garters, girdles, and clothing with elastic groin bands.

    Avoid prolonged periods of standing. Alternate position by standing on the toes and then the heels.

    Elevate the legs above the level of the heart when sitting.

Avoid dangling the legs.

Avoid positions that restrict venous blood flow; do not use a knee gatch or cross legs.

Avoid nicotine and smoking.

Avoid trauma to the extremities.

For female patients: avoid the use of estrogen-based oral contraceptives.

—Encourage the patient to initiate a walking program. Provide referral to monitored exercise programs.

FOLLOW-UP CARE

- Stress the importance of regular follow-up visits. Make sure the patient has the necessary names and telephone numbers.
- Encourage the patient to obtain a MedicAlert bracelet and identification card listing medications, such as anticoagulants.

REFERRALS

- Stress the importance of smoking cessation and weight loss. Provide referral to appropriate community resources.
- Obtain referrals for home health care services as necessary.

Home Care Procedures

Aerosol Therapy

—**Aerosol therapy:** delivery of medication as nebulized particles suspended in a gas or air into the air passages.

—*Metered dose inhaler (MDI):* handheld pocket-sized pressurized canister that delivers an aerosol-containing medication.

—*Small-volume nebulizer (SVN):* nebulizer that is powered by an external gas source such as compressed air or oxygen.

INDICATIONS
- Asthma
- Bronchitis
- Chronic obstructive pulmonary disease (COPD)

ADVERSE EFFECTS
- Dyspnea, wheezing
- Agitation, anxiety
- Insomnia
- Headache
- Nausea
- Foul taste in mouth
- Tremors
- Tachycardia, palpitations

HOME CARE
- Give both the patient and the caregiver *verbal* and *written* instruction. Provide them with the name and telephone number of a physician or nurse to call if questions arise.
- Review the purpose and type of aerosol therapy to be used; stress the importance of using only the prescribed number of inhalations.
- Discuss medications to be delivered and any side effects of the aerosol medications to expect and report.
- Using placebo equipment, permit time for practice and demonstration.
- Assist the patient to obtain the necessary equipment and supplies.

HOW TO USE A METERED DOSE INHALER

1. Remove the mouthpiece and cap from the inhaler. Insert the metal stem of the inhaler into the small hole on the side of the mouthpiece, and then shake the device 5 to 10 times.
2. Purse your lips and exhale fully. Hold the inhaler upside down, and close your lips and teeth around the mouthpiece. Tilt your head back slightly; take a slow, deep breath. As you do, firmly press the inhaler against the mouthpiece only once to release one dose of medication. Breathe in until your lungs feel full of air.
3. Remove the mouthpiece from your mouth, and hold your breath for a count of 3 to 5. Purse your lips and exhale slowly. Note: your heart may beat faster or you may feel slightly dizzy for a few minutes the first few times you use the inhaler, but this should pass. If it persists, notify your physician or a nurse.
4. If 2 puffs are recommended, wait 1 to 3 minutes between puffs. Do not exceed the number of puffs without checking with the physician or nurse.
5. Clean your inhaler once a day. Take it apart and rinse the mouthpiece and cap under warm, running water for 1 minute. Allow the parts to dry completely, and then reassemble them.

Metered Dose Inhaler

- *General information*
  —Provide instructions on inhaler:
    Each inhaler contains approximately 200 puffs.
    To determine the amount of medication left in an MDI, place the canister in a pan of water: an empty canister floats; a full canister sinks to the bottom. (See Figure on p. 648.)
    Provide instruction on use of an MDI (see box above).

A

PRODUCING AN EFFECTIVE COUGH

General guidelines

1. Sit upright and erect to provide maximum ventilation.
2. Take an analgesic before exercise as ordered; pain limits chest expansion.
3. Splint an affected area such as the abdomen or chest to reduce pain; the patient may splint the area with gentle hand pressure or by "hugging" a pillow. Flexing the knees also can support abdominal muscles.
4. Use ice chips or sips of water to make coughing easier.

Procedure

Take a deep breath (maximum inhalation) to increase force of the cough.

Hold breath for 2 seconds to distribute inhaled air to small airways.

Cough twice or until you feel there is no air left in lungs; this moves the secretions forward.

Pause long enough to gain control.

Repeat the procedure as ordered.

Small-Volume Nebulizer

- *General information*
  —Instruct the patient to inhale slowly through the mouth during treatment.
  —Encourage the patient to cough and breathe deeply to produce and expel mucus and secretions during and after the treatment (see box above).
  —Explain that nebulizer treatment is often followed by chest percussion or postural drainage to loosen secretions, which is done by the home health care nurse.

Method to determine the amount of medication left in a metered dose inhaler. (From Beare PG, Myers IL: *Principles and practice of adult health nursing,* ed 2, St Louis, 1994, Mosby.)

Anticoagulation Therapy

—Anticoagulation therapy: use of anticoagulant medications in the prevention or treatment of arterial or venous thrombosis (blood clots) for a number of medical diseases and disorders. The types of anticoagulants are warfarin, administered orally; heparin and enoxaparin, administered by subcutaneous injection. Also included is antiplatelet therapy such as aspirin, ticlopidine, and clopidogrel. The time a patient remains on anticoagulation therapy depends on the underlying condition for which it is prescribed; it can be lifelong or of short duration.

INDICATIONS

- Pulmonary embolism
- Cerebral embolism
- Valvular heart disease
- Following placement of heart valve prosthesis

- Presence of mural thrombus
- Following myocardial infarction (heart attack)
- Use of vascular stents
- Inherited hypercoagulable states
- Prophylaxis after major orthopedic surgery

SIDE EFFECTS/COMPLICATIONS

- Bleeding
  —Nosebleeds
  —Bleeding gums
  —Hemoptysis (spitting up blood)
  —Hematemesis
  —Increased menstrual flow
  —Hemoccult positive
  —Hematoma, bruises, bleeding under the skin
- Pain in the abdomen, flank, or joints
- Symptoms of stroke or transient ischemic attacks, associated with noncompliance with medication

🏠 HOME CARE

- Give both the patient and the caregiver *verbal* and *written* instructions. Provide them with the name and telephone number of a physician or nurse to call if questions arise. Use visual aids to assist in instruction.
- Initiate the teaching plan as soon as it is known that the patient will be discharged while receiving anticoagulant therapy.
- *General information*
  —Review the explanation of the condition that requires anticoagulation; the type of anticoagulant (warfarin or heparin) that is prescribed; the benefits, dosage, time of administration, and side effects; the importance of taking the medication at the same time each day and never skipping a dose; and what to do if a dose is missed.
- *Warning signs*
  —Review signs and symptoms of bleeding the patient should report to a physician or nurse.
    Spontaneous bleeding of nose or gums
    Bleeding hemorrhoids
    Bloody stools
    Reddish or purplish spots on skin
    Vomiting, diarrhea, and fever that last longer than 24 hours

- *Special instructions*
  —Instruct the patient to monitor all bruises by drawing a line around the margin of the bruise and notifying the physician or nurse if it begins to extend beyond the margins. For cuts, instruct the patient to apply firm pressure to the cut for 10 minutes; if the arm or leg is cut, elevate it above the level of the heart. If bleeding does not stop, seek immediate help.
  —Discuss safety precautions to prevent injury that might lead to bleeding.
    Avoid vigorous nose blowing and toothbrushing. Avoid use of water-jet tooth cleaners. Use a soft-bristled toothbrush or electric toothbrush. Do not put a toothpick or sharp object in mouth.
    Wear shoes and slippers at all times to prevent injury to the feet; see a podiatrist to trim calluses and corns.
    Wear gloves while gardening.
    Use an electric shaver instead of a safety blade or use hair removal cream.
    Avoid working or playing with sharp instruments or power tools.
  —For women:
    Monitor menstrual flow if excessive (more than normal pattern) and notify physician or nurse of abnormally heavy flow.
    Advise the patient *to avoid pregnancy* while taking warfarin, since it can cause serious birth defects. Stress the importance of consulting a physician or nurse if pregnancy is desired or suspected.
    Consult with a physician or nurse as to appropriate type of contraception; avoid use of an intrauterine device.
  —Instruct the patient or caregiver in the procedure for administration of a subcutaneous injection.
    Give the patient or caregiver sufficient time to practice the procedure.
    Discuss the importance of rotating the injection site with every dose to prevent bleeding, infection, and soreness. If the site becomes sore, apply warm (not hot) dry heat.
    Instruct the patient or caregiver to wash hands and use aseptic technique when handling the syringe and needle.
    Demonstrate withdrawal of the correct amount of heparin.

Demonstrate and explain each step of the procedure.

○ Select the injection site. Check for redness, bruising, pain, or drainage. If noted, avoid the site and report to the health care provider.

○ Use subcutaneous fatty tissue; avoid bruised areas, hematomas, incisions, or scarred tissue; and avoid area within 2 inches of the umbilicus.

○ Cleanse skin with alcohol.

○ Hold the syringe filled with the correct heparin dose like a pencil or dart.

○ Pinch up skin, forming a fat roll between the fingers.

○ Insert the needle at a 45-degree angle and quickly push into subcutaneous tissue up to the hub or syringe; do not pull back on the plunger. Inject the medication, slowly withdraw the needle, and press the skin gently; avoid rubbing or massaging the area.

○ Enter date, time, site, and dosage of each injection on the home record.

Leave the equipment at bedside for practice. Arrange to have equipment that will be used at home available. Advise the patient where to purchase equipment.

—Instruct the patient or caregiver in the oral administration of warfarin.

Explain to the patient that the medication comes in different dosages and that each dose is a different color.

Review the prescribed dose and the schedule for administration.

Avoid consistently large intakes of foods high in vitamin K, such as leafy green vegetables, tomatoes, bananas, and fish, which can decrease the effect of warfarin.

Advise the patient to limit alcohol intake because alcohol can increase the effect of drugs.

• *Medications*

—Explain the purpose, dosage, schedule, and route of administration of the prescribed medications, as well as side effects to report to a physician or nurse.

—Discuss the importance of not taking over-the-counter medications that contain aspirin or salicylate. Instruct the patient to read labels of all medications and to check with a physician, nurse, or pharmacist for appropriate medications (e.g., cold remedies, vitamins, analgesics).

—Instruct the patient to refill medication prescriptions 1 to 2 weeks before supply runs out; store medication in a cool place, avoiding extremes of hot and cold.

—Advise the patient to obtain extra medication before traveling and to arrange for laboratory tests at the place of the visit.

—Instruct the patient to notify all health care providers of medication before any procedures or surgeries.

- *Activity*

—Tell the patient to refrain from dangerous hobbies or contact sports that can cause bodily trauma or injury. Encourage questions regarding activity allowances and limitations on occupational and leisure activities.

FOLLOW-UP CARE

- Stress the importance of regular follow-up visits. Make sure the patient has the necessary names and telephone numbers.
- Stress the importance of having laboratory work done as ordered. Explain that frequent periodic blood tests will be required to monitor and adjust drug dosages. Once the desired level is reached, blood testing will decrease, although routine laboratory work will be needed for as long as anticoagulant therapy is prescribed.

—Therapeutic serum levels

Warfarin: prothrombin time 1.5 to 2 × control

International Ratio (INR): 1:3

○ For prosthetic valves: 2.5 to 3.5

○ For deep vein thrombosis/pulmonary embolism: 2.0 to 3.0

Heparin: partial thromboplastin time 2 to 3 × control

- Help the patient obtain a MedicAlert bracelet and identification card listing the diagnosis and medications.

Cancer: General Care

—Cancer: general care: the patient may experience loss of appetite, nausea and vomiting, or stomatitis as a result of cancer or its treatment. Both the patient and caregiver should know what problems may develop and how to manage them.

LOSS OF APPETITE

Loss of appetite can be a serious problem, leading to malnutrition and severe weight loss. Eating enough of the right kinds of food can be difficult when the patient has little or no appetite.

- Take a walk before mealtime; mild exercise can stimulate appetite.
- Avoid drinking liquids before meals, since fluids are filling. If a drink is desired, drink something nutritious such as juice or milk.
- Eat with family or friends if possible. Eating will seem less of a chore if it is a social event.
- Eat a variety of foods. Make food more appealing with herbs, spices, and sauces. Use butter, bacon bits, croutons, wine sauces, and marinades.
- Do not fill up on salads or "diet" foods. Eat vegetables and fruits with meat, poultry, and fish to ensure enough calories and proper nutrition.
- Eat smaller meals and eat more often.
- The physican may recommend dietary supplements that can be added to milk, soup, or pudding.

NAUSEA AND VOMITING

Nausea and vomiting are common side effects of cancer chemotherapy and radiation therapy. Physicians often prescribe an antiemetic before treatment and every 3 or 4 hours after treatment for 1 or 2 days.

- Eat soda crackers and suck on sour candy balls during the day to relieve queasiness.
- Choose cold or room-temperature foods instead of hot ones, since hot and warm foods seem to cause nausea.
- Avoid salt, fatty and sweet foods, or any food with a strong odor. Choose bland, creamy foods such as cottage cheese and mashed potatoes or other bland foods such as toast.
- Stay away from nauseating odors, sights, and sounds. Get as much fresh air as possible; a leisurely walk can help relieve nausea.
- Eat lightly before treatment and for a few hours after treatment.
- Try relaxation therapy, self-hypnosis, or imagery to relieve nausea-inducing tension.
- Encourage distraction with a book, television, or activity.
- Sleep during episodes of nausea, if possible.

- If vomiting occurs, eat or drink nothing until the stomach is settled, usually a few hours after the last vomiting episode. Then begin sipping clear liquids or sucking on ice cubes. If liquids are tolerated, begin eating bland foods a few hours after starting liquids.
- Take an antiemetic as prescribed.

STOMATITIS

Inflammation of the lining of the mouth may occur 7 to 14 days after the beginning of cancer chemotherapy or radiation therapy to the mouth or may begin earlier if other problems are present. A dentist should assess the status of the mouth and teeth before treatment begins.

- Stomatitis can be prevented or alleviated by using a soft-bristled toothbrush and rinsing with a solution of 1 pint of water with ½ teaspoon of salt and ½ teaspoon of baking soda after meals and at bedtime. Flossing with unwaxed dental floss, drinking water or nonacidic juice, eating artificially sweetened candy, chewing artificially sweetened gum, and using artificial saliva sprays for dry mouth may also help.
- Apply petroleum jelly or cocoa butter to the lips and an artificial saliva preparation to the oral cavity.
- Watch for signs and symptoms of stomatitis: burning feeling in the mouth; red, irritated oral lining; swollen, inflamed tongue; sores in mouth.
- Treatment is based on the extent and seriousness of the stomatitis. Measures include rinsing with the solution described above; loosening thick mucus and crusted drainage with milk of magnesia, Maalox, or another antacid; or using an analgesic rinse before meals to lessen the pain of swallowing.
- Drink cool beverages and eat Popsicles to soothe the oral cavity.
- Wear dentures only during meals.
- Avoid spicy, acidic, and crusty or rough foods and hot or cold foods and beverages.
- Report signs of infection to the physician or nurse: soft, white patches; dry, brownish yellow ulcers with well-defined edges; or open areas on the lips or mouth.
- Maintain good oral hygiene.

Differences between benign and malignant tumors

Characteristic	Benign tumor	Malignant tumor
Structure and differentiation	Typical of tissue origin	Atypical of tissue origin
Rate of growth	Usually slow	May be slow, rapid, or very rapid
Progression	Slowly progressive (may remain stationary; may regress); rarely fatal if treated	Usually progressive; almost always fatal if untreated
Mode of growth	Expansion (encapsulated)	Infiltration and/or metastasis
Tissue destruction	No	Common (ulceration and necrosis)
Recurrence	Rare	Common
Prognosis	May be fatal if inaccessible	Fatal if uncontrolled

From Belcher AE: *Cancer nursing*, St Louis, 1992, Mosby.

TERMINOLOGY

- Benign versus malignant: see table above
- Doubling time: mean length of time for division of all tumor cells present; it has been calculated that approximately 30 doubling times are required for a tumor to reach 1 centimeter in diameter
- Direct invasion of contiguous organs or local spread: tumor cells can invade a structure such as the uterus; spread from one organ to another, such as from the colon to the liver; or implant in surrounding serous cavities such cancer of the ovary that spreads to the peritoneal surface (also called seeding)
- Metastasis: spread of cancer from a primary site of origin to distant organs by lymphatics or blood vessels, for example, the spread of lung cancer to the brain; common sites of metastasis are the lungs, liver, bones, and brain
- Types of cancer:
  Carcinomas: cancers of epithelial cells
  Sarcomas: cancers of bone, muscle, or connective tissue
  Leukemias: cancers of blood-forming organs
  Lymphomas: cancers of infection-fighting organs

Cast Care

—Cast care: maintenance of a cast, a plaster- or synthetic-coated bandage that comes in strips or rolls. Casts are applied to immobilize musculoskeletal tissues after trauma or surgery. They are made of plaster, synthetic materials such as fiberglass or plastic, or cast tape. Fiberglass, plastic, and cast tape have some advantages over plaster because they may get wet without being seriously damaged, are lightweight, and last longer. In addition, x-rays can be taken with the cast on to evaluate the healing process, whereas the x-rays do not penetrate plaster well. The cast bandage, which comes in strips or rolls, is dipped in water and applied to the injured body part. It molds to the shape and then hardens as it dries. Types of casts include extremity casts (short arm, long arm, short leg, long leg), body casts (chest and abdomen), hip spica or spica casts (cover hips and one or both legs), cervical casts, and Minerva casts (cover chest, neck, and hand).

PREPROCEDURAL TEACHING

- Review the physician's explanation of the procedure and the reason for it; encourage the patient to ask questions and to discuss any fears or anxieties.

Review of Preprocedural Care

- Explain the need for x-rays to ascertain the extent of trauma and assess bone alignment (before and after reduction).
- Describe how casts are applied.
  - —A sedative, narcotic, or anesthetic may be given before application. The skin surface is checked for open lesions and blisters, then the skin is cleansed and rubbing alcohol is applied to dry the skin surface to be casted.
  - —Soft padding is applied to the skin to protect it and underlying bones from direct contact with or pressure from the cast.
  - —The cast is applied to fit snugly so that the injured bones are held immobilized and in the correct position. Explain that the cast will be looser after swelling of the injury subsides.

SIDE EFFECTS/COMPLICATIONS

- Neurovascular impairment
- Fever
- Infection
- Skin impairment
- Compartment syndrome
- Cast syndrome

HOME CARE

- Give both the patient and the caregiver *verbal* and *written* instructions. Provide them with the name and telephone number of a physician or nurse to call if questions arise.
- *Cast care*
  —Instruct the patient on the importance of protecting the cast until it dries: 2 to 3 days for plaster; usually less than a day for synthetic material.
  > While the cast is still damp, elevate it on firm pillows without plastic covers to prevent it from becoming deformed.
  >
  > Explain that the skin underneath the cast will feel warm until it dries. However, warm areas after the cast has dried may indicate infection, which should be reported to the physician.
  >
  > While the cast is drying, it should be handled as little as possible. When necessary the cast is lifted by supporting it under two joints using the palms of the hands. Avoid pressing fingers into the cast, which would put pressure on the skin inside.
  >
  > The cast should be left uncovered to facilitate drying. Fans placed 18 to 24 inches from the cast may be used to speed drying except after open reduction. Heat lamps should not be used because they could burn the skin under the cast.
  —Review daily care once the cast is completely dried.
  > Plaster casts must be kept dry; use plastic bags when bathing, using the toilet (for spica cast), or going out in rain or snow.
  >
  > A damp cloth and scouring powder can be used to clean soiled spots.
  >
  > For a synthetic cast such as fiberglass, immersion in water may be permitted if there are no wounds under the cast.

The cast should be rinsed inside and out to flush out dirt and chemicals. The cast and stockinette should be dried thoroughly to avoid excess moisture on skin. A hair dryer set on the cool setting can be used.

—Instruct the patient on the importance of maintaining good skin care under and around the cast.

Do not insert objects such as coat hangers under the cast, since this could scrape the skin and cause infection.

Powders and lotions should be used only outside the cast so that the skin stays clean and soft.

Explain the importance of keeping dirt, sand, and powder away from the inside of the cast, since they can cause sore areas.

Instruct the patient to massage the skin distal to the cast.

Instruct the patient to notify the physician if skin irritation develops: redness, swelling, breaks in skin.

—Explain how to reduce swelling.

Elevate the injured part above the heart by propping it up on pillows or some other support (tell the patient to recline if the cast is on the leg).

Apply ice to the cast over the fractured area; ice should be put into a dry plastic bag or ice pack and should go halfway around the cast.

Advise the patient that swelling or edema around the site of injury is common at first and creates pressure against the inside of the cast. Advise the patient that for the first 48 hours or so after the cast is applied, it will feel tight.

As swelling subsides and the cast becomes loose, it may be necessary for the physician to replace the cast to ensure that broken bones do not move out of place.

- *Warning signs*

—Review the signs and symptoms that should be reported to a physician or nurse.

If soft spots or cracks develop in the cast or if it feels too loose

Pain or soreness under the cast, especially around bony prominences, such as the wrist or ankle, that is not relieved by repositioning of the body

Red, blue, or white color of the skin; when a finger or toe protruding from the cast is squeezed until it is white, the pink color should return within 4 to 6 seconds

Fingers or toes that are cool and do not warm up after 20 minutes of being covered

Increased swelling

Tingling or burning sensation

Inability to move the muscles around the cast

Foul odor around the cast edges

Any breaks in the cast

For spica or body casts: shortness of breath, nausea, vomiting, abdominal distention (cast syndrome) caused by air swallowing

- *Activity*
  —Advise the patient not to walk on a leg cast for the first 48 hours unless otherwise instructed by the physician. Once allowed to walk on the cast, the patient should be sure to use a walking heel if weight bearing is permitted.
  —Describe and demonstrate the proper use of ambulatory aids, such as crutches, a cane, or a walker.
  —Instruct the patient on transferring techniques to move from bed to a chair, to get into a car, and to use the toilet as indicated.
  —Discuss the need for active range-of-motion exercises to unaffected extremities and show the patient how to perform them.
- *Diet*
  —Encourage at least 3000 ml of fluids per day to maintain skin turgor.

REFERRALS

- Provide referrals for home health care services as indicated.
- Refer the patient to a physical therapist as needed.

Catheter Care: External Venous, Central Venous, Hickman, and Broviac

—**Catheter: convenient way to deliver medications and withdraw blood samples without having to insert a needle in the patient's vein. The catheter is a soft plastic tube. One end of the tube is placed in a large vein, the other stays outside the** body. The catheter has a cap that can be removed when blood samples are needed or drugs must be given. The venous catheter is inserted percutaneously into the superior vena cava through the subclavian or external jugular vein.

INDICATIONS

- Administration of anticancer drugs
- Frequent blood drawing
- Administration of blood products

SIDE EFFECTS/COMPLICATIONS

- Infection at the site of insertion of the catheter
- Venous thrombosis
- Catheter migration
- Occlusion of catheter

HOME CARE

- Give both the patient and the caregiver *verbal* and *written* instructions. Provide them with the name and telephone number of a physician or nurse to call if questions arise. Use visual aids and permit time for return demonstration of procedures before discharge.
- *Warning signs*
  —Review the signs and symptoms that should be reported to a physician or nurse.
    Pain, redness, and puffiness around the catheter site
    Drainage from the catheter site
    Temperature above 100° F
    Catheter slippage
    Blood in the catheter
    Inability to flush the catheter
    Difficulty breathing
    Sudden chest pain at insertion site
- *Special instructions*
  —Review the purpose of catheter insertion. If for infusion of medication:
    Discuss the type and amount of solution to be infused.
    Discuss proper storage of medication; if refrigerated bring to room temperature before administration.

Advise and assist the patient to obtain medications and supplies for infusion.

Instruct the patient not to microwave medications.

—Review dressing change and catheter care procedures per prescribed protocol (see the following two sections).

Instruct the patient to inspect the insertion site daily.

Teach proper handwashing techniques; instruct the patient to wash hands before changing dressings.

Dressing on the catheter must be changed frequently, at least every other day, until the wound site has healed.

After the site has healed, the patient may be allowed to clean around the wound site with soap and water while showering and then dry the area and apply a small gauze pad or adhesive bandage to the exit site.

Before changing the dressing, assemble the following equipment: hydrogen peroxide (some protocols may recommend Betadine), small container in which to pour the hydrogen peroxide, alcohol wipes, antibiotic ointment, dressing, tape, cotton-tipped ear swabs.

Wash hands.

Remove the old dressing and wash hands again.

Pour hydrogen peroxide into the container, and dip a cotton swab into the hydrogen peroxide. Starting at the wound site and using a circular motion, clean the skin around the wound site, working outward. Use a new cotton swab whenever more hydrogen peroxide is needed.

Clean the length of the catheter with an alcohol wipe.

Apply the antibiotic ointment to the wound site with a cotton swab.

Tape the new dressing over the wound site.

—Review the procedure for changing the catheter cap.

Cap should be changed every 7 days.

Assemble the following equipment: catheter cap, catheter clamp, alcohol wipes.

Wash hands.

Clamp the catheter.

Unscrew the old cap; wipe around the end of the catheter with alcohol wipes.

Screw on the new cap. Unclamp the catheter.

—Review the procedure for flushing the catheter.

Catheter is flushed based on policy (as often as once a day) to prevent blood clots from forming inside it.

Assemble the following equipment: vial of heparin-saline solution, disposable syringe and needle, alcohol wipes.

Wash hands.

Open the bottle of heparin-saline solution; wipe the vial opening with an alcohol wipe.

Remove the needle guard from the syringe and pull back the plunger; insert the needle into the vial, turn the vial upside down, and pull back on the syringe to fill it. Tap on the side of the syringe to remove the air bubbles.

Clean the catheter cap with an alcohol wipe, insert the needle into the cap, and push down on the plunger to inject solution into the catheter.

Remove the needle; carefully discard it and the syringe.

—Review the procedure for catheter maintenance.

Have a catheter repair kit to use when a leak occurs.

Call the physician or nurse if the catheter continues to leak even after repair.

- *Medications*
—Explain the purpose, dosage, schedule, and route of administration of any prescribed drugs, as well as side effects to report to a physician or nurse.

FOLLOW-UP CARE

- Stress the importance of regular follow-up visits. Make sure the patient has the necessary names and telephone numbers.

Catheter Care: Implanted Port

—Implanted (infusion) port: catheter and port placed under the skin to provide vascular access for patients requiring repeated infusions of drugs, solutions, and blood products and to take blood samples needed without accessing or damaging veins. The port consists of a soft plastic catheter and port with a metal base and rubber top through which medications are given and blood is drawn. There are no external parts. The port is surgically placed in the chest or abdomen. The catheter is threaded into the superior vena cava or right atrium via the subclavian or internal jugular vein.

INDICATIONS

- Administration of
  —Anticancer drugs
  —Total parenteral nutrition
  —Blood, blood products
- Repeated blood drawing

🏠 HOME CARE

- Give both the patient and the caregiver *verbal* and *written* instructions. Provide them with the name and telephone number of a physician or nurse to call if questions arise. Use visual aids and permit time for the patient and caregiver to return demonstrate the procedure before discharge.
- *Warning signs*
  —Review the signs and symptoms that should be reported to a physician or nurse.
  > Redness, pain, or puffiness around port
  > Drainage from incision site or from needle insertion
  > Temperature above 100° F
  > Shortness of breath
  > Chest pain
- *Special instructions*
  —Review the purpose of the port insertion, how long it will stay in, and how frequently it will be changed.
  —Discuss protection of the skin over the port.
  > Instruct the patient not to wear bra straps or clothing that may rub the port site and to adjust the car seat belt if it rubs the port site.
  > Unless receiving an infusion the patient may shower, bathe, and swim without worry.
  > When receiving an infusion the patient should keep the site dry and protected.
  —Review the procedure for changing the drug reservoir bag.
  > Directions for changing the bag vary with the type of pump.
  > Provide the patient with a diagram and complete instructions.
  > Advise and assist the patient to obtain the necessary medical supplies. Explain how to order the medicine and total parenteral nutrition solution. Remind the

patient to renew the prescription before medicine or supplies run out.

—Review procedures for administration of drugs or solutions.

If treatment is needed for an extended period, a bent needle (Huber needle) is inserted into the port and connected to an ambulatory infusion pump. The needle is changed every 7 days or until treatment is finished.

The pump is attached to the body by a belt or pouch and worn for the duration of treatment.

The dressing is taped over the needle and must be checked to ensure that the tape is holding the dressing and the needle has not slipped. The dressing may need to be changed periodically according to the protocol.

—Review the infusion of medications.

Discuss the type, amount, and preparation of solution to be infused.

Teach the patient how to use the infusion pump if ordered.

Discuss the proper storage of medication.

Review any side effects of medication that should be reported.

—Review the administration of total parenteral nutrition solution.

Review the preparation, schedule of infusion, and use of infusion pump as indicated.

Instruct the patient on storing total parenteral nutrition solution and the need to inspect the solution for contamination.

Instruct the patient on measuring and recording intake and output and testing urine for sugar and acetone as ordered.

Review the signs and symptoms to report: rapid weight loss or gain, glucose in urine.

Discuss the procedure for discarding cytotoxic drugs appropriately following OSHA regulations.

FOLLOW-UP CARE

• Stress the importance of regular follow-up visits. Make sure the patient has the necessary names and telephone numbers.

Catheter Care: Peripherally Inserted Central Venous Catheter

C

—Peripherally inserted central venous catheter (PICC): catheter inserted into the vein at or above the antecubital space with the tip terminating in the distal superior vena cava. This catheter is usually made of silicone. The insertion of the catheter facilitates access to the venous system to provide a route for intermittent or continuous infusion of IV therapy without damaging veins. A PICC can be inserted in the outpatient setting without anesthesia or sedation. The veins used for venipuncture and insertion of the PICC include the cephalic, basilic, median cephalic, or median basilic.

INDICATIONS
- Administration of anticancer drugs
- Administration of blood products
- Repeated blood drawings
- Continuous infusion of medications such as opioids for pain management

HOME CARE
- Give both the patient and the caregiver *verbal* and *written* instructions. Provide them with the name and telephone number of a physician or a home health care nurse to call if questions arise. Use visual aids and permit time for the patient and caregiver to return demonstrate the procedure before discharge.
- *Warning signs*
  —Review the signs and symptoms that should be reported to a physician or a nurse.
    Catheter site
    O Redness, pain on the site or above the site of insertion or at the shoulder level
    O Swelling and redness of the arm
    O Drainage at the site of insertion
    O Inability to flush the catheter or obtain blood from the catheter

General symptoms
- ○ Temperature above 100° F
- ○ Shortness of breath
- ○ Chest pain

—Review potential complications to report: catheter embolism, catheter malposition, arrhythmia, and potential postinsertion complications such as catheter-related infections, thrombo-phlebitis, and catheter occlusion.

- *Special instructions*
—Review dressing change and catheter care procedures (protocol per institution or as prescribed by the physician).
—Identify the type of catheter in place. The care and flushing procedure of the catheter vary according to the type of catheter (Abbot, Groshong, Cook, etc.). Provide specific instructions in writing.
—Review the purpose of catheter insertion.
—Explain that medications are usually administered by the home health care nurse or at a clinic visit. If patient is to self-administer medication, instruct the patient to allow the medication to warm to room temperature before administration. Advise and assist the patient to obtain medications and supplies for infusion. Instruct the patient that PICC lines are not to be used for high-pressure injections such as emergency drugs.
—Review catheter care.
  Instruct the patient to apply moist heat to the area above the site of insertion for 20 minutes three to four times per day for the first 48 hours after catheter insertion to decrease the risk of phlebitis. If the catheter has been sutured in place, provide instruction for the care of the sutures.
  Assess the catheter site daily for signs of inflammation and infection. Also observe for loose sutures that may permit the catheter to migrate out.
—Review the procedure for cap changing (see institutional protocol or care of a Hickman or Broviac catheter).
—Review the procedure for flushing the catheter according to protocol and catheter type. (A Cook catheter requires a heparin flush whereas a Groshong catheter requires a normal saline flush.)
—Review the procedure for catheter maintenance and permit time for the patient and caregiver to return demonstrate and practice.

  —Instruct the patient to have a catheter repair kit available in the home and to call the physician or nurse if the catheter begins to leak or continues to leak after repair.
- *Medications*
  —Explain the purpose, dosage, schedule, and route of administration of any prescribed drugs, as well as side effects to report to a physician or nurse.
  —Discuss the procedure for discarding cytotoxic drugs appropriately following OSHA guidelines.

FOLLOW-UP CARE

- Stress the importance of regular follow-up visits. Make sure the patient has the necessary names and phone numbers.
- *Activities*
  —Instruct the patient to bathe but cover the PICC line dressing with plastic. If the dressing gets wet, instruct the patient to change the dressing immediately.
  —Instruct the patient to avoid lifting heavy objects with the arm where the PICC was inserted.
  —Discuss activity allowances and limitations.

Chemotherapy

—Chemotherapy: systemic cancer treatment using cytotoxic drugs to destroy malignant cells; used for widespread disease or when there is high risk of recurrence in the body. Chemotherapy may be used alone as a curative measure or can be used as an adjuvant to surgery or radiation therapy. As a palliative treatment, it is used to relieve obstruction or pain.

CANCER CHEMOTHERAPEUTIC AGENTS

- Alkylating agents: chlorambucil, cyclophosphamide, ifosfamide, mechlorethamine, melphalan
- Nitrosoureas: carmustine, lomustine, streptozocin, busulfan, carboplatin, cisplatin, thiotepa
- Antimetabolites: cytarabine, floxuridine, fluorouracil, mercaptopurine, methotrexate, thioguanine

- Antibiotics: bleomycin, dactinomycin, daunorubicin, doxorubicin, mitomycin, plicamycin
- Plant alkaloids: etoposide, vincristine, vinblastine, taxanes
- Miscellaneous drugs: asparaginase, dacarbazine, levamisole, procarbazine
- Hormones and antihormonal drugs: androgens, estrogens, progestins, corticosteroids, antiestrogens
- Biologic response modifiers: interferons, interleukins, erythropoietin, colony-stimulating factors

CONTRAINDICATIONS/PRECAUTIONS

- Based on patient's pretreatment condition, stage of disease, response to therapy, and allergies or sensitivities
- Patient's functional status may be used to monitor tolerance to therapy

ROUTES OF ADMINISTRATION

- Oral
- Intravenous
- Vascular access: central venous catheter (Hickman; see p. 660), implantable port devices (see p. 662), peripherally inserted catheter (see p. 665)
- Intraarterial
- Intracavitary: intraperitoneal, intrapleural
- Intrathecal via Ommaya reservoir (reservoir placed in ventricle of the brain)
- Intramuscular and subcutaneous routes used less frequently

LABORATORY TESTS

- Specific to each type of chemotherapeutic agent used
- General: serum: complete blood count, electrolytes, cultures; liver function test: urinalysis, Hematest
- Bone marrow biopsy
- Pulmonary function studies
- Electrocardiogram

PREPROCEDURAL TEACHING

- Review the physician's explanation of the type of chemotherapy and the reason for it. Discuss when it will be scheduled, where it will be administered (hospital versus outpatient), route of administration, frequency of treatments, and length of time required to complete the treatment. Encourage the patient to ask questions and to discuss any fears or anxieties.

- Assess the patient's financial and insurance resources to assist in planning home care.

Review of Postprocedural Care

- Review the side effects associated with the type of drug to be used and explain that medications will be used to reduce the effects of chemotherapy.
- Inform the patient about possible hair loss and the need to buy a wig or wear a hat, scarf, or turban. Women should have hair cut short before treatment begins, purchase a wig, and have their natural hair styled to resemble the wig.

SIDE EFFECTS/TOXICITY

- Specific toxic side effects and problems depend on the type of medication.
  —Gastrointestinal disturbances: anorexia, nausea, vomiting, diarrhea
  —Bone marrow suppression
  —Hair loss, skin rash, stomatitis
  —Electrolyte and chemical imbalance
  —Hematologic abnormalities
  —Hepatic toxicity
  —Renal dysfunction
  —Cardiac and pulmonary dysfunction

HOME CARE

- Give both the patient and the caregiver *verbal* and *written* instructions. Provide them with the name and telephone number of a physician or nurse to call if questions arise. Use visual aids to assist in instruction.
- Discuss the chemotherapeutic agent(s) ordered, any side effects, route of administration, and necessary equipment and supplies required for treatment.
- Review specific side effects and signs of toxicity to report.
  —Instruct the patient and the caregiver on emergency actions to take (see Anaphylaxis, p. 44) if allergic reactions occur.

- *General information*
  —Explain that fatigue and other side effects begin during the first week of therapy and gradually disappear 2 to 4 weeks after therapy ends.
  —Teach the patient the importance of oral hygiene (see stomatitus discussion in Cancer: General Care, p. 654).
  —Advise the patient on skin care. Instruct the patient to inspect the skin and report any signs of abrasions or skin breaks. Use mild soap and warm water on irritated areas and pat dry.
  —Avoid sun exposure; wear soft, loose clothing over irritated areas.
- *Warning signs*
  —Review the signs and symptoms that should be reported to a physician or nurse.
      Infection: pain, swelling, redness, drainage
      Excessive nausea, vomiting, diarrhea
      Bleeding
      Excessive fatigue
      Shortness of breath
      Palpitations
      Mucositis
      Difficulty with urination
      Paresthesias
      Confusion, memory loss
      Itching, burning
- *Special instructions*
  —Discuss immunosuppression and the need to monitor the blood count. If the white blood cell count is low, the patient should avoid persons with infections or colds, large crowds, and recently vaccinated children.
  —For specific problems see Bone Marrow Suppression (p. 109) and Cancer (p. 150).
- *Medications*
  —Explain the purpose, dosage, schedule, and route of administration of any prescribed drugs, as well as side effects to report to a physician or nurse.
  —Demonstrate the use of equipment and permit time for return demonstration and practice.
  —Assist the patient to obtain the necessary equipment and supplies in time to have at home upon discharge.

- *Activity*
  —Encourage the patient to continue work and other activities of daily living as tolerated, including regular exercise.
  —Teach the patient how to manage fatigue and maintain mobility, for example, by planning important activities before treatment and after treatment based on energy level.
  —Stress the need to take measures to avoid injuries: do not use safety razors and hard toothbrushes, do not strain at defecation, do not play contact sports.
- *Diet*
  —Teach the patient the importance of a high-protein, high-carbohydrate diet and avoidance of hot and spicy foods.
  —Encourage small, frequent meals if the patient is nauseated. Advise the patient to take an antiemetic ½ hour before meals.
  —Instruct the patient to maintain a weight and food diary if nausea and vomiting persist.
  —Encourage a fluid intake of 1000 to 3000 ml/day.

FOLLOW-UP CARE

- Stress the importance of keeping all scheduled treatment, laboratory, and medical follow-up appointments. Make sure the patient has the necessary names and telephone numbers.

REFERRALS

- Assist the patient to obtain necessary referrals for home health care and social services as indicated.
- Refer the patient to a support group and other community resources as needed.

Crutch Walking

—Crutch walking: use of ambulatory aids to limit or eliminate the amount of weight on the lower extremities. Use of crutches permits the patient to be mobile while the extremity is healing from traumatic injury or surgery.

PREPROCEDURAL TEACHING

- Discuss the selection of proper crutches.
  - —Underarm crutches with double uprights and hand bars are the most commonly used. Crutches may be made of wood or aluminum.
  - —Shoulder pieces must have a rubber cover to prevent axillary pressure from hard wood or aluminum.
  - —Rubber suction tips over each crutch base prevent slipping.
- Measure the patient for crutches.
  - —Crutch length is measured from the anterior fold of the axilla to the lateral side of the heel, and 2 inches is added.
  - —The level of the hand piece is in a position that allows a slight bend at the elbow (25 to 30 degrees).

SIDE EFFECTS/COMPLICATIONS

- Reinjury caused by falls
- Axillary nerve damage

HOME CARE

- Give both the patient and the caregiver *verbal* and *written* instructions. Provide them with the name and telephone number of a physician or nurse to call if questions arise.
- *General information*
  - —Review the physician's explanation of the use of crutches.
- *Warning signs*
  - —Review the signs and symptoms that should be reported to a physician or nurse.
    - Numbness and tingling down the arms to the thumb that do not go away quickly when leaning on the crutch tops is stopped
  - —Explain that leaning too long or putting too much pressure in the axillary (armpit) area can injure nerves and cut off circulation down the arms.
- *Special instructions*
  - —Review the specific walking procedures, permitting time to practice before discharge.
    - For crutch walking with some weight bearing on both legs: move one foot and leg and the crutch in the opposite hand forward at the same time, then move the other crutch and opposite foot and leg forward.

For crutch walking with no weight bearing on one leg (i.e., one leg in cast with no weight bearing allowed): move both crutches and the affected leg forward about 8 to 10 inches. Shift weight to the wrists and hands and step forward with the unaffected leg. Always move crutches, foot, and leg forward at the same time.

—Review safety measures.

Keep the crutches even as they are advanced ahead a comfortable and stable distance, approximately 10 to 12 inches.

Pressure (weight) goes on the hands and not the armpits.

Keep elbows into sides of the body to help stabilize the crutches under the arms.

Do not walk with the crutches too close to the feet, since this may result in tripping on them. Crutches should be placed 2 to 3 inches out to the side of the feet.

Remove loose throw rugs, electrical cords, toys, and other objects on the floor at home to prevent falls.

Avoid walking on slick or wet floors to prevent falls.

Keep crutch tips clean, since dirt and dust can build up on them and make them slippery. Advise the patient of the importance of replacing worn tips.

—Discuss and demonstrate sitting and rising with crutches.

Sitting down in a chair with crutches: walk up close to the chair. Turn, then back up until the chair touches the back of the legs. Hold the handgrips of both crutches with one hand, and with the other hand reach for the arm or seat of the chair. Bearing weight on the handgrips of the crutches and the arm or seat of the chair, lower into the chair. Slide the affected leg forward.

Getting up from a chair with crutches: slide forward in the chair as far as possible. Position the unaffected foot slightly farther back than the affected foot. Both crutches should be on the affected side. Holding on to the handgrips of the crutches, use the other hand to push from the edge or armrest of the chair when leaning forward to stand.

Stress the importance of not sitting down with crutches under the arms, since this can cause damage to the axillary nerve from undue pressure.

—Discuss and demonstrate walking up and down stairs.

> Walking up stairs with one crutch in each hand: walk close to the bottom of the steps. Put all weight on the handgrips and step up to the next step with the unaffected leg and foot. Bring the body, affected leg, and crutches up to the same step, making sure the crutches are centered on the step.

> Walking down stairs with one crutch in each hand: walk to the edge of the top step. Bend the hips and place both crutches and the affected leg on the next lower step. Put weight on crutches and bring the unaffected leg down to the same step.

> Walking up stairs with railing: place both crutches under the arm opposite the banister and grasp both handgrips. Grasp the railing with the free hand. Put all weight on the hands and lift the unaffected foot and leg up to the next step. Bring crutches, body, and affected leg up to the same step.

> Walking down stairs with railing: put both crutches in one hand, holding them together at handgrips and under the arm. Put the other hand on the railing. Move the affected leg and crutches down to the next step. (Do not put any weight on the affected leg if it should not bear weight.) Put all weight on handgrips of the crutches and the railing, and step down with the unaffected leg. Avoid axillary pressure.

Dialysis
(Hemodialysis, Peritoneal Dialysis)

—Dialysis: a temporary or permanent process that artificially replaces the excretory function of the kidney. Dialysis is used to remove excessive amounts of drugs, fluids, or toxic waste products from the body and to correct serious electrolyte and fluid imbalances.

—Hemodialysis: removal of toxins from the body by shunting the patient's blood from the body through a machine for filtration and diffusion and then returning the blood to the patient's circulation. Hemodialysis requires access to the patient's bloodstream by special vascular catheters called shunts. An external shunt involves two cannulas from an artery and vein connected outside the body, usually on the arm. An internal arteriovenous fistula is a connection made between an artery and vein or an artificial graft implanted between the artery and vein. This is done on the arm or thigh. Hemodialysis may be a temporary measure, as for acute renal failure or hepatic coma, or a permanent measure, as for chronic renal failure or end-stage renal disease. The sessions last 3 to 5 hours and take place three or four times a week.

—Peritoneal dialysis: instillation of dialyzing solution directly into the abdominal cavity through a silicone catheter (Tenckhoff). The body tissue acts as a filter to remove the toxins. The fluid is left in for a specified time and then drained. Peritoneal dialysis can be performed by machine or manually by gravity. There are three types: intermittent, continuous ambulatory, and continuous cycling. Intermittent peritoneal dialysis is performed in 8- to 10-hour sessions four or five times a week. It can be done manually or by a cycling machine. The patient is restricted to the bed or chair during the procedure. In continuous ambulatory peritoneal dialysis, exchanges take place every 4 hours during the day and every 8 hours at night. The patient can be up and about, continuing daily activities. After fluid instillation, the bag remains connected and is placed under the clothing until time to drain and change it. Continuous cycling peritoneal dialysis is a combination of the other types. Three exchanges are done at night by a cycling machine and one cycle is done during the day. The patient is ambulatory during the day and confined to bed at night.

INDICATIONS

- Acute poisoning (aspirin, methanol, phenobarbital)
- Acute renal failure
- Chronic renal failure
- End-stage renal failure

- Hepatic coma
- Hyperkalemia
- Metabolic acidosis

PREPROCEDURAL TEACHING

- Review the physician's explanation of the type of procedure, the reason for it, and whether it is permanent or temporary. Encourage the patient to ask questions and to discuss any fears or anxieties.

Review of Preprocedural Care

- Discuss preprocedural tests.
  —Blood studies: to determine drug and electrolyte levels and kidney function
     Blood urea nitrogen
     Creatinine
     Protein
     Clotting levels
     Platelets
  —Urine studies
     Creatinine clearance
     Urinalysis
     Culture and sensitivity
  —Diagnostic scans
     X-ray of kidneys, ureter, bladder (KUB)
     Intravenous pyelogram
     Renal ultrasound
     Renal computed tomography
  —Renal biopsy
- Discuss the specific type of *hemodialysis*.
  —For temporary hemodialysis: written consent for insertion of the catheter into a large vein in the shoulder or groin area; procedure performed under local anesthetic
  —For permanent hemodialysis: written consent for insertion of the arteriovenous shunt; procedure done as same-day surgery under general anesthetic; patient may stay in hospital overnight or longer; nothing by mouth (NPO) status from midnight of the night before
- *Peritoneal dialysis:* written consent needed for surgery and local anesthesia; same-day surgery with overnight or longer stay; small incision made on the abdomen below the umbilicus

to insert a Silastic catheter; procedure may be performed at the bedside under certain conditions

Review of Postprocedural Care

- Stress the need to protect the operative site from compression.
- For hemodialysis, explain that the extremity will be elevated and monitored for pulses, excessive bleeding, and temperature.
- For peritoneal dialysis, see Abdominal Surgery, p. 6.

SIDE EFFECTS/COMPLICATIONS

- After insertion of shunt
  —Clot formation
  —Bleeding
  —Anemia
  —Infection of operative site: redness, warm to touch, tenderness, purulent drainage
- During or after hemodialysis
  —Hypotension
  —Hypertension
  —Dysrhythmias
  —Muscle cramps (potassium imbalance)
  —Air embolus
  —Hemorrhage from heparinization
  —Hepatitis B
  —Dialysis disequilibrium syndrome
  —Restless leg syndrome
  —Mechanical problems
- During or after peritoneal dialysis
  —Peritonitis
  —Catheter displacement
  —Catheter plugging
  —Shortness of breath
  —Hyperglycemia
  —Hypoglycemia
  —Bowel adhesions
  —Leakage and extravasation of dialysate
  —Mechanical cycling problems

HOME CARE

- Give both the patient and the caregiver *verbal* and *written* instructions. Provide them with the name and telephone number

of a physician or nurse and the dialysis center to call if
questions arise. Use visual aids to assist in instruction.
- *General information*
  —Explain the disease, the underlying cause for dialysis, and the
  type of dialysis treatment to the patient and family.

Hemodialysis

- *Warning signs*
  —Review the signs and symptoms that should be reported to a
  physician or nurse or the dialysis center.
    Swelling and pain over the access site
    Numbness or tingling in the extremity
    Coolness in the extremity distal to the access site
    Loss of thrill or bruit
    Blood that is cool to touch in the external shunt
    Disconnection of the external shunt
    Infection at the site: redness, tenderness, swelling, warm to
    touch, possible drainage
- *Special instructions*
  —Discuss shunt care: clean with hydrogen peroxide solution
  (or other solution as prescribed) daily until completely healed
  and sutures are removed (10 to 14 days); keep site clean and
  dry; wash site with mild soap and water between dialysis
  treatments; keep sterile dressing over site.
  —Tell the patient to avoid infection by not showering, bathing,
  or swimming for several hours after dialysis.
  —Instruct the patient to watch the access area for bleeding or
  bruising under the skin after dialysis starts; demonstrate how
  to monitor vascular access, including palpating thrill
  (vibration) and auscultating for bruit daily or as ordered.
  —Review precautions to take with the shunt: avoid lying,
  tugging, or pulling on the affected extremity; avoid wearing
  tight clothing or jewelry over the access site; do not lift heavy
  objects or strain with the affected extremity; never permit
  blood drawing, blood pressure monitoring, or injection on the
  affected extremity.
  —For an external shunt:
    Explain the need to have a bandage wrapped loosely
    around the area to prevent accidental removal or
    disconnection.

Emphasize the importance of having clamps attached to the bandage at all times. Discuss what to do if the shunt connection comes loose or is disconnected.

—For an internal shunt:

Show the patient how to check pulsations.

Peritoneal Dialysis

- *Warning signs*

  —Review the signs and symptoms that should be reported to a physician or nurse.

  Infection of cannula insertion site: redness, swelling, warmth to touch, tenderness, possible drainage

  Increase in abdominal girth, abdominal distention or pain, absence of bowel movements or inability to pass gas

- *Special instructions*

  —Discuss the need for and teach the peritoneal dialysis procedure. Permit time for practice. Refer the patient to a dialysis nurse for specific instructions. Stress that the procedure is done with sterile technique.

  —Review skin and peritoneal catheter care.

  Change dressing daily or whenever wet or soiled.

  Inspect site carefully.

  Cleanse area with hydrogen peroxide or prescribed solution, using sterile applicators; pat area dry.

  Apply a sterile dressing over the site, taping all sides securely.

  Protect the catheter from damage. Keep the sterile cap in place.

  Stress the importance of maintaining sterile technique when opening and closing catheter connections.

  —Discuss the procedure for peritoneal dialysis infusion.

  Review the signs and symptoms that should be reported to a physician or nurse.

  ○ Shortness of breath or trouble breathing

  ○ Slow outflow even after repositioning or no outflow

  ○ Abdominal pain

  ○ Leakage around catheter

  ○ Outflow solution foul smelling, cloudy, fecal colored, or bloody (new site will have blood-tinged outflow for the first or second day after catheter insertion)

  ○ Presence of fibrin (clear or white strands) in outflow

Review self-administration technique. Refer the patient to the dialysis nurse for a specific demonstration.

Discuss the need for the following:

○ Urinate before the procedure.

○ Wash hands.

○ Check the solution for intact bag and clarity.

○ Warm the solution slightly if desired (with warming pad at lowest setting, never in microwave).

○ Put on a surgical mask and use sterile gloves.

○ Prepare all materials necessary for exchange.

○ Clean the connections per protocol and connect the solution bags.

Discuss the amount of dialysis solution to be infused and the number of exchanges required (infusion + dwell + drain = 1 exchange).

Review common symptoms with infusion: fullness of abdomen or rectum; cramping; shoulder aching; aching in penis, scrotum, or vagina, especially at the beginning (should decrease during the dwell).

General Care

- *Special instructions*
  - —Peritoneal dialysis: instruct the patient to monitor and maintain the following:

    Dialysis record (number of exchanges, dwell time, beginning and ending times, amount of solution infused and drained)

    Daily log of weights, using the same scale, clothing, and time of day when weighing; report changes in weight of 2 pounds or more

    Blood pressure, pulse, temperature

    Intake and output
  - —Refer the patient to the dialysis nurse for assistance in obtaining appropriate equipment and supplies.
- *Medications*
  - —Explain the purpose, dosage, schedule, and route of administration of any prescribed drugs, as well as side effects to report to a physician or nurse.

—Instruct the patient to omit hypertensive medications before hemodialysis as instructed.

—Instruct the patient to avoid using over-the-counter medications without checking with the physician or nurse.

- *Activity*

—Encourage the patient to discuss allowances and limitations with respect to occupation, recreation, and activities.

—Tell the patient to avoid lifting heavy objects or straining of the extremity with access. Inform the patient of the need to avoid contact sports (football, soccer, basketball) or unusually strenuous exercise.

—Explain the need for frequent rest periods, especially after dialysis.

- *Diet*

—Discuss the diet prescribed by the physician for the underlying condition.

—Refer the patient to a dietitian as indicated.

—Explain the need to restrict liquids and define the limits.

PSYCHOSOCIAL CARE

- Encourage verbalization of concerns and fears about how dialysis may affect lifestyle and activities.
- Encourage participation in planning home care.
- Assist the patient, family, and significant others to obtain counseling if needed.

FOLLOW-UP CARE

- Stress the importance of keeping regular follow-up medical and laboratory appointments. Remind the patient to bring the daily log to appointments. Make sure the patient has the necessary names and telephone numbers.
- Encourage or assist the patient to obtain a MedicAlert bracelet and identification card listing the diagnosis and medication.

REFERRALS

- Assist the patient to obtain home health care referral services through the social worker and discharge planner.

Diarrhea

—Diarrhea: frequent passage of loose stools (>200 g/day) containing 70% to 90% water. Stools may contain mucus, pus, or blood. Diarrhea is usually a symptom of some underlying disorder or is a side effect of treatment, such as chemotherapy or radiation therapy.

CAUSES/CONTRIBUTING FACTORS

- Acute diarrhea
  - Diet alteration
  - Improper cooking
  - Spoiled food
  - Drug reaction
  - Infection
  - Ingestion of toxins
- Chronic diarrhea
  - Lactase insufficiency
  - Laxative abuse
  - Stress and anxiety
  - Inflammatory bowel syndrome
  - Irritable bowel syndrome
  - Cancer of the colon
  - Chemotherapeutic agents
  - Radiation
  - Gastrointestinal surgery
  - Malabsorption disease

SIGNS/SYMPTOMS

- Abdominal pain
- Cramping
- Increased stool frequency
- Loose, liquid stools
- Urgency
- Change in color of stool

COMPLICATIONS

- Dehydration
- Electrolyte imbalance

🏠 HOME CARE

- Give both the patient and the caregiver *verbal* and *written* instructions. Provide them with the name and telephone number of a physician or nurse to call if questions arise.
- *General information*
  —Explain the disease and the underlying cause.
- *Warning signs*
  —Review the signs and symptoms that should be reported to a physician or nurse.
    - Uncontrolled diarrhea lasting longer than 24 hours
    - Stools with blood, pus, or mucus
    - Increasing fatigue or weakness
    - Abdominal pain or severe discomfort that accompanies diarrhea and is not relieved by passage of stools or gas
    - Fever of 101° F or greater
    - Chills, vomiting, or fainting
    - Excessive thirst
- *Special instructions*
  —Instruct the patient to maintain a record of stools, including the number per day, time, color, amount, consistency, odor, and presence of mucus, blood, or pus.
  —Teach the patient to perform perianal and perineal skin care after every bowel movement, including washing gently with mild soap and warm water, applying protective ointment and gels, and drying the area by gently patting with a soft towel. Sitz baths may be used as necessary.
  —Discuss the need for good hygiene: wash hands after each stool, clean bathroom after each stool if bathroom is shared with others.
- *Medications*
  —Explain the purpose, dosage, schedule, and route of administration of any prescribed drugs, as well as side effects to report to a physician or nurse.
  —Explain the need to avoid use of antidiarrheal agents if the diarrhea is due to gastrointestinal infection (e.g., *Shigella*) without checking with a physician.
  —Tell the patient to avoid use of antacids that contain magnesium, which aggravates diarrhea.
- *Diet*
  —Discuss the need to rest the stomach and increase fluid intake up to 3000 ml/day. Encourage clear fluids: water, diluted

broth, decaffeinated tea, carbonated liquids served flat, gelatin, or sports drinks a sip at a time until the stomach can handle a larger amount. Tell the patient to avoid fluids that are too hot or cold, since these increase peristalsis.

—Tell the patient to avoid irritating foods until all symptoms have disappeared: spicy, fatty, or fried foods; milk; caffeine; raw fruits and vegetables; alcohol.

—Encourage a low-fat, low-fiber diet: bananas, toast, apple-sauce, soda crackers. Once stools begin to firm, food as tolerated can be increased: chicken, mashed potatoes, cottage cheese.

Dying at Home

—Dying at home: over the past years, there has been a dramatic growth in the number of individuals with chronic illnesses who wish to "stay home to die." Led largely by the increased number of elderly persons, both patients and families may request discharge to home to die in familiar surroundings. The hospice movement has also fostered a desire to "die at home" for those with terminal illnesses. A patient and family may choose a hospice program or a traditional home care agency for support in this final phase of life. Provide patients and their families with information to plan for an expected death in the home setting, which will assist them to make a decision about accepting this responsibility.

TERMINOLOGY

- *Planned/expected death:* a gradual decline of physical systems in patients with an incurable condition. Care provided at home is focused on ensuring that the patient remains comfortable and pain free until the end. Planned, expected death, coordinated with the physician, does not usually require notification of paramedics or coroner, depending on state and local regulations.
- *Unexpected death:* a sudden collapse/death of an individual who has no known terminal disease or who has a disabling

disease for which death is not imminently expected. Depending on state and local regulations, such an event requires notification of the physician and a call to the police/coroner or paramedics for transport to a local emergency room.

CONSIDERATIONS WHEN PLANNING FOR AN EXPECTED DEATH AT HOME

- Provide *verbal* and *written* instruction specific to the patient's needs. Provide the name and telephone number of a physician or nurse to call for any questions.
- Provide referrals to home health care services as required.
- Review state and local regulations regarding procedures involving expected death in the home.

Essential Planning

- Assist the family in the decision-making process by arranging a family conference to discuss necessary requirements and procedures for caring for the patient at home. Include social and home health care services.
  - —Advise the patient and family that if the patient does not wish to go to the hospital when his or her physical condition worsens, they will need a "do not resuscitate" (DNR) order from the physician.
  - —In some jurisdictions a formal procedure for patients at home exists that allows paramedics and other health professionals to recognize a legal DNR order. Such a procedure may include the wearing of an official "DNR bracelet" and/or the posting of a DNR order near the patient. Advise the patient and family that this is a decision that may be reversed at any time by the patient.
  - —Advise the patient and family that it is helpful to have a living will or advance directive to clearly spell out the patient's wishes. It is also very helpful to designate someone to have a durable power of attorney so that the patient can transfer fiscal and legal responsibilities when no longer able to handle them.
  - —Advise the family to select and make arrangements with a funeral home. Making decisions about the type of funeral service, music, readings, and location for and type of burial may be more easily done early in the dying process. Advise the family to include the patient in these discussions

whenever possible to ensure that they are following the patient's wishes.

—Discuss withdrawal of life-sustaining care openly with the patient's family because this may be an uncomfortable issue for them. Involve other health professionals or spiritual leaders to assist with this difficult decision. Discuss the need to adhere to state laws and regulations in making decisions about what life support may be withdrawn.

—Encourage the family to identify one or two individuals who will serve as primary caregivers and a plan to provide respite for them, especially if there is only one primary caregiver.

Clinical Support

- Explain that assistance from other health care professionals such as home care and hospice agencies is available. Personal care may be provided by a home health aide to promote physical comfort, depending on specific needs.

  —Explain that a social worker or spiritual counselor can often help the patient and family cope with their feelings about the impending death and make decisions. Advise and provide referrals whenever there are unresolved feelings or a lack of clarity about a death at home. Explain that not every situation is amenable to home care throughout the dying process.

  —Instruct caregivers in the use of any necessary equipment such as oxygen, a hospital bed, commode, and IV supplies.

  —Advise the caregiver about ways to make the home more convenient for delivery of care (e.g., creating a bedroom downstairs to facilitate easier access by the caregiver).

  —Instruct the caregiver in any needed care such as a Foley catheter, gastrostomy tube, tracheostomy, etc., as needed. If the patient becomes incontinent of urine or stool, teach the family about the use of adult diapers and/or under-hip pads, such as Chux. If the family cannot afford these products, teach them how to use a draw sheet and towels as padding.

  —Instruct the caregiver in the use of medications: develop a written schedule. Stress the importance of following the medication regimen as ordered and of calling the nurse or physician if side effects or problems arise.

  —Stress the importance of ongoing assessment of pain and maintaining the patient's level of comfort with appropriate interventions (see Pain Management, p. 708).

Advise caregivers to monitor for signs of increasing pain: frowning, restlessness, agitation, or irritability. For patients with chronic pain, however, no additional signs and symptoms may be present, so asking is important.

Explain that if the prescribed medication is insufficient to control or significantly alleviate the pain, the nurse or physician should be notified.

Explain that using a pain management log is helpful in identifying what works most effectively, especially if pain is difficult to control.

—Discuss the importance of keeping the patient as pain free and alert as possible.

—Instruct the patient and family that increasing disinterest in food and liquid is expected and that the patient should not be forced to eat or drink. Advise the family that this may be due to anorexia or a desire to be "done with living." Provide small frequent feedings as tolerated. Using a straw with one finger held over the end is an easy way to provide small amounts of liquid to prevent a dry mouth and provide some fluid intake.

Impending Death

- Instruct the family in signs of impending death. These may vary depending on diagnosis, but often include the following:
  —Patient sleeps most of the time
  —Restlessness or confusion
  —Unresponsiveness or loss of consciousness
  —Labored, irregular breathing or short periods of apnea
  —Cooling of the extremities, mottling, purplish color or darkening of the skin
  —Increasing fluid retention
- Advise the family to call the nurse or physician at this time, especially if they are unsure of symptoms or need support.
- Instruct the family in signs of death:
  —Breathing has stopped.
  —There is no heartbeat.
  —Eyelids are partially open, but eyes are in a fixed stare.
  —Bladder and rectum relax and release contents.
- Instruct the family to notify the physician or nurse (who notifies physician) once signs of death are present. In some states a home health care or hospice nurse may pronounce death at home; in others it must be a physician. For an expected death

the physician collaborates with the home health care nurse to avoid the need to transport the patient to the emergency room for pronouncement. This permits direct transport to the funeral home.

Postmortem Care

This is performed only for an expected death at home. For unexpected deaths, the coroner's office requires that the body not be touched.

- Determine that there are no signs of life (no pulse or respirations for 1 to 3 minutes) and notify the physician; note on paper the time of death. Advise the family to notify the mortuary to arrange for transport.
- Explain the procedure for postmortem care. Advise the family that they may perform some or all of these activities or wait until home health care nurse or mortuary personnel arrive.
  —Wash hands and put on gloves.
  —Place dentures in the patient's mouth and close the mouth.
  —Remove all tubes, intravenous lines, or other supportive devices. If instructed, family may do this or they may wait for the nurse or mortuary personnel to arrive.
  —Place the patient's body in good alignment.
  —Close the patient's eyes.
  —Cover the patient's body with a sheet.
- Advise family members where to return any rented medical equipment as needed. (If requested, advise the family where they may donate any purchased medical equipment, such as the American Cancer Society or Easter Seals.)

Glucose Monitoring, Blood
(Fingerstick)

—Glucose monitoring: determine fasting or random levels of blood glucose with capillary blood; used for regulating blood glucose levels and adjusting medication dosages per blood glucose level.

INDICATIONS

- Diabetes mellitus
- Patients receiving total parenteral nutrition (TPN) to monitor for hyperglycemia

 HOME CARE

- Give both the patient and caregiver *verbal* and *written* instructions. Provide them with the name and telephone number of a physician or nurse to call if questions arise. Use the patient's own glucose monitoring machine, if available, to tailor teaching to the patient's specific needs and equipment.

EQUIPMENT/SUPPLIES

- Blood glucose–monitoring machine
- Lancets (disposable)
- Lancet injector
- Cotton balls
- Depending on the type of monitor used: alcohol pads or a bottle of alcohol; a watch with a second hand or a kitchen timer if the monitor does not time itself
- Needle/lancet disposable container

PREPROCEDURAL TEACHING

- Advise the patient and family in the selection of equipment that accommodates the patient's cognitive and visual status and manual dexterity if the patient has not purchased a glucose monitor.
  —Assess and identify any financial hardship of the patient before recommending a glucose monitor and supplies because health insurance may not pay for a machine and/or test strips.
- Advise the patient that often there are coupons or rebates available for some machines.

PROCEDURAL TEACHING

- Review reasons for the need to evaluate and monitor blood glucose levels regularly.
  —High blood glucose levels often cannot be determined by the way the patient feels.
  —Regular testing provides the patient, nurse, dietitian, and physician with information needed to regulate the medication

dosage, diet, and exercise regimen. For example, during an illness increased monitoring may be necessary.

—Blood glucose levels kept under control minimize or prevent complications that affect vision, nerves, kidneys, and blood vessels.

• Advise the patient of the importance of following the manufacturer's instructions, because each glucose monitor has different steps and requirements to provide accurate results.

• Provide instruction in calibration of the glucose monitor; allow time for return demonstration and practice. Stress the importance of performing the procedure as outlined in the manufacturer's directions.

• Advise the patient to identify a clean area in the home to store testing supplies and equipment.

• Discuss the importance of keeping a log of blood glucose readings. Assist the patient to set up a log if one is not included with monitor (see p. 692). Log parameters should include the date, time of testing, and length of time since last meal and/or medication.

• Provide instruction and observe the patient performing the procedure.

—Identify a convenient place to do the test and lay out equipment on a clean surface area. Wash hands with soap and warm water; dry them thoroughly with a clean towel.

—Collect all supplies and prepare the equipment. Remove the test strip from the container and place face up near monitor.

—Clean the finger with an alcohol swab or alcohol-soaked cotton ball unless alcohol is contraindicated by the glucose-monitoring system. (Note that some glucose-monitoring strips may give erroneous readings if alcohol is used.)

—Open and clench the fist several times to promote blood flow.

—Load the lancet injector with a lancet, if used.

—Turn on the glucose monitor.

—Prick the finger with the lancet.

—Dispose of the lancet in the needle disposal container, if the point is exposed. If the point is covered, dispose of the lancet after testing is completed.

—Firmly squeeze the finger with the forefinger and thumb of the other hand to aid in blood flow and reduce any pain.

—Allow a full, hanging blood droplet to form and drop onto a test strip, covering the whole target area without touching the strip. Depending on the glucose monitor some strips are placed in the machine before the blood drop is placed and some after. Follow the manufacturer's instructions. Some newer systems allow strips to be touched without affecting the results.

—Avoid "milking" the finger is the blood flow is slow. If it is necessary to start over, wrap the hand in a warm, clean cloth for 1 to 3 minutes to improve the blood flow.

—Apply gentle pressure with a cotton ball to the fingerprick until bleeding stops.

—Advise the patient that the blood glucose reading appears on the monitor's display window within 15 to 60 minutes depending on the type of system. If an older machine is used, time the reading of results with the second hand of a watch or a kitchen timer according to the manufacturer's directions.

- Record results in the log. (Take the log along to appointments with the physician.)
- Return equipment and supplies to the selected storage area.
- Stress the importance of testing blood glucose as ordered (e.g., patients taking insulin test their blood glucose levels four times per day, at least until well stabilized). Recommended times for testing are usually before each meal and at bedtime.
- Discuss the importance of keeping scheduled medical and laboratory follow-up visits. Discuss the need to compare home monitoring results to venipuncture results done in the laboratory if home fasting values differ significantly from laboratory fasting values.

Log of Blood Glucose Test Results
Target range for blood glucose (sugar): _____   Name: _____

Date	Meds/ insulin	Before breakfast	Meds/ insulin	Before lunch	Meds/ insulin	Before dinner	Meds/ insulin	At bedtime	Other	Notes: diet, exercise, illness, stress, etc.
Sun		Time: Results:		Time: Results:		Time: Results:		Time: Results:	Time: Results:	
Mon		Time: Results:		Time: Results:		Time: Results:		Time: Results:	Time: Results:	
Tues		Time: Results:		Time: Results:		Time: Results:		Time: Results:	Time: Results:	

		Time: Results:		Time: Results:		Time: Results:	Time: Results:
Wed		Time: Results:		Time: Results:		Time: Results:	Time: Results:
Thurs		Time: Results:		Time: Results:		Time: Results:	Time: Results:
Fri		Time: Results:		Time: Results:		Time: Results:	Time: Results:
Sat		Time: Results:		Time: Results:		Time: Results:	Time: Results:

Comments: _____

Ostomy
(Ileostomy, Colostomy)

—Ostomy: a temporary or permanent opening into the bowel that allows fecal materials to be expelled at the skin surface. The opening onto the skin is called a stoma.

—Ileostomy: permanent ileostomy is removal of the colon and rectum and closure of the anus (proctocolectomy). The terminal ileum is brought through the abdominal wall, and an external pouch is worn. Continent ileostomy (Kock pouch) is surgical removal of the rectum and colon with construction of an internal ileal reservoir, nipple valve, and stoma. Fecal waste collects in the nipple-valved pouch until the patient drains the pouch through the stoma with a catheter. No external pouch is worn. The internal pouch is emptied several times a day. The stoma is flat with the skin surface. The ileostomy effluent is liquid.

—Colostomy: surgical removal of the entire rectum and affected colon and closure of the anus; if the rectum is left intact, the colostomy may be temporary. The location of the stoma and the effluent consistency depend on the section of colon resected: ascending (liquid effluent), transverse (loose semiformed effluent), descending, or sigmoid colon (effluent close to normal).

INDICATIONS
- Ileostomy
  - —Ulcerative colitis
  - —Crohn's disease
  - —Small bowel obstruction
  - —Polyposis
- Colostomy
  - —Colon cancer
  - —Diverticulitis
  - —Fistula
  - —Ulcerative colitis

PREPROCEDURAL TEACHING

- Review the physician's explanation of the procedure and the type of ostomy. Describe how the ostomy will function, its location, and the appearance and smell of fecal drainage. Use simple descriptions and illustrations.
- Describe and allow the patient to see equipment and supplies such as the pouch.
- Explain the stoma selection process, asking the patient's preference. Permit the patient to wear a stoma pouch over the area to ensure comfort at the selected site.
- Arrange for a visit from the enterostomal therapist and an ostomy patient from the United Ostomy Association.

Review of Preprocedural Care

- Review preoperative procedures (see Abdominal Surgery, p. 6), including bowel preparation.
- Permit time for questions. Encourage verbalization and expression of fears and feelings regarding changes in body image, sexuality, and role function.

SIDE EFFECTS/COMPLICATIONS

- Leakage under the appliance
- Signs of wound infection
- Electrolyte imbalance
- Dehydration
- Obstruction
- Prolapse
- Hemorrhage
- Stricture
- Retraction
- Necrosis

HOME CARE

- Give both the patient and the caregiver *verbal* and *written* instructions. Provide them with the name and telephone number of a physician, nurse, or enterostomal therapist to call if questions arise. Use visual aids to assist in instruction and permit time for return demonstration and practice.

- *General information*
  —Describe the type and location of the ostomy created, reviewing indications. Explain that drainage depends on food ingested.
  —Explain that an ostomy requires special attention, including diet modifications and restriction and meticulous skin care.
- *Warning signs*
  —Review the signs and symptoms that should be reported to a physician or nurse.
    Infection of stoma: redness, purulent drainage, swelling, pain, warm to touch, fever
    Prolapse of stoma, bloody drainage, persistent diarrhea through stoma, excessive flatus, lack of fecal material, or change in usual pattern of elimination
    Bowel obstruction, nausea, vomiting, diarrhea, and abdominal pain
    Ileostomy: inability to intubate stoma, abdominal distention, nausea, vomiting, abdominal pain, nipple valve dysfunction, incontinence of stool, flatus, high-volume watery stool, pouch full within 20 to 30 minutes
    Erosion of skin
- *Special instructions*
  —Discuss and demonstrate skin care around the stoma. Permit time for return demonstration and practice.
    Instruct the patient to inspect the skin daily for signs of irritation or infection.
    Each time the pouch is changed, clean the skin with soap and water. Apply a skin barrier to the clean, dry skin before the new pouch is attached.
    Place a pectin-based wafer in the pouch.
    If a rash occurs, use a heat lamp or hair dryer to dry the skin.
    Sprinkle a small amount of powder (e.g., karaya, Stomahesive) on the skin, wipe off the excess, and blot with a skin sealant to seal the powder to the skin.
    Explain that the skin barrier opening should be the size of the stoma to prevent contact of stool with the skin.
    Powder the skin after the pouch has been applied.

—Demonstrate emptying of a fecal ostomy pouch. Explain that the pouch should be emptied when it is about one third full. Provide time for return demonstration and practice.

> Have the patient sit on the toilet with the pouch between the legs or sit on a chair with the pouch opening in the toilet.
>
> While holding up the end of the pouch, remove the clamp and let the contents of the pouch drain into the toilet. Putting some toilet paper on the surface of the water helps to prevent splashing.
>
> Squeeze the remaining contents out of the pouch.
>
> Hold up the end of the pouch and pour a cup of water into the pouch through the opening. Swish the water around to clean out the inside of the pouch. Do not get the stoma or the seal around the stoma wet.
>
> Use toilet paper to clean around the opening of the pouch. Clamp the pouch shut again.

—Demonstrate removal of an ostomy pouch. Permit time for return demonstration and practice.

> Instruct the patient to inspect the stoma for signs of injury and to change the ostomy pouch every 5 to 7 days and whenever the pouch first begins to leak. Gather the following equipment before beginning: adhesive solvent, gauze pads, powder (if desired), towel, and scissors.
>
> While standing, hold the skin around the stoma taut and begin peeling off the adhesive square that holds the pouch to the skin. Peeling from top to bottom works best. If the pouch cannot be peeled off, use adhesive solvent to loosen the edges.
>
> Wipe excess drainage around the stoma with gauze pads.
>
> Wash the area around the stoma with soap and water. Dry thoroughly. Apply powder if the skin is irritated. Apply a skin barrier if desired.

—Demonstrate application of an ostomy pouch. Permit time for return demonstration and practice.

> Peel back the paper from the adhesive faceplate.
>
> Center the pouch opening over the stoma, and press all around the faceplate to ensure that it is firmly attached to the skin.

Attach the belt if the patient wishes to wear it.

Press the air out of the pouch and clamp the bottom.

—Explain the emptying of a continent ileostomy (Kock pouch).

To remove stool and flatus, place a large-bore tube into the stoma several times a day.

- *Medications*

—Explain the purpose, dosage, schedule, and route of administration of any prescribed drugs, as well as side effects to report to the physician or nurse.

- *Activity*

—Encourage the patient to resume activities of daily living as soon as able.

—Explain that regular exercise will build the patient's strength. Inform the patient of the need to avoid activities that cause abdominal strain (e.g., weight lifting) or contact sports (e.g., football, ice hockey).

—Encourage questions regarding specific allowances and limitations for occupation, recreation, or activities.

—Assure the patient that a preosteotomy lifestyle can be resumed once the stoma has healed. Provide examples and guidelines.

—Explain that showers and baths are permissible because the stoma will not be hurt by soap or direct water. The patient may wear a disposable/temporary pouch if concerned about leakage.

—Advise the patient to avoid wearing tight, constrictive clothing (e.g., girdle, belt) directly over the stoma.

—Suggest measures to take before traveling.

Purchase enough ostomy supplies for the entire trip or find out where to buy supplies en route.

If the usual pouch is reusable, purchase disposable pouches as a precaution.

Carry supplies in hand luggage to prevent loss. For long air travel, arrange with the airline to have special meals ordered.

Notify the physician about the travel and request prophylactic medication for diarrhea or constipation. If traveling to a foreign country, drink only potable water.

—Discuss the effect an ostomy may have on the patient's sexual activity. Provide information and encourage counseling if the patient or partner is unable to discuss sexuality.

The presence of an osteotomy usually does not interfere with sexual function, except that men with bladder or rectal cancer may have temporary or permanent impotence.

Pregnancy is possible but should be planned. The female patient should talk with a physician or nurse before becoming pregnant and should be given information regarding contraception.

Sexual activity may resume when the stoma is healed and the patient and partner are ready.

Verbalization and communication between the patient and partner are important.

The stoma cannot be injured by close physical contact.

The pouch should be emptied before intercourse. The patient may wish to use a pouch cover.

- *Diet*
  —Review dietary restrictions for preventing stoma blockage and diarrhea, flatus, and odor. Provide written information and refer the patient to a dietitian for additional information and counseling.
  —Encourage fluid intake to maintain fluid and electrolyte balance, especially on hot days or during bouts of diarrhea. Advise the patient to avoid use of laxatives and diuretics, which increase fluid loss.
  —Explain how diet can affect ostomy output (see Appendix E).
  —Instruct the patient to avoid gas-producing foods such as broccoli, cabbage, beans, onions, radishes, carbonated drinks, and beer. When eating such foods, the patient should use a product such as Beano to reduce gas formation.
  —Suggest that the patient prevent odor by avoiding eggs, fish, onion, garlic, asparagus, cheese, and alcohol.
  —For ileostomy, instruct the patient to buy odor-absorbing tablets to place in the ostomy bag or a commercial gas release valve.
  —Explain how to prevent blockage of the stoma by avoiding high-fiber foods such as celery, lettuce, nuts, and corn.
  —Inform the patient that diarrhea can be avoided by not eating highly spiced foods or raw fruits and vegetables (e.g., green beans, broccoli).
  —Instruct the patient to have meals at regular times, to eat slowly and chew well, to have moderate-sized portions, and

to try new foods in small servings in case they have ill effects.

—Explain that gas formation can be prevented by avoiding the use of straws, gum chewing or chewing with the mouth open, and smoking.

PSYCHOSOCIAL CARE

• Permit time for emotional adjustment. Encourage the patient to ask questions and express feelings about body image and lifestyle changes.

• Encourage the patient to seek psychosocial support and counseling as indicated.

FOLLOW-UP CARE

• Stress the importance of regular medical and laboratory follow-up visits. Make sure the patient has the necessary names and telephone numbers.

REFERRALS

• Provide referrals for enterostomal therapy, home health care services, dietary management, supplies, and medical social services as indicated.

• Refer to support groups, and the United Ostomy Association.

Oxygen Therapy

—Oxygen therapy: provision of oxygen to the tissue so that normal metabolism can occur; used to relieve hypoxemia and prevent hypoxia. Oxygen may be delivered as a liquid, by means of an oxygen concentrator, or from a cylinder as compressed gas.

COMPLICATIONS

• Atelectasis

• Oxygen toxicity: sore throat, cough, nausea, anxiety, numbness, muscular twitching, chest pain with deep inspiration

▢ HOME CARE

- Give both the patient and the caregiver *verbal* and *written* instructions. Provide them with the name and telephone number of a physician or nurse to call if questions arise.
- *General information*
  —Explain the purpose of oxygen therapy and how it will be delivered.
- *Warning signs*
  —Review the signs and symptoms that should be reported to a physician or nurse.

      Irregular, shallow, or slow breathing; difficulty in breathing
      Restlessness or anxiety
      Tiredness, drowsiness, trouble waking up
      Persistent headache
      Slurred speech
      Confusion, difficulty in concentrating
      Bluish fingernails or lips
- *Special instructions*
  —Work with the social service or home health care agency to find equipment and a supplier near the patient's home. Include the patient and caregiver in decision making.
  —Assist the patient to obtain a home health care referral for follow-up at home.
  —Review the oxygen concentration delivery that was ordered. Explain the importance of maintaining the appropriate flow rate, since high flow rates in patients with chronic obstructive pulmonary disease can suppress the respiratory drive.
  —Teach the patient how to remove and reposition the oxygen equipment to permit wiping off and drying the face, nose blowing, and eating.
  —For a patient who requires humidity and aerosol therapy, provide instructions.
  —Explain that humidification and adequate hydration are important because oxygen dries the mucous membranes.
  —Demonstrate the use of equipment and how to fill humidifiers and nebulizers.
  —Demonstrate the administration of medication via handheld nebulizers.
  —Instruct the patient on clearing secretions, which can interfere with oxygenation.

—Show the patient how to care for the skin and mucous membranes, since with prolonged wear, oxygen devices can cause skin irritation and breakdown, which can provide an additional route for microorganisms.

—Instruct the patient to use cotton balls or moleskin around the tubing to avoid skin irritation over the ears.

—Demonstrate the use, care, and cleaning of equipment.

—Teach the patient how to use the oxygen source, oxygen delivery device, and humidification source.

—Demonstrate how to check water in the humidifier and nebulizer every 8 hours to maintain an adequate level and how to refill as needed.

—Explain the importance of maintaining the temperature of humidifiers between 95° and 97.8° F.

—Ensure that the humidifier is placed on a table at least 2 feet from walls and furniture, with the steam directed into the room.

—Provide instruction on oxygen management when traveling around town with oxygen: plan ahead before travel. Call the oxygen supply company and ask what equipment is needed and how long to allot for travel between refills. Allow for a 20% to 25% safety margin of oxygen supply to cover unexpected delays. Use a watch with an alarm function to remind you that the oxygen tank is running low. Practice operating the oxygen equipment before travel.

—Inform the patient that liquid oxygen is available in a small, lightweight container similar in size to a thermos bottle; advise that it be reserved for trips outside the home, since it is expensive to use continuously.

—Discuss oxygen management when traveling by automobile.

Demonstrate how to secure the oxygen unit with a seatbelt and shoulder harness.

Instruct the patient or caregiver to keep the oxygen container upright at all times to avoid rapid release of oxygen. Slight tipping of liquid oxygen tanks during loading and unloading is not dangerous.

Advise the patient to store extra tanks in the trunk of the car, since tanks are too large to stand upright.

Instruct the patient to keep the car window partly open while using oxygen.

Tell camper or motor home owners to contact the oxygen supply company for installation of a liquid oxygen reservoir.

—If the patient is planning to travel by local public transportation, advise contacting the city's transportation department to check restrictions on oxygen equipment on local transportation systems.

—Stress the importance of not smoking or allowing others to smoke near the patient because of the possibility of combustion, fire, or explosion.

—Explain the necessity of checking all electrical equipment used in the same room with oxygen administration for frayed cords or the potential for sparking to avoid combustion and fire or explosion.

—Tell the patient not to place carpet, clothing, or furniture over the tubing, since a leak could result.

—Demonstrate the use of an all-purpose fire extinguisher and instruct the patient to keep one near the equipment.

—Advise the patient to notify the local fire department of the presence of oxygen in the house and to request free safety inspections, if available.

• *Medications*

—Explain the purpose, dosage, schedule, and route of administration of any prescribed drugs, as well as side effects to report to a physician or nurse.

• *Activity*

—Encourage walking and other activities as tolerated. Advise the patient to use a portable oxygen source because continuous oxygen therapy can limit mobility.

—Suggest that the patient use oxygen, as ordered, during meals, showers, or sexual activities.

FOLLOW-UP CARE AND REFERRALS

• Stress the importance of regular follow-up visits. Make sure the patient has the necessary names and telephone numbers.

• Discuss with the patient and caregiver the need to notify the local fire department and electric and gas utility companies of the presence of oxygen in the home.

• Instruct the patient to keep emergency numbers by the telephone.

Pacemaker Care

—Pacemaker care: use and maintenance of an electronic device that stimulates the myocardium to control or maintain the heart rate. The pacemaker can be a temporary or permanent mode of treatment. The battery-powered pulse generator and lead system senses heart function and stimulates the myocardium to contract.

INDICATIONS

- Sinus node dysfunction
- Conduction blocks
- Bradyarrhythmias
- Tachyarrhythmias

PREPROCEDURAL TEACHING

- Review the physician's explanation of implantation of the pacemaker and the reason for it; encourage the patient to ask questions and to discuss any fears or anxieties. Explain the need for informed consent.

Review of Preprocedural Care

- Instruct the patient not to eat or drink for 6 to 8 hours before the procedure.
- Explain that the procedure will be done under local anesthesia and sedation and will last for 1 to 3 hours.
- Explain that the patient's head will be positioned to one side and draped.
- Inform the patient that some pressure may be felt during the procedure.
- Explain that the lead(s) will be threaded into the right atrium through the subclavian vein via fluoroscopy.
- Tell the patient that an incision will be made under the collarbone.
- Explain that the patient will be continuously monitored during and after the procedure.
- Inform the patient that there may be some pain at the insertion site.

Review of Postprocedural Care

- Tell that patient that bed rest will be maintained for the first 4 to 6 hours to prevent lead dislodgment.
- Explain that stiffness and soreness will be felt at the insertion site.
- Inform the patient that the arm on the side of the incision may be immobilized in a sling.
- Explain that postoperative electrocardiographic monitoring will continue for 24 hours.

SIDE EFFECTS/COMPLICATIONS

- Pacemaker dysfunction
- Catheter dislodgment
- Stokes-Adams syndrome
- Cardiac dysrhythmia
- Infection
- Bleeding
- Perforation
- Cardiac tamponade

HOME CARE

- Give both the patient and the caregiver *verbal* and *written* instructions. Provide them with the name and telephone number of a physician or nurse to call if questions arise.
- *General information*
  —Explain the underlying rhythm disorder, type of pacemaker (temporary or permanent), and care.
- *Warning signs*
  —Review the signs and symptoms that should be reported to a physician or nurse.
    Pacemaker dysfunction: syncope, pallor, fatigue, shortness of breath, palpitations or irregular pulse, pulse out of range of programmed settings, chest pain
    Catheter dislodgment: hiccups, twitching of chest and abdominal muscles
    Stokes-Adams syndrome: vertigo, syncope, convulsions, coma
    Infection: fever, redness, warmth, pain, swelling, discoloration, bleeding, or drainage at incision site
- *Special instructions*
  —Teach the patient how to measure a pulse radially; explain that it should be done each day at rest.

—Instruct the patient to inform all dentists and physicians of the pacemaker before any procedures.

—Instruct the patient to inform airport security personnel of the pacemaker before passing through the metal detector to avoid triggering the alarm.

—Reassure the female patient that pregnancy is not contraindicated. Instruct her to inform her physician that she is planning a pregnancy so that the pacemaker can be adjusted to rate changes associated with pregnancy.

—Teach the patient how to take his or her pulse. Stress the importance of taking and recording pulse daily, resting 5 minutes before taking the pulse, and taking it for 1 full minute. Instruct the patient to report to the health care provider any significant deviation from the pacemaker setting.

—Teach the patient signs and symptoms to report: irregular pulse, dizziness or fainting spells, shortness of breath, ankle swelling, signs of infection at the insertion site (redness, swelling, tenderness).

—Discuss electrical safety.

Tell the patient to avoid working with radar or electrical equipment such as diathermy or electrocautery devices, arc welding, electrical smelting furnaces, large electrical generators, CB radios with high-power linear amplifiers, radio or television transmitters while they are operating, and magnetic resonance imaging devices.

Instruct the patient to ground home appliances.

Stress the importance of using caution around strong magnetic fields, microwave ovens, and blow dryers.

Instruct the patient to move away from any fields that interfere with pacemaker function; the pacemaker will resume normal programmed function.

Provide the patient and caregiver with written information on the pacemaker model, date of insertion, location of generator, and pacer programming.

Explain that the expected life of a pacemaker battery is 5 to 10 years, depending on the type of battery.

Explain that the part of the pacemaker system that may need changing is the generator.

- *Medications*
  —Explain the purpose, dosage, schedule, and route of administration of any prescribed drugs, as well as side effects to report to a physician or nurse.
  —Stress the importance of avoiding use of over-the-counter medications without consulting a physician.
- *Activity*
  —Encourage the patient to discuss allowances and limitations with respect to occupation, recreation, and activities.
  —Explain activity limitations as directed by the physician. Advise the patient to avoid heavy lifting (>10 pounds) and vigorous arm or shoulder activity. Explain that sexual activity may be resumed as tolerated.
  —Demonstrate range-of-motion exercises for the affected shoulder, and tell the patient to begin them after the first 24 hours.
  —Tell the patient not to drive for the first 4 weeks.
  —Stress the importance of avoiding contact sports.
  —Instruct the patient to avoid traveling for 3 months after pacemaker insertion.
  —Advise the patient not to wear restrictive clothing over the pacemaker site.
  —Tell the patient to avoid direct contact with or blows to the pacemaker site.

PSYCHOSOCIAL CARE

- Encourage the patient to verbalize fears and concerns about the underlying rhythm disorder, the need for a pacemaker, changes in lifestyle, and pacemaker management.

FOLLOW-UP CARE AND REFERRALS

- Stress the importance of regular follow-up visits, including the pacemaker clinic. Make sure the patient has the necessary names and telephone numbers. If telephone monitoring is available, discuss this option with the patient.
- Instruct the patient to schedule an appointment soon before the expiration date of the battery.
- Assist the patient to obtain a MedicAlert bracelet and an identification card listing the type of pacemaker, set rate, date of implantation, and name of physician.

Pain Management

—Pain management: dealing with the state in which a person experiences and reports severe discomfort or an uncomfortable sensation. Pain can be influenced by a variety of physiologic, psychologic, and sociologic factors. *Tolerance* is the ability to endure pain intensity. *Threshold* is the amount or degree of discomfort the patient can tolerate before terming the sensation painful. *Acute pain* is intense, has an end point, warns of actual or potential tissue damage, and resolves when healing occurs. *Chronic pain* lasts longer than 6 months and may be continuous or intermittent. Chronic pain does not serve as a warning of tissue damage.

HOME CARE

- Give both the patient and the caregiver *verbal* and *written* instructions. Provide them with the name and telephone number of a physician or nurse to call if questions arise.
- *General information*
  —Explain the relationship of pain to the disease process. Assist the patient to understand the source of pain.
- *Special instructions*
  —Assist the patient to identify factors or actions that trigger pain, such as activity, movements, and temperature extremes.
  —Discuss past effective and ineffective pain relief measures. Explore the past effect of pain relief measures on the patient, such as sleepiness, lethargy, and decreased energy or sexual activity.
  —Assist the patient to localize and describe the intensity of pain using a scale (e.g., 0 to 10, with 0 meaning absence of pain and 10 being intense pain) and to identify any alleviating or aggravating factors.
  —Encourage use of a log to record pain rating and management strategies.
  —Discuss interventions other than taking medications for intractable pain.
      Anesthetic procedures such as nerve blocks, trigger point injections, and use of nitrous oxide

Neuroablative procedures such as cordotomy

Physiatric supportive measures such as using a prosthesis, physical therapy, and occupational therapy

—Discuss alternative strategies patients can use to relieve pain without taking prescribed drugs, and explain that these techniques may also augment the effect of pain medication (see box on p. 710).

Sensory interventions—*massage such as back and foot massage:* to relax muscular tension and increase local circulation; *range-of-motion exercises (passive, assistive, or active):* to relax muscles, improve circulation, and prevent pain related to stiffness and immobility; *cold application:* used initially to decrease tissue injury response (swelling) and decrease pain; *heat application:* used after cold to aid in clearance of tissue toxins and mobilize fluids; *transcutaneous electrical nerve stimulation (TENS):* pocket-size battery-operated device used to send mild continuous electrical impulses through the skin by means of electrodes placed on the body (see discussion on pp. 712-713)

Emotional interventions to increase pain threshold by controlling or reducing anxiety, fatigue, or depression—*prevention or control of anxiety:* to reduce muscle tension and increase pain tolerance through relaxation exercises and slow, controlled breathing; *promotion of self-control:* to reduce feelings of helplessness and lack of control that contribute to anxiety and pain; *pacing of activities*

Cognitive interventions—*distraction:* focus on something unrelated to pain (e.g., conversing, watching television or videos, listening to music), humor; *guided imagery:* use of images to alter a physical or emotional state, promote relaxation, and decrease pain sensation

—Discuss the need to identify body positions of comfort; encourage attention to proper posture and body alignment. Advise the patient to immobilize or rest the affected area.

—Tell the patient to relieve pressure areas by turning or using pressure reduction devices such as an air-fluidized support system.

PAIN MANAGEMENT TECHNIQUES

Relaxation

Relaxation relieves pain by easing muscle tension. This can also help you feel less tired and nervous and help other pain-relieving methods work better.

How to Relax

Sit or lie down in a quiet place. Be sure you are comfortable. Do not cross your legs or arms. Take a deep breath, and tense your muscles (you may tense up your whole body or concentrate on one set of muscles at a time, such as your facial muscles or those in your arms and hands).

Hold your breath and keep your muscles tense. Release your breath and your muscles at the same time. Let your body go limp (repeat for other muscle areas if you are concentrating on one set at a time).

You can add imagery or music to help you relax. Relaxation tapes are available from your health care agency or local music store.

Do not be discouraged if relaxation does not help immediately. Practice the relaxation technique for at least 2 weeks before you give it up. If you find that it aggravates your pain, try another method.

Imagery

Imagery involves using your imagination to create mental scenes that use all your senses: sight, sound, touch, smell, and taste. You can imagine exotic locations or revisit one of your favorite places. You can create stories and characters to add to your scenes. Imagery can take your mind off your fear, boredom, and pain.

How to Use Imagery

Close your eyes. A few moments of the relaxation technique (see above) will help your body and mind prepare for imagery. Let your mind begin forming its image. The following is an example of

Continued

PAIN MANAGEMENT TECHNIQUES—cont'd

imagery. Imagine that you are at the seashore. You are sitting in the wet sand; the afternoon sun is warm on your shoulders. The ocean rolls into the shore in gentle waves, and the water laps teasingly at your toes. A hungry pair of seagulls cry overhead and take swift, darting dives at a dog that is scavenging along the shore. Your tension lessens with each wave that touches your toes and retreats. You close your eyes and take a deep, slow breath of air. You are completely relaxed. Stay on the beach as long as you like. To end the image, count to three and open your eyes. Resume your regular activities slowly.

Distraction

A distraction is any activity that takes your mind off your pain and focuses your attention elsewhere. Doing crafts, reading a book, watching television, or listening to music through headphones can distract your mind. Distraction works well when you are waiting for drugs to take effect or if you have brief bouts of pain. Sometimes people can take their minds off their pain for long periods, especially if the pain is mild.

Skin Stimulation

Skin stimulation is used to block pain sensation in the nerves. Pressure, massage, hot and cold applications, rubbing, and mild electrical current are all ways to stimulate the skin. If you are having radiation therapy, consult your physician before applying any skin stimulation. You can do the stimulation at the site of the pain, near it, or on the side opposite the pain. For example, stimulating the left wrist when the right wrist is in pain can actually ease the pain in the right wrist.

Pressure

Using your entire hand, the heel of your hand, your thumb, your knuckles, or both hands, apply

Continued

PAIN MANAGEMENT TECHNIQUES—cont'd

pressure for at least 15 seconds at the point where you feel pain. Keep trying spots around the painful area if you find no relief the first time. You may extend the time you apply pressure to 1 minute.

Massage

You or someone else can perform the slow, circular motions of massage. The feet, back, neck, and scalp can be massaged to relieve tension and pain anywhere in the body. Some people prefer to use oils or lotions during the massage. If deep massage is too uncomfortable, try light stroking. Do not massage red, raw, or broken skin.

Heat and Cold

Some people prefer cold; others prefer heat. Use whichever works better for you. A convenient way to use cold is to freeze gel-filled packs and wrap them in towels. Ice cubes can also be used. Heat can be applied with a heating pad; hot, moist towels; or a hot water bottle or by taking a hot bath. Be careful not to burn your skin with water that is too hot or to go to sleep with a heating pad on. Do not expose your skin to intense cold for long.

Transcutaneous Electrical Nerve Stimulation (TENS)

TENS can be used to eliminate or ease pain. A TENS unit is a pocket-sized, battery-operated device that provides a mild, continuous electrical current through the skin by the use of two to four electrodes taped to the skin. Lead wires connect the electrodes to the device. It is this mild electrical current that blocks or modifies the pain messages and replaces them with a buzzing, tingling sensation. TENS is also thought to stimulate the body's production of endorphin, a natural pain reliever.

—Discuss the use of TENS. Explain that the mild electrical current blocks or modifies pain messages before they reach the brain and replaces them with a buzzing or tingling sensation. Inform the patient that TENS may stimulate the body's production of endorphin, a natural pain reliever. Instruct the patient in the use and home care of the TENS unit.

   Apply a thin coat of gel over each entire electrode.

   Place the electrodes securely on the skin with tape.

   Place the electrodes close to the site of pain.

   Turn the intensity knob until a slight tingling or buzzing sensation is felt on the skin. Increase the intensity if the pain is still felt or decrease the intensity if the tingling sensation causes discomfort.

   Turn the TENS unit off before removing it.

   Wipe the electrodes with an alcohol and water mixture after removing them from the skin.

   Do not allow the unit to get wet. If it does get wet, allow it to dry thoroughly before using it again.

   Replace the electrodes if the adhesive surface separates from the backing or if they no longer adhere firmly to the skin.

   Replace the battery pack or recharge as needed. If there is no tingling sensation when the intensity is turned up, the batteries are weakening.

   Use hypoallergenic tape to secure the electrodes to prevent redness or rash, cleanse the skin well after removing the electrodes, and apply lotion to the placement sites.

• *Medications*

—Explain the purpose, dosage, schedule, and route of administration of any prescribed drugs, as well as side effects to report to a physician or nurse.

—Give the patient general guidelines for the use of pain medications.

   Provide information on the Agency for Health Care Policy and Research (AHCPR) guidelines for patients.

   Explain that a variety of pain relief measures may be necessary for some types of pain.

   Instruct the patient to use pain relief measures before pain becomes severe. Determine the patient's ability or willingness to participate actively in use of pain relief measures, and suggest pain relief measures the patient believes will be helpful.

Rely on patient behavior that indicates pain severity rather than relying on known physical stimuli.

Encourage the patient to try a pain relief measure at least twice before abandoning it as ineffective. Instruct the patient to keep an open mind as to what may relieve pain.

Urge the patient to keep trying to relieve the pain and not to become discouraged.

—Discuss the use of nonnarcotic analgesics.

Inform the patient that nonnarcotic analgesics include acetaminophen, aspirin, and nonsteroidal antiinflammatory drugs such as ibuprofen, indomethacin, and naproxen.

Explain that these medications are generally well tolerated but have the potential to cause gastrointestinal ulceration, renal and hepatic toxic effects, and inhibition of platelet aggregation.

Tell the patient that if the nonnarcotic does not have a therapeutic effect initially, the dosage should be increased before another type of drug is tried.

—Discuss the use of narcotics, which are indicated for severe postoperative pain or intractable pain such as that associated with cancer.

Inform the patient that narcotics include morphine, hydromorphone, and methadone and that these may be administered by intravenous drip, intrathecally, or epidurally to enhance the analgesic effect.

Explain that fixed dosage schedules with adequate doses for pain relief provide more constant blood levels and predictable pain relief. Suggest that additional doses may be needed for breakthrough pain.

Discuss the side effects of narcotic analgesics: constipation, vomiting, and respiratory and central nervous system depression.

Review the use of narcotic agonists and antagonists: nalbuphine (Nubain), butorphanol (Stadol), pentazocine (Talwin), and buprenorphine (Buprenex).

—Explain the use of analgesic potentiators.

Inform the patient that these include hydroxyzine (Vistaril); diazepam (Valium); lorazepam (Ativan); diphenhydramine (Benadryl); and phenothiazine derivatives such as promethazine (Phenergan), prochlorperazine (Compazine), and chlorpromazine (Thorazine).

—Discuss the use of stimulants.

Inform the patient that these include cocaine, methylphenidate (Ritalin), dextroamphetamine, and caffeine.

—Discuss other types of drugs used in pain control, including tricyclic antidepressants such as amitriptyline (Elavil), imipramine (Tofranil), and doxepine (Sinequan), as well as butyrophenones such as droperidol (Inapsine) and haloperidol (Haldol).

—Discuss and demonstrate the use of equipment for administering pain relief medications.

External and implantable pumps for intravenous, epidural, and intrathecal administration of narcotic analgesics

Patient-controlled analgesia (PCA), particularly for the management of acute pain such as postoperative pain

Continuous subcutaneous infusion with an ambulatory infusion pump

TENS

Discuss the side effects of narcotics. For example, constipation requires the use of laxatives and stool softeners (e.g., senna [Senokot]).

Pressure Ulcer Sores
(Decubitus Ulcers)

—Pressure ulcers: an area of tissue necrosis, usually over a bony prominence, that results from tissue hypoxia caused by pressure. Patients at risk include the elderly, patients with spinal cord injuries, and debilitated patients who are increasingly immobile.

STAGES OF PRESSURE ULCER

- Stage I: erythema only; no break in skin
- Stage II: partial thickness; loss of skin involving epidermis, often into dermis
- Stage III: full thickness; involves epidermis extending into dermis and involves subcutaneous tissue
- Stage IV: deep tissue destruction extending to subcutaneous tissue and into fascia, muscle, and bone

RISK FACTORS

- Old age
- Immobility
- Impaired sensation
- Incontinence
- Malnutrition
- Skin shearing

SIGNS/SYMPTOMS

- Redness
- Warmth at pressure area
- Disruption of skin integrity with pain, swelling, heat, induration, drainage, tissue necrosis

COMPLICATIONS

- Infection: bacteremia, septicemia
- Further tissue necrosis

DIAGNOSTIC TESTS

- Describe each procedure, its purpose, and the normal feelings or sensations that are likely, as well as any preprocedural and postprocedural care.
  —Wound cultures
  —Serum albumin

TREATMENT
Medical

- Therapy
  —Diet, vitamins, mineral supplements
  —Pressure relief devices: pads, mattresses, bed
- Drugs
  —Systemic and topical antibiotics

Surgical

- Debridement (surgical or chemical [mechanical]): to remove necrotic tissue
- Surgical repair and grafting

 HOME CARE

- Give both the patient and the caregiver *verbal* and *written* instructions. Provide them with the name and telephone number of a physician or nurse to call if questions arise.
- *General information*
  —Explain the underlying cause or contributing factors. Identify and review the patient's stage of ulcer development, discussing specific procedures to prevent further progression.
  —Explain that treatment depends on the stage of healing. Instruct the caregiver to recognize and record the signs of healing.
- *Warning signs*
  —Review the signs and symptoms that should be reported to a physician or nurse.
      Weight loss
      Elevated temperature
      Increased drainage from the ulcer
      Foul odor from the dressing
      Further necrosis around the ulcer and reddened areas at other pressure points
- *Special instructions*
  —Ulcer care, stages I and II
      Eliminate causative factors.
      Cleanse the skin every 8 hours with mild soap. Pat dry.
      Massage the skin gently to increase circulation. Avoid vigorous rubbing. Do not massage reddened areas.
      Protect the skin surface of the affected area with protective skin gels, ointment, and porous dressings as ordered. Avoid using tape directly on the skin. Demonstrate proper application techniques. If necessary, tape lightly. Use special protective pads and mattresses.
      If the patient is on bed rest, turn every 1 to 2 hours. Show the patient how to use a turn sheet; instruct the patient not to slide on the sheets. Keep bedsheets wrinkle free; change linens frequently if the patient is diaphoretic or incontinent.

P

Encourage the patient to position self on unaffected areas.

If the patient is incontinent, encourage frequent use of the commode. Tell the patient to avoid use of heavy or excessive incontinent pads, which can increase perspiration and irritate skin.

—Ulcer care, stages III and IV

After debridement, inspect the wound for size, color, odor, and drainage and record information. Cleanse the wound using prescribed procedure. Provide the caregiver with written instruction. Review the signs and symptoms to report: elevated temperature, increased drainage, foul odor.

Explain debridement or skin grafting procedures as indicated.

Discuss with the caretaker the importance of daily hygiene to prevent infection and skin breakdown. Stress the importance of regular (three times a day or more) inspections of bony prominences and maintaining skin integrity by keeping skin clean and dry. Use mild soap and water. Provide perineal care after voiding or bowel movement.

Avoid use of skin-damaging products: harsh soaps, alcohol-based lotions, tincture of benzoin, hexachlorophene.

Instruct the patient and caregiver not to use a heat lamp because it increases the metabolic rate of the tissues, resulting in increased demand for blood flow in an area with impaired perfusion. As a result, ulcer diameter and depth can be increased.

Instruct the patient and caregiver to gently massage the area around the bony prominence (not on it) and administer gentle back rubs with a bland emollient; remove any excess and avoid use of alcohol.

Instruct the patient and caregiver in protecting the heels, elbows, back of head, iliac crests, sacrum, and coccyx against skin breakdown by using foam rubber pads.

Demonstrate wound care, including cleansing procedure and application of medication and dressing changes.

Arrange to obtain equipment, such as pressure-reducing mattress, footboard, bed cradle, and wound care supplies, that will be used at home. Explain the function of pressure relief devices and demonstrate how to use the equipment properly. Advise the patient and caregiver on where to buy equipment, such as drugstores and medical supply stores.

Consult with an enterostomal therapist for specific wound care instruction if necessary.

- *Medications*
  —Explain the purpose, dosage, schedule, and route of administration of any prescribed drugs, as well as side effects to report to a physician or nurse.
- *Activity*
  —Explain the importance of increasing activity as tolerated, changing positions every 2 to 3 hours while in bed or in chair, and avoiding pressure on affected area.
  —Instruct the caregiver in assisting the patient out of bed and into a chair.
  —Teach active and passive range-of-motion exercises for all extremities and explain that they should be performed every 4 hours.
- *Diet*
  —Encourage a high-calorie, high-protein diet with adequate fluid intake (2 liters/day), unless contraindicated, to maintain body weight and promote healing.
  —For the debilitated patient, instruct the patient to eat small, frequent meals that include protein- and calorie-rich supplements.

FOLLOW-UP CARE

- Stress the importance of regular follow-up visits for medical and laboratory evaluation. Make sure the patient has the necessary names and telephone numbers.

Pulse Taking

—Pulse taking: measurement of the pulse, the regular contraction and expansion of an artery as the wave of blood passes through the blood vessel. Common sites for taking arterial pulses are the wrist (radial), neck (carotid), forehead (temporal), back of knee (popliteal), and inside of elbow (antecubitus). The most common sites for patients to take their own pulse are the wrist and neck.

HOME CARE

- Give both the patient and the caregiver *verbal* and *written* instructions. Provide them with the name and telephone number of a physician or nurse to call if questions arise.
- Explain what the pulse is, why the patient needs to take his or her pulse, and what to do if the pulse is too fast, too slow, or irregular.
- Explain that a number of factors can affect the pulse rate: exercise; stress; stimulants such as tobacco, caffeine, recreational or illicit drugs, and alcohol; cold or allergy medication; and imbalances of electrolytes such as sodium and potassium.
- Instruct the patient in taking the pulse, and permit time for return demonstration and practice.
  —Use two fingers, the pointer and middle fingers (the thumb is not suitable because it contains a pulse).
  —Place the two fingers *lightly* at the point of throbbing and pulsation. Explain that firm pressure may obliterate the pulse.
    Radial pulse (on the inside of the wrist): start at the outside of the wrist; slide the two fingers slightly inward until the pulse is felt.
    Carotid pulse (to the right or left of the throat area): start at the center of the throat just under the chin; slide the two fingers to the right or left about 1 inch until a pulsation is felt.
- Instruct the patient to count the pulses for 30 seconds and multiply by 2. Explain that this is the pulse rate per minute.
- Instruct the patient to record the pulse rate and indicate what he or she was doing or eating if the rate is slower, faster, or irregular compared with his or her normal rate. See the table on p. 721 for a sample pulse-taking diary.

Pulse-taking diary

My heart rate should be: _____

Date	Time	Heart rate	Notes

Radiation Therapy

—Radiation therapy: the major treatment modality in cancer care. Radiation therapy involves the use of gamma rays to disturb proliferation of cells by decreasing the rate of mitosis or impairing DNA synthesis, thereby reducing tumor mass. Radiation is used at all phases of the cancer trajectory: curative, adjuvant, and palliative.

TYPES OF RADIATION DELIVERY SYSTEMS

- External beam/teletherapy: the patient lies on a table at a distance from the source and is exposed to a prescribed dose of radiation on a daily basis. The radiation field usually includes the tumor and draining lymphatics.
- Implant therapy/brachytherapy (closed therapy): sealed sources implanted directly into the tumor or cavity surrounding the tumor. The sources used (cesium, iridium) are nonpenetrating and deposit most of the dose in a small area. The goal is to deliver a high dose to a small volume of tissue. The patient is

radioactive for the time the source is in place (usually 3 to 5 days). Precautions (time, distance, shielding) are necessary.
- Radiopharmaceutical/isotope therapy: use of unsealed sources such as liquids to treat cancers. The most commonly used is iodine-131 for thyroid cancer; the half-life is 8 days.
- Interstitial thermoradiotherapy: combination of heat with radiation. The dose can be delivered locally, regionally, or systemically (whole body) by electromagnetic, radiofrequency, or ultrasound techniques.
- Intraoperative radiation therapy: provides direct visualization and treatment of tumors to control local recurrences.
- Combination of chemotherapy and radiation therapy: to treat residual disease after surgery.
- Radiosensitizers: nonhypoxic or hypoxic agents used to increase lethal effects of radiation.

SIDE EFFECTS/COMPLICATIONS
- Acute (during treatment to 6 months), subacute (after 6 months), or chronic (with variable time to expression). Side effects are seen sooner in the skin, mucous membranes, and hair follicles and later in the vascular system and muscles. Early side effects are believed to be reparable; late effects are more often permanent.
- General effects: fatigue, anorexia
- Transient erythema: as early as first treatment; dry or wet desquamation in the second or third week
- Pulmonary effects: increased cough that is productive or nonproductive; dyspnea; pneumonitis (dyspnea, cough, fever, night sweats); late effect is fibrosis, usually asymptomatic
- Gastrointestinal effects: vomiting, anorexia, diarrhea, gastric distention
- Toxic effects: depend on site of irradiation, volume of tissue irradiated, total dosage delivered, time frame

DIAGNOSTIC TESTS
- Describe each procedure, its purpose, and the normal feelings or sensations that are likely, as well as any preprocedural and postprocedural care.
  —Complete blood cell count
  —Electrolytes
  —Urinalysis

TREATMENT
Medical

- Drugs
  —Antiemetics
  —Antibiotics
  —Antidiarrheals
  —Blood products
  —Pain management

🏠 HOME CARE

- Give both the patient and the caregiver *verbal* and *written* instructions. Provide them with the name and telephone number of a physician or nurse to call if questions arise.
- *General information*
  —Reinforce the physician's explanation of therapy: the type to be delivered, frequency and length of treatment (weeks), and expected side effects versus toxic effects.
  —Explain that high-dose radiation therapy causes sterility.
  —Discuss issues of fertility and sexual function including sperm banking and erectile dysfunction (p. 278) as indicated.
  —For women undergoing radiation therapy for endometrial cancer, explain that vaginal shrinkage may occur.
  —*Warning signs*
  —Review the signs and symptoms that should be reported to a physician or nurse.

    Skin reactions: redness, itching, swelling, dry or moist desquamation, pain
    Mucositis
    Nausea, vomiting
    Diarrhea
    Tachycardia
    Dyspnea
    Xerostomia
    For women undergoing radiation therapy for endometrial cancer: vaginal or rectal bleeding, foul-smelling discharge, abdominal pain, hematuria

- *Special instructions*
  —Discuss the need to prevent infection by avoiding large crowds and persons with upper respiratory tract infections.
  —Instruct patient and caretaker to inspect radiation sites daily.

R

—Instruct the patient in skin care, including maintenance of dye markings and the need to avoid use of soap and other ointments, sunbathing, and heat applications (see box on p. 725).

—Teach the patient the importance of oral hygiene if receiving oral, head, or neck radiation therapy (see Cancer, p. 150).

—Instruct the patient to avoid tight or constricting clothing around the radiation site. Instruct women receiving irradiation to the breast to avoid underwire bras and instead to use a loose sport bra for support.

• *Activity*

—Teach the patient how to manage fatigue and maintain mobility, for example, planning activities before and after treatment based on energy level.

—Encourage the patient to continue working and other activities of daily living as tolerated, including regular exercise.

• *Diet*

—Teach the patient the importance of a regular diet with small, frequent feedings as necessary.

—Advise the patient to avoid eating several hours before and after treatment to prevent nausea.

—Encourage fluid intake of up to 3000 ml/day.

FOLLOW-UP CARE

• Stress the importance of keeping all scheduled treatment, laboratory, and medical follow-up appointments. Make sure the patient has the necessary names and telephone numbers.

REFERRALS

• Provide referrals for home health care, social services, and a skilled nursing facility as indicated.

• Refer the patient to support groups and other community resources as needed.

SKIN CARE DURING EXTERNAL BEAM THERAPY

External beam radiation therapy can cause mild to severe skin reactions, based on how much radiation is given and how often, how much skin area is treated, and the type of radiation used. Usually in the first 2 weeks of treatment, the patient experiences **erythema** where the skin over the area being treated with radiation turns pink or red, becomes sensitive to sunlight, loses hair, or develops a rash. With more treatments, a condition called **dry desquamation** may develop; the skin may peel and become painful and weepy. Patients most likely will notice a skin reaction 10 days to 2 weeks after treatment has been completed. Hair loss from the treated scalp begins about 10 days after the first treatment.

Prevention of skin reactions

To prevent skin reactions or make them less severe, instruct the patient to do the following.

- Clean the skin with warm, not hot, water.
- After washing, rinse with tepid water and pat dry with a soft towel.
- Do not soak in a tub. Do not remove the treatment field markings during bathing. Avoid soap as much as possible. If soap is needed for adequate cleansing, use Aveeno, Dove, or some other mild, unscented soap that will not dry the skin.
- Do not use heating pads, hot packs, or ice on the area being treated.
- Do not use perfumed or powdered products on the treated skin. Do not use ointments or menthol rubs.
- Shave with an electric razor.
- Protect the skin from heat, cold, and sunlight by using a sunscreen with a sun protection factor of 15 or higher. Shield the face and neck with a scarf or wide-brimmed hat.
- Wear loose-fitting clothing. Tight clothes and belts rub and irritate already sensitive skin.

Continued

SKIN CARE DURING EXTERNAL BEAM THERAPY—cont'd

Prevention of skin reactions—cont'd
- Do not put adhesive bandages, such as Band-Aids, on treated skin.
- Use a light dusting of cornstarch to prevent itching and to remove moisture in neck creases and armpits and beneath the breasts.

Treatment of skin reactions

For dry desquamation, use pure aloe vera gel, vitamin A and D ointments, Lubriderm, or other water-soluble, nonirritating substances.

For moist desquamation, apply cool compresses moistened with water or normal saline. Special ointments may be prescribed. Moisture vapor-permeable film or other sterile dressings, such as Op-Site or Tegaderm, may be applied to the area to protect it while it heals. Instruct the patient to expose the area to air for 10 to 15 minutes two or three times per day. Moist desquamation usually heals 1 to 2 weeks after treatment ends.

For pain in the treated area, an over-the-counter analgesic such as aspirin, acetaminophen (e.g., Tylenol), or ibuprofen (e.g., Motrin, Advil) may be used. After the skin heals, it may still be sensitive to heat, cold, and sunlight. Some chemotherapy drugs cause "radiation recall," which is a return of the previous skin reaction, usually seen as redness in the treated area.

For hair loss, discuss with the patient that this is likely to occur during treatment. Instruct the patient to select scarves, hats, wigs, or hairpieces before treatment. Have the stylist match the real hair style to the wig so that the difference is less obvious when the patient begins to wear the wig. Hair loss is usually temporary but depends on the amount of radiation received, gender, age, and whether the patient also receives cancer chemotherapy.

Discuss the signs and symptoms to report to the physician or nurse: rash; dry, itchy, flaky areas; peeling and weeping; pain.

Tracheostomy Care

—**Tracheostomy: insertion of a tube into the trachea through a surgically created incision (tracheotomy).**

INDICATIONS

- Presence of tumor
- Upper airway obstruction by foreign body, edema, or mucus
- Conjunction with laryngectomy or neck resection
- Ventilator dependency
- Inability to maintain airway or clear secretions

HOME CARE

- Give both the patient and the caregiver *verbal* and *written* instructions. Provide them with the name and telephone number of a physician or nurse to call if questions arise.
- *General information*
  - —Explain the underlying cause and contributing factors.
  - —Describe and demonstrate the type of tracheostomy tube that has been inserted and permit time for the patient to practice removing and reinserting the outer and inner cannula.
- *Warning signs*
  - —Review the signs and symptoms that should be reported to a physician or nurse.
    - Stomal irritation
    - Infection: elevated temperature, purulent secretions, redness, bleeding
    - Persistent cough
    - Inability to remove secretions
    - Respiratory distress
- *Special instructions*
  - —Demonstrate skin care around the stoma: use soap, rinse with water, and pat dry. Avoid the use of hydrogen peroxide and Betadine, which may enhance skin breakdown.
  - —Discuss the need to shower daily: cover the tracheostomy with a stoma shield; when using a shower hose, direct the spray below the neck and avoid getting soap into the stoma.
  - —For male patients, discuss the need to shave with an electric razor or safety razor and to avoid getting lather into the stoma.

—Inform the patient of the need to keep the stoma covered at all times. Suggest wearing clothing with high necklines and scarves to protect against foreign materials.

—Teach the patient and caregiver how to use oxygen and other respiratory equipment at home. Advise them on where to obtain equipment (e.g., pharmacy, medical supply company).

—Instruct the patient in handwashing technique, stressing the importance of washing the hands before cleaning the tracheostomy after suctioning.

—Instruct the patient in disposal of soiled dressings and supplies.

—Demonstrate suctioning technique: take three or four deep breaths before and after suctioning if breathing spontaneously.

—Demonstrate insertion of the suction catheter until resistance is felt.

—Instruct the patient to apply suction when the catheter is pulled out. Limit suction to 10 seconds only.

—Demonstrate cleaning and storage of suction catheters: rinse the catheter thoroughly with running water, soak it in hydrogen peroxide for 5 minutes, rinse thoroughly, place it in boiling water for 10 to 15 minutes, allow it to air dry on a clean towel, and store in a clean plastic bag. Inform the patient that catheters may be used for multiple days and discarded when secretions cannot be removed completely.

—Demonstrate care of the tracheostomy tube. Stress the importance of using clean technique when cleaning the tracheostomy. Tracheostomy dressings are not necessary unless secretions are excessive. Emphasize the importance of covering the stoma when coughing.

—Teach and demonstrate procedures for cleaning cannulas, changing tracheostomy ties, and changing dressings.

—Instruct the patient to sit upright or in a semireclining position with the neck hyperextended.

—Teach the caregiver how to clear a plugged tracheostomy.

—Discuss the need to use a commercial humidifier or pan of water on the stove to add comfort and prevent encrustation. Instruct the patient to avoid extremes of temperature because they can irritate the tracheal mucosa.

—Discuss the need to avoid persons with respiratory infections and respiratory irritants (e.g., smoke, dust, fumes, aerosols, powder).

—Instruct the patient to carry some means of communication (e.g., pad and pencil, magic slate).

—Assist the patient in organizing an emergency kit containing an extra tube (same size or smaller) and supplies.

• *Medications*

—Explain the purpose, dosage, schedule, and route of administration of any prescribed drugs, as well as side effects to report to a physician or nurse.

—Discuss the need to avoid taking over-the-counter medications without first checking with a physician.

• *Activity*

—Advise the patient of the importance of exercising to tolerance and planning rest periods.

—Tell the patient that swimming is not permitted.

• *Diet*

—Explain that a regular diet should be followed unless contraindicated.

—Instruct the patient with a tracheostomy tube with a cuff to inflate the tube while eating and deflate after meals.

—Advise the patient to drink at least 3000 ml daily unless contraindicated.

—Explain the administration of tube feedings if ordered (see Tube Feeding, p. 734).

—Instruct the patient to sit in an upright position during meals or tube feeding administration.

FOLLOW-UP CARE

• Stress the importance of regular follow-up visits. Make sure the patient has the necessary names and telephone numbers.

• Assist the patient to obtain a MedicAlert band identifying the patient as a neck breather for emergency situations.

• Stress the importance of not smoking or using tobacco products and of avoiding passive smoking.

REFERRALS

• Assist the patient to obtain referrals for home care services, equipment, supplies, and social services as needed.

• Provide a referral for a speech pathologist.

• Provide community support resources and phone numbers for psychologic counseling and respite care.

Transfer Techniques

—Transfer techniques: procedures used to prevent injury to patients and caregivers when patients are unable to move about independently or require assistance to change position or with ambulation. Utilized correctly, these techniques promote the use of good body mechanics by the caregiver and maximize the patient's functional ability.

🏠 HOME CARE

- Give both the patient and caregiver *verbal* and *written* instructions tailored to the patient's specific needs and equipment.
- Provide them with the name and telephone number of a physician or nurse to call if questions arise.
- *General information*
  —Stress the importance of using good body mechanics by all family members and caregivers.
  —Encourage the patient to assist as much as is physically possible.
  —Demonstrate the technique to be used for the patient.
  —Permit time for practice.

ASSISTIVE DEVICES/EQUIPMENT

- Discuss devices and equipment available to prevent unnecessary strain on the lower back.
- Advise the caregiver where to obtain the following equipment.
  —Transfer belt
  —Quad cane
  —Walker
  —Wheelchair

BED TO CHAIR TRANSFER
Preprocedural Care

This technique is used for chairs, wheelchairs, commodes, or shower chairs.

- Instruct the caregiver to secure equipment before beginning the transfer procedure.
  —Bed: secure wheel locks and lower the bed to its lowest setting if the patient is in a hospital bed.

—Wheelchair: fold up the foot rests and lock the wheels, if moving the patient to a wheelchair.

—Chair: cover the chair seat with a pad, blanket, or cushion if appropriate.

—Commode: raise the lid of the commode, if moving the patient to a commode.

• Place a chair next to the bed facing either the head or foot of the bed. Place the chair on the side of the bed that is the patient's strongest side.

• Adjust the head of the bed according to the patient's condition, needs, and preference.

• Lower the side rail.

Procedure

• Instruct the caregiver to:

—Assist the patient to sit up with the feet dangling over the side of the bed for a few minutes before transfer.

—Assess the patient for signs of distress: paleness, difficulty breathing, weakness, dizziness/lightheadedness, or perspiration.

—Assist the patient to put on nonskid shoes or slippers, as desired.

—Put a transfer belt on the patient if used, and assist the patient to move to the edge of the bed.

Stand with the neck, shoulders, back, hips, and feet in as straight a line as possible, placing the feet flat and apart to provide a broad base of support.

Face the patient, standing close, flex the knees and hips, and instruct the patient to place hands on the caregiver's shoulders. Place the caregiver's knees against the patient's knees or just outside patient's knees.

Place hands under the patient's shoulders against the ribcage, or if a transfer belt is used, grasp the belt with both hands behind the patient.

—Tell the patient when ready to move, so that the patient can assist. Help the patient to stand at the agreed-upon signal (e.g., "on three; one, two, three!").

—Once the patient is standing, help the patient turn so that the backs of the legs are touching the chair seat.

—Ask the patient to place hands on the chair arms if appropriate for the type of chair.

—Slowly lower the patient onto the chair seat.

T

—As appropriate, lower the foot rests of the wheelchair.

—Remove the transfer belt if used.

—Ensure that the patient is comfortable with appropriate body alignment.

CHAIR TO BED TRANSFER
Preprocedural Care

This technique may be used for hospital beds or personal home-style beds.

- Place the wheelchair next to the bed facing either the head or foot of the bed. Fold up the foot rests and lock the wheels.
- Secure the bed wheel locks and lower the bed to its lowest setting if the patient is moving to a medical bed.
- Adjust the head of the bed according to the patient's condition, needs, and preference.
- Raise the side rail on the far side of the bed.

Procedure

- Instruct the caregiver to
  —Put a transfer belt on the patient if used, and assist the patient to move to the edge of the chair.
  —Stand with the neck, shoulders, back, hips, and feet in as straight a line as possible, placing the feet flat and apart to provide a broad base of support
  —Face the patient, standing close, flex the knees and hips, and instruct the patient to place hands on the caregiver's shoulders. Place the caregiver's knees against patient's knees or just outside patient's knees.
  —Place hands under the patient's shoulders against the ribcage, or if a transfer belt used, grasp the belt with both hands behind the patient.
  —Tell the patient when ready to move, so that the patient can assist at the agreed-upon signal.
  —If necessary, rock the patient three times, increasing the momentum on the third rock to raise the patient to standing (often necessary if the patient is rising from an easy chair).
  —Once the patient is standing, help the patient turn so that the backs of the legs are touching the bed.
  —Ask the patient to place hands on the bed.
  —Slowly lower the patient onto the bed.
  —Remove the transfer belt if used.
  —Assist the patient into a comfortable position.

SITTING TO STANDING
Preprocedural Care

- Use the procedures outlined above up to the point of standing if the patient is ambulatory.
- Position assistive devices such as a walker, cane, or quad cane.
- Instruct the caregiver to have the patient wear well-fitting, comfortable shoes. Before the patient stands, position the assistive device for easy grasping.

Procedure

- Support the patient until he or she is able to stand steadily.
- With the patient standing, instruct the caregiver to have the patient stand straight, but not place all of weight on the walker or cane.
  —Walker: assist the patient to take the walker and:
      Stand close to, but not touching, the front of the walker.
      Pick up the walker and move it forward, placing all four legs of the walker down.
      Step into the walker with a normal step, using the arms to help support and steady balance.
      Ensure that the patient leans slightly forward, not backward.
  —Cane: assist the patient to take the cane on the stronger side and hold it with straight wrist about 5 inches from the outside of the small toe.

CAR TRANSFER FROM WHEELCHAIR
Preprocedural Care

- Fully open the car door and position the seat as far back as it will go.
- Roll down the window to provide a stable surface to hold, if necessary.

Procedure

- Follow the appropriate transfer procedure.
- Remove both foot rests from the wheelchair.
- Instruct the caregiver to stand slightly to one side and assist from over, rather than around, the patient.
- Protect the patient's head while getting in or out of the car.
- Assist the patient to fasten the safety belt.

Tube Feeding
(Enteral Feeding)

—Tube feeding: nutritional support provided by the enteral route for the treatment or prevention of malnutrition. Enteral products are composed of standard and modular formulas and are used for tube feeding. A gastric feeding tube or a gastrostomy tube may be used. The gastric feeding tube is placed through the naris (nasogastric) or mouth (orogastric) into the stomach. The gastrostomy tube is inserted through an opening created in the stomach. It is indicated for patients who require prolonged nutritional support. A gastrostomy button has been shown to decrease many of the disadvantages of the gastrostomy tube (e.g., leakage, mobility, catheter occlusion and expulsion).

INDICATIONS
- Debilitated comatose patient
- Strictures of esophagus
- Malignant neoplasms

SIDE EFFECTS/COMPLICATIONS
- Pulmonary aspiration (nasogastric tube)
- Mechanical problems: obstruction, displacement
- Metabolic problems (e.g., diarrhea, dehydration, hyperglycemia, electrolyte imbalances, vitamin and trace element deficiencies, high gastric residuals)
- Gastrostomy: skin irritation, breakdown

▦ HOME CARE
- Give both the patient and the caregiver *verbal* and *written* instructions. Provide them with the name and telephone number of a physician or nurse to call if questions arise.
- *General information*
  —Discuss the purpose and indication for and type of enteral feedings.

- *Warning signs*
  - —Review the signs and symptoms that should be reported to a physician or nurse.
    - Gastrointestinal intolerance: nausea, vomiting, abdominal distention, cramping, diarrhea
    - Wound infection with gastrostomy: fever, redness, drainage, swelling, tenderness, odor
- *Special instructions*
  - —Advise the caregiver on how and where to obtain formula, equipment, and supplies (e.g., drug store, medical supply company).
  - —Teach care of the feeding tube.
    - For a nasogastric tube, wash gently with soap and water and pat dry. Secure the tube to prevent tension on the patient's tissue and skin.
    - For a gastrostomy, teach the patient how to change the tube. Explain that the tube can be removed after several weeks and reinserted for feedings. The skin around the tube should be inspected daily and the skin washed gently and patted dry. Cotton-tip applicators may be used to clean around the stoma site.
  - —Instruct and demonstrate how to avoid nausea and vomiting: avoid rapid infusion and adjust rate as ordered.
  - —Discuss the need to flush the tube with 50 to 150 ml of water after each feeding or medication administration. Blocked tubes should be flushed with proteolytic enzyme papain (Adolph's Meat Tenderizer), pancreatic enzyme (Viokase), cola, or cranberry juice using a syringe.
  - —Demonstrate preparation and administration of the feeding. Demonstrate use of a pump if the patient will receive continuous feedings. Permit time for practice by the caregiver.
  - —Instruct the caregiver to keep a record of the amount, time, and frequency of and patient tolerance to feedings.
- *Medications*
  - —Explain the purpose, dosage, schedule, and route of administration of any prescribed drugs, as well as side effects to report to a physician or nurse.
  - —Instruct the caregiver to substitute a liquid preparation for pills or to crush the pill into a fine powder and dissolve in 30 ml of water after consulting with a physician or pharmacist.

- *Diet*
  —Discuss the prescribed type and amount of feeding. Instruct the patient to elevate the head of the bed more than 30 degrees during feeding and for an hour after feeding to prevent regurgitation or aspiration. Show the caregiver how to check for tube feeding residual before each feeding.
  —Demonstrate irrigation of the feeding tube with 50 ml of warm water before administering feeding. Explain that if the patient coughs or appears to be choking, the feedings should not be administered and the physician should be notified.
  —Explain that only enough formula for 24 hours should be prepared and that formula must not hang for more than 8 hours (without an ice pouch).
  —Tell the caregiver to administer the feeding formula at room temperature. Instruct the caregiver to refrigerate all opened products and discard after 24 hours, to use clean technique when handling the feeding tube and enteral products, and to change the feeding equipment every 24 hours.

FOLLOW-UP CARE

- Stress the importance of regular follow-up medical and laboratory evaluations. Make sure the patient has the necessary names and telephone numbers.

Urinary Catheter
(Foley, Suprapubic Catheter)

—Urinary catheter: indwelling catheter inserted through the urethra or through the abdomen (suprapubic) into the bladder to drain the urine into a drainage bag.

INDICATIONS

- Total incontinence
- Neurogenic bladder
- Inability to urinate because of enlarged prostate

PREPROCEDURAL TEACHING

- Review the physician's explanation of the procedure and the reason for it; encourage the patient to ask questions and to discuss any fears or anxieties.
- Review catheter insertion.
    —Urethral approach: a thin flexible tube/catheter with a balloon is inserted through the urethra into the bladder. Once inserted, the balloon is inflated to prevent it from slipping out and is connected to a drainage bag. The catheter is taped to the thigh to prevent pulling.
    —Suprapubic or abdominal approach: the procedure may be done under local or general anesthesia and requires written consent. A urinary bladder catheter is inserted through the skin about 1 inch above the symphysis pubis and is sutured to the abdominal skin.

Review of Postprocedural Care

- Explain that the catheter is taped in place securely and a different site is used every day.
- Instruct the patient to keep the drainage bag below the level of the bladder.
- Explain that the abdominal dressing is changed every day; the area is cleansed with Betadine and sterile gauze is taped in place.

SIDE EFFECTS/COMPLICATIONS

- Urinary tract infection
- Catheter obstruction
- Pyelonephritis
- Urinary tract stones
- Difficulty in urinating after removal
- Infection at site of insertion of suprapubic catheter

🔲 HOME CARE

- Give both the patient and the caregiver *verbal* and *written* instructions. Provide them with the name and telephone number of a physician or nurse to call if questions arise.
- *General information*
    —Explain the underlying reason for the procedure.

- *Warning signs*
  —Review the signs, symptoms, and problems that should be reported to a physician or nurse.

  Lack of urine output longer than 4 hours (check for kinks)

  Infection: low back pain or flank pain; cloudy, foul-smelling urine; bloody urine; fever; chills; poor appetite; lack of energy; sediment in urine

  Persistent leakage around the catheter

  Pain, tenderness, or swelling around the catheter

  Break in the catheter

  Catheter falls out

- *Special instructions*
  —Explain that a *urethral catheter* may create the urge to urinate. Stress the importance of not trying to remove the catheter.

  —Explain that urethral catheter anchoring sites should be alternated daily (the inner thigh for women and the upper thigh or abdomen for men) and taped securely to prevent accidental pulling.

  —Instruct a patient with a *suprapubic catheter* to cleanse the "new" insertion or stoma site with a Betadine solution (if the patient is not sensitive to iodine) and cover it with a gauze dressing. Crusting may be cleaned with a Q-tip and hydrogen peroxide and rinsed with water.

  —Discuss daily care of a suprapubic catheter.

  Explain that a "seasoned" stoma may be washed with unscented soap and water.

  Inspect the peristomal site for redness or drainage; gently clean the area with mild soap and water.

  If the catheter accidentally comes out, instruct the patient to cover with a clean 4 × 4 gauze square, secure it with tape, and notify the physician or nurse.

  Tell the patient that a suprapubic catheter may be taped to the abdomen if necessary.

  —Instruct the patient to monitor and record urine output for amount and color of urine.

  —Explain that the catheter should be connected to a drainage bag and the bag should be below the level of the bladder to prevent flow back into the bladder whether the patient is lying, sitting, or standing. Inform the patient that the drainage bag may be carried in a shopping bag while the patient is walking or the catheter may be connected to a leg bag.

—Discuss the types of drainage bags, and advise the patient where to obtain supplies.

> Leg bag: usually used during the day. The tubing attaches directly to the catheter, and the bag holds about 500 ml (½ quart). Advise the patient to choose a bag that does not bulge when full. The leg bag is attached to the leg with cloth or Velcro straps or fits into a cloth sleeve. It should not show under clothing. Rubber straps should not be used, since they irritate the skin. The drainage valve or cap should be accessible and easily opened.

> Drainage bag: a larger drainage bag is used for night and should hold about 1500 ml (1½ quarts). The bedside bag should have plenty of tubing to allow movement in bed. The bag should be placed on a stand below the level of the catheter. The drainage valve or cap should be accessible and easily opened.

—Demonstrate how to empty the drainage bag and tell the patient it should be emptied every 8 hours or when filled.

> Hold the bag over the toilet.

> Free the drain tip, loosen the clamp, and drain the bag into the toilet or collection container. Reclamp the tube and clean the tip of the drain tube with Betadine solution.

> Do not touch the tip of the drain tube or let the drain tube touch the toilet or collecting container.

—Demonstrate how to change drainage bags.

> Wash hands.

> Wipe the connection with alcohol.

> Protect the ends of the catheter and tubing with a clean gauze square when disconnecting the catheter and before reconnecting it to the drainage system.

—Explain that bags may be reused after careful cleansing.

> Rinse the inside of the bag with soapy water and then rinse well with clear water. Fill the bag with one part vinegar to four parts water and soak the inside for 30 minutes.

> Empty the bag and let it air dry.

> Store in a clean, dust-free place until ready to use again.

—Stress the importance of perineal care and demonstrate.

> Wash around the urethral catheter to prevent crusting. Wash with unscented soap and water twice a day and dry gently.

> Wash around the rectal area with soap and water twice a day or after each bowel movement.

- *Medications*
  —Explain the purpose, dosage, schedule, and route of administration of any prescribed drugs, as well as side effects to report to a physician or nurse.
- *Activity*
  —Encourage the patient to discuss allowances and limitations with respect to occupation, recreation, or activities.
  —Explain that showering or bathing may be done on instructions from the physician (depending on the underlying reason for catheter placement).
- *Diet*
  —Inform the patient that the diet is regular or as prescribed by the physician according to the underlying condition.
  —Stress the importance of drinking 10 to 15 glasses of clear fluids and juices per day unless restricted by the underlying condition. Cranberry, plum, and prune juices help prevent urinary tract infection.
  —Inform the patient that consumption of caffeine and alcohol should be kept to a minimum.

FOLLOW-UP CARE

- Stress the importance of regular follow-up visits. Make sure the patient has the necessary names and telephone numbers.

REFERRALS

- Provide referrals for home health care services, including information on where to obtain the necessary supplies as indicated.

Urinary Diversion
(Ileal Conduit)

—Urinary diversion: surgical procedure performed to provide an alternative route for urine excretion. A number of procedures may be done to divert urinary flow through a new opening on the abdomen. In an *ileal conduit* (Bricker), a segment of ileum is cut away to create a receptacle or pouch to which the ureters are connected. One end is sewn closed, and the other is brought to an opening in the abdominal wall to form a stoma (opening) through which urine flows continuously into a special bag strapped to the body. An external bag must be worn at all times. In a *continent urinary diversion* (Kock pouch), a segment of ileum is cut away to form a reservoir (internal pouch) for urine to which the ureters are attached. Two natural valves or "nipple valves" are created, one to prevent backflow and the other to maintain continence. Self-catheterization is required. The *hemi-Kock pouch* is a neobladder made of the intestinal pouch (see above). It is used only in men because the female urethra is too short, and strong abdominal muscular pressure against the bladder is needed to urinate through the penis.

INDICATIONS

- Cystectomy
- Severe neuropathic bladder
- Severe interstitial cystitis

PREPROCEDURAL TEACHING

- Review the physician's explanation of the procedure and the reason for it; encourage the patient to ask questions and to discuss any fears or anxieties. Explain the need for informed consent for surgery, anesthesia, blood transfusions, and photographs if needed.

Review of Preprocedural Care

- Explain that the patient will be admitted to the hospital 1 day before surgery.
- Explain that the enterostomal nurse will come to interview the patient, show appliances, and mark the abdomen for the ostomy site.
- Discuss bowel preparation.
  —Two days before surgery the patient should ingest only clear fluids and possibly a laxative.
  —The day before surgery the patient is asked to drink at least 4000 ml (1 gallon) of specially prepared solution (GoLYTELY) over a 6-hour period (antiemetics are given beforehand).

U

—After bowel movements are clear, oral antibiotics are given to "sterilize the intestines."

- Tell the patient that the pubic hair may be clipped the night before and the patient may be shaved from the nipple line to midthigh, including the perineum.
- Discuss the need to shower with bactericidal soap (e.g., Hibiclens).
- Inform the patient of the need for nothing by mouth (NPO) status from midnight the night before.
- Explain that intravenous hydration and intravenous antibiotics will be started.

Review of Postprocedural Care

- See general care under Abdominal Surgery, p. 6.
- Tell the patient that the procedure takes 3 to 4 hours or more and is performed with the patient under general anesthesia.
- Review the drainage tubes that may be used: urethral catheter (usually removed after 2 or more days except with a hemi-Kock procedure); two drainage tubes through the stoma from the new reservoir ("pouch"); flat Penrose drain and/or Jackson-Pratt drain near the incision; ureteral stents from kidneys.

COMPLICATIONS

- Urine leakage at internal connections
- Hemorrhage
- Paralytic ileus
- Wound infection
- Impotence (temporary or permanent)
- Obstruction at ureteral junction sites
- Dyspareunia
- Peristomal hernia
- Stomal prolapse, retraction, necrosis
- Deep vein thrombosis
- Pulmonary embolism
- Prolonged diarrhea or bowel dysfunction
- Fistula
- Metabolic acidosis
- Electrolyte imbalances

🏠 HOME CARE

- Give both the patient and the caregiver *verbal* and *written* instructions. Provide them with the name and telephone number of a physician or nurse to call if questions arise.
- *Wound/incision care*
  - —Provide instruction on wound care and dressing changes.
  - —Discuss the care of drainage tubes. Explain that catheters remain in the stoma about 4 weeks and that a "Kock-o-gram" or "pouch-o-gram" (contrast material instilled into the pouch and x-rays taken) will be performed to confirm healing of all suture lines before catheters are removed.
- *Warning signs*
  - —Review the signs and symptoms of perforation that should be reported to a physician or nurse.
      - Infection: redness, swelling, warm to touch, tenderness, purulent drainage
      - Change in appearance of stoma: protruding, receding, bluish tint, excoriation, redness
      - Acute abdominal pain or persistent pain
      - Change in bowel habits: constipation, diarrhea, flatulence (gas)
      - Urinary tract infection: cloudy urine, fever, malaise
      - Difficulty in self-catheterization
      - No urine output after 4 hours and after irrigation
      - Hematuria
- *Special instructions*
  - —Advise and assist the patient in obtaining supplies. Provide a list of the supplies needed, including size and type of appliance.
  - —Emphasize the importance of having enough supplies and carrying supplies when traveling.
  - —Stress the importance of maintaining free flow of urine (mucus will always be present in urine because the intestine normally sheds mucus; occasional flecks of blood may also be present).
  - —Demonstrate catheter irrigation.
      - Gather supplies: saline solution and piston syringe. Saline solution may be made by adding 1 tablespoon of salt to 1 quart of distilled water, mixing, and refrigerating, or by placing 1 quart of water in a clean pan on the stove, bringing to a boil, removing and allowing to cool to

U

room temperature, pouring the water into a clean quart-size container, adding 1 tablespoon salt and mixing, covering with a lid, and refrigerating. Any remaining solution should be discarded after 2 days.

Wash hands.

Draw up 30 ml of saline solution in the syringe and set it aside.

Clean the connection with soap and water; then rinse. Disconnect the catheter from the drainage tubing.

Insert the tip of the syringe into the catheter and inject the solution slowly (do not force).

Pull back on the syringe to remove the saline solution and mucus and discard into the toilet.

If the fluid does not return, attach the catheter to the drainage tubing and let it drain by gravity. (If it does not drain within 5 minutes, repeat the preceding steps using 15 ml of solution.)

If the catheter is not draining well between irrigations, irrigate it an extra time.

After the catheter is removed, another catheter will be inserted for daily irrigations.

The 60 ml (cc) piston syringe may be used again. Separate the parts, wash with unscented soap and water, rinse, and let air dry. Store in a clean, dry place.

—Review the technique for self-catheterization.

Gather all supplies: paper towels, special catheter, water-soluble lubricant, piston syringe, and saline solution.

Wash hands.

Remove the dressing or bag from the stoma.

Lubricate the tip of the catheter.

Insert the catheter into the stoma until urine flows. When it stops, insert a few more inches until flow stops completely. Irrigate as described above.

Remove the catheter. Cleanse the area and reapply the dressing or ostomy bag.

Keep a catheter and supplies available even when going out.

Stress the importance of maintaining a self-catheterization schedule after the catheter is removed (a different schedule may be advised).

Week	Day	Night
1	Every 2 hours	Every 3 hours
2	Every 3 hours	Every 4 hours
3	Every 4 hours	Every 5 hours
4	Every 5 hours	Every 6 hours

The goal is to reach a schedule of 4 or 5 times a day, allowing for at least 7 hours of uninterrupted sleep per night. This is influenced by the size of the pouch and amount of fluids taken in. Explain that almost all men leak urine from the penis after removal of the catheter. Kegel exercises (see Urinary Incontinence, p. 749) will decrease leakage after several weeks, but the patient may still have some leakage at night.

—Teach the patient how to change the appliance, using instructions provided by the enterostomal nurse.

Gather all supplies: paper towels, gauze, washcloth, or tampon; selected appliance with precut opening; powder (e.g., karaya or Stomahesive); skin sealant; tape; plastic bag for used items.

Wash hands.

Remove the old pouch, using adhesive solvent if necessary to loosen the seal. Since the solvent is flammable, do not smoke or be near flames when removing the pouch.

Wash the stoma with warm water and let dry. A paper towel, gauze, washcloth, or tampon may be used as a wick over the stoma until the new bag is placed.

Inspect the skin and stoma for discolored (bluish) areas, redness, irritation, excoriation, excessive swelling, or excessive hair. For mild irritation, dust the skin lightly with karaya or Stomahesive. Severe irritation may necessitate a skin barrier (wafer cut to fit around the stoma).

If no irritation is present and the skin needs shaving, shave it dry over karaya powder.

Put skin sealant on over the powder and let dry (change wick if needed).

Put the wafer in place without creases and centered around the stoma. Remove the paper.

Place the pouch or ostomy plate over the wafer or, if there is no wafer, directly on the skin. Avoid making wrinkles or creases.

Close the spout on the bag.

Place tape around all edges of the ostomy pouch to increase wearing time.

Connect the appliance to a leg bag or let it drain into an ostomy bag, but empty the bag when half full so as not to break the skin seal.

—Instruct the patient to connect the appliance to continuous closed-gravity drainage at night. Keep the drainage appliance lower than the tube.

—Stress the importance of daily inspection of the stoma, noting color and size (should be pink; size will decrease after 6 months but stoma will not be flush with the abdomen).

—Discuss sexual activity. Explain that normal activity can be resumed unless a male patient has had a cystectomy. For impotent men, discuss other methods of sexual expression and procedures available (see Erectile Dysfunction, p. 278). Advise women to use extra lubricant.

—Inform the patient that showering and bathing may be resumed as recommended by the physician.

• *Medications*

—Explain the purpose, dosage, schedule, and route of administration of any prescribed drugs, as well as side effects to report to a physician or nurse.

• *Activity*

—Encourage the patient to discuss allowances and limitations with respect to occupation, recreation, or activity (see Abdominal Surgery, p. 6).

• *Diet*

—Inform the patient that a regular diet or one prescribed by the physician for the underlying condition should be followed.

—Explain that some foods (e.g., asparagus, fish, eggs, spicy foods) cause a strong urine odor but that drops or tablets may be placed in the pouch to decrease odors.

—Encourage the patient to drink 10 to 12 glasses of clear fluids a day. Tell the patient that cranberry juice helps cut down on mucus. Advise decreasing fluid intake in the evening to permit uninterrupted sleep.

PSYCHOSOCIAL CARE

- Encourage the expression of feelings about the changes in body image and sexual function. Assist the patient, family, and significant other to obtain counseling if necessary.

FOLLOW-UP CARE

- Stress the importance of follow-up visits. Make sure the patient has the necessary names and telephone numbers.
- Encourage or assist the patient to obtain a MedicAlert bracelet and identification card listing diagnosis, medication, and other data.

REFERRALS

- Assist the patient to obtain referrals for home health care services, supplies, equipment, and medical social services as needed.
- Assist the patient to identify community-based resources and support programs.
- Direct the patient to the United Ostomy Association as a source for further information.

Urinary Diversion Care

—Urinary diversion care: The most common type of urinary diversion is the ileal conduit, in which a piece of small bowel is used as a passage (conduit) for urine to the surface of the skin. This piece of bowel is closed at one end. The other end is brought to the surface of the abdomen to form a stoma (opening). The ureters are attached inside the abdomen so that urine drains through the ileal conduit and out through the stoma. Other urinary diversions include colon conduit (the sigmoid colon is used as the passage), ureterostomy (the ureters are brought through the abdominal wall to form a stoma), and vesicotomy (an opening into the bladder).

U

APPLYING AN OSTOMY POUCH

- Peel back the paper from the adhesive faceplate. Center the pouch opening over the stoma, and press all around the

faceplate to ensure that it is firmly attached to the skin. Attach the belt for additional security if you wish.
- Press the air out of the pouch. Clamp the bottom.

REMOVING AN OSTOMY POUCH

Explain the need to change the ostomy pouch every 5 to 7 days. Instruct the patient to gather the following equipment before beginning: adhesive solvent, gauze pads, powder (if desired), towel, and scissors. Describe the procedure.

- While standing, hold the skin around the stoma taut and begin peeling off the adhesive square that holds the pouch to the skin. Peeling from top to bottom works best. If the pouch does not peel off, use adhesive solvent to loosen the edges.
- Wipe away excess drainage from around the stoma with gauze pads.
- Wash the area around the stoma with soap and water. Dry thoroughly. Apply powder if the skin is irritated. You may also want to apply a skin barrier.

COLLECTING URINE FOR CULTURE AND SENSITIVITY

- The nurse or physician will remove the external pouch and insert a sterile catheter into the stoma to collect a sterile specimen.

SPECIAL ASPECTS OF CARE

- Use a skin barrier or liquid film to protect the skin from irritation.
- Drink at least 8 glasses of water a day.
- Test urine pH regularly, using a freshly voided specimen before a meal. The pH should be 4.5 to 8. Test sticks are available at drugstores. Vitamin C works well for keeping an acid urine. Odor may indicate an alkaline urine, which can cause stones to form or a urinary tract infection to develop.
- *General information*
  —Review the type of procedure performed and the drains and catheters left in place.
- *Warning signs*
  —Review the signs and symptoms that should be reported to a physician or nurse.
  Blockage of catheter
  Fever, chills

Continued bright red blood in the urine after several days

Leakage of urine around the catheter

Wound infection (redness, tenderness, warm to touch, possible drainage of pus)

Onset of or increased vaginal discharge or bleeding

- *Special instructions*
  —Review the care of catheters: indwelling or suprapubic catheter (see Urinary Catheter, p. 736).
  —Explain the postvoid residual technique.

    Establish a time schedule (usually every 4 hours, or more often if needed).

    Sit on the toilet for at least 5 minutes and urinate normally (may take 2 or more days before normal urination).

    After urination, measure the postvoid residual by opening the suprapubic catheter and emptying into a receptacle.

    Amount of urine from the suprapubic catheter should decrease as normal urination amount increases.

    Keep a record of the amounts voided and postvoid.

  —Teach the patient how to unplug the suprapubic catheter.

    Wash hands.

    Wipe the connection with alcohol.

    Grasp the plug with one hand and the catheter end with the other hand.

    Gently twist the plug to loosen and remove it while squeezing the catheter with the other hand (thumb and index finger).

    Place the catheter end over the receptacle and open to drain.

    Replace the plug.

  —Discuss the importance of cleansing the perineum at least twice a day.

  —Stress the importance of cleansing the rectal area at least twice a day or after every bowel movement.

Urinary Incontinence

—**Urinary incontinence: frequent or constant involuntary loss of urine control. It commonly occurs in older people, but may** occur in people of all ages. Urinary incontinence also may occur as result of disease, injury to the spinal cord, fatigue, or confusion. *Stress incontinence* is leakage of urine during laughing, coughing, sneezing, or exercise. It occurs when bladder pressure exceeds urethral pressure and is the most common type of incontinence. *Functional incontinence* is associated with diseases and injuries (head injury, dementia, or impaired mobility); there is no physical impairment. *Reflex incontinence* is a lack of impulse sensed by bladder fullness. It occurs as a result of spinal injury or other neurologic abnormality. *Urge incontinence* (instability incontinence) is the sensation of a full bladder and the inability to reach the toilet in time. It occurs in patients with conditions such as diabetes, stroke, dementia, Parkinson's disease, and multiple sclerosis. *Overflow* or *total incontinence* is the constant leakage of urine in the presence of a large residual (retention) due to bladder obstruction (e.g., prostate enlargement) or loss of bladder function.

CAUSES/CONTRIBUTING FACTORS

- Neurologic factors
  —Spinal cord injury and neurogenic bladder
  —Dementia
  —Stroke
  —Diseases: multiple sclerosis, Parkinson's disease
- Women
  —Anatomy
  —Childbearing: weakens pelvic muscles and causes sphincter incompetence
- Urologic factors
  —Procedures/surgery
  —Urinary tract infection; urinary tract obstruction
- Environmental/extraneous factors
  —Drugs: diuretics, cardiac medications, sleeping pills
  —Radiation therapy

SIGNS/SYMPTOMS

- Imcomplete bladder emptying
- Incontinence
  —Dribbling of urine
  —Loss of urine with increased intraabdominal pressure (e.g., cough, sneeze)

—Involuntary urination
- Frequency, urgency
- Large amounts of urine output

COMPLICATIONS

- Urinary tract infection
- Pyelonephritis
- Septic shock
- Implantation devices
    —Erosion of scrotum, labia, or bladder-urethra junction
    —Mechanical failure
    —Dysreflexia (see Neurogenic Bladder, p. 459)

DIAGNOSTIC TESTS

- Describe each procedure, its purpose, and the normal feelings or sensations that are likely, as well as any preprocedural and postprocedural care.
    —Urine studies: urinalysis; culture and sensitivity
    —Urodynamic studies: to determine cause and extent of incontinence
        Cystometrogram: to measure pressure-volume relationship of bladder
        Voiding cystourethrogram and pressure-flow studies: to measure pressure of various areas and flow rates of urine
        Uroflowmetry: to provide information about bladder strength and ability of the urethral sphincter to open
        Urethral pressure profile: use of a special catheter inserted into the urethra to measure the closing pressure of the urethra to stop the urine flow
        Sphincter electromyography: to evaluate the urinary sphincter and compare the results with those from cystometry
    —Intravenous pyelogram/urogram
    —Postvoid residual: to measure how much is left in the bladder after normal voiding (>100 ml indicates retention problem)
    —Cystoscopy: to determine loss of muscle elasticity
    —Blood studies: to evaluate kidney function

TREATMENT
Medical

- *Therapy*
  —Behavioral techniques: to help the patient sense bladder filling and delay voiding until he or she can reach the toilet with the goal of reducing small voidings

    Pelvic muscle exercises (Kegel exercises)

    Biofeedback: electrical stimulation of muscles around urethra

    Bladder training: teach patient to resist urge to void and delay voiding for a set time

  —Devices

    Females: vaginal cones to improve pelvic muscle tone; pessaries

    Males: external condom catheter or penile clamp

  —Catheterization: continuous or intermittent (see Urinary Catheter, p. 736)

- *Drugs*
  —Anticholinergics and smooth muscle relaxants for urge incontinence: oxybutynin, imipramine
  —α-Adrenergic drugs for stress incontinence: norephedrine, pseudoephedrine (Sudafed)

Surgical

- Procedures to restore the bladder-urethral structure
  —Urethral suspension (Marshall-Marchetti-Krantz; Stamey)
  —Pubovaginal sling urethroplexy
  —Artificial urinary sphincter: a hydraulically activated sphincter device placed around the bladder neck or urethra to allow the bladder to empty; the device is activated by manually squeezing the bulbs implanted in the labia or scrotum
  —Bladder pacemaker: implantation of electrodes into the sacral nerves to provide stimulation to the bladder to empty; the electrodes are connected to a device under the skin and are controlled by the patient using an external transmitter

HOME CARE

- Give both the patient and the caregiver *verbal* and *written* instructions. Provide them with the name and telephone number of a physician or nurse to call if questions arise.

- *General information*
    —Review and discuss care of surgically implanted devices. Instruct the patient to notify the physician or nurse of wound infection, mechanical failure of the device, or urinary tract infection.
    —Encourage the patient to notify the nurse or physician if the incontinence management program is not working.
- *Special instructions*
    —Discuss the various urinary containment devices available to protect clothing (adult diapers, pads, or undergarments; drip collector for males) and bedding. Assist the patient to choose and obtain appropriate devices from pharmacies, medical supply stores, or supermarkets.
    —Instruct the patient on the importance of skin care.
        Wash regularly with soap and water, completely dry the skin, and apply a protective skin sealant or moisture barrier.
        Change the protective undergarments as directed by the manufacturer.
        Change clothing or bedding immediately if they get wet; wash the perineal area.
        If using plastic pads or a sheet, avoid direct skin contact with the plastic.
        Keep the perineal area clean and change pads and undergarments to prevent odors. Inspect the area regularly.
    —Discuss the importance of establishing a bladder training program for the specific type of incontinence problem.
        Help the patient identify usual voiding patterns. Tell the patient to keep a record of the times each day he or she urinates, measure the amount of urine at each voiding, and record the number of times and when incontinence or leakage occurs.
        Stress the importance of scheduling a regular timed schedule of voiding patterns based on the voiding record (i.e., every 2 to 3 hours, after sitting for extended periods) or self-catheterization.
        Review measures to facilitate urination at the scheduled times of the day or night: finding a private location, assuming a comfortable position, listening to running water, gently pulling the pubic hair, stroking the inner

---

PELVIC MUSCLE (KEGEL) EXERCISES FOR STRESS INCONTINENCE

- Schedule times and select a place for the exercises.
- Do the exercises while seated (watching TV, working at your desk, driving), standing (in line at the store), or lying down.
- Begin the sessions with 10 complete cycles, building up to 30 to 50 repetitions as advised.
- To complete one cycle:
  —tighten and hold the pelvic muscles for 10 seconds
  —relax the pelvic muscles for 10 seconds. Repeat.
- Each session should take up to 10 minutes.
- Do the exercises every other day (up to three times a week) as part of a maintenance program.

---

thigh lightly or with ice, pouring warm water over the perineum or placing hands in warm water.

—Advise the patient to limit fluids with meals to 8 ounces, to spread the intake of fluids between meals, limiting the amount to sips (2 to 3 ounces), and to avoid drinking more than 2 to 3 ounces of fluid 2 hours before bedtime.

—Discuss the purpose of pelvic muscle (Kegel) exercises (to strengthen sphincter and urethral muscles) and assist the patient to initiate the exercise program.

—Instruct the patient on the correct muscle groups to exercise (those around the urethra and vagina). If a *female* patient has difficulty locating the muscles, place a finger or probe in the vagina and ask her to tighten the muscles around it, then do the same for the rectum. If a *male* patient has difficulty locating the muscles, place a finger or probe in the rectum and ask him to tighten the muscles around it.

—Explain the technique (see box above).

—Explain that pelvic muscle exercises should not be done routinely with each voiding because of possible damage to the urethra.

—Discuss biofeedback procedures available and permit a practice session to ensure proper techniques such as inserting a probe into the vagina (women) or rectum (men). Patches around the rectum may also be used. Lights and graphs on the recorder provide visual feedback when the patient is using the correct muscle group. Each session is 20 to 30 minutes long; four to six sessions are required.

—For a *female patient,* discuss additional procedures available to strengthen pelvic muscles. Provide instruction on insertion and cleaning of devices and allow time for practice. A vaginal cone (wide end first) is inserted into the vagina initially. The patient is instructed to hold it in place for 15 minutes twice a day. Progressively heavier cones are used. Pessaries and vaginal rings may be inserted into the vagina for bladder support and to prevent leakage. Advise the patient to obtain a bedside commode as indicated.

—For a *male patient,* discuss the use of an external condom catheter. If it is used, instruct the patient in the importance of inspecting the penis daily and maintaining good hygiene to prevent skin breakdown. Explain that care must be taken to use the correct size condom, apply tape or adhesive correctly, and change the catheter every day. Advise the patient to obtain and keep a urinal at the bedside.

—Discuss the need to make changes in the home environment such as keeping a night light on to avoid falls or sleeping nearer to a bathroom.

—Teach the patient and the caregiver how to perform intermittent catheterization or self-catheterization as ordered.

—Teach the patient how to insert and care for an indwelling catheter as indicated.

• *Medications*

—Explain the purpose, dosage, schedule, and route of administration of any drugs prescribed for stress incontinence, as well as side effects to report to a physician or nurse.

—Advise the patient to take drugs such as diuretics early in day to avoid interference with bedtime.

• *Diet*

—Discuss weight control as indicated, explaining that excess weight can lead to loss of bladder control.

—Advise the patient to drink up to 1½ quarts of fluid each day to avoid infection and formation of stones, unless fluid intake is restricted. Encourage drinks such as cranberry juice that leave an acid ash in the urine, which minimizes the occurrence of urinary tract infections.

—Tell the patient to limit fluid intake a few hours before bedtime or when planning a long trip on which bathroom stops will not be possible.

—Tell the patient to avoid carbonated beverages, drinks with caffeine (e.g., colas), and alcohol.

PSYCHOSOCIAL CARE

• Encourage verbalization about feelings and frustrations over incontinence, disruption to lifestyle, odor, and discomfort.

• Refer the patient to advocacy and support groups for incontinence, such as Incontinence Restored, Inc., Help for Incontinent People (HIP), Inc., and the Simon Foundation for Continence.

REFERRALS

• Advise and assist the patient to obtain supplies and equipment.

• Obtain referrals for home care services and equipment for patients with total incontinence to perform bladder catheterizations.

Urinary Incontinence Surgical Repair, Female
(Bladder Neck Suspension)

—Urinary incontinence surgical repair: surgical procedure to restore urinary continence. In the Marshall-Marchetti-Krantz procedure, the bladder neck and urethra are sutured to the perichondrium of the symphysis pubis or the periosteum of the superior pubic ramus using an extraperitoneal abdominal approach. In the Pereyra bladder neck suspension, a vaginal dissection and small suprapubic incision are used to access the bladder and urethra for suspension. In the Raz procedure, the bladder is elevated and suspended using tissue or inorganic material for support. The Raz procedure is performed transvaginally.

INDICATIONS

- Urinary incontinence (see p. 749)

PREPROCEDURAL TEACHING

- Review the physician's explanation of the specific type of procedure and the reason for it; encourage the patient to ask questions and to discuss any fears or anxieties.

Review of Preprocedural Care

- Explain that admission is usually on the day of surgery, that the procedure lasts 2 to 3 hours, and that it may be done under general anesthesia or spinal anesthesia.
- Discuss the diagnostic studies for urinary incontinence (see p. 749).
- Inform the patient about the routine preoperative studies: blood and urine tests, chest x-ray, and electrocardiogram.
- Tell the patient that a clear liquid diet is usually necessary for 2 days before surgery.
- Explain that a laxative should be taken 2 nights before and an enema the night before surgery.
- Tell the patient undergoing a vaginal procedure that a vaginal douche will be inserted during surgery and removed within 24 hours after the procedure.
- Discuss the need for a shower and shampoo with bactericidal soap (e.g., Safeguard, Dial, Hibiclens) the night before surgery.
- Inform the patient that the pubic hair may be shaved before the operation.
- Discuss the need for nothing by mouth (NPO) status the night before surgery.

Review of Postprocedural Care

- Explain that depending on the procedure, the patient will remain in the hospital for 2 to 5 days after the procedure.
- Inform the patient that she will be required to move, turn, and deep breathe the day of surgery and will probably get out of bed the day after surgery.
- Review the drainage tubes that may be used: a urinary catheter, which is usually removed the day after surgery if a suprapubic catheter is present (may remain longer for some procedures), and a suprapubic catheter, which is usually plugged on the day after the surgery.

- Describe the purpose of the vaginal pack, which is usually removed the morning after the operation. Explain that some vaginal bleeding is possible after surgery but usually stops within a few days.
- Explain that intravenous fluids are usually stopped on the day after surgery and fluid is limited to approximately 5 glasses of clear fluid a day.
- Describe the technique of postvoid residuals (see Home Care below).

COMPLICATIONS

- Urinary tract infection
- Pyelonephritis
- Septic shock
- Deep vein thrombosis
- Wound infection
- Urinary retention

HOME CARE

- Give both the patient and the caregiver *verbal* and *written* instructions. Provide them with the name and telephone number of a physician or nurse to call if questions arise.

Appendixes

APPENDIX A
Desirable Weights for Men and Women

BODY MASS INDEX (BMI)*

$$BMI = \frac{Weight\ (kg)}{Height^2\ (m)}$$

Normal range:
    Male   21.9-22.4
    Female 21.3-22.1

---

*See calculations on pp. 762-763.

IDEAL BODY WEIGHT
Adults (>18 years):
Male IBW (kg) = 50 + 2.3 for each inch over 60 inches
Female IBW (kg) = 45.5 + 2.3 for each inch over 60 inches
Children:
Age 1 to 18 years, height <60 inches:
$$IBW\ (kg) + [1.65 \times height^2\ (cm)]/1000$$

From Ellsworth AJ, et al: *Mosby's medical drug reference,* 1999-2000, St Louis, Mosby.

BODY MASS INDEX (BMI) CALCULATIONS

Weight (lb)	Height (ft, in)																
	4'10"	4'11"	5'0"	5'1"	5'2"	5'3"	5'4"	5'5"	5'6"	5'7"	5'8"	5'9"	5'10"	5'11"	6'0"	6'1"	6'2"
125	26	25	24	24	23	22	22	21	20	20	19	18	18	17	17	17	16
130	27	26	25	25	24	23	22	22	21	20	20	19	19	18	18	17	17
135	28	27	26	26	25	24	23	23	22	21	21	20	19	19	18	18	17
140	29	28	27	27	26	25	24	23	23	22	21	21	20	20	19	19	18
145	30	29	28	27	27	26	25	24	23	23	22	21	21	20	20	19	19
150	31	30	29	28	27	27	26	25	24	24	23	22	22	21	20	20	19
155	32	31	30	29	28	28	27	26	25	24	24	23	22	22	21	21	20
160	34	32	31	30	29	28	28	27	26	25	24	24	23	22	22	21	21
165	35	33	32	31	30	29	28	28	27	26	25	24	24	23	22	22	21
170	36	34	33	32	31	30	29	28	28	27	26	25	24	24	23	22	22
175	37	35	34	33	32	31	30	29	28	27	27	26	25	24	24	23	23

Weight (lb)																	
180	38	36	35	34	33	32	31	30	29	28	27	27	26	25	25	24	23
185	39	37	36	35	34	33	32	31	30	29	28	27	27	26	25	24	24
190	40	38	37	36	35	34	33	32	31	30	29	28	27	27	26	25	24
195	41	39	38	37	36	35	34	33	32	31	30	29	28	27	27	26	25
200	42	40	39	38	37	36	34	33	32	31	30	30	29	28	27	26	26
205	43	41	40	39	38	36	35	34	33	32	31	30	29	29	28	27	26
210	44	43	41	40	38	37	36	35	34	33	32	31	30	29	29	28	26
215	45	44	42	41	39	38	37	36	35	34	33	32	31	30	29	28	27
220	46	45	43	42	40	39	38	37	36	35	34	33	32	31	30	29	28
225	47	46	44	43	41	40	39	38	36	35	34	33	32	31	31	30	28
230	48	47	45	44	42	41	40	38	37	36	35	34	33	32	31	30	30

BMI: What it means to your health (adults ages 20-65 years)

18.5-24.9   Good weight for most people

≥25   Risk for cardiovascular and other diseases increases

≥30   Risk of death increases

1983 METROPOLITAN LIFE INSURANCE HEIGHT AND WEIGHT TABLE

Height	Small frame	Medium frame	Large frame
Men*			
5′2″	128-134	131-141	138-150
5′3″	130-136	133-143	140-153
5′4″	132-138	135-145	142-156
5′5″	134-140	137-148	144-160
5′6″	136-142	139-151	146-164
5′7″	138-145	142-154	149-168
5′8″	140-148	145-157	152-172
5′9″	142-151	148-160	155-176
5′10″	144-154	151-163	158-180
5′11″	146-157	154-166	161-184
6′0″	149-160	157-170	164-188
6′1″	152-164	160-174	168-192
6′2″	155-168	164-178	172-197
6′3″	158-172	167-182	176-202
6′4″	162-176	171-187	181-207

*Weights at ages 25 to 59, based on lowest mortality. Weight in pounds according to frame (in indoor clothing weighing 5 lb, shoes with 1″ heels).

1983 METROPOLITAN LIFE INSURANCE HEIGHT AND WEIGHT TABLE—cont'd

Height	Small frame	Medium frame	Large frame
Women†			
4'10"	102-111	109-121	118-131
4'11"	103-113	111-123	120-134
5'0"	104-115	113-126	122-137
5'1"	106-118	115-129	125-140
5'2"	108-121	118-132	128-143
5'3"	111-124	121-135	131-147
5'4"	114-127	124-138	134-151
5'5"	117-130	127-141	137-155
5'6"	120-133	130-144	140-159
5'7"	123-136	133-147	143-163
5'8"	126-139	136-150	146-167
5'9"	129-142	139-153	149-170
5'10"	132-145	142-156	152-173
5'11"	135-148	145-159	155-176
6'0"	138-151	148-162	158-179

†Weights at ages 25 to 59, based on lowest mortality. Weight in pounds according to frame (in indoor clothing weighing 3 lb, shoes with 1" heels).

APPENDIX B
Caloric Needs of Healthy Adults and Hospitalized Patients

Healthy Adult (Resting State)
30 kilocalories per kilogram of ideal body weight

Hospitalized Adult
2000-3000 calories per day

APPENDIX C
Therapeutic Diets

MODIFICATION OF PROTEIN INTAKE

Daily protein intake	Food limitations*	Practicality
150-200 g	Meat, cheese, eggs; >10 oz/day (1 egg = 1 oz meat); starches: 5 or more servings/day; vegetables: 4 or more servings/day; fruits: 3 or more servings/day; milk, casein, shakes, eggnogs, protein supplements added	High-protein, high-fat diet
100-140 g	Meat, cheese: 10 oz/day; starches: 5 to 6 servings/day; vegetables: 4 to 5 servings/day; fruits: 3 to 4 servings/day; milk included	Average American diet; relatively high in fat
60 g (10% of total calories)†	Meat, cheese: 6 oz/day; starches: <5 servings/day; vegetables: <4 servings/day; fruits: <3 servings/day; milk in limited amounts; calories increased with sugar and fat	Generally acceptable for home use; diet fairly easily manipulated according to patient preferences

40 g (6% of calories)†	Meat, cheese: 4 oz/day; starches: 3 servings/day; vegetables: 4 servings/day; fruits: 3 servings/day; calories increased with sugar and fat	Difficult to follow at home unless patient is unusually cooperative
20 g (3% of calories)†	Meat, cheese: essentially none; eggs: 2/day; starches: 2 servings/day; fruits: 2 servings/day; vegetables: 2 servings/day; calories increased with sugar and fat	Should be limited to hospital use
8 to 10 g (trace)	Meat, cheese, eggs, milk: essentially none; starches, vegetables: severely limited (low-protein bread only); calories mostly as fruits, juices, sugar, and fat	For hospital use only

*Serving sizes: most vegetables = ½ cup; most fruits = 1 piece or ½ cup; starches = 1 slice bread or approximately ⅓ to ½ cup of cooked starch.

†Percent of calories based on 2400 calories/day.

MODIFICATION OF SODIUM INTAKE

Daily sodium (Na) intake*	Food limitations	Practicality
5-6 g Na (= 12.5-15 g salt)	Includes table salt, heavily or visibly salted items	Average American diet
4 g Na (= 10 g salt)	No additional salt on tray or at table	Practical for home use
3 g Na (= 7.5 g salt)	Food only lightly salted in preparation; restrict heavily or visibly salted items (potato chips, pretzels, crackers, pickles, olives, relishes, sauces, most soups); no salt on tray	Practical for home use
2 g Na (= 5 g salt)	Above limitations plus no salt in food preparation; avoid most processed foods (canned foods, dry cereals, luncheon meats, bacon, ham, cheese) unless calculated into diet; regular bread, butter, milk in limited amounts	Fairly practical for home use with cooperative patient
1 g Na (= 2.5 g salt)	Above limitations plus use of only salt-free bread	Practical for home use only with unusually cooperative patient
0.5 g Na (= 1.25 g salt)	Above limitations plus limitation of meat (4 oz/day), eggs, some vegetables; milk (1 pt/day) and salt-free butter allowed	Not practical for home use

*1 g Na = 43 mEq; 1 mEq Na = 23 mg; 1 g NaCl = 2.5 g Na; 1 g Na = 0.4 g NaCl.

HIGH-SODIUM FOODS TO OMIT
ON A SODIUM-RESTRICTED DIET
Condiments

Pickles, olives, relishes, salted nuts, meat tenderizers, commercial salad dressings, monosodium glutamate (Accent), steak sauce, ketchup, soy sauce, Worcestershire sauce, horseradish sauce, chili sauce, commercial mustard, onion salt, garlic salt, celery salt, butter salt, seasoned salt

Breads

Salted crackers

Meat, Fish, Poultry, Cheese, and Substitutes

Cured, smoked, and processed meats such as ham, bacon, corned beef, chipped beef, weiners, luncheon meats, bologna, salt pork, regular canned salmon and tuna; all cheese except low sodium and cottage cheese; TV dinners, pizza, frozen Italian entrees, imitation sausage and bacon

Beverages

Commercial buttermilk, instant hot cocoa mixes

Soups

Commercial canned and dehydrated soups (except low-sodium soups), bouillon, consommé

Vegetables

Sauerkraut, hominy, pork and beans, canned tomato and vegetable juices

Fats

Gravy, regular peanut butter

Potato or Potato Substitutes

Potato chips, corn chips, salted popcorn, pretzels, frozen potato casseroles, commercially packaged rice and noodle mixes, dehydrated potatoes and potato mixes, bread stuffing

MODIFICATION OF FOOD CONSISTENCY
Clear Liquid Diet

This diet provides clear fluids that leave little residue and are absorbed with a minimum of digestive activity. It includes only broth, gelatin, strained fruit juices, clear beverages, and low-residue supplements. Since some of these have high osmolality, they may not be well tolerated by some patients. Clear liquids generally do not provide the Recommended Dietary Allowance (RDA) for any nutrients except perhaps for vitamin C. They should not be used for more than 2 or 3 days without supplementation.

Full Liquid Diet

This diet includes foods that liquefy at room temperature; many foods such as whole milk, custard, pudding, strained cream soups, eggnog, and ice cream contain fat and lactose, which some patients do not tolerate well. Complete enteral supplements may be preferred for such patients or may be added to increase calories and protein. This diet can meet the RDA for all nutrients, except iron for women of childbearing age.

Soft Diet

The soft diet contains foods that are tender but are not ground or pureed. Whole meats, cooked vegetables, and fruits of moderate fiber content are allowed. This generally excludes dried foods, most raw fruits and vegetables, and very coarse breads and cereals and is fairly low in fiber and residue.

Pureed or Ground Diet

This diet includes foods that are especially easy to masticate and swallow. It is useful in patients who have dysphagia or dental problems.

Bland Diet

This is designed for patients with peptic ulcer disease. A bland diet eliminates foods suspected to be gastric irritants or to stimulate gastric secretions. It generally excludes highly spiced foods, pepper, caffeine, and alcohol.

Low-Fiber, Low-Residue Diet

Intended to reduce fecal bulk, this diet is restricted in milk, certain vegetables, fruits, and whole-grain breads and cereals.

High-Fiber Diet

This diet includes unrefined starches (whole-grain bread, brown rice, potatoes, corn, beans), raw fruits, and vegetables. Bran may be added if desired.

Appendix C from Weinsier RL, Heinburger DC, Butterworth CE: *Handbook of clinical nutrition,* ed 2, St Louis, 1989, Mosby.

APPENDIX D
Food Sources of Selected Nutrients

FOODS HIGH IN SODIUM

Processed foods: canned foods (meats, sauces, fish, vegetables), luncheon meats, dry cereals, cheese, ham, bacon, smoked or cured fish
Prepackaged foods
Salted crackers
Pickles, olives, relishes
Salty nuts, chips
Bouillon cubes
Yeast

FOODS HIGH IN POTASSIUM

Fruits: apricots, avocado, bananas, rhubarb, melons (cantaloupe, watermelon), oranges, grapes, coconut, dried fruits, fruit juices
Vegetables: artichokes, raw carrots, tomatoes, cooked spinach, cooked potatoes, pumpkin, swiss chard, cooked sweet potato, dried beans, peas, mushrooms
Bouillon cubes
Cider, beer, wine
Nuts
Chocolate
Chili powder
Turmeric
Packaged soups
Canned spaghetti, vegetables, soups

FOODS LOW IN POTASSIUM

Fruits: applesauce, grapefruit, canned pear, canned pineapple, plums, frozen strawberries, tangerines, cranberries, lemons

Vegetables: cooked or raw cabbage, cooked cauliflower, corn, cucumber, cooked eggplant, cooked green beans, cooked green peas, cooked onion, cooked summer squash

FOODS HIGH IN PHOSPHORUS

Meats: brain, kidney, liver, beef (lean round, cooked), lean pork

Fish: cod, halibut

Poultry

Dairy products: milk, cheese

Whole grains: oatmeal, bran, barley

Nuts: roasted peanuts, brazil nuts, peanut butter

Vegetables: beans (kidney, white, lima), cooked green peas, dried beans and peas, cooked artichokes, white potatoes, cooked brussels sprouts

Eggs

Carbonated drinks with phosphoric acid added

FOODS LOW IN PHOSPHORUS

Most fruits

Most vegetables

FOODS HIGH IN CALCIUM

Dairy products: milk, cheese, ice cream

Vegetables: greens (collard, mustard, turnip), cooked spinach, cooked broccoli, cooked beans (kidney, lima, white), raw cabbage, raw carrots

Fruits: prunes, oranges, tangerines

FOODS HIGH IN IRON

Meats: calf liver, beef liver, chicken

Boiled eggs

Vegetables: spinach, cooked beans (kidney, white, lima), asparagus, iceberg lettuce, mustard greens, cooked green peas, raw cauliflower

Fruits: watermelon, prunes, dried dates, dried apricots, raisins, blueberries, strawberries

FOOD SOURCES OF MAJOR VITAMINS
Vitamin A

Food	Portion size	Amount of vitamin	
		RE/portion	**RE/100 g**
Meats			
Beef liver, fried	3½ oz	10640	10640
Calf liver, cooked	3½ oz	8116	8116
Chicken liver, cooked	2 livers	7806	12880
Vegetables			
Potatoes, sweet, baked	1 medium	2488	830
Carrots, raw	1 large	2025	1100
cooked	½ cup	800	1050
Spinach, raw	3½ oz	810	810
cooked	½ cup	737	657
Pumpkin, cooked	½ cup	800	640
Collard greens, cooked	½ cup	540	540
Squash, winter	½ squash	420	420
Turnip greens, cooked	½ cup	396	630
Mustard greens, cooked	½ cup	212	212
Lettuce, romaine	4 leaves	190	190
iceberg	¼ head	97	97
Broccoli, cooked	½ cup	110	250
Asparagus, cooked	5-6 medium	90	90
Tomatoes, raw	1 small	90	90
Fruits			
Watermelon	10″ × 16″ slice	531	59
Cantaloupe	¼ melon	430	430
Apricots, raw	3 medium	277	277
dried	4 halves	101	109
Papaya, raw	⅓ medium	175	175
Nectarines, raw	1 medium	165	165

One RE (retinol equivalent) = 3.33 IU from animal sources and 10 IU from plant sources.

Thiamin (B$_1$)

Food	Portion size	Amount of vitamin	
		mg/portion	mg/100 g
Meats			
Pork chops, cooked	3½ oz	0.98	0.98
Ham, fresh, cooked	3½ oz	0.96	0.96
Beef liver, fried	3½ oz	0.26	0.26
Nuts			
Brazil	¼ cup	0.82	1.09
Pecans	¼ cup	0.18	0.73
Cashew	¼ cup	0.11	0.44
Cereal products			
Barley cereals	½ cup	0.22	0.23
Wheat germ	1 tbsp	0.15	1.68
Oatmeal, cooked	½ cup	0.13	0.11
Vegetables			
Green peas, cooked	½ cup	0.28	0.28
Soybeans, cooked	½ cup	0.21	0.26
Asparagus, cooked	5-6 medium	0.16	0.16
Beans, cooked			
Lima	½ cup	0.14	0.18
Kidney	½ cup	0.14	0.11
Corn on cob, cooked	4″ ear	0.12	0.12
Miscellaneous			
Brewer's yeast	1 tbsp	1.25	15.61

Riboflavin (B$_2$)

Food	Portion size	Amount of vitamin	
		mg/portion	mg/100 g
Meats			
Beef liver, fried	3½ oz	4.10	4.10
Calf liver, fried	3½ oz	4.10	4.10
Chicken liver, cooked	3½ oz	1.75	1.75
Veal roast, cooked	3½ oz	0.44	0.44
Beef, ground, cooked	3½ oz	0.21	0.21
Egg, boiled	1 large	0.14	0.28
Cereal products			
Barley cereals	½ cup	0.12	0.13
Dairy products			
Milk, whole	1 cup	0.42	0.17
Ice cream (1 scoop)	½ cup	0.17	0.25
Cheese, cottage, low-fat, 2%	⅓ cup	0.14	0.14
Blue or Roquefort	1 oz	0.11	0.39
Cheddar	1 oz	0.11	0.39
Brick	1 oz	0.10	0.36
Vegetables			
Collard greens, cooked	½ cup	0.20	0.20
Spinach, raw	3½ oz	0.20	0.20
Broccoli, cooked	½ cup	0.20	0.20
Asparagus, cooked	5-6 medium	0.18	0.18
Brussels sprouts, cooked	½ cup	0.14	0.14
Mustard greens, cooked	½ cup	0.14	0.14
Spinach, cooked	½ cup	0.13	0.14
Miscellaneous			
Brewer's yeast	1 tbsp	0.43	4.30

Niacin (B$_3$)

Food	Portion size	Amount of vitamin	
		mg/portion	mg/100 g
Meats			
Calf liver, fried	3½ oz	16.5	16.5
Beef liver, fried	3½ oz	14.4	14.4
Chicken, cooked	3½ oz	6.6	6.6
Beef, ground, cooked	3½ oz	5.7	5.7
Chicken liver, cooked	3½ oz	4.5	4.5
Haddock, cooked	3½ oz	2.1	2.1
Nuts			
Peanuts, roasted	1 oz	5.6	2.0
Peanut butter	2 tbsp	4.8	15.8
Vegetables			
Green peas, cooked	½ cup	1.7	2.3
Potatoes, white, baked	1 medium	1.7	1.7
Asparagus, cooked	5-6 medium	1.4	1.4
Corn on cob, cooked	4″ ear	1.4	1.4
Peas, black-eyed	½ cup	1.1	1.4
Collard greens, cooked	½ cup	1.2	1.2
Lima beans, cooked	½ cup	1.0	1.3
Miscellaneous			
Brewer's yeast	1 tbsp	3.8	38.0

Pyridoxine (B$_6$)

Food	Portion size	Amount of vitamin	
		mg/portion	mg/100 g
Meats			
Salmon, broiled	3½ oz	0.70	0.70
Chicken, baked	3½ oz	0.52	0.52
Beef, ground	3½ oz	0.39	0.39
Pork chop, broiled	3½ oz	0.35	0.35
Beef liver, fried	3½ oz	0.35	0.35
Tuna, canned	3 oz	0.34	0.40
Turkey, baked	3½ oz	0.27	0.27
Vegetables			
Potato, baked	1 medium	0.70	0.70
Spinach, cooked	½ cup	0.22	0.14
Broccoli, cooked	½ cup	0.15	0.14
Turnip greens	½ cup	0.13	0.13
Asparagus	½ cup	0.13	0.13
Fruits			
Banana	1 medium	0.66	0.58
Figs, dried	10	0.42	0.23
Watermelon	1 cup	0.23	0.14
Cantaloupe	1 cup	0.18	0.11
Orange	1 medium	0.08	0.07
Miscellaneous			
Brewer's yeast	1 tbsp	0.40	4.00

Vitamin B$_{12}$

Food	Portion size	Amount of vitamin	
		mg/portion	mg/100 g
Meats			
Beef liver, fried	3½ oz	31-120	31-120
Beef round	3½ oz	3.4-4.5	3.4-4.5
Ham	3½ oz	0.9-1.6	0.9-1.6
Haddock	3½ oz	0.6	0.6
Egg, whole	1 large	0.6	1.3
Dairy products			
Milk, whole	1 cup	1.3	0.6
Cheese, Swiss	1 oz	0.5	1.7
American	1 oz	0.2	0.7

Folic acid

Food	Portion size	Amount of vitamin	
		µg/portion	µg/100 g
Meats			
Chicken liver	3½ oz	770	770
Beef liver, fried	3½ oz	175	175
Vegetables			
Spinach, cooked	½ cup	131	131
Asparagus, cooked	5-6 medium	89-140	89-140
Turnip greens, cooked	½ cup	86	106
Kale, cooked	½ cup	34	51
Endive, raw	20 long leaves	27-63	27-63
Broccoli, cooked	½ cup	26	34
Escarole, raw	4 large leaves	26	26
Okra, cooked	8-9 pods	24	24
Brussels sprouts, cooked	½ cup	20	27
Mustard greens, cooked	½ cup	17-38	17-38
Acorn squash, cooked	½ medium	17	17
Cauliflower, cooked	½ cup	16	29
Nuts			
Walnuts	8-10 halves	12	77
Filberts	10-12 nuts	10	67
Peanuts	1 tbsp	9	57
Almonds	12-15 nuts	7	46
Pecans	12 halves	4	27

Tables from Weinsier RL, Heinburger DC, Butterworth CE Jr: *Handbook of clinical nutrition,* ed 2, St Louis, 1989, Mosby.

APPENDIX E
Foods for Specific Conditions

HIGH-FIBER FOODS FOR DIVERTICULOSIS
- Whole-grain cereals and breads
- Beans
- Peas
- Fresh vegetables
- Fresh fruit
- Broccoli/brussels sprouts
- Potatoes/potato skins, wild rice

FOODS TO AVOID FOR DIVERTICULOSIS
- Popcorn, corn on cob, whole corn
- Celery
- Fresh vegetables
- Wild rice, whole grains
- Chinese vegetables
- Coconut, dried fruit, fruit peels
- Meat with casings
- Nuts and kernals

FOODS THAT CAUSE STOMA ODOR
- Broccoli
- Baked beans
- Onions, asparagus, cabbage
- Eggs, fish
- Blue and cheddar cheese
- Alcohol and beer
- Turnips

FOODS THAT THICKEN OUTPUT
- Bananas
- Rice, pasta
- Cheese

FOODS THAT LOOSEN OUTPUT
- Raw fruits
- Vegetables
- Greasy food

Modified from Beare PG, Myers JL: *Adult health nursing,* ed 3, St Louis, 1998, Mosby, p 1545.

APPENDIX F
Patient Resources

Phone numbers for local offices and divisions are listed in the white pages of the telephone book.

Acoustic Neuroma Association
P.O. Box 12402
Atlanta, GA 30355
(404) 237-8023
www.anausa.org

Agency for Health Care Policy and Research (AHCPR)
P.O. Box 8547
Silver Spring, MD 20907-8547
1-800-358-9295
www.ahcpr.gov

AIDS Clinical Trials Information Service
P.O. Box 6421
Rockville, MD 20849
1-800-874-2572 (English/Spanish)
1-800-243-7012 (hearing impaired)
www.actis.org

AIDS Treatment Information Service
P.O. Box 6303
Rockville, MD 20849
1-800-448-0440 (English/Spanish)
1-800-243-7012 (hearing impaired)
www.hivatis.org

Alcoholic Center for Information and Drug Dependency
c/o National Council on Alcoholic and Drug Dependency
12 W. 21st St.
New York, NY 10010
(212) 206-6770
1-800-nca-call
www.ncadd.org

Alcoholics Anonymous World Services
P.O. Box 459
Grand Central Station
New York, NY 10163
(212) 870-3400
www.alcoholics-anonymous.org

ALS (Amyotrophic Lateral Sclerosis) Association
27001 Agoura Rd., Suite 150
Calabasas Hills, CA 91301-5104
(818) 880-9007
1-800-782-4747
www.alsa.org
www.alsinfo@alsa.national.org

Alzheimer's Association
919 N. Michigan Ave, Suite 1100
Chicago, IL 60611
(312) 335-8700
1-800-272-3900
www.alz.org

American Academy of Ophthalmology
Eye Net
P.O. Box 7424
San Francisco, CA 94120-7424
(415) 561-8500
www.eyenet.org

American Brain Tumor Association
2720 River Rd.
Des Plaines, IL 60018
(847) 827-9910
1-800-886-2282
www.abta.org

American Cancer Society
National Center
1599 Clifton Rd. NE
Atlanta, GA 30329
(404) 320-3333
1-800-227-2345
www.cancer.org

American Diabetes Association
National Center
1660 Duke St.
Alexandria, VA 22314
1-800-232-3472 (general information)
1-800-DIABETES (patient literature)
www.diabetes.org

American Heart Association
National Center
7272 Greenville Ave.
Dallas, TX 75231
1-800-AHA-USA1
1-800-242-1793
www.americanheart.org

American Heart Association
(AHA Stroke Connection)
National Center
7272 Greenville Ave.
Dallas, TX 75231
1-800-AHA-USA1
www.stroke.org

American Liver Foundation
1425 Pompton Ave.
Cedar Grove, NJ 07009
1-800-GO-LIVER (465-4837)
www.sadieo.ucsf.edu/alf/alffinal

American Lung Association
National Headquarters
1790 Broadway
New York, NY 10019-4374
(212) 315-8700
1-800-LUNG-USA
www.lungusa.org
www.lalung.org

American Parkinson's Disease Association
1250 Hylan Blvd., Suite 4-B
Staten Island, NY 10305-1943
1-800-223-2732
www.apdaparkinson.com

American Red Cross
National Headquarters
2131 K St. NW
Washington, DC 20006
(202) 728-6401
www.redcross.org

Arthritis Foundation
1330 W. Peachtree St.
Atlanta, GA 30309
(404) 872-7100
1-800-283-7800 (patient information)
www.arthritis.org

Bone Marrow Transplant Family Support Network
P.O. Box 845
Avon, CT 06001
1-800-826-9376
www.ai.mit.edu/people/laurel/Bmt-talk/bmt-talk.html

The Brain Injury Association
105 N. Alfred St.
Alexandria, VA 22314
(703) 236-6000
www.biausa.org

Cancer Care, Inc.
1180 Avenue of the Americas
New York, NY 10036
(212) 302-2400
1-800-813-HOPE
www.cancercare.org

Cancer Information Service
So. California Regional Office
10940 Wilshire Blvd., Suite 1710
Los Angeles, CA 90024
(310) 794-0545
1-800-4-CANCER (Spanish available)
1-800-638-6070 (Alaska)
1-800-524-1234 (Hawaii)
www.nci.nih.gov

CDC National AIDS Hotline
P.O. Box 13827
Research Triangle Park, NC 27709
1-800-342-AIDS
1-800-344-7432 (Spanish)
1-800-243-7889 (TTY/TDD)
www.ashastd.org

Christopher Reeve Paralysis Foundation
500 Morris Ave.
Springfield, NJ 07081
(973) 379-2690
1-800-225-0292
www.paralysis.org

Crohn's and Colitis Foundation of America
444 Park Ave. S
New York, NY 10016-7374
(212) 685-3440
1-800-343-3637
www.ccfa.org

Cystic Fibrosis Foundation
6931 Arlington Rd., Suite 200
Bethesda, MD 20814
(301) 951-4422
1-800-FIGHT CF
www.cff.org

Epilepsy Foundation of America
4351 Garden City Dr.
Landover, MD 20785
(301) 459-3700
1-800-EFA-1000
www.efa.org

The Glaucoma Foundation
33 Maiden Lane
New York, NY 10038
1-800-GLAUCOMA
www.glaucoma-foundation.org/info

Guillain-Barré Syndrome Foundation International
P.O. Box 262
Wynnewood, PA 19096
(610) 667-0131
www.webmast.com/gbs

Information Center for Individuals with Disabilities
P.O. Box 750119
Arlington Heights, MA 02175-0119
(617) 450-9888
www.realprogress.com/icid/index.html

International Association of Laryngectomees
c/o American Cancer Society
1599 Clifton Rd. NE
Atlanta, GA 30329-4251
(317) 570-4578
www.larynxlink.com

Leukemia Society of America, Inc.
Home Office
600 Third Ave.
New York, NY 10016
(212) 573-8484
1-800-955-4572
www.leukemia.org

Lupus Foundation of America
So. California Chapter
17985 Sky Park Circle, Suite J
Irvine, CA 92614
(301) 670-9292
1-800-558-0121 (to request an information packet only)
www.lupus.org

Lymphedema International Network
www.lymphedema.com

Lymphoma Research Foundation
8800 Venice Blvd., #207
Los Angeles, CA 90034
(310) 204-7040
www.lymphoma.org

Meals-on-Wheels
2254 San Diego Ave., Suite 200
San Diego, CA 92110
(619) 260-6110
1-800-677-1116
www.meals-on-wheels.org

MedicAlert
2323 Colorado Ave.
Turlock, CA 95382
(209) 668-3333
1-800-344-3226
www.medicalert.org

The Mended Hearts, Inc.
7272 Greenville Ave.
Dallas, TX 75231
(214) 706-1442
www.mendedhearts.org

Multiple Sclerosis Association of America
National Headquarters
706 Haddonfield Rd.
Cherry Hill, NJ 08002
1-800-LEARN-MS
www.msaa.com

Multiple Sclerosis Society
National Headquarters
(212) 986-3240
1-800-FIGHT MS
1-800-344-4867
www.nmss.org

Muscular Dystrophy Association
National Headquarters
3300 E. Sunrise Dr.
Tucson, AZ 85718-3208
1-800-572-1717
www.mdausa.org
e-mail: mda@mdausa.org

Myasthenia Gravis Foundation
123 W. Madison, Suite 800
Chicago, IL 60602-4503
(312) 258-0522
1-800-541-5454
www.myasthenia.org

National Adrenal Disease Foundation
505 Northern Blvd.
Great Neck, NY 11021
(516) 487-4992
www.medhelp.org/nadf

National Amputation Foundation
38-40 Church St.
Malverne, NY 11565
(516) 887-3600
(516) 887-3667 FAX
www.va.gov/vso/naf.htm

National Arthritis and Musculoskeletal and Skin Diseases
    Information
Clearinghouse, National Institute of Arthritis and Musculoskeletal
    and Skin Diseases
Building 31, Room 4C05
31 Center Dr., MSC 2350
Bethesda, MD 20892-2350
(301) 496-8188
(301) 587-4352 FAX
www.nih.gov/niams

National Association for Home Care
228 7th St. SE
Washington, DC 20003
(202) 547-7424 (ask for Public Information Line)
www.nahc.org

National Association of People with AIDS
1413 K St. NW
7th Floor
Washington, DC 20005
(202) 898-0414
(202) 898-0435 (FAX)
www.napwa.org

National Cancer Institute
1-800-4-CANCER
9000 Rockville Pike
Bethesda, MD 20892
www.nci.nih.gov

National Diabetes Information Clearing House
1 Information Way
Bethesda, MD 20892
(301) 654-3327
www.niddk.nih.gov/health/diabetes/ndic.htm

National Heart, Lung, and Blood Institute
Information Center
P.O. Box 30105
Bethesda, MD 20824
(301) 251-1222
(301) 496-4236 (for general public)
www.nhlbi.nih.gov

National Hemophilia Foundation
110 Greene St., Suite 303
New York, NY 10012
(212) 219-8180
1-800-42-HANDI (Spanish available)
www.hemophilia.org

National Hospice Organization
1901 N. Moore St., Suite 901
Arlington, VA 22209
(703) 243-5900
www.nho.org

National Information Center on Deafness
31 Center Dr., MSC 2320
Bethesda, MD 20892-2320
www.nih.gov/nidcd

National Institute of Allergy and Infectious Diseases
Building 31, Room 7A50
31 Central Drive, MSC 2520
Bethesda, MD 20892-2520
(301) 496-5717
www.niaid.nih.gov

National Institute of Diabetes and Digestive and Kidney Diseases
  Project Officer
2 Information Way
Bethesda, MD 20892
(302) 468-6344
www.niddk.nih.gov

National Institute of Neurological Disorders and Stroke
Office of Scientific and Health Reports
Building 31/RM 8A16
31 Center Drive, MSC 2540
Bethesda, MD 20892-2540
(301) 496-5751
(pamphlets on stroke)
www.ninds.nih.gov

National Jewish Medical and Research Center
Lung, Allergic, and Immune Diseases
1400 Jackson St.
Denver, CO 80206
(303) 398-1477
Lung Disease Hotline
1-800-222-LUNG
www.nationaljewish.org

National Kidney Foundation
30 E. 33rd St., 11th Floor
New York, NY 10016
(212) 889-2210
1-800-622-9010
www.kidney.org

National Marrow Donor Program
3433 Broadway St. NE, Suite 500
Minneapolis, MN 55413
(414) 257-8325
1-800-654-1247
www.marrow.org

National Multiple Sclerosis Society
733 3rd Ave., Third Floor
New York, NY 10017
(212) 986-3240
1-800-FIGHT-MS
www.nmss.org

National Osteoporosis Foundation
National Headquarters
1232 22nd St. NW
Washington, DC 20037-1292
(202) 223-2226
www.nof.org

National Osteoporosis Foundation
Chicago Office
C/O AMA
515 North State St.
Chicago, IL 60610
(312) 464-5110
(312) 464-5863 FAX
www.nof.org

National Parkinson Foundation, Inc.
1501 N.W. 9th Ave.
Miami, FL 33136
1-800-327-4545
www.parkinson.org

National Prostate Cancer Coalition
1156 15th St. NW, Suite 905
Washington, DC 20005
(202) 463-9455
www.4npcc.org/base/doc2.html

National Rehabilitation Information Center
1010 Wayne Ave., Suite 800
Silver Spring, MD 20910-5633
(301) 562-2400
www.naric.com

National Spinal Cord Injury Association
8300 Colesville Rd., Suite 551
Silver Spring, MD 20910
(310) 588-6959
Spinal Cord Injury Hotline
1-800-526-3456
www.spinalcord.org
www.healthfinder.gov

National Stroke Association
96 Inverness Dr. E, Suite I
Englewood, CO 80112-5341
(303) 771-1700
1-800-787-6537
www.stroke.org

Osteoporosis and Related Bone Disease National Resource Center
National Institute of Arthritis and Musculoskeletal and Skin
  Diseases
1150 17th St., NW, Suite 500
Washington, DC 20036
(202) 223-0344
1-800-624-BONE
www.osteo.org

Parkinson Disease Foundation
710 W. 168th St.
New York, NY 10032-9982
1-800-457-6676
www.pdf.org

Project Information (for AIDS patients and clinicians)
205 13th St., Suite 2001
San Francisco, CA 94103
1-800-822-7422
www.projectinform.org

Public Health Service's Agency for Health Care Policy and
  Research
Publications Clearinghouse
P.O. Box 8547
Silver Spring, MD 20907
1-800-358-9295
(patient guidelines for urinary incontinence in adults, angina
  pectoris, heart failure; available in English or Spanish)
www.ahcpr.gov

Self Help for Hard of Hearing People
National Office
7910 Woodmont Ave., Suite 1200
Bethesda, MD 20814
(301) 657-2249
www.shhh.org

Simon Foundation for Continence
P.O. Box 835
Wilmette, IL 60091
(708) 864-3913
1-800-23-SIMON

Stroke Clubs International
805 12th St.
Galveston, TX 77550
(409) 762-1022

Symptoms in Terminal Illness: A Research Workshop. September
    22-23, 1997.
Accessed 8/15/99
www.nih.gov/ninr/end-of-life.htm

United Ostomy Association
19772 MacArthur Blvd., Suite 200
Irvine, CA 92612-2405
(949) 660-8624
1-800-826-0826
www.uoa.org

United Parkinson Foundation
1501 N.W. 9th Ave.
Miami, FL 33136
(800) 327-4545

The Wellness Community
65 Ceramic Dr.
Columbus, OH 43214-3063
(614) 263-5012
www.wellnesscolumbus.org

Bibliography

Aegerter E, Kirkpatrick JA: *Orthopedic diseases,* Philadelphia, 1975, WB Saunders.

Beare PG, Myers JL: *Adult health nursing,* ed 3, St Louis, 1998, Mosby.

Belcher AE: *Mosby's clinical series: cancer nursing,* St Louis, 1992, Mosby.

Benedict LA, Tennant JK, Morrison KL et al: *Telephone triage for home care,* Gaitherburg, MD.

Bradley M, Pupiales M: Essential elements of ostomy care, *Am J Nurs* 97:38-45, 1997.

Brundage D: *Mosby's clinical series: renal disorders,* St Louis, 1993, Mosby.

Canobbio MM: *Mosby's clinical series: cardiovascular disorders,* St Louis, 1990, Mosby.

Cheitlin MD, Sokolow M, McIlroy MB: *Clinical cardiology,* ed 6, Norwalk, Conn, 1993, Appleton & Lange.

Chipps E, Clannin N, Campbell V: *Mosby's clinical series: neurologic disorders,* St Louis, 1992, Mosby.

Durham E, Weiss L: How patients die, *Am J Nurs* 97:41-46, 1997.

Eutsey DE: *Geriatric patient education resource manual,* ed 2, Gaithersburg, Md, 1999, Aspen.

Ferri FF: *Practical guide to the care of the medical patient,* ed 4, St Louis, 1998, Mosby.

Garrick JG, Webb DR: *Sports injuries,* ed 2, Philadelphia, 1999, WB Saunders.

Giloth BE: *Managing hospital-based patient education,* Washington, DC, 1993, American Hospital Publishing.

Gray M: *Mosby's clinical series: genitourinary disorders,* St Louis, 1992, Mosby.

Griffith H, Dambro M: *The five minute clinical consultant,* Philadelphia, 1993, Lea & Febiger.

Grimes DE: *Mosby's clinical series: infectious diseases,* St Louis, 1991, Mosby.

Groenwald SL, Frogge MH, Goodman M et al: *Cancer nursing: principles and practice,* ed 3, Boston, 1993, Jones & Bartlett.

Handbook of medical surgical nursing, Springhouse, Penn, 1994, Springhouse.

Hodgson B: *Illustrated guide to home health care,* Springhouse, Penn, 1995, Springhouse.

Holloway N: *Medical surgical care planning,* ed 2, Springhouse, Penn, 1993, Springhouse.

Home health nursing pocket consultant, St Louis, 1995, Mosby.

Ignatavicius DD, Hausman KA: *Pocket companion for medical-surgical nursing,* ed 2, Philadelphia, 1995, WB Saunders.

Isselbacher K, Braunwald E, Wilson J, et al: *Harrison's principles of internal medicine,* ed 13, New York, 1994, McGraw-Hill.

Jaffe MS, Skidmore-Roth L: *Home health: nursing care plans,* ed 3, St Louis, 1998, Mosby.

Johnson JY, Smith-Temple J, Carr P: *Nurses' guide to home health procedures,* Philadelphia, 1998, Lippincott.

Kniesl CR, Ames SW: *Adult health nursing: a biopsychosocial approach,* Reading, Mass, 1986, Addison-Wesley.

Korinko AM, Yurick A: Maintaining skin integrity during radiation therapy, *AJN* 97:40-44, 1997.

Langford RW, Thompson JM: *Mosby's handbook of diseases,* St Louis, 1996, Mosby.

Leboeuf G: *Home health care handbook,* Great Falls, Va, 1996, Noel Press.

Macklin D: How to manage PICCS, *Am J Nurs* 97:26-32, 1997.

Marrelli TM: *Hospice and palliative care handbook,* St Louis, 1999, Mosby.

McCue JD: The naturalness of dying, *JAMA* 273:1039-1043, 1995.

Miaskowski C, Buchsel P: *Oncology nursing: assessment and clinical care,* St Louis, 1999, Mosby.

Mosby's patient teaching guides, St Louis, 1996, Mosby.

Mourad LA: *Mosby's clinical series: orthopedic disorders,* St Louis, 1991, Mosby.

Mudge-Grout CL: *Immunologic disorders,* St Louis, 1992, Mosby.

Narayan MC et al: Dying and death in the home, telephone triage for home care, Gaithersburg, Md, 1998, Aspen.

Nurses desk reference: diagnostics: a comprehensive manual of laboratory tests and diagnostic procedures, Springhouse, Penn, 1994, Springhouse.

Onion D: *The little black book of primary care: pearls and references,* New York, 1993, WW Norton.

Otto SE: *Oncology nursing,* ed 2, St Louis, 1994, Mosby.

Pagana K, Pagana T: *Mosby's diagnostic and laboratory test reference,* St Louis, 1998, Mosby.

Palandri MK, Sorrentin CR: *Pocket companion: Luckmann and Sorensen's medical surgical nursing,* ed 4, Philadelphia, 1993, WB Saunders.

Pocket companion for home health nurses, Springhouse, Penn, 1997, Springhouse.

Professional guide to diseases, ed 4, Springhouse, Penn, 1992, Springhouse.

Redman BK: *The practice of patient education,* ed 8, St Louis, 1997, Mosby.

Rice R: *Handbook of home health nursing procedure,* St Louis, 1995, Mosby.

Rutherford RB: *Vascular surgery,* ed 4, Philadelphia, 1995, WB Saunders.

Ryder MA: Peripherally inserted central venous catheters, *Nurs Clin North Am* 28:935-971, 1993.

Stillwell S: *Mosby's critical care nursing reference,* ed 2, St Louis, 1996, Mosby.

Swearingen PL: *Manual of medical-surgical nursing care,* ed 4, St Louis, 1999, Mosby.

Taber's cyclopedic medical dictionary, Philadelphia, 1993, FA Davis.

Thelan LA, Urden LD, Lough ME et al: *Critical care nursing: diagnosis and management,* ed 3, St Louis, 1998, Mosby.

Thompson J, McFarland G, Hirsch J et al: *Clinical nursing,* ed 3, St Louis, 1998, Mosby.

Tucker SM, Canobbio MM, Paquette EV et al: *Patient care standards,* ed 7, St Louis, 2000, Mosby.

Visiting Nurse Associations of America, ed: *Caregiver's handbook,* New York, 1998, DK Publishing.

Wagner MM: Pathophysiology related to peripheral vascular disease, *Nurs Clin North Am* 21:195-206, 1986.

Weinsier RL, Heimburger DC, Butterworth CE: *Handbook of clinical nutrition: clinician's manual for prevention, diagnosis, and management of nutritional problems,* ed 2, St Louis, 1989, Mosby.

Whitman NI et al: *Teaching in nursing practice: a professional model,* ed 2, Norwalk, Conn, 1992, Appleton & Lange.

Wilson SF, Thompson JM: *Respiratory disorders,* St Louis, 1993, Mosby.

Youngkin EQ, Wawin KJ, Kissinger JF et al: *Pharmacotherapeutics: a primary care clinical guide,* Norwalk, Conn, 1999, Appleton & Lange.

Index

797